1 MONTH OF
FREE
READING

at

www.ForgottenBooks.com

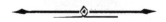

By purchasing this book you are eligible for one month membership to ForgottenBooks.com, giving you unlimited access to our entire collection of over 1,000,000 titles via our web site and mobile apps.

To claim your free month visit:

www.forgottenbooks.com/free786042

ISBN 978-0-266-51858-7
PIBN 10786042

TWENTIETH CENTURY
PRACTICE

AN INTERNATIONAL ENCYCLOPEDIA

OF

MODERN MEDICAL SCIENCE

BY

LEADING AUTHORITIES OF EUROPE AND AMERICA

EDITED BY

THOMAS L. STEDMAN, M.D.

NEW YORK CITY

IN TWENTY VOLUMES

VOLUME XX

TUBERCULOSIS, YELLOW FEVER, AND MISCELLANEOUS

GENERAL INDEX

192304
11. 11. 24

NEW YORK
WILLIAM WOOD AND COMPANY
1900

PRESS OF
THE PUBLISHERS' PRINTING COMPANY
82, 84 LAFAYETTE PLACE
NEW YORK

PREFACE TO VOLUME XX.

THE Twentieth Century Practice, with this twentieth volume, reaches its appointed end, and its editor cannot relinquish his task without a word of gratitude to those whose labors have created these volumes, and of explanation to those who possess them. As far as possible the work has appeared in accordance with the original plan, but occasionally events have conspired to force a rearrangement of the articles in the several volumes. Distance, sickness, and death have each intervened with their several prohibitions. Semmola, Leloir, Dujardin-Beaumetz, Oertel, Ernest Hart, Kerr, Grainger Stewart, O'Dwyer, and Whittaker have here given the world their last words, the final results of their lifework. Others who had promised their co-operation passed away before their tasks were completed, and for this and other reasons it has, in several instances, been found necessary to invoke the aid of new writers, or to hasten or delay the preparation of certain subjects. Any inconvenience arising from this unavoidable deviation from natural sequence will be obviated by means of the very full analytical index. In the preparation of this index the needs of the consulter have been kept constantly in view. Special note has been made of the symptomatic indications of disease and of the points in differential diagnosis, thereby, it is hoped, widening the usefulness of the series as a work of reference. Most valuable assistance in this part of the work has been rendered by Dr. Emma E. Walker, of New York. The editor desires to thank the contributors for the promptness with which they have met their obligations, often at great personal inconvenience, and for the painstaking care exercised in the preparation of their treatises. To those who so satisfactorily discharged the difficult task of translation from the German, French, Spanish, Italian, Russian, and Japanese he is also much indebted. And finally he would acknowledge with gratitude the unfailing courtesy and the patience with him and with events which the publishers have evinced from the very inception of the undertaking. T. L. S.

CONTENTS.

CONTRIBUTORS TO VOLUME XX.

HENRY W. BERG, M.D., New York.

Attending Physician to the Willard Parker and Riverside Hospitals; Adjunct Attending Physician to Mt. Sinai Hospital.

JOHN T. BOWEN, M.D., Boston.

Physician for Diseases of the Skin, Massachusetts General Hospital; Instructor in Dermatology at Harvard University.

THOMAS R. BROWN, M.D., Baltimore.

Chief of Clinic, Johns Hopkins Hospital Medical Dispensary.

S. ADOLPH KNOPF, M.D., New York.

Physician to the Lung Department of the New York Throat and Nose Hospital; Formerly Assistant Physician to Professor Dettweiler, at the Falkenstein Sanatorium, Germany; Vice-President of the Pennsylvania Society for the Prevention of Tuberculosis.

AUGUST JEROME LARTIGAU, M.D., New York.

Tutor in Pathology, College of Physicians and Surgeons, Columbia University, New York; Assistant Pathologist to Roosevelt Hospital, New York City; Late Assistant in the Bender Hygienic Laboratory, Albany, N. Y.

WOLFRED NELSON, C.M., M.D., F.R.G.S., New York.

Member of the College of Physicians and Surgeons, Quebec; Formerly Member of the State Board of Health, Panama.

JAMES E. NEWCOMB, M.D., New York.

Attending Laryngologist to the Out-Patient Department of the Roosevelt Hospital and to the Demilt Dispensary; Instructor in Laryngology in Cornell University Medical College.

BEAUMONT SMALL, M.D., Ottawa.

Attending Physician to St. Luke's General Hospital; Consulting Physician to the Children's Hospital; Ex-examiner in Materia Medica and Pharmacy, College of Physicians and Surgeons of Ontario.

FRANCIS WARNER, M.D., F.R.C.P., London.

Physician to the London Hospital; Lecturer on Therapeutics, London Hospital Medical College.

TUBERCULOSIS.

(BACTERIOLOGY, PATHOLOGY, AND ETIOLOGY.)

BY

AUGUST JEROME LARTIGAU,

NEW YORK.

TUBERCULOSIS.

(BACTERIOLOGY, PATHOLOGY, AND ETIOLOGY.)

Definition.—Tuberculosis is an infectious disease common to man and certain animals. It is incited by the bacillus tuberculosis and is characterized by an exudative and productive inflammation in which necrosis of the affected tissues is commonly observed. The typical morphological feature of the tissue-reaction consists of small nodular bodies called *tubercles.*

History.

Surely since all progress of mind consists for the most part in differentiation, in the resolution of a complex object into its component aspects, any large apprehension of a theme begins with its earliest history. The progress of the world is, it has been said, a progress by reaction. It has never been a steady advance towards higher and higher perfection, but, rather an interrupted progression —marked now by long intervals of apparent apathy, now by periods of enthusiastic activity. And the transition from the teachings of early Greek medicine to those of cellular pathology and bacterial toxicology was essentially a movement of reaction. From the time of its rudest conception to the present, advancement of the knowledge of tuberculosis has been a parallel movement.

The development, in its most precise sense, of the conception of tuberculosis as a pathological entity is one of comparatively recent origin. A disease with such a striking clinical presentation as phthisis could hardly have escaped that fine keenness of observation so markedly predominant in some of the past observers of medical science. Indeed, so long ago as the fourth and fifth centuries before the Christian era this malady attracted attention. Naturally, in the absence of any definite morphological criterion, and with the knowledge of them depending solely upon external signs, diseases not of that order were often confounded with phenomena of a tuberculous character. In fact, the expression *phthisis* was primarily applicable to all disorders which brought on wasting; later its limitations were narrowed to cachectic disturbances of the respiratory system.

Fix where we may the early origin of our cognizance of tuberculosis, critical inquiry will still be able to find us some earlier apprehension of the subject. In the works of Hippocrates, perhaps, may be found the most remote and best rudimentary anticipation of the clinical nature of consumption. His description certainly sums up some of the most striking clinical manifestations of the disease. Some measure of the same forethought may to a less degree be discovered in the works of Aristotle, Dioscorides, the physician of Cleopatra, and Celsus, while the clinical picture of phthisis given by Aretæus has remained classic from the elegance of its descriptions. Under the name *phthæ* the latter recognizes consumption in its most genuine form, and to him most likely belongs the credit of having first clearly described the disease as a special pathological manifestation.

Any acquaintance of the anatomical side of tuberculosis seriously begins only in the latter part of the seventeenth century; nevertheless, the clinical comprehension of pulmonary tuberculosis made an imperfect and vacillating progression through the labors of Galen, Cælius Aurelianus, Oribasius, Aetius, Alexander Trallian, Paulus Ægineta, Maimonides, and the Arabian physician, Rhazes. Although possessed of not a little renown in former times it cannot be said that the writings of Avicenna, Paracelsus, and Alexander Benedictus contributed to progress in this direction. Forrestus in 1653 published his "Observationum et curationum opera omnia" at Rouen, in which he distinguishes himself by giving a detailed recital of a variety of cases founded on extensive practical observations.

The evolution of the knowledge of tuberculosis from this period becomes largely centred in the study of pathological anatomy.

In the history of medicine there is perhaps no other chapter so rich in interest as that which treats of the development of the conception of the tubercles as the fundamental anatomical lesion. The earliest serious indication of this is found in the writings of Platerus, Bennet, Bonetus, and Sylvius. According to Hoffmann the works of Aretæus showed evidences of a recognition of tuberculous nodosities in the lungs. The compilation of Bonetus, which is considered one of the classical works regarding the changes produced by diseases, contains the clinical histories of several cases of pulmonary phthisis with notes of the autopsy findings, describing cavities and the "sebaceous" contents of "granulations."

In tracing the history of these pathological studies it is interesting to note that Sylvius seems to have been the first to recognize the existence of lymph nodes in connection with ulcerations and suppurations of the lungs. Although having a place in the Greek nosology, chronic enlargements of the superficial lymphatic glands received little study for many centuries thereafter. It was not until the close of the seventeenth century that attention was directed to the close similarity between scrofulous lymph nodes and the caseous nodules in phthisical lungs. This early association of scrofula and tuberculosis, the result of the investigations of Sylvius, possesses considerable historical interest in that the changes in phthisical lungs, it was afterwards conceived, were the manifestations of scrofula in assumed pulmonary lymphatic glands, a view in which Sylvius was supported by numerous contemporary and later writers.

So long ago as 1646, and fully twenty-five years before the observations of Sylvius, there appeared a work by Fabricius Hildanus in which are recorded a number of dissections in consumptive cases in which a mesenteric and pulmonary affection were combined. From the publications of Lieutaud, Stark, Mangetus, and other investigators of the eighteenth century, it is evident that post-mortem studies had become more frequent. In a revised edition of Bonetus' works Mangetus recorded his own observations in forty-nine cases of miliary tuberculosis. He states that in one case (that of a young man who died from phthisis) he made a post-mortem examination and found "grandines" (miliary tubercles) in the lungs, liver, spleen, kidneys, mesenteric glands, and intestines. Likening these bodies to millet-seed—*semen milii*—and regarding them as tuberculous in their nature, he, too, assumes that they arise from lymphatic glands; and furthermore remarks that they are found not only in the tissues of man but also in those of animals. Further additions to this subject were made by the writings of Hoffmann, Van Swieten, and Morgagni, thus giving the tubercle a more important position in the conception of the time. If we may credit some authors, Morton in the early seventeenth century is said to have believed that no form of pulmonary phthisis could develop without tubercles.

One notable step was made by Th. Reid in 1785. Instead of regarding "tubercles" or "grandines" as enlarged lymphatic glands, he conceived the idea that they were products of exudation. The chief value of this belief lay not so much in its intrinsic worth as because the severance from the traditional conceptions gave new impetus to closer investigation. But notwithstanding the evidences of some advance in the understanding of consumptive maladies, the labors of men just preceding Reid—Sauvages, Raulin, Marx, Kortum, Ryan, Cullen, Portal, etc.—can hardly be said to have contributed much to the elucidation of the pathological problem.

The year 1793 was distinguished by the publication of a variety of medical works of considerable interest, at the head of which the "Morbid Anatomy of Some of the Important Parts of the Human Body" of Dr. Baillie holds a prominent position as indicating a new attitude toward and interest in the more exact objective study of morbid phenomena. "Tubercles," the author says, "are firm white bodies interspersed through the substance of the lungs, and apparently formed in the cellular structure; for nothing like a gland is to be discovered in the cellular membrane of the lungs in a healthy state; and the follicles of the bronchiæ are not converted into tubercles; they are first very minute; the clusters probably unite and form larger masses; the most common size is that of a garden pea; they are firm in their consistence, and often contain a portion of thick, curdy pus. . . ."

The notion of tuberculosis as a general disease characterized by multiple localizations in various organs is really of relatively recent date. The physicians of antiquity developed the symptomatology of phthisis; with those of the seventeenth and eighteenth centuries arose the school of anatomopathologists. From the birth of the present century may be traced the fundamental conception of tuberculosis in its most general sense.

To Bayle, the precursor and teacher of Laennec, incontestably belongs the credit of having for the first time attempted a classification of pulmonary phthisis on a strict anatomical basis. In his book, published in 1810, may be found the records of one hundred and nine post-mortem examinations of tuberculous subjects. As a result of these observations he recognizes six types of phthisis distinguished by purely morphological differences, and his wealth of cases enabled him to develop the conception of tuberculosis as a process affecting different parts of the body.

Investigations of this character culminated in the studies of Laennec, who subordinated the whole conception to the unity of tuberculous processes. In 1811 Laennec published in the "Dictionnaire des Sciences médicales" the findings of his first studies in the pathological anatomy of tubercle, and subsequently completed them in the famous "Traité de l'auscultation médiate et des maladies des poumons et du cœur," which appeared in 1819. For him pulmonary phthisis was a pathological entity characterized by a unique lesion, the tubercle. Regarding the tubercle as an accidental product foreign to the normal state and having no prototype in the healthy body, Laennec saw only "tuberculous material" in all the pathological lesions which conformed to the fundamental characters of this tissue, howsoever dissimilar in other respects. This material occurred either in the form of isolated, sharply circumscribed bodies or as infiltrations: "The tuberculous material presents at the start the appearance of a grayish and semi-transparent substance, which little by little becomes opaque, yellow, and very dense; it subsequently softens and acquires a fluidity almost equal to that of pus. . . . This softening begins in the centre of each mass, where the tuberculous substance becomes from day to day more soft and humid, *caséiforme,* or at least unctuous to the touch like soft cheese; the softening gains little by little the circumference and becomes finally complete."

For one born in this day of exacter and larger knowledge it is difficult adequately to estimate the triumph and magnitude of this *tour-de-force* of objective analysis. The ulterior consequences of such an elucidation greatly dominate our entire pathology of this disease at the present time. Laennec, sealing the pathological unity of tuberculosis, had foreclosed many a problem in the sphere of practice.

The greatness of any advance has often been measured by the violence of the opposition to it; with this index alone an estimate of the work of Laennec must place him in the foremost rank of the heroes of medicine. Wholly absorbed in the doctrine of chronic phlegmasia of the lungs Broussais recognized two orders, one entertained by inflammation of the blood-vessel capillaries and the other the resultant of that of the lymphatic vessels. The second type constituted *tuberculization,* which was always preceded by phlegmasia of the first order; thus tuberculosis necessarily always became for him the expression of some anterior chronic inflammation of the respiratory system—pneumonia, bronchitis, laryngitis, pleurisy, etc. Impassioned in his belief, he became a formidable giant of opposition to the doctrine of unity, and with the rise of the school of Broussais — Lepecq, La Cloture, Gendrin, Lobstein, Bouillaud, and Lombard—truth became overshadowed by the tyranny of error, expressions of which we shall later find in the arguments of Virchow and Foerster.

The investigations of Baillie, Bayle, and Laennec, culminating in the discovery of the miliary tubercle, established the vexed relations of scrofula to tuberculosis by the subordination of scrofulous lesions to the latter. In place of the cheesy gland the tubercle became the pathological unity, and wherever caseous deposits were found they were regarded as originating from the miliary tubercle. As the former were more readily recognized than the latter, the occurrence of caseation became the criterion of tuberculosis. Thus to Laennec and such of his followers as Velpeau, Rokitansky, and Cruveilhier the enlarged lymph glands with their caseous centres presented in a characteristic fashion the anatomical manifestations of tuberculosis.

Conclusions essentially similar to those of Laennec resulting from the investigations of Louis, Andral, Cruveilhier, Carswell, and others did much to extend the sphere of influence of this school. In less than thirty years, with the work of Bayle, Laennec, Broussais, Louis, Cruveilhier, and Andral the ideas concerning the nature of pulmonary tuberculosis had undergone important changes, and knowledge in this direction had made more progress than since the first ages of medicine. Apparently the final word had been uttered on a question which had seemed likely to divide medicine for a long time into two rival sects.

With the passing of the first half of the nineteenth century microscopical investigations were coming into vogue. Of those earliest in this field may be cited Lebert, who was soon carried away with the idea that he had discovered the "corpuscle tuberculeux," a specific element, he believed, different from all known structures. What he considered pathognomonic of tubercle were but nuclei and epithelial cells in various stages of degeneration.

The doctrine of Laennec at this time was generally accepted in France; in England Hughes Bennett had adopted it without restriction, and in Vienna the teaching of Rokitansky was practically the same. But dissenting voices were heard now and again—doubts having been excited by the remarkable researches of Reinhardt in 1850, and those of Virchow which quickly followed. In addition to depriving the corpuscles of Lebert of their specific nature, by showing that they may arise from pus cells, etc., the former of these observers fancied that tuberculous material was identical with the product of other inflammations. The ensuing confusion, however, was more directly dependent upon the writings of Virchow. Limiting the term tubercle solely to miliary tubercle, he held that "almost all that is produced in the course of tuberculosis, and which has not the form of a nodule, is a thickened inflammatory product and has no direct relation to tubercle." To him tuberculous material was not so much a special product of tubercles as a termination of diverse processes of neoplastic, purulent, catarrhal, or phlegmasic nature. But Virchow like Laennec regarded the tubercle as a special product, a tumor rich in cells, of a very unstable nature, and readily susceptible to caseation. This interpretation of Virchow, adopted by Foerster, Pawlicki, Niemeyer, Villemin, Morel, Vulpian, and others, soon spread widely, and the dualistic theory became the current conception of the day.

The concurrence of true tubercles with caseous pneumonia must have been so frequent that it could not have escaped observation or been considered a mere coincidence. Explanation of such a coexistence was readily found in the views of Dittrich and Buhl, who believed that tubercles were secondary and consecutive to the absorption of the caseous material. Deeply imbued with the dualistic theory of Virchow, Niemeyer contributed most perhaps to its popularization, and especially from the viewpoint of the clinician. "The greatest danger to which a phthisical patient is exposed is that of becoming tuberculous"—this was the formula of the hour.

So powerful was the teaching of the genius of cellular pathology that the few dissenting voices raised in favor of the unity of phthisis produced little effect. Turning from Germany, where pathologist and clinician alike were dualists, to France, we find there many who still proclaimed the unity of caseous pneumonia and miliary tubercle, the principal of whom were Cornil, Herard, Chauffard, Pidoux, Barth, Behier, and Briquet. In England the same opinion was entertained by Wilson Fox and Green.

From the time of the microscopical studies of Lebert and Reinhardt, it had become even more clearly apparent that the key to many problems must be sought in histological researches. Resolving such investigations to their final analysis—cellular research—Virchow inaugurated a new era in the history of pathology by showing that all the functions of the body in health and in disease are but the manifestations of cell activities. At this period tubercle was regarded in the sense that Virchow had given it—as a mass of small round cells made up of a small amount of protoplasm, resembling lymphoid cells of the lymph nodes and spleen. Such masses of cells, disposed in a fine reticulated stroma, converted the tubercle into a product analogous to lymphoma. Langhans, Koster, and Schüppel, on the other hand, defined tubercle in its most typical and characteristic form as composed of three types of cells—the giant cell of Langhans, epithelioid, and small round cells.

This was the attitude of both pathologist and clinician five decades after the introductory studies of Laennec. However, one observer at least, Villemin, then professor at Val-de-Grace, was endeavoring to prove on new lines the doctrine of unity.

The first effort to produce tuberculosis experimentally dates back in all probability to the year 1789. Kortum inoculated a boy in the region of the neck with "scrofulous pus." Fortunately the result was negative. Experiments of a similar nature were made on dogs three years later by Hébréard; also by Lepellier on guinea-pigs in 1830. In no instance were the animal inoculations successful. The last-named experimenter, and Goodlaad and Deygallières even went so far as to inoculate themselves, without, however, producing tuberculosis. Systematic investigations, undertaken by Cruveilhier in 1826, did much to discredit the views of Laennec. He injected mercury into the trachea and into the veins of animals, and observed as a result abundant nodular formations in the lungs, liver, and mesentery. The tubercles often contained in their centres one or more particles of mercury surrounded by cheesy pus. Cruveilhier came to the conclusion that tubercles are not specific pathological products. Using other substances Richard Vines interpreted his results in the same manner.

In the year 1843 Klencke announced that, after the inoculation of rabbits with miliary tubercles and other tuberculous matter, the animals became tuberculous. The importance and significance of these experimental results were lost for many years afterwards. Notwithstanding the fact that Klencke discovered the experimental inoculability of tuberculosis, the complete demonstration of the communicability, specific character, and unity was none the less the creation of Villemin. At a time when attention was focussed on other themes of vexatious discussion Villemin, at a meeting of the Académie de Médecine on the fifth day of December, 1865, announced the results of his experiments on the inoculability of tuberculosis, the far-reaching significance of which was not fully realized for some time by the scientific world: "Tuberculosis is the effect of a specific causal agent, a virus. This morbid agent like its congeners must reside in the morbid products, which it has determined by its direct action upon the normal elements of the affected tissues. Introduced into an organism susceptible to its impressions this agent must reproduce and reproduce itself during the same time as the disease of which it is the essential principle and determining cause. Experimentation has confirmed these results of induction." Summing up his conclusions he says: "Tuberculosis is a specific affection. Its cause resides in an inoculable agent. Tuberculosis belongs then to the class of virulent maladies and in the nosological scheme must take place beside syphilis, but more close to glanders." These were the conclusions upon which our whole modern conception stands. Hostile objections were raised on almost every side, many speculative, others based on poorly conducted experiments, and finally some due to erroneous interpretation, but Villemin by intelligent elaboration of his experiments produced link by link the complete chain of indubitable evidence now accepted for all time.

Repetition of the inoculation experiments by Herard and Cornil, Roustan, Verga and Biffi, Mantegazza, and others gave results similar to those of Villemin. Over against this Lebert and Wyss, Burdon Sanderson, Wilson Fox, Waldenburg, Cohnheim, and B. Fraenkel claimed to have produced experimentally lesions similar to tuberculosis with tuberculous material, and likewise with substances frankly non-tuberculous in nature. For instance, the two last-named investigators claimed even to reproduce the same condition by the introduction of such bodies as gutta-percha, cinnabar, etc. Conclusions of this kind from so eminent an authority as Cohnheim for a moment seemed to have dealt the final blow to the doctrine of specificity.

The discrepancy in the experimental results of Cohnheim and Fraenkel, and those of Villemin and such of his followers as Herard, Cornil, and Constantin Paul was explained in large part by the researches of Klebs, who did much to draw attention to differences in the evolution and microscopical characters of processes more or less similar to tuberculosis. With the investigations of Chauveau, Gerlach, and Bollinger upon ingestion tuberculosis, the inoculability of the disease was firmly established. Thus the teaching of Laennec is now become the foundation stone of the conception of tuberculosis.

By means of corneal inoculations with tuberculous substances Armanni further confirmed the specificity of tuberculosis. It is interesting to note that Cohnheim, in repeating the earlier experiments of himself and Fraenkel, failed to obtain their first results. This was followed by a remarkable series of investigations by Cohnheim and Solomonsen upon tuberculosis of the iris, subsequently repeated by Hänsell, Baumgarten, and Schuchardt.

Concomitant with the development of the purely experimental side, histological researches led to he same conclusion. Investigators were not slow to appreciate that the giant cell as such could not be considered the microscopical characteristic of tubercle; indeed, Ziegler and Barmgarten demonstrated its presence in other inflammations. Moreover, the last-named observer pointed out structures histologically similar to the tubercles of Langhans which were the result of simple mechanical irritation. More comprehensive in his study, Hip. Martin, in addition to verifying the observations of Ziegler and Baumgarten, established a fact of more importance in its ultimate applications: The inoculation of the foreign-body tubercle, such as Ziegler experimented with, produced no lesion whatsoever when introduced into animals; in contradistinction to this, true tubercles invariably excited the same disease in its typical manifestations.

Once the unity and infectious character of tuberculosis were accepted, the trend of thought naturally directed itself to the intimate nature of its exciting agent. It has already been seen with what fine intuitive sense Villemin denied that the cells or elements of tuberculous material were of themselves the infecting principle, but held that this was simply contained in them. This was verily an anticipation of subsequent realizations.

Klebs announced in 1877 that the inoculation of animals with cultures from tuberculous products upon the white of eggs produced lesions similar to those following the injection of tuberculous tissues themselves. This "monas tuberculosum" of Klebs was verified by Schüller and Reinstadler some time afterwards. But neither these investigations nor those of Toussaint did anything to solve this *question du jour*.

The announcement of the discovery of the bacillus tuberculosis was made by Koch before the Physiological Society of Berlin on the twenty-fourth day of March, 1882, the complete memoir appearing two years later. The subsequent history of this disease constitutes the whole theme of the remainder of what follows on tuberculosis.

BACTERIOLOGY.

As a natural outcome of the discovery of the tubercle bacillus much attention has been given to the bacteriology of tuberculosis, both clinical and experimental. There is scarcely another subject of equal magnitude which has witnessed the same development and perfection of study. The new field made possible by the investigations of Villemin, and opened up with results so brilliantly realized by Koch, has been assiduously cultivated by a host of workers. The wealth of contributions to this knowledge may well be taken as the criterion of a research activity the equal of which has hardly been known in any other department. Such labor has been inestimable in its ulterior consequences. Withal, the greater amount of the information derived therefrom has related mainly to details and cannot truly be said to have extensively modified the fundamental conclusions enunciated by Koch.

Tinctorial Reactions.

In the history of the discovery of many microorganisms direct observation has played a most prominent part. With tuberculosis, however, special difficulties presented themselves, as might have been inferred from the futility of previous attempts to identify the infecting agent. Attempts to stain fresh material or hardened tissues soon demonstrated the inefficiency of the tinctorial methods then in vogue. So evident was it that any success would be the direct outcome of improved technique that Koch undertook researches in this direction. His earliest experiments were made with the diseased tissues of animals hardened in alcohol. Utilizing a previous observation that the coloration of bacteria with simple aqueous solutions of basic aniline dyes was much facilitated if these solutions were made slightly alkaline, Koch, by submitting cover-slip specimens from various tuberculous lesions for so long a time as twenty-four hours to an alkaline solution of methlyene blue, ultimately succeeded in staining certain fine rods.   With the introduction of this improvement the history of the bacillus tuberculosis begins.   Appreciation of the value of studying the tubercle bacillus in sections led Koch perforce to develop modifications in the tinctorial procedures, inasmuch as the methods employed were inefficient to demonstrate both the bacillus and histological features of the section.   The action of a concentrated aqueous solution of vesuvin until the preparations were brown, after they had first been stained with methylene blue for twenty-four hours, accomplished the desired result.

The communication of Baumgarten several weeks after the announcement of the discovery of the tubercle bacillus possesses considerable interest.   During the course of an experimental research on tuberculosis in rabbits this observer had occasion to examine freshly hardened and unstained tissue from these animals in a weak solution of caustic potash.   Examining them under these conditions he detected bacilli which did not stain by Weigert's method.   Basing his opinion on this "negative reaction," he considered them "pathognomonic of tuberculosis."   Shortly after this Baumgarten had the opportunity at one of the meetings of the Medical Society of Berlin to submit his preparations to Koch, who pronounced the bacilli identical with his bacillus tuberculosis.

In the present state of improved technique the original method of Koch for staining the tubercle bacillus can present at most but an interest of a purely historical character.   Quickly following the note of Koch, Ehrlich made known a more certain and convenient procedure.   In lieu of the alkaline mixture an aqueous solution of aniline methyl violet or fuchsin was substituted.   After staining for fifteen to twenty minutes with the aniline dyes the preparations were decolorized with a moderately strong watery solution of nitric acid, and thus the tubercle bacilli took the violet or red stain while the remaining elements were unstained.   As a more or less direct derivative of this procedure many other modifications were developed—the methods of Ziehl, with Neelsen's modification of the same, of Fraenkel, Gabbet, Gibbes, Kühne, and others.   As decolorizing agents a great number of substances have been used.   Thus, Petri recommended glacial acetic acid, Watson Cheyne, formic acid, and the use of oxalic acid was urged by Cornil and by Alvarez and Tavel.   More recently Hauser has tried lactic and citric acids in five to ten per cent. aqueous solution or two to three per cent. alcoholic solution; alcoholic or aqueous solutions of picric acid are also lauded by Hauser because they decolorize the tissues readily without affecting the coloration of the tubercle bacillus.

Such a variety of methods for staining the tubercle bacillus is in vogue that the selection of any method necessarily depends largely on questions of certainty, adaptation, and preference. The principle of all differential stains is based on the fact that when once stained the tubercle bacillus offers considerable resistance to decolorizing agents generally, while other microorganisms lose their stain when exposed to the same conditions. To this there are several exceptions —the bacillus of leprosy, the smegma bacillus, and certain other bacteria which have been isolated from timothy grass, cow dung, milk, butter, etc.—all of which possess tinctorial reactions very similar to that of the tubercle bacillus. Lustgarten has described a bacillus in syphilitic lesions which reacts to stains like the tubercle bacillus. The specific relationship of this organism to syphilis has, however, been very much discredited in recent years. The differential stains of the important members of this group will be considered in the section on Bacteriological Diagnosis.

The following methods have given me excellent results:

DEMONSTRATION OF THE BACILLI IN FLUIDS.

For the coloration of the bacillus tuberculosis in fluids, such as sputum, exudates, urine, etc., the material should be spread in a thin layer over a cover glass, dried in the air, and then passed three times through the flame.

Ziehl-Neelsen's Stain.—The cover glass is preferably floated in a watch glass with the specimen side down on the carbolic-fuchsin solution, then gently heated almost to ebullition for three or four minutes. Some hold the cover glass or slide in the forceps with the specimen side up and thoroughly cover with carbolic-fuchsin solution. It is warmed over a flame for one to two minutes, preferably avoiding ebullition. Drying of the stain on the specimen should be prevented by adding from time to time a little fresh carbolic fuchsin.

The fuchsin mixture is made by adding to a five-per-cent. watery solution of carbolic acid about one-tenth its volume of saturated alcoholic solution of fuchsin. After heating, the excess of dye is washed off with water and the specimen is placed in five-per-cent. aqueous or alcoholic solution of sulphuric acid (fifteen per cent. nitric acid may also be used). When the color disappears the specimen is thoroughly rinsed in two or more portions of sixty or seventy per cent. alcohol, and finally in water. This will to a certain extent restore the red color. The next step is to counterstain with a one- or two-per-cent. aqueous solution of methylene blue for about one minute, the excess of which is washed off with water. Partial or complete decolorization of the tubercle bacilli should be avoided by not exposing the specimen too long to the action of the acid. A little experience will determine the time required for the action of the decolorizing agent. The examination is then made, after drying of the specimen, with an oil-immersion lens. If a slide be used to spread the material on, the intervention of a cover glass is not necessary. The tubercle bacilli will be stained red and the other bacteria blue.

Gabbet's Method.—The writer has found this method most convenient for general practical purposes. It has the advantage of decolorizing and counterstaining in one step. Stain in carbolic fuchsin for about one minute, steaming the preparation and adding more staining-fluid as it evaporates. Wash in water, and then cover with the sulphuric-methylene blue; wash in water thoroughly and mount. Generally thirty seconds to one minute is long enough for the acid methylene blue mixture. In this way the bacillus tuberculosis is stained red and the other bacteria and cell nuclei blue, the decolorization and contrast staining being effected in one operation. The methylene blue solution consists of two parts of the blue stain in one hundred parts of a twenty-five-per-cent. solution of sulphuric acid.

DEMONSTRATION OF THE BACILLI IN SECTIONS.

For staining tubercle bacilli in sections a number of reliable methods exist, of which the following have given satisfaction. Alcohol hardened specimens give the best results.

Ziehl-Neelsen's Method.—Sufficiently thin sections of tissue are left in the carbolic-fuchsin solution for about twenty-four hours. Heating the fluid for one hour at a temperature of 45° to 50° C., or placing in the incubator at the body temperature over night or less time answers equally well. Decolorize in five-per-cent. sulphuric acid for a few seconds, then in seventy-per-cent. alcohol. Stain for one to two minutes in an aqueous solution of methylene blue, wash in water, dehydrate with absolute alcohol, clear up in xylol or oil of cedar, and mount in Canada balsam.

Hodenpyl recommends a modification which prevents shrinkage of the section and is quicker. Frozen sections, or those cut in celloidin or paraffin, are placed in albumin solution; then transferred to the cover glass or slide and gently blotted with washed cheese-cloth used in several layers, and again immediately transferred to strong alcohol to fix the sections to the glass. The specimen is then placed in the watch glass containing carbolic fuchsin and heated for about five minutes. It is decolorized in one-per-cent. alcoholic hydrochloric-acid solution for about a minute or two, then passed into a saturated solution of lithium carbonate to neutralize, and finally into ninety-five-per-cent. alcohol. The specimen may be counterstained by leaving it in a weak alcoholic solution of methylene blue. It should be cleared in xylol or oil of origanum and mounted in Canada balsam.

The albumin solution recommended is prepared by adding the white of two eggs to 300 c.c. of distilled water and slightly alkalinizing the whole by the addition of a small amount of salicylate of sodium. The mixture may be kept for some time by the addition of a little camphor.

For simple detection of the bacilli in tissues it is usually better to have no color in the specimen other than that which the bacilli take up. A method which has given the writer eminently satisfactory results with double staining is that of Kühne and strongly recommended by Borrel.

Kühne's Method.—Stain paraffin sections with alum-hæmatoxylin or hæmatein; two minutes suffice for good nuclear coloration. Wash in water. Stain in carbolic fuchsin for ten to fifteen minutes and wash again in water. Submit to the action of a two-per-cent. aqueous solution of aniline hydrochlorate (salzsaures Anilin) for about ten to fifteen seconds. Wash in water, then in absolute alcohol, and finally in xylol. Mount in xylol balsam. Protoplasm and blood cells may also be stained with an aqueous solution of aurantia employed after the alcohol.

PRINCIPLE OF THE DIFFERENTIAL STAIN.

This resistance of the stain to acids, at one time believed absolutely characteristic of the tubercle bacillus, has received varying explanations at different times, none of which did more than satisfy the exigencies of the moment. Comparative studies of the bacillus tuberculosis and the smegma bacillus of Alvarez and Tavel demonstrated similar tinctorial reactions for both organisms, and it was thought once that certain dissimilarities explained the selective tinctorial attributes considered specific. Assuming that both bacilli owed their staining peculiarities to fatty envelopes, which at once resisted the penetration of stains and prevented the action of acids, Bienstock some years ago undertook some investigations with a view to proving this hypothesis. By cultivating various saprophytic species in media containing butter he ascertained that these bacteria when treated with a warm fuchsin solution for ten minutes resisted the action of strong acid mixtures.   Gottstein soon afterwards found bacteria in the cerumen of the ear, which offered the same reactions as the smegma bacillus.   Repeating Bienstock's experiments on a more extensive scale, using media containing various substances, such as butter, lanolin, wax, paraffin, etc., he convinced himself of the accuracy of the other's results.   And, moreover, another important point was brought to light by these investigations.   If these bacilli from the ear or the smegma bacilli be submitted to the action of a hot solution of caustic soda to which five per cent. alcohol has been added and are then washed in water and finally in alcohol, it will be found that the fatty capsule has been completely removed, and this manipulation destroys the characteristic staining reaction.   Similar treatment of the tubercle bacillus produces no change in tinctorial behavior.   The theory of the protective fatty envelope is obviously insufficient to explain the specificity of this reaction.

Hammerschlag found that the alcoholic and ethereal extracts of dried bacilli treated with potash solutions no longer stained after Ehrlich's manner, but still took up aniline gentian violet or carbolic fuchsin, and resisted decolorization by strong acids.   The action of sodium hydroxide upon tubercle bacilli, according to Weyl, gives a yellow liquid which consists of two layers, the lower of which behaves in a characteristic manner to acids.   He thinks that this represents the envelope of the bacilli.   Not very long ago Aronson made known the results of his studies into the chemical constitution of the tubercle bacillus, from which we learn that he considers a reddish-brown material, giving the reactions of wax, enveloping the organism, but not in it, as the substance which is so strongly resistant to decolorizing methods.   It is evident that at the present time we are not able to explain with any measure of confidence the underlying principle of the behavior of the bacillus tuberculosis to stains.

The first belief that the tubercle bacillus does not take the simpler staining-fluids was necessarily modified in time.   In 1883 Lichtheim and Giacomi discovered that the action of simple concentrated aqueous solutions of fuchsin or gentian violet if continued for several hours answered the purpose very well, and these observations were confirmed by Baumgarten and Ehrlich.   The latter pointed out this curious fact, that when stained under these conditions the bacilli were less resistant to acids than when aniline or carbolic solutions had been employed.   This has been confirmed by Straus, who found that not only cold but even warm aqueous or hydroalcoholic solutions gave less resistant stains.

It is possible to stain tubercle bacilli by Gram's method, but this procedure and that of Weigert possess so few advantages and so many disadvantages that their employment must indeed be very infrequent.

Morphological Characters.

In stained specimens the tubercle bacilli are generally fine slender rods, measuring from 1.5 to 3.5 μ in length. Sometimes larger forms up to 5 or even 8 μ are met with not only under artificial conditions

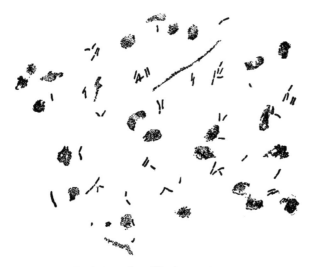

Fɪɢ. 1 —Tubercle Bacilli in Sputum (Straus).

of growth but likewise in tissues. Contrasting strikingly with the variations of length is the more fixed and regular thickness of the organism with a given method of staining. It is quite slender, frequently not exceeding 0.2 or 0.3 μ in thickness. Some observers mention forms as thick as 0.5 μ. The thickness, which is so generally uniform, at times shows apparent irregularities, appearing as a series of contractions as though the bacillus were a chain of ovoid bodies.

Slightly curved forms make up the greatest number; in some rare instances the curving is so considerable that they are in the form of a U. In addition, bacilli are not uncommonly observed, which appear as if formed of articulated segments joined at a wide angle and giving one the impression that they are broken bacteria. For the most part the arrangement of the rods is discrete, often in pairs, either joined end to end or parallel; now and again more or less aggregated clumps, or chains of variable lengths—strepto-forms—may be present.

It is very common to see a peculiar beaded appearance in the stained tubercle bacilli, although specimens from young cultures generally show even and uniform staining. The beading is due to an irregularity in staining of the protoplasm visible at greater or less intervals. In unstained specimens these appear as clear, refractive dots in the protoplasm. These are viewed by the majority of bacteriologists as portions of fragmented protoplasm, but some insist that they are spores. The assumption that these highly refractive portions of protoplasm are spores—endogenous spores—appears to be based on insufficient evidence. If tubercle bacilli are strongly stained with carbolic fuchsin and then submitted to the action of bisulphite of sodium, the whole protoplasm will be unstained except some oval portions which retain the fuchsin. Such bodies Ehrlich thought were spores. Looking at them in the same way Nocard and Roux described "grains" which to them had entirely the aspect of spores. The interpretation of these as spores presents certain difficulties, and most notable, as Metchnikoff points out, is the fact that the clear spaces do not take the stain after exposure for long periods to warm solutions, a procedure which, on the other hand, is successful in demonstrating the spores of other bacteria, such as anthrax bacilli.

A method of double staining with Ziehl's solution and carbolic methylene blue has, in the experience of Czaplewski, brought out in specimens from old cultures small oval portions seen as bright red bodies in the blue protoplasm of the bacilli. Despite observations of this kind the trend of recent investigations of these suggestive spore-like bodies leans to a negative rather than to a positive answer. Certainly these portions of protoplasm do not represent spores in the sense generally given to that term. Critical estimation, however, should not lose sight of the fact that while no definite differences in reaction to heat, desiccation, or antiseptics have been established between forms of tubercle bacilli containing these refractive portions and those free from them, repeated observations have shown that old cultures of human or avian bacilli consist, instead of bacillary forms, largely of small round bodies taking the stains deeply. Transplantation of these cultures on suitable media gives new growth consisting of typical bacilli. Forms of this kind Straus looked upon as more resistant, and yet not of the nature of spores as the expression is generally accepted.

VARIATIONS IN FORM.

Babes, Petrone, and Nocard and Roux were among the first to note significant variations in the morphology of the tubercle bacillus; but it was only in 1888 that Metchnikoff called particular attention to the pleomorphic forms. In old serum or glycerin-agar cultures he found bacilli remarkable for their small size and resemblance to cocci.

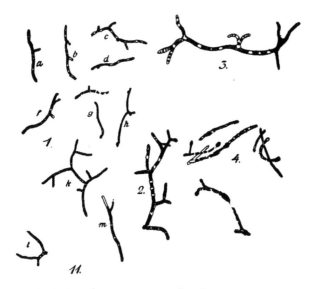

FIG. 2.—Branching Form of the Tubercle Bacillus (Coppen Jones)

Sometimes they were oval or lancet shaped; certain cultures were made up exclusively of these short forms. But Metchnikoff's paper related more especially to those large varieties found in cultures which had been incubated at high temperatures (43.6° to 44° C.) for about twenty days on glycerin-agar. In the midst of ordinary types there were seen long and thick bacilli with swollen ends and which stained very deeply. Still older growths contained branching organisms and intermediate forms.

Shortly thereafter Klein published a report of filamentous club-shaped and branching bacilli in old cultures. Further and fuller studies of the uncommon morphological variations were made by

Marfucci, Fischl, Babes, Bruns, Coppen Jones, Ledoux-Lebard, and Craig.

The long filamentous microorganisms described by Fischl, Coppen Jones, and others often presented elementary branching at almost right angles with vacuoles and metachromatic granules similar to those observed in actinomycosis by Babes. Dichotomous division has been repeatedly mentioned by investigators; indeed, Coppen Jones described in tuberculous sputum forms of the tubercle bacillus showing very characteristic features of the actinomyces-group of microorganisms.

Suggestive results along the lines of experimental morphology have led investigators to regard the bacillus tuberculosis as closely related to a higher group of organisms, and naturally any similarities of appearance have been studied with considerable interest. In 1897 Babes and Levaditi published some results which have done much to excite new interest in the subject. At the end of thirty days rabbits that had received subdural inoculations of tubercle bacilli presented foci which had a radiated appearance consisting of elongated, branched, and clubbed bacilli, the clubs taking the methylene blue stain once the rest of the organism had been stained deeply by Ehrlich's method.

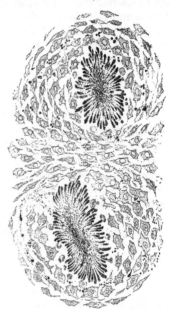

Fig. 3.—Actinomycotic Form of the Tubercle Bacillus (Babes and Levaditi).

Practically the same results were obtained by Friedrich from intraventricular injections into the heart of rabbits. A variant of this same method is found in the experiments of O. Schultze. Following direct inoculations into the kidney, liver, testicle, and mamma of rabbits, usually in from fourteen to fifty days, the tubercle bacillus, when the process remained localized, was partly in bacillary form, in part also in actinomycotic form. It was found impossible to demonstrate the club formation by the use of Ziehl-Neelsen stain, but with Gram-Weigert or Birch-Hirschfeld's actinomyces stain they could be well studied. More recently Friedrich and Nösske have again gone over the same ground with results largely confirmatory of previous researches.

It is important to point out that much of the work upon the pleomorphic types of the bacillus tuberculosis, especially the earlier observations, were made with bovine and avian tuberculosis, although similar investigations with bacilli of human origin are not lacking. It would seem that change of environment is one of the most potent factors in altering the morphological characters. So Kráhl and Dubar have completely changed the tubercle bacillus of human and avian origin in its morphological appearance by growth in cold-blooded animals. Differences have been insisted upon by Theobald Smith between bovine and human bacilli. According to him bovine bacilli tend to remain short while the others are more slender.

Biology.

Study of the life history of the bacillus tuberculosis has supplied us with a large number of facts of the highest degree of practical importance. Ordinarily the tubercle bacillus is a strict parasite, and its biological characters are of such a nature that it scarcely finds appropriate conditions outside the living organism for its multiplication. Saprophytic growth probably does not occur naturally, but attention has been directed to the fact by Nocard and Roux that prolonged cultivation in artificial media containing glycerin so modifies it that after a time cultures may be obtained in simple bouillon in which it would not grow when introduced from a fresh culture recently grown from infected tissues. Later investigations by Proskauer and Beck, Kimla, Poupé and Vesely exhibit this saprophytic adaptability in a more striking degree still. The possibility of cultivation in so simple fluids as those containing only inorganic salts without either glycerin or albumin is indeed full of interest.

In contradistinction to the bacillus tuberculosis of human derivation that of avian sources or from cold-blooded animals very quickly adapts itself to saprophytic modes of existence as shown by the experiments of Straus, Nocard, Ferran, Dubard, and others. This would seemingly indicate that at some remote time it was a true saprophyte. Observations by Nuttall point to an actual multiplication of the bacilli in sputum outside the body; and from analogy it seems highly probable that it takes place in a limited degree in the mucopurulent secretion, which accumulates in pulmonary cavities in tuberculous patients. Under such conditions its development might in a certain sense be regarded as saprophytic.

Viability.—The length of life of the tubercle bacillus depends upon many conditions, one of the most important of which is its source. If subcultures be made from growths of human bacilli five or six months old, cultivation is occasionally successful; with older cultures attempts almost invariably fail. Such a test is inconclusive, however, by reason of its crudeness. Animal experimentation in matters of this kind must always be the basis of conclusion, for often living tubercle bacilli culturally give negative results while animal inoculations will frequently prove successful. Hence much of the earlier work must perforce be discarded.

Dried tuberculous sputum has been found to contain still virulent bacilli, and similar results are obtained when the bacilli are kept for several weeks in distilled water. Chantemesse and Widal kept tubercle bacilli alive in sterile water at a temperature varying from 8° to 18° C. for fifty and seventy days. Treated in the same way, but at a higher temperature, Straus and Dubarry found the avian bacillus still alive at the end of one hundred and fifteen days. Portions of lung from a tuberculous cow dried and pulverized produced tuberculosis in guinea-pigs at the end of one hundred and two days (Cadéac and Malet). The viability of avian tubercle bacilli in a general way is stated to be longer than that of mammalian bacilli. Subcultures are possible with cultures over one year old. Indeed, Marfucci successfully transplanted a culture at least two years old.

Multiplication.—Like most bacteria the bacillus tuberculosis multiplies by transverse fission. Observations of W. Hesse with his new medium incline this investigator to regard longitudinal division as a possible additional mode of growth, but repeated examinations by myself and my colleague Hiss have afforded no direct evidences of such a form of multiplication. Further and fuller investigation would be required for confirmation of Hesse's view.

Relation to Oxygen.—The fact that the tubercle bacillus does not grow in the depths of solid media and that even in liquids, in which diffusion of oxygen is easier, the growth more readily develops on the surface is proof that it is frankly aérobic in its tendencies. Growth in an anaérobic atmosphere, however, is quite possible; thus Fraenkel classifies it as a facultative anaérobic microorganism.

Motility.—Opinion has been unanimous until recently that the bacillus tuberculosis is a non-motile organism. Schumowski, however, made observations in Uschinsky's laboratory which led him to believe that it is not infrequently a motile bacillus. If a particle of culture be taken from the growing pellicle and examined, he says, it will be found to consist of a central filamentous network in which numerous bacilli exhibit more or less motility of an active vibratory kind. When drying is prevented, this movement may continue for forty-eight hours, after which time it ceases, an occurrence which certainly indicates that it is independent of Brownian movement. Schumowski attributed the motility to flagella, although he was unable to demonstrate them. Ferrán, of Barcelona, made similar observations under somewhat different circumstances. Finally Dubard, in his report at the congress for the study of tuberculosis in 1898, stated that in the course of an investigation of fish tuberculosis he also had observed motile forms of the tubercle bacillus.

Conclusions of this kind are to be accepted with some reserve at the present time; more extended study alone can decide the accuracy of these observations.

Behavior Under Various Physical and Chemical Influences.

The tubercle bacillus reacts to different physical and chemical influences in various ways. Knowledge of this behavior with regard to certain conditions has great practical value.

Temperature.—The bacillus tuberculosis of man and mammals grows best at 37° or 38° C. At a temperature exceeding 42° C. growth ceases; with temperatures below 30° C. multiplication is very feeble. Indeed, Koch found that at 28° or 29° C. development is completely arrested. The microorganism of avian tuberculosis on the other hand shows adaptation to wider ranges of temperature. While it grows actively between 30° and 43° and even 45° C., Marfucci states that after acclimatization a slow growth may also be obtained at a temperature of 20° C.; the maximum temperature of cultivation is about 50° C. The habitat of the bacillus in fish, as well as its parasitic life in other cold-blooded animals, generally makes it possible to obtain active vegetation at so low a degree as 10° C. (Dubard).

Experimental studies of Galtier upon the resistance of tubercle bacillus to low temperatures gave interesting results. Alternating congelation at −3° to −8° C. and thawing at +3° to + 8°C. for several weeks did not kill the bacilli. Similar observations by Cadéac and Malet proved the correctness of these facts.

Investigations of more practical significance were made long ago by Toussaint. In order to determine whether the heat obtained when roasting meat was sufficient to destroy the virulence of tuberculous meat, experiments were made which showed that the central part of such meat was still infective. The report of the Royal Commission on Tuberculosis contains identical conclusions by Woodhead. Analogous researches by Galtier demonstrated that infected milk or

extract of tuberculous meat when brought to the boiling temperature
was incapable of producing animal tuberculosis; after a less degree
of heat, however, inoculations gave positive results. The effect of
heat on tuberculous milk formed the subject only a few years ago of
an elaborate research by Woodhead. He seems to accept as proved
that raising milk to 100° C. even for a single instant will completely
kill the tubercle bacilli contained in it. Although the character of
the disease produced was perhaps modified, and although in some
cases the proportion of test animals affected was small, tuberculosis
was nevertheless produced in guinea-pigs by intraperitoneal inoculation of milk which had been heated but for a moment at 90° C., heated
for twenty-two minutes at 75° C., for thirty minutes at 70° C., three
hours at 65° C., and twelve hours at 50° C. After heating for longer
periods at each of the mentioned temperatures the milk was incapable
of inciting tuberculosis in any of the animals.

The resistance of tubercle bacilli in sputum to dry and moist heat
has been the subject of a number of studies. Dried tuberculous sputum placed in an oven at 100° C. (dry heat) for one hour was still
virulent to guinea-pigs; similar sputum submitted to the same temperature of moist heat for fifteen minutes still showed living organisms in two out of three inoculations; this degree of moist heat continued for thirty minutes was thoroughly effective in killing them.
The action of steam at 100° C. on fresh undried sputum for fifteen
minutes gave similar results. Sputum of this kind boiled for two,
five, and ten minutes respectively was found infective to guinea-
pigs only after the boiling for two minutes. Repeating these experiments of Schill and Fischer, Voelsch arrived at apparently contradic-
tory results, concluding that just bringing to the boiling-point once,
or even twice, is insufficient to destroy the tubercle bacillus. These
conclusions cannot be accepted in the light of our knowledge of the
action of dead tubercle bacilli as shown by Prudden and Hodenpyl
and Straus and Gamaleïa. Doubtless Voelsch's animal lesions were
of this same nature.

Working with old cultures supposedly containing spores Yersin
compared the effects of heat from 55° to 110° C. for ten minutes upon
such cultures to those from a fresh spleen, presumably free from
spores. At the end of fifteen days growth was obtained from the
culture (free from spores?) submitted to 55° C.; in thirty-seven days
a culture was grown from those submitted to 60° C., and finally heating at 70° C. gave no results. The memoir of Grancher and Ledoux-
Lebard contains parallel experiments upon human and avian tubercle
bacilli with both dry and moist heat with the following results: Diluted cultures of avian bacillus tuberculosis heated in a water-bath

for fifty minutes at 50° C. still gave subcultures, but after sixty minutes no development could be obtained. At 60° C. development occurred after ten minutes' exposure, but after twenty minutes they were sterile. Exposure from 70° to 100° C. for one minute or even one-half minute at 100° C. gave negative results. In similar investigations upon human tubercle bacilli after an exposure of ten and even fifteen minutes at 50° C. growth could still be obtained; for one minute at 70° C. the culture was sterile. Accordant with other investigators Grancher and Ledoux-Lebard find that dried bacilli resist heat better than moist cultures.

Having in mind the influence of heat in so-called pasteurization of milk Forster made some observations on the effect of moist heat upon tuberculous milk, crushed tuberculous tissue, and sputum in water. The results showed that heating to 60° C. for forty-five minutes or to 70° C. for five to ten minutes sterilized the material. The action of a temperature of 50° C. for twelve hours did not suffice to accomplish this result. The experience of Bonhoff in the main coincided with the above results.

De Man in Forster's laboratory made a series of tests with tuberculous tissue. The thermal death points established by him are now generally published in text-books. He used chiefly disintegrated, semi-fluid, cheesy matter from tuberculous udders. After an exposure at 60° C. for fifteen, thirty, and forty-five minutes the material was still infective; the application of this heat for sixty minutes, however, completely destroyed the bacilli. Sputum equally exposed for sixty minutes was innocuous. From these results it has been generally assumed that when exposed to this temperature for one hour tubercle bacilli will be killed.

Woodhead fed guinea-pigs with infected milk which had been subjected to 60° C. for one-half hour, without producing tuberculosis. On the other hand, milk heated to the same point for fifteen minutes and injected into animals gave positive results in two out of three trials; of three guinea-pigs inoculated with similar milk for thirty minutes lesions developed in one. In a recent article on the thermal death point of the tubercle bacillus in milk and other fluids Theobald Smith concludes that tubercle bacilli, when suspended in distilled water, normal salt solution, bouillon, and milk, are destroyed at 60° C. in fifteen to twenty minutes. The larger number are destroyed in five to ten minutes. When they were suspended in milk he found that the pellicle which forms during the exposure at 60° C. might contain living bacilli after sixty minutes.

Desiccation.—Recognition of the importance of sputum as a means of dissemination of the infectious agent long ago led Villemin to undertake some studies with a view to finding out how far desiccation influences the viability of the bacillus tuberculosis. The results proved that dried sputum still retained its virulence at the end of several weeks. Koch allowed phthisical sputum to dry for four to eight weeks at room temperature, at the end of which time he found the material still virulent. Alternate desiccation and moistening for a period of twelve hours was shown by Malassez and Vignal not to abolish the virulency. Sputum dried for four months was demonstrated to contain virulent bacilli, and about the sixth month Schill and Fischer found that a few virulent organisms still remained, but about the seventh month all the tubercle bacilli were dead. Galtier, Cadéac and Malet, and Sawizky similarly attest the long persistence of virulence in dried tuberculous material. Cadéac and Malet produced tuberculosis with dried material one hundred and fifty days old.

Putrefaction.—Inoculations of tuberculous tissues, allowed to undergo putrefaction for fifteen, seventeen, or more days, gave positive results in the hands of Galtier. Putrefaction of material in the air, water, or earth does not seem to destroy its infectiousness for a considerable time. The same writer obtained positive results under these conditions at the end of thirty days. For instance, a tuberculous rabbit which was buried in the ground and exhumed twenty-three days later in a high degree of putrefaction still contained virulent tubercle bacilli. Equally interesting were the investigations of Cadéac and Malet, who buried portions of tuberculous lungs and determined their infectivity at the end of seventy-seven, one hundred and twenty-four, one hundred and fifty-nine, and one hundred and sixty-seven days. Schottelius makes the statement that after "several years" the lungs of buried phthisical subjects still contain tubercle bacilli capable of producing tuberculous lesions.

Sunlight.—A careful review of the literature shows that there are reported but few series of experiments with reference to the effect of direct sunlight on the viability of the bacillus tuberculosis. Since the experiments of Downes and Blunt with mixed cultures and Arloing with pure cultures of various germs direct sunlight has been regarded as one of the most potent natural agencies in annihilating the virulence of bacteria. It seems not unreasonable then that considerable stress should have been laid upon this question in its application to tuberculosis. Koch showed that the direct solar rays killed the bacillus in from several minutes to several hours, according to the thickness of the layer exposed. Moreover, he found that diffuse light when prolonged produces the same effect. Cultures placed in broad daylight but protected from the direct solar rays perish in five to seven days.

In a similar manner Straus destroyed cultures of the same organism by placing them for two hours in the direct sunlight of summer. Dried cultures under the same circumstances were destroyed in one-half hour.

Feltz, after exposing to the direct rays of the sun for one hundred and thirty-seven days a mixture of soil and tuberculous sputum, found it still capable of inducing an experimental tuberculosis; after this time it had lost its virulence. This author asserts that a portion of the same mixture, when exposed to the changing climatic and atmospheric conditions as they occur naturally, retained its virulence only a little over two months. An investigation to determine the direct influence of sunlight conducted by Migneco led him to the following conclusions: (a) Sunlight exercises a deleterious influence upon the tubercle bacillus, just as it does upon other bacteria; (b) tubercle bacilli, as found in tuberculous sputum and spread on linen or woollen cloths, are not able to withstand the influence of direct sunlight for more than twenty-four to thirty hours, provided the sputum is not spread in too thick a layer; (c) the virulence of the tubercle bacillus diminishes gradually during exposure to the sun, and eventually, at the end of from ten to fifteen hours, entirely loses its virulence.

More recently Mitchell and Crouch, from a study of the influence of sunlight on tuberculous sputum in Denver, came to the conclusion in the first place, that the tubercle bacillus, as expectorated on a sandy soil, is still virulent after thirty-five hours' exposure to the direct rays of the sun, and that such sputum has suffered but little diminution in virulence after twenty-four hours' exposure; in the second place, in from twenty-four to thirty-five hours' exposure the virulence is gradually diminished and finally lost if the exposure extends beyond the last-mentioned time. Finally, G. Lucibelli found that tubercle bacilli in dried sputum were killed in eighteen days when exposed to diffused light, but not so in sixty or eighty days in the dark.

X-Rays.—The question whether the Roentgen rays exert any influence on bacterial life has not as yet been very exhaustively studied. J. Brunton Blaikie, Francis Pott, and E. Ausset, who have made a number of investigations with a view to determine this question, are unanimous in their conclusion that the *x*-rays do not affect the growth of the tubercle bacillus in cultures.

Chemical Substances.—The action of many chemical substances upon the tubercle bacillus has been very fully studied mostly in relation to utilitarian practices. Careful investigation of the disinfecting properties of these various substances has been made by Schill and Fischer. Thus sputum submitted to the action of alcohol for ten

hours lost its virulence; but its infectivity was not destroyed by exposure for twenty-four hours to one-per-cent. creosote solution, arsenious acid, saturated aqueous solution of naphthalin (one-per-cent.), solution of iodide of potassium, bromide of potassium, bromine water, iodine water (1 : 500), saturated aqueous iodoform solution, vapor of iodoform, or essence of turpentine. One- and two-per-cent. solutions of carbolic acid were equally inefficacious; to be effectual in twenty hours a three-per-cent. solution was found necessary. Investigating the action of sulphurous acid upon virulent tubercle bacilli Vallin demonstrated that an exposure of fourteen hours killed them, provided 30 gm. of sulphur was burned to the cubic metre of space; dried tuberculous material exposed during twenty-four hours with 20 gm. to the cubic metre still remained infective. Thoinot, in addition to confirming the higher resistance of dried bacilli to sulphurous acid, advocates the burning of at least 60 gm. to the cubic metre for twenty-four hours; a less quantity he thinks gives a less constant security. Parrot and Hip. Martin with the use of 1 : 500 salicylic-acid solutions, or 1 : 1,000 corrosive sublimate, failed to abolish the virulence of the sputum with a twenty-four hours' exposure.

Yersin (1888) carried out some experiments of the same nature with cultures of the tubercle bacillus of the same age and virulence. These experiments were extremely interesting. The table of results is herewith appended:

	Parts per 1,000.	Exposure necessary to kill.
Carbolic acid	50	30 seconds.
Carbolic acid	10	1 minute.
Absolute alcohol	1,000	5 minutes.
Iodoform-ether	10	5 minutes.
Ether	1,000	10 minutes.
Bichloride of mercury	1	10 minutes.
Thymol	3	2 hours.
Saturated aqueous solution of creosote	....	
Saturated aqueous solution of β-naphthol	....	
Salicylic acid	2.5	6 hours.
Boric acid	40	

Similar researches by P. Villemin to determine the amount necessary to inhibit growth were made with many substances. Thus nutrient agar-agar, with which finely powdered iodoform had been incorporated, gave feeble but always evident subcultures. Nor do the vapors of creosote, benzene, nitrobenzene, terpin, etc., arrest growth. Vapors of ammonia, on the other hand, completely kill the cultures.

So much benefit was at one time reported from the use of iodo-

form in tuberculous foci that Baumgarten determined to investigate this problem from the experimental side.   Cultures of bacillus
tuberculosis were mixed with ten to forty parts of iodoform and
the whole was inoculated beneath the skin of guinea-pigs; the animals
died in the same manner that the control ones did.   Hence Baumgarten concluded that iodoform exerted no antiseptic action on this
organism.   In Salamonsen's laboratory, Rovsing arrived at the same
conclusion.   The injection of tuberculous material with eight to ten
times its weight of iodoform into the anterior chamber of the eye
produced tuberculosis as certainly as if no iodoform were added.
The good effects, then, of this drug could not be attributed to any
direct inhibitive action upon the tubercle bacillus.   Catrin, Filleau,
and Le Petit confirmed the observations of Rovsing.

Gosselin (of Caen) varying the experiment gave daily inoculations
to rabbits of three drops of iodoform-ether for two months and then
inoculated them with tuberculosis.   But the evolution of the disease was apparently unaffected, or possibly slightly retarded.   Jean-
nel came to the same practical conclusion.   Investigations were recently carried out in Baumgarten's laboratory by Troje and Tangel
which showed that iodoform exerts a mild inhibitive action on the
bacillus tuberculosis; these investigators claim to have produced
with bacilli attenuated in this way divers tuberculous lesions of a
chronic nature.   A series of interesting investigations by Stchégoleff
made in Straus' laboratory threw a flood of light on this important
subject.   The addition of five per cent. iodoform to glycerin bouillon
uniformly prevented growth of the tubercle bacillus.   Inoculation
experiments with virulent cultures emulsified in a liquid containing
ten per cent. iodoform produced a mild tuberculous infection.

New facts were added to the understanding of the action of iodoform in practical medicine by a series of comparative studies with
pyogenic cocci.   A culture of the staphylococcus pyogenes aureus
in iodoform-bouillon injected into rabbits determines no appreciable
lesions, while a filtrate from such a culture free from iodoform uniformly kills the inoculated animal.   If now a portion of this toxic
filtrate, which is so fatal to animals, be mixed with ten per cent. iodoform, inoculation of the mixture remains without effect.   Results
of this kind explain the beneficial effects so long pointed out, especially by surgeons; the toxic bacterial products seemingly are merely
rendered inert.   It is not impossible that the good results with tuberculons foci are brought about in the same way.

Working with some of the essential oils (oils of cinnamon and
peppermint) Murray could see no effect on the growths after long ex-
posures.   The vapor of formalin (six-per-cent. solution) acting on

cultures for forty and ninety-six hours was efficient in destroying them.

Courmont has added an interesting fact in the observation that tuberculous exudates have a distinct bactericidal action on the tubercle bacillus.

The question which has aroused much interest in connection with ingestion tuberculosis is the action of the gastric juice upon tubercle bacilli. Experiments by Falk and Wesener were made by introducing tuberculous material into an artificial gastric juice and leaving it there for some hours, after which it was inoculated into animals and shown not to have lost its virulence. In lieu of an artificial gastric juice Straus and Wurtz utilized for their researches that obtained from a young dog. They subjected pure cultures of the bacillus tuberculosis (avian) to this secretion for from eight to twelve hours and found that after that length of time the germs were still able to incite a local tuberculosis when inoculated into animals. Straus later expressed his belief that this was only the effect of dead tubercle bacilli and not the result of incitation by living bacilli. The same author has shown that the action of the gastric juice on the bacillus is due to its acidity and not to any digestive action, for a simple aqueous solution (1 to 3 : 1,000) of hydrochloric acid has the same effect. It can be easily understood that the conditions of the experiments are more rigorous than in the stomach, where the gastric juice would be diluted by admixure with food, and the bacilli protected by the substances containing them.

CHEMICAL CONSTITUTION AND PRODUCTS OF METABOLISM.

Chemical studies have not been wanting upon the composition of the tubercle bacillus or the nature of the products of its elaboration. The great mass of these investigations naturally relate to tuberculin, notwithstanding which the exact composition of this important substance still remains obscure.

Chemistry of the Body of the Tubercle Bacillus.—If investigations upon the products be eliminated, the paucity of studies upon the chemical nature of the body of the tubercle bacillus is surprising. Hammerschlag, among the first to make a systematic analysis, found that dried masses of bacilli on being treated with alcohol and ether lost as much as twenty-seven per cent. of their weight, a loss fully three times greater than that for most bacteria under similar conditions. Examination of the extract demonstrated fatty substances and lecithin without cholesterin; moreover, it contained a toxic principle which when injected into animals caused convulsions and

death. The part insoluble in ether and alcohol, in addition to an
undetermined albuminous substance, contained cellulose. As stated
elsewhere, Weyl found that the action of sodium hydroxide solution upon tubercle bacilli resulted in a yellow solution which separated into two layers, the lower of which was particularly interesting
in that it behaved in a characteristic manner tinctorially by resisting
acids. He assumed that this represented the envelope of the bacteria. The material of the upper layer contained a toxalbumin, which
when injected beneath the skin of animals produced local necrosis.
The analysis made by E. A. de Schweinitz and Marion Dorset
showed that the amount of crude fat is very large, about thirty-seven
per cent. of the weight of the dried germs, and consists of palmitic
acid, probably arachidic acid, and some undetermined volatile acid.
A further and most important contribution to the chemistry of the
tubercle bacillus has recently been made by Ruppel, who finds that
sixty-four per cent. of the dried bacilli consists of deuteroalbu-
moses. The main point which he established is that the bacillus
tuberculosis possesses a tryptic faculty by virtue of which it is
capable of acting on albuminous substances, forming peptones and
coincidently tryptophan. Of the fats he obtained three classes, according to treatment. Cold alcohol extracts about eight per cent. of
the total weight of the bacilli, becoming at the same time of a deep
red color; the coloring principle, which is a chromogen, is formed by
the action of alcohol and oxygen. Analysis demonstrates that the
fat belongs to the higher alcohol series. The residue after extraction with cold alcohol yields with hot alcohol a substance which
begins to melt at 65° C., but at 200° C. is still not completely clear.
The ether extract melts at 65° to 70° C. and smells like beeswax.
The quantity of material extracted with alcohol and ether varies, according to the age of the culture, from eight or ten per cent. up to
twenty-five or twenty-six per cent. of the total weight. According to
Ruppel, no solutions give clearly marked albumin reactions. Bacilli
purified of fat and exposed to superheated steam show eighteen to
twenty per cent. of their weight of an albumose-like substance analogous to the atmidalbumoses of Neumeister. The peculiar substances
which cannot again be dissolved seem to contain in several cases the
chief proportion of the active material of the free bacilli.

A substance which forms one-fifth or one-fourth of the weight
of dried tubercle bacilli has been recently studied by Aronson,
who declared that it is not fat, as Unna and Klebs believed, but
wax. According to him the specific color reaction is due to· it.
Moreover, it is a dark reddish-brown substance with a smell not
unlike that of ordinary beeswax; its resistant properties to ordi-

nary solvents are characteristic, for it is insoluble in even the stronger acids.

Metabolic Products, Tuberculin.—Before 1890 some activity had already been shown in the study of the products of the bacillus tuberculosis, but investigations of a systematic nature are of more recent origin. On the 4th of August, 1890, Koch announced that he had found a substance which immunized animals against tuberculosis, but withheld its derivation until the following year when he indicated its source and mode of preparation. This was tuberculin—a name subsequently given it by Bujwid. The discovery seemed to promise so much that medical interest for a time naturally centered itself upon studies calculated to give a fuller knowledge of the nature of this product. In the course of experimental researches Koch made the observation that the subcutaneous injection of a culture of tubercle bacilli into an already tuberculous guinea-pig produced a tuberculous ulcer at the point of inoculation, which healed in a short time, contrary to what occurs in a previously healthy animal. In the latter the ulcer persists to the end of the disease. The injection of dead bacilli also produced only a local process which healed soon. Moreover, the introduction of small doses repeated every day or two resulted in general amelioration of the animal's condition; and the ulcer at the point of inoculation healed, something which never occurred in the untreated animals. Continuing the research Koch finally determined that such effects were due to the soluble products of the tubercle bacillus which he extracted in glycerin. This constituted the original tuberculin of Koch.

Consequent upon the investigations of Koch chemical studies of the products of metabolism of the bacillus tuberculosis were stimulated to such an extent that the literature reached astounding proportions. Researches of this kind referred to the determination of the composition of tuberculin as well as to related problems of immunity, for so intimately have the two been linked that it is difficult to disassociate them.

If a well-developed glycerin-bouillon culture of tubercle bacilli be evaporated over a water-bath to one-tenth its original bulk and then filtered through chemically pure filter paper, a brownish liquid is obtained; this is the crude tuberculin. It contains between forty and fifty per cent. of glycerin and various mineral salts, coloring-substances, and extractives of uncertain nature. The active principle is insoluble in absolute alcohol and may thus be obtained by precipitation in an impure state. The coloring-matter may be removed, and in that way a dry colorless substance may be obtained containing the essential principle, which is much more powerful than the glycerin extract. Koch estimated that tuberculin probably contained one per cent. of the active body. It did not take very long to show that the use of tuberculin was attended often with considerable danger. Therefore numerous attempts were made to obtain a preparation containing the essential principle free from the toxic substances. Finally, precipitation with sixty-per-cent. alcohol was found to give a white material, which if dried at 100° C. is changed to a powder of a slightly grayish color. This "purified tuberculin" is easily soluble in water, but the solution rapidly deteriorates; solutions made in fifty-per-cent. glycerin are on the other hand very stable. Chemically this tuberculin gives reactions common to albuminoid substances; it gives the biuret reaction, reacts to Millon's and Adamkiewicz's reagents, etc. The chemical analysis of the purified tuberculin made by Brieger and Proskauer gave the following results:

Ash..................... .... 16.00 to 20.00 per cent.
Carbon................................ 47.20 to 48.73   "
Hydrogen............................ 7.06 to 7.55   "
Nitrogen............................ 14.45 to 14.73   "
Sulphur............................ 1.14 to 1.17   "

In April, 1897, Koch announced his new tuberculin, "T. R.," which is an aqueous extract of the soluble constituents of the pulverized bacilli. Glycerin is added to prevent contamination. For diagnostic purposes the old tuberculin is generally preferred.

Passing over the work of several investigators of this subject to the important contribution made by Hunter in 1891, we find that his analyses were of the crude tuberculin. He concluded that it consisted of (1) albumoses, chiefly protoalbumose and deuteroalbumose, along with heteroalbumose, and occasionally a trace of dysalbumose; (2) alkaloidal substances, two of which can be obtained in the form of the platinum compounds of their hydrochlorate salts; (3) extractives, small in quantity, and of unrecognized nature; (4) mucin; (5) glycerin and coloring-matter. In addition organic and inorganic salts were found.

Hunter carried his researches still further and tried the effects on tuberculous patients of the different products, which he extracted from the crude tuberculin. Substances precipitated by alcohol, he thought, exercised a distinct curative action on the affected tissues, whilst the soluble products in alcohol (albumoses principally) had a pyretogenic as well as curative action. By precipitating all the albumoses in crude tuberculin with ammonium sulphate and removing certain salts by dialysis, Hunter believed he obtained a product which would excite a local inflammatory reaction of tuberculous tissues without any disagreeable general effects.

Notwithstanding the previous researches of Hammerschlag, Koch, Proskauer, and Brieger, Hueppe and Scholl, Hunter, and Weyl, studies made by Kühne marked a distinct advance in our knowledge of this subject. In the main he confirmed the chemical analysis of Hunter, except that he found peptone. Furthermore, he isolated an albumose not previously described and which was named acroalbumose. Comparative studies showed him that the same ingredients could be found when uninoculated glycerin broth was incubated. The relative amounts present in cultures varied, but in a series of experiments with media containing the higher albumoses Kühne showed that in inoculated media there appeared a larger proportion of the lower albumoses—antecedents of peptone. Other experiments seemed to show that the several principles isolated are simply carriers of the essential toxic agent. By growing tubercle bacilli in media in which no proteid substances were present, analysis showed only an albuminate and no albumoses or peptones. Injected into animals this had the same effect as tuberculin. Studies of this kind point to the fact that the toxic products are probably not of the nature of albumoses. Of their exact nature we can say very little at present. From these and the researches of Hoffman, Matthes, de Schweinitz, Maragliano, and Trudeau and Baldwin, it is evident that cultures of tubercle bacilli contain poisonous albuminous substances, which are products of bacterial growth and have chemical reactions like the albumoses, albuminates, and nucleoproteids.

Recently Behring has reported the separation of a more active poison than any hitherto obtained. De Schweinitz and Dorset have prepared small quantities of a necrotizing substance. Other investigations by Maragliano have proved the existence of a toxalbumin exercising a hypothermic action on tuberculous guinea-pigs, an action which it loses when heated to 100° C. A little later De Schweinitz and Dorset confirmed the existence of this body by its action on healthy animals; and finally quite recently Ledoux-Lebard and Bezançon and Gouget have obtained results essentially similar to those of Maragliano.

Man, whether healthy or not, is incomparably more susceptible to the action of tuberculin than the guinea-pig. In a healthy man 25 cgm. suffice to produce an intense reaction—chills, vomiting, and fever. So small a dose as 1 cgm. provokes a feeble general reaction in the way of slight fever and greater or less malaise. On the other hand, in man the subject of tuberculosis, doses so small as from a few milligrams to 1 cgm. determine remarkably striking local and general effects. Ordinarily the reaction begins with a chill, then the temperature rises to 39° or 40° C. (100.2°-104° F.), at the same time pain in the extremities, cough, systemic depression, and often vomiting occur. The effects begin generally four or five hours after the injection, and last from ten to fourteen or more hours. Tissues affected with tuberculosis—lupus, etc.—become the seat of a local inflammatory process when tuberculin is introduced into the body.

So striking is the local reaction in subjects suffering from some external form of tuberculosis, and more especially in those the victims of lupus, that it is remarkably characteristic. In a lupus patient, for example, several hours after the injection it is evident that the affected areas have become red and swollen, frequently before the onset of the chill. During the febrile stage the redness and swelling augment. This is so marked in some instances that the diseased portions take on a deep reddish-brown or necrotic aspect. The swelling disappears at the end of several days while the areas of disease may be covered with crusts or scabs formed by the exuded serum. Finally these fall away leaving a glossy and red cicatrix. The reactions in tuberculous lymph glands and joints, while naturally less striking, are nevertheless quite distinct. The manifestations of reaction in pulmonary tuberculosis, on the other hand, are indicated by increased cough and expectoration.

In a healthy guinea-pig two or more cubic centimetres of this substance may be injected without any apparent untoward effects; not so, however, in the case of a tuberculous animal which may die from subcutaneous inoculation of only 1 cgm. A dose of 5 cgm. is regularly fatal, even when the animal is only slightly tuberculous. Death may occur in from six to thirty hours, or sooner, according to the severity of the disease. The lesions consist of a congestion of the tissue in the vicinity of the point of inoculation, of the lymph nodes, liver, and spleen; the intestine is also generally much congested.

On the one hand, it is now fairly well known that other products than those of the tubercle bacillus may excite similar phenomena to those of tuberculin in tuberculous animals. For instance, Matthes proved that peptones and albumose isolated from ordinary peptic digestion of various albumins give rise to reactions not unlike those of tuberculin in tuberculous guinea-pigs. Similarly the injection of milk, ricin, and lactic acid produces reactions in diseased animals. Buchner also showed that a series of albuminous bodies (proteins) extracted from the anthrax bacillus, the bacillus of glanders, and the bacillus prodigiosus gave rise to the same manifestations. Again, it has been found that such reactions may occur in other diseases characterized by a local deposition of new tissue in the body.

Similar phenomena have been obtained in lepra with tuberculin.

Joseph, Arning, Goldschmidt, and Babes and Kalendero have contributed some reports of this kind. Netter claims to have gotten characteristic reactions with tuberculin in twenty-seven out of one hundred patients suffering from other diseases. Phenomena of the same nature were incited by tuberculin in syphilitic subjects (Neumann, Straus, and Teissier); Billroth and von Eiselsberg observed it in actinomycosis, and Trasbot in a case of cancer. Stockman has recently shown that animals injected with large quantities of dead tubercle bacilli afterwards give the tuberculin reaction.

It is very clear from the result of recent investigations that the underlying principles of the tuberculin reaction are far from being well understood.

Cultural Characteristics.

At first a number of difficulties for a time made cultivation often uncertain. Until 1887 the principal medium used was blood serum. With the introduction of other nutrient substances, among the most important of which are media containing from five to eight per cent. of glycerin, chiefly as glycerin agar-agar, serum, and broth, renewed activity was shown on all sides in the study of tuberculosis. Distinctive differences of growth may be noted on artificial media, depending on the source of the bacilli, whether mammals, birds, or cold-blooded animals.

For purposes of convenience and clearness the descriptions of cultural characters will be understood to refer to mammalian tuberculosis, unless specifically stated to the contrary. Cultural features of tubercle bacilli of other origin will be treated of under a separate heading.

General Methods of Obtaining Cultures.

A culture may be conveniently obtained from a guinea-pig inoculated with tuberculous material and killed at the end of three or four weeks. If solidified blood serum be well inoculated with thoroughly teased or crushed fragments of the liver, spleen, or infected lymphatic glands, a growth may be obtained in two weeks or more. The writer has always succeeded in obtaining a good growth from the glands of the groin following inoculation beneath the skin, just below this point. Thus it is not necessary to wait for the development of a generalized tuberculosis. It is always advisable to inoculate a considerable number of tubes, because sometimes only a limited number of cultures will give successful results. The greatest care is required to prevent contamination by other microbic species. Drying of the serum may be prevented by covering the top of the tube with a rubber cap.

For purposes of cultivation directly from tuberculous tissues Straus states that glycerin agar-agar is not so suitable as blood serum or even glycerin potato; culture upon glycerin agar-agar is frequently impossible before the fifth or sixth generation upon blood serum (Straus).

Kitasato in 1892 described a method by which pure cultures could be secured from tuberculous sputum. After the mouth has been well cleansed the expectoration is received into a sterilized Petri dish, and a small amount of the more dense portion is carefully washed in ten or more successive portions of sterilized water. This manipulation removes the microorganisms accidently attached to the mass of sputum in its passage through the mouth. In the last washing the specimen is torn apart with sterile instruments and cultures are made upon blood serum or glycerin agar-agar from the interior of the mass. In about two weeks or more evidences of growth will appear. The method of washing the sputum used by Kitasato has been simplified by Czaplewski and Hensel, who found in their investigations upon whooping-cough that instead of washing the sputum in water in dishes, shaking it in tubes containing simple peptone media or sterile water a few times removed the bacteria quickly. Three or four washings were often sufficient for this purpose.

Rapid growths of tubercle bacilli may be obtained in three or four days from tuberculous sputum upon a new medium recently introduced by W. Hesse (*Zeitschrift für Hygiene*, 1899, Bd. 31, p. 502). This consists of the following ingredients:

Nahrstoff Heyden	5 gm.
Sodium chloride	5 "
Glycerin	30 "
Agar-agar	10 "
Normal sodium-hydrate solution	5 c.c.
Distilled water	1,000 "

The nutrient composition is melted and poured into Petri dishes, where it is allowed to solidify. Then the sputum, which should be as fresh as possible, is spread in thin streaks with a platinum loop over the surface of the medium. Washing the sputum after the manner of Czaplewski and Hensel, and then taking only the central parts of the mass as in Kitasato's method, has given good results in the writer's experience.

Cultures on Blood Serum (Solidified).—When the surface of solidified blood serum is inoculated with material from tuberculous tissue and incubated at 37° or 38° C., there appear from the tenth to the fifteenth day minute points of growth of dull, whitish color, generally somewhat irregular in size and slightly elevated above the surface of the serum. Such colonies ordinarily reach a comparatively small size, and remain discrete, becoming confluent only when many are closely aggregated. Koch compared the appearance of these to that of small dry scales. Although the culture goes on developing the growth is rarely very abundant. Cultures prepared directly from animal sources sometimes show little tendency to grow well, and it may not be until the fourth or fifth generation that the culture becomes more luxuriant. Tendencies of this kind are probably explicable upon the ground of habit and environment.

Cultural variations depending on transplantation are not uncommon. In sub-cultures the growth is luxuriant and forms a wrinkled membrane of gray or whitish color, which may cover the whole surface of the medium. The growth which frequently extends to the water of condensation at the bottom of the tube does not cloud it, but instead forms a thin grayish-white pellicle over the surface. The growth is often of such a character that it is difficult to dissociate a portion completely in a drop of water. Modifications of appearance to a certain extent also occur with variations in the degree of consistence of the serum. When this is very firm the dry membranous appearance is more marked, whereas with softer media the culture becomes more irregular, thicker, and verrucoid, as well as adherent to the underlying surface. At the end of one month development on serum usually reaches its maximum of growth; such cultures may acquire a brownish color. Successive transplantations for long periods produce inappreciable changes. Thus for more than nine years Koch maintained cultures of tubercle bacilli without any passage through animals, and at the end of this time they still possessed all their characteristics save a slight diminution in virulence.

Cultures not infrequently take an unusual color, such as yellowish and reddish, especially in media which are not particularly favorable, such as the serum of the horse or dog.

With a magnification of sixty to eighty diameters the early thin surface growth presents a characteristic appearance. The bacilli, arranged in parallel rows, form peripherally sinuous streaks which radiate outwards; the central portions are composed of similar figures closely interwoven. Impression preparations, made by applying a dry cover glass to the surface edges of growing masses, show this arrangement very well. Koch, with this so-called " *Klatschpräparat*," described a disposition in the form of undulated meshes in serum; Fischl, on the other hand, in examining the margins of unstained specimens recognized the existence of filaments and dendritic vegetation. Furthermore, in sections of agar cultures Coppen-Jones described not a heterogeneous mass of rods, but bundles arranged for the most part perpendicularly to the surface. But more particularly the investigations of Ledoux-Lebard added most interesting points to our knowledge of the development of colonies of the tubercle bacillus. Following step by step the growth of such colonies he saw the bacilli elongate into ramified filaments which formed anastomosing fasciculi.

Fluid Serum.—Koch long ago succeeded in growing tubercle bacilli in this medium. On the surface the culture forms a thin, dry, very fragile membrane, which is broken on the slightest agitation, when it sinks to the bottom of the tube, but the serum remains indefinitely clear.

Glycerin Agar.—With the introduction by Nocard and Roux, in 1887, of glycerinated media comparatively facile cultivation of the tubercle bacillus was made possible. As pointed out by Straus and others, however, such media are sometimes not satisfactory for obtaining cultures directly from infected tissues. The addition of six to eight per cent. of glycerin to peptone agar-agar was found to enhance the growth activity to a remarkable extent, so much so that its application has been extended to blood serum, broth, potato, and many nutritive solutions. The advantage in the use of glycerin agar lies in the fact that sub-cultures show earlier growth, which progresses more rapidly than on coagulated serum; on coagulated glycerin serum a visible culture may appear as early as the fourth day.

The appearance of cultures upon glycerin agar or coagulated serum differs from that of the solidified blood serum by being more luxuriant, but otherwise the general characters remain essentially the same. Stab inoculations show growth only in the uppermost portions of the line of inoculation; on the surface the culture grows in the form of a thick white mass with sinuous margins. The color subsequently changes to yellowish. Cultures on glycerin media, solid or liquid, develop a strong odor suggesting fruit.

The addition of rabbit's or dog's blood to glycerin agar-agar liquefied by heat, which is then allowed to solidify in slants, is a modification strongly recommended recently by Bezançon and Griffon. They have not only found this nutrient mixture very useful for sub-cultures, but have easily obtained direct cultures from animal tissues and tuberculous exudations in man.

Glycerin Broth.—After the method of Straus and Gamaleïa, a rapid and abundant growth may be secured by floating on the surface of bouillon, containing five or six per cent. of glycerin, thin bits of culture derived from solid media. At the end of two or three weeks abundant development will have taken place in the form of a thick and dry, wrinkled, whitish membrane, frequently rising to a certain height on the sides of the tube or flask.   Sometimes the bacilli grow

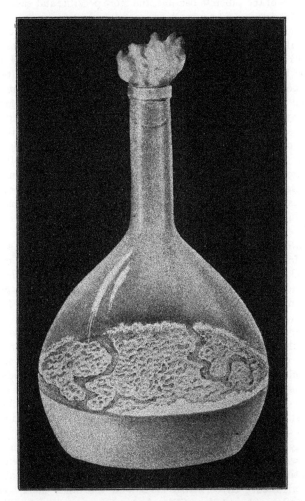

Fig. 4.—Culture of the Tubercle Bacillus (Human) in Glycerin Bouillon (Straus).

in little white masses which fall to the bottom and form a powdery layer.   Hip. Martin obtained excellent cultures in bouillon made from the flesh of various fish (more especially the herring), to which **six** per cent. of glycerin had been added.   By replacing broth with **a** decoction of yeast to which five per cent. of glycerin was added ·Hammerschlag also obtained good results. The two last-named media may be utilized with agar-agar. The more marked the saprophytic tendencies of the tubercle bacillus, the more possible and easier is its growth in simple peptone broth.

Potato.—When transferred from glycerin agar or bouillon cultures the bacillus tuberculosis grows very well on potato. Attempts by Koch to cultivate it on this vegetable medium were uniformly unsuccessful; but essays by Powlowsky gave more satisfactory results. To insure good growth it is especially important to have the infectious material well penetrate the substance of the medium. Before the tenth day little can be observed, but about the twelfth dull, grayish areas may be noted on the surface; and by the twentieth, the surface is covered with a characteristic dry, easily removable white growth. With age the culture thickens and may present small grayish-white points of elevation. Moreover, the reaction of the medium will have become faintly alkaline. The addition of five per cent. glycerinated water seems to favor the cultural activity somewhat. Spreading the potato surface with a thin layer of glycerin agar equally enhances the value of the medium.

Gelatin.—Ordinary simple agar-agar and gelatin media are unsuited for the cultivation of the tubercle bacillus. Growth may be obtained in gelatin to which glycerin has been added, but as development ordinarily necessitates a temperature of 37.5° C. gelatin (liquid under these conditions) is of little practical utility for the purpose.

Other Nutrient Media.—Numerous experiments by Sander have shown that cultivation is possible not only on serum, potato, etc., but also on other widely different substances, such as carrot, radish, macaroni, and so on; in the same way growth has been studied in infusions of these substances, to which glycerin had been added.· What is quite important in its practical application is his observation that cultures from tissues can be more readily obtained on potato than on glycerin agar-agar.

Studying the influence of reaction Sander showed that an acid reaction was more favorable to growth. Potato medium, generally acid at the start, becomes alkaline in time and then multiplication is finally arrested. Glycerinated media, on the other hand, remain persistently acid, and the utility of glycerin, according to this experimenter, rests in this fact. Another interesting point brought out is that under such conditions of growth the virulence not only diminishes very greatly, but, as elsewhere stated, circumstances of this kind so lessen the parasitic nature of the bacillus tuberculosis that in course of time it can be induced to grow feebly upon ordinary agar-agar.

Further researches into the biological behavior of this organism

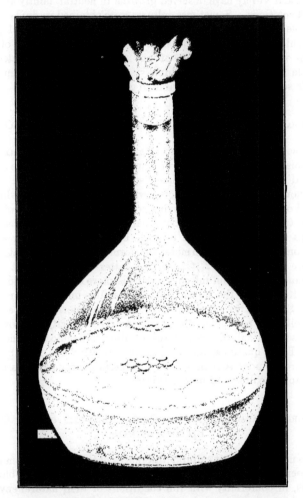

Fig. 5 —Culture of the Tubercle Bacillus (Avian) in Glycerin Bouillon (Straus).

have shown the ability to cultivate it in fluids of extremely simple composition. Comparative experimental studies by Proskauer and Beck illustrate this point. For instance, cultures of greater or less luxuriance have been obtained in non-albuminous solutions containing asparagin and in mixtures of commercial ammonium carbonate, primary potassium phosphate, magnesium sulphate, glycerin, and water. Carrying experiments of this kind still further, Kimla, Poupé, and Vesely have observed growths in neutral, faintly alkaline, or acid solutions. Sometimes cultures were obtained in fluids of considerable acidity. In simple solutions of mannite, tartrate of potassium, chloride of sodium, potassium phosphate, and sulphate of magnesium without the addition of any glycerin they cultivated the tubercle bacillus, but in Uschinsky's, Rollin's, or Lehmann-Neumann's solutions they were unable to get any cultures.

CULTURAL CHARACTERISTICS OF TUBERCLE BACILLI OF AVIAN ORIGIN.

On solid media the avian tubercle bacillus gives a more luxuriant and moister growth than that of mammalian origin. At the second or third generation the inoculated surface becomes covered with a continuous, quite thick and moist, white, glistening layer, which at the end of a month becomes a wrinkled membrane. Cultures of mammalian tuberculosis are coherent, hard, and difficult to break up, whereas the culture of avian tubercle bacilli is much softer and of little consistence. Furthermore, the former cease to grow at a temperature higher than 42° C., but the latter still develop at 45° C. Direct inoculation from infected organs is more successful and easier than cultivation of the human tubercle bacillus under similar conditions. Sub-cultures of avian origin are characterized by a facile adaptability to new environment and marked activity of growth as compared with sub-cultures of the bacillus tuberculosis from mammals. These qualities, however, are but relative and not absolute, and there are none that may not under certain circumstances be observed in the cultures of human origin.

CULTURAL CHARACTERISTICS OF TUBERCLE BACILLI OF THE COLD-BLOODED ANIMALS.

The most prominent cultural differences of these bacilli from those just described lie in the fact that cultures derived from cold-blooded animals, in conformity with the conditions of their natural environment, give active growth between 10° and 30° C. At higher temperatures than 34° C., growth ceases or becomes very sluggish, unless frequent transplantation be made and the rise of temperature be very slow and progressive. Beyond this and the saprophytic tendencies of the bacilli, cultures of this kind resemble in the main those derived from avian sources. Bataillon, Dubard, and Terre found that the optimum temperature for tubercle bacilli, which they isolated from a diseased carp, was about 25° C. At 23° C. the growth was still most luxuriant.

The Position of the Tubercle Bacillus Among Micro-organisms.

Some years ago Metchnikoff formulated the doctrine that the tubercle bacillus as commonly seen represented only a phase in the developmental cycle of a filamentous fungus, a view which has latterly received more widespread acceptance. We have in the researches of Fischl, Bruns, Coppen Jones, Kruse, Lehmann and Neumann, and Schultze and Lubarsch a marked growth of this conception that it is really a member of a higher group of organisms, a view still further extended by the studies of Babes and Levaditi, Friederich, Schultze, and Friederich and Nösske. Thus Klein suggests that the branching is a reversion to an ancestral type which presented mycelial growth; Fischl pointed out analogies to the actinomyces, and Coppen Jones holds that both belong to the same group, but he leaves undecided whether or not this is among the hyphomycetes or some other class. He thinks there may be some as yet unknown saprophytic mode of existence of the bacillus, and suggests the name tuberculomyces (hominis, avium, etc., as the case may be). Bruns, taking the view of Fischer, modifies it by saying "they pertain to the saprophytic growth form of a higher organism, which as a parasite in the animal body appears in the form of rods." Graf, who oversaw Bruns' preparations, was of the opinion that the appearance looked much like the branching of the "Nostaceen." They are a group closest to the Cladothriceæ. Marpmann in the light of Bruns' interpretation designates it mycobacterium tuberculosis, a designation which finds acceptance by Lehmann and Neumann.

With the finer distinctions in latter years of the Cladothriceæ, Streptothriceæ, etc., some writers have endeavored to class the tubercle bacillus among the latter. Kruse brings the organism into close relation with a certain group of organisms (including the ray fungus) which has been extensively widened by the discovery of a considerable number of different forms, of which the pathogenic have the capacity to produce inflammatory phenomena, chronic in duration, and of the type of infectious granulomata. Johan-Olsen and some others apparently accept this classification. Ledoux-Lebard bases an attempt at the same thing largely upon a study of the development of colonies, but he brings this microorganism under the Cladothriceæ and names it accordingly the Sclerothrix Kochii or Sclerothrix Marfuccii (mammalian or avian).

Contrary to the belief of those who regard the branching and filament formation as an expression of higher development, some have considered it as simply a degeneration of pathogenic forms without any significance as to classification. This is a view advocated by A. Fischer, who places these types of the bacillus tuberculosis as well as similar ones of the diphtheria bacillus in the group of involution forms. There are several objections to this interpretation, of which it will suffice to mention that the forms in question are not limited to old cultures and unfavorable conditions of environment. The opinion more generally entertained is that the occurrence of these morphological types necessitates some change of formerly accepted views as to the classification of the microorganisms concerned; yet with Craig we would say that "further investigations are needed in order to enable us to come to any definite conclusion of the significance of the branched forms . . . and for the present it would seem to be premature to adopt any radical change in the accepted classification of the tubercle bacillus and the diphtheria bacillus."

Experimental Tuberculosis.

No single side of tuberculosis has been more fully investigated than this one. Beginning with the experiments of Villemin the evolution of this subject has been far more rapid than that of any other phase of tuberculosis.

The inoculation of pure cultures of the tubercle bacillus into receptive animals, such as the guinea-pig or rabbit, incites the same phenomena that the introduction of tuberculous tissue does; the classical lesions so admirably defined by Villemin are reproduced in their entirety. The evolution of experimental tuberculosis is necessarily modified by the channel of infection; and inasmuch as different tissues are vulnerable in different degrees, the pathological presentation naturally follows the order of tissues primarily incited to these changes. Again, other determining conditions obviously affect more or less the evolution of the disease. For instance, susceptibility constitutes one of the most potent conditions of infection; indeed, everything may depend on this single factor.

We have reason to believe that the category of animals in which an experimental tuberculosis can be induced must be very large, much more comprehensive than heretofore believed. With some animals this is naturally an easier matter than with others, the pig or rabbit being more susceptible than the goat, for example. And then the important question of the source of the tubercle bacilli is one which must always be taken into consideration. The introduction of fowl tubercle bacilli into the rabbit would ordinarily scarcely induce tuberculosis, although this animal is quite susceptible to bacilli of mammalian derivation.

Within the scope of a limited article it is impossible to do other than picture tuberculosis in some of its experimental variations, so as to give some idea of the main type forms.

General Results of Inoculation.

As a result of the introduction of tubercle bacilli into receptive animals multiplication of the bacilli occurs in the tissues, and after a variable time the tissues are incited to the development of tuberculosis in one or more of its many forms, depending on a whole series of conditions which are more or less clearly understood. If the conditions be appropriate the bacilli extend from the point of inoculation to the tissues of the body elsewhere. In some instances the dissemination is through the blood, in others the spread takes place by way of the lymphatics. Depending on the route taken, two great types of infection are produced, as will be seen later.

Anatomically, experimental tuberculosis, as the spontaneous disease in man, manifests itself in some instances by exudative inflammation, in others by proliferation of the tissue elements. Both are often associated in this disease. Cheesy degeneration is common in tuberculous inflammation, and to a large extent gives the process certain distinctive features which permit its more or less easy recognition. Productive inflammation in tuberculosis is characterized by the formation of variously sized small nodular bodies called tubercles.

Variations in Virulence.

Virulence is but a relative term and depends upon many conditions—some peculiar to the bacilli, others to the tissues infected. In the same measure that variations of pathogenic activity occur among bacteria generally, so like differences have been noted with the bacillus tuberculosis. Age is an important factor in modifying virulence; but this is only the application of a general biological formula. Schill and Fischer, Chantemesse and Widal, and others have well shown this attenuating influence for the tubercle bacillus. Temperature, light, desiccation, putrefaction, etc., constitute a whole series of physical, chemical, and other conditions, causing differences of activity, and this is modified also to some degree by less understood inherent peculiarities of the organism.

As the above-named factors widely modify the virulence, so it is important to appreciate dissimilarities of pathogenic power depending on the animal source—natural environment—of the tubercle bacillus. It is now generally known that many of the lower animals are frequently as receptive to the tubercle bacillus as man. It is probable that modifications occur through a long series of transfers from one animal to another of the same character, in consequence of which the germ acquires a certain selective adaptation for a particular host. For example, the bacillus of avian tuberculosis, which is extremely pathogenic for birds, may excite even in considerable amounts nothing but local inflammatory phenomena in mammals without any generalization of the process; or a culture which is unusually virulent for rabbits when inoculated into cold-blooded animals may be wholly or largely innocuous.

Passing to tuberculosis as it is found in the human subject we are confronted by the problem of variation in its restricted sense. It is obvious that dissimilarities of this nature are less likely to occur in bacterial species which are parasitic upon individuals of the same species. The development of any variations, if they occur at all, is naturally feeble as compared with some already cited. Koch believed that tubercle bacilli from different sources possess the same degree of virulence. But differences in the termination of certain forms of tuberculosis—visceral tuberculosis contrasted with like infection of the joints, or tuberculous meningitis and tuberculous peritonitis—have not entirely escaped notice. Heretofore we have taken into consideration the soil with little or no reference to the inciting factor of tuberculosis. Preoccupied with considerations of this nature S. Arloing, of Lyons, was among the first to survey this field of experimental medicine. So long ago as 1883 he showed that differences exist beween bacilli removed from scrofulous surgical lesions and those obtained from a phthisical lung. Thus infectious material from pulmonary lesions or sputum when inoculated sûbcutaneously resulted in tuberculosis in both' the guinea-pig and rabbit, but in experiments with material taken from bone scrofula, strumous glands, etc., the guinea-pigs alone died, the rabbits almost always escaping. These conclusions were contested by Nocard, di Renzi, Straus, and Auclair, mainly on the ground that any differences of results were referable to a paucity of bacteria on the one hand or to the fact that tissues experimented with contained dead tubercle bacilli. Notwithstanding contrary conclusions the accuracy of Arloing's views is still to be refuted by convincing experimental investigation. Courmont and Denis, in a comparatively recent study of pulmonary tuberculosis with attenuated bacilli, conclude that visceral tuberculosis is due to virulent bacilli in contradistinction to scrofulous tuberculosis, so called. As in some measure lending support to the results of Arloing and his pupils might be mentioned the studies of Theobald Smith, which though somewhat limited, nevertheless lead him to believe in the existence of minor variations in the virulence of tubercle bacilli. As this experimenter remarks, the outcome of studies of the pathogenic power of the tubercle bacillus upon animals must not be taken too literally. It should be borne in mind that results at the most are but comparative. The exhibition of an increased virulence towards certain animals should not be regarded as synonymous with exalted virulence for the human subject.

F. Craven Moore last year published the results of some experiments similar to those of Arloing, bearing on the same problem. He says that it is at once obvious that his results confirm the contention of Arloing that while scrofulous glands are capable of producing a progressive tuberculosis in the guinea-pig, they signally fail to overcome the natural resistance of the rabbit to infection, under the same experimental conditions. The writer believes that he has abundantly confirmed these views in a series of experiments carried out during the past year. A full account of these experiments will be published later, but it need only be said that striking differences in virulence were observed in human tubercle bacilli obtained under different clinical conditions.

The differences, latterly accentuated by Theobald Smith and Dinwiddie, in relative virulence for the domestic animals of human and bovine tuberculosis had already been noted by Villemin: "None of the rabbits inoculated with human tubercle gave so rapid and so completely generalized a tuberculosis as was obtained by inoculating them from the cow." Variations of pathogenicity are also shown in the subsequent labors of Siedamgrotzky, Klein and Gibbes, and Frothingham. Experimental evidence collected by Dinwiddie convinces him that bovine tubercle is more virulent than the human variety for cattle, sheep, goats, and rabbits, while no distinction can be established in the case of horses, pigs, cats, and dogs.

EXPERIMENTAL TUBERCULOSIS IN MAMMALS.

All mammals are not equally susceptible to experimental tuberculosis. It is less easily produced in carnivora than in herbivora. In no animal can so many favorable conditions be found as in the guinea-pig. Rabbits respond less readily to the stimulus of tuberculous infection. Pigs and calves are quite easily infected.

Subcutaneous Inoculations.—The introduction of a small bit of infected tuberculous tissue or a portion of a pure culture of mammalian tuberculosis beneath the skin of the groin of a *guinea-pig* will usually be followed in nine or ten days by a more or less evident tumefaction—a local lesion which by microscopical examination will be seen to be tuberculous. At the end of several weeks the abscess which will have formed discharges a caseous pus, giving rise to an ulcer. Once formed the ulcer exhibits little tendency to close. In this connection certain observations made by Koch are not without interest. Experiments which served as the basis for the introduction of tuberculin demonstrated that the inoculation of a culture into an already tuberculous rabbit produced at the point of inoculation necrosis of the skin, and then the dry eschar which was thrown off left a non-tuberculous ulceration, which gradually healed without there having been any appreciable changes in the corresponding lymphatic glands. Straus made observations of a similar kind.

Concomitant with the development of the local lesion the glands of the groin become swollen and hard, and finally undergo caseous transformation. But going hand-in-hand with these phenomena an irregular fever is set up; the animal loses in weight, this progressive emaciation continuing until the termination of the disease, which commonly occurs in six to eight weeks or only in six months, according to the amount and virulence of the inciting agent as well as the receptivity of the inoculated animal. The main autopsy findings limit themselves to a generalized tuberculous process affecting the spleen, liver, and the lymphatic glands. Implication of the lungs, which ordinarily is less extensive than elsewhere, occurs principally in the form of disseminated gray tubercles. Whenever the evolution of the disease is hurried and death occurs in five or six weeks, the liver and spleen will frequently contain but a few discrete miliary tubercles; but if longer, the aspect of the spleen and liver is very different. The spleen may often be quite large and firm in consistence, and on section present a surface of a brownish-red color. Variously sized, irregular, grayish-yellow areas are often present in the organ. The latter are hard, dry masses of coagulation necrosis which have not passed into caseation properly so called. The liver presents a varying likeness to this in appearance; it is augmented in size and shows yellowish-white areas of necrosis alternating with zones of a deep reddish-brown color. Here again it is essentially a process of necrosis.

On the other hand, caseation is the rule in the infected glands. Strangely, the kidneys escape wholly or only rarely contain a few miliary tubercles. The more chronic the progress of the disease the more likely will these organs be involved, the cortical rather than the pyramidal regions of the kidneys. Rabbits, however, often will present lesions of this tissue. The serous membranes sometimes show miliary tubercles.

To this evolution of the experimental infection in the guinea-pig the French give the name "type Villemin."

The spread of the infectious agent by means of the lymphatics has been especially studied by Arloing. Subcutaneous inoculation into the thigh is followed in about fifteen days by tumefaction of the lymph glands of the groin of the corresponding side; by the twentieth day the lumbar glands of the same side will have become involved, the entire lymphatic system of the opposite side remaining intact. Beginning splenic involvement will be noted at the end of the fourth week as well as commencing swelling of the retrohepatic lymphatic glands. From this time lesions of the bronchial glands and lungs become manifest and the dissemination tends to lose its unilateral character. In about two months the process is general. If the disease be of longer duration tuberculous changes will be noted in the nodes of the groin and lumbar region on the opposite side. This series of changes is so constant that frequently, as Arloing showed, it is possible to determine in a general way the time of infection from the extent of lymphatic involvement. Should the inoculation be made at the base of the ear, then the infection becomes descending with the same characteristic unilateral progression: first the preauricular, then the prescapular nodes of the same side, followed by the lungs and bronchial lymphatic glands. Subsequently universal infection takes place.

To summarize, then, it is evident that subcutaneous infection is essentially lymphatic in its propagation, the landmarks in the progression of which are sharply marked by the successive glandular involvements.

The evolution of the disease in the *rabbit* follows a very different course, not only with reference to the distribution of the lesions, but also with respect to the channel of dissemination. While glandular involvement sometimes occurs, nevertheless conditions in the animal spare this anatomical tissue, so much so that even the glands immediately in relation to the point of inoculation frequently present no external or gross signs of disease. When the animal dies at the end of two or three months, the abdominal lymphatic system may be wholly intact, on one side as well as on the other. At the seat of inoculation the lesion consists of a caseous abscess. Often the various viscera, but more prominently the lungs, are affected with tuberculous eruptions from the earliest period. Manifestations of this kind led Arloing to conclude that the tubercle bacilli in the guinea-pig, as already stated, elect the lymphatic route in contradistinction to the blood channel by which the spread is usually effected in the rabbit.

Intraperitoneal Inoculation.—This form of inoculation produces a more rapid infection with earlier generalization of the lesions. Injection of tubercle bacilli into the peritoneal cavity is soon followed by an intense peritonitis. The omentum is infiltrated with tubercles within a few weeks, which results in considerable thickening. Both layers of the peritoneum are studded with miliary tubercles. Processes of this intensity will generally be noted at the end of the twelfth day. Progressing, the disease manifests itself in the lumbar, cœliac, and anterior and posterior mediastinal glands. From this time on the lesions begin to appear in the liver, spleen, and lungs, so that by the end of the third week the lesions might be said to be widespread. The gastrointestinal tract is usually free from tuberculosis. Preceded by more or less cachexia, death occurs in from two to six weeks. The peritoneal infiltration may be so diffuse that the appearance is that of a compact caseous mass. The introduction of large numbers of bacilli kills the animal in a few days; at the autopsy a hemorrhagic exudate is observed in the peritoneal and pleural cavities, but no visible tubercles will be found in the organs (Koch, Straus and Gamaleïa).

Intravenous Inoculation.—The realization of acute experimental miliary tuberculosis is well secured by the injection of tubercle bacilli into the veins of a rabbit. Apart from the acuity and rapid generalization of the process, the lesions differ in few respects from those obtained with the previous methods. The inoculation incites in all the vascular organs, lungs, liver, spleen, bone-marrow, etc., an eruption of fine miliary tubercles. In some cases the animals succumb in fifteen to twenty days, having lost one-third, two-fifths, or one-half of their weight.

Inoculation into the Anterior Chamber of the Eye.—Introduced by Armanni and fully investigated by Cohnheim and Salomonsen, this method gives interesting results. A small fragment of fresh tuberculous tissue or a small amount of culture is introduced into the anterior chamber of the eye of preferably an albino rabbit. The absence of pigment in the iris interferes less with observation. If the experiment has been properly conducted, signs of traumatic interference disappear in a few days, and the introduced bit of tissue can be well seen in front of the crystalline lens. After a time the inoculated fragment almost or entirely disappears; finally, about the twenty-fifth day there will be seen on the surface of the iris a number of very fine miliary tubercles which become larger and caseous. Later the cornea may become infected, and so in some cases a general panophthalmia is established. At the autopsy varying involvement of the lymph nodes, lungs, and other viscera is commonly noted.

Inhalation Experiments.—Lesions of tuberculosis can be caused in guinea-pigs by making them breathe in an atmosphere containing dust contaminated with tubercle bacilli. Shortly following his discovery Koch took up this subject and found that some animals showed dyspnœa at the end of a week or more; some died on the twenty-fourth or twenty-fifth day, and those still living were sacrificed on the forty-eighth day. All the rabbits and guinea-pigs showed tubercles in the lungs, the lesion being more extensive the longer the duration of the pathological process. In the sacrificed animals the liver and spleen also contained tubercles. The appearance of the pulmonary lesions recalled that of caseous pneumonia in man, or again that seen in spontaneous tuberculosis in these animals. The process in the lungs often affects the bronchopneumonic type.

Ingestion Experiments.—Intestinal tuberculosis has been experimentally produced in guinea-pigs, rabbits, dogs, cats, calves, monkeys, sheep, and other animals. Pigs are readily susceptible to this mode of infection. As pointed out long ago by Chauveau, ingestion tuberculosis is characterized by special features of localization. The initial lesions manifest themselves primarily in the lymphatic apparatus of the intestine (solitary follicles and Peyer's patches), and later (in about four weeks) in the mesenteric and cæcal lymphatic glands. Guinea-pigs fed with tuberculous material show the earliest lesion in the form of a local process generally in the small intestine and cæcum. This appears very often towards the eighteenth to twenty-second day. The frequency with which the small gut or cæcum is involved is variable. Thus, of twenty animals studied, Sydney Martin found the small intestine involved in all but one; the cæcum showed tuberculosis in all but three. The frequency with which the cæcum is infected in guinea-pigs is explained by the fact that in them it contains large and numerous Peyer's patches and so differs greatly from this organ in man or the carnivora.

The intestinal ulcerations which are far from constant may be totally absent. Dobroklonski some years ago, as well as the writer more recently, showed that guinea-pigs which had been fed with pure cultures of the bacillus tuberculosis sometimes presented at the end of five or six days bacilli in the mesenteric glands and in the thickness of the intestinal wall without any detectable lesion of the epithelium.

Tuberculosis of the intestine is followed by that of the mesenteric and cæcal glands in about twenty-eight days; from these tissues the infection passes to the cœliac glands, liver, spleen, bronchial and posterior mediastinal glands, and lungs. When the disease lasts a longer time, the anterior mediastinal glands may become involved as well as the lumbar glands or those of the lesser omentum.

Inoculation of pigs after this manner is followed by practically the same phenomena; from the local disease of the intestine the process extends to the neighboring glands and so on. Curiously in pigs the tonsil is an important point of absorption of the tuberculous virus. In calves we again have the same picture, except that in these animals extensive tuberculosis of the pleura may occur without necessarily any lung implication. Infection through the pharynx must often occur in calves also.

Inoculation with Dead Tubercle Bacilli.—A few critical minds before 1890 had already realized the limitations of existing conceptions explaining the cellular reactions encountered in tuberculosis. About this time Marfucci had observed that the introduction of dead bacilli (avian) into eggs which were afterwards incubated resulted in cachectic chickens without any tuberculous lesions. Specific knowledge of the action of dead bacteria in the living body dates back to the striking researches of Prudden and Hodenpyl. In a comprehensive piece of original work these investigators successively studied the effects of subcutaneous, intraperitoneal, pleural, and intravenous injections of dead tubercle bacilli. Prolonged boiling, they found, while causing a considerable breaking up of the tubercle bacillus, did not interfere with its characteristic staining, nor did it alter the morphology of many of the individuals of a culture. Thus the bacilli could be easily detected at their seat of lodgment. Most important, however, was the determination that dead tubercle bacilli, separated from such of their metabolic products as are set free in the media or are removed by boiling in water or fifty-per-cent. glycerin, were capable of inducing effects upon the tissues of the rabbit with which they were brought in contact. The dead bacilli possessed marked chemotactic properties. Injected in considerable amounts into the subcutaneous tissue or into the pleural or peritoneal cavities they exhibited pyogenic power, an observation previously noted by Koch. Moreover, under these conditions the body cells are excited to the production of tissue resembling that of a tuberculous nature. And they demonstrated that the introduction of small numbers of tubercle bacilli into the blood-vessels of rabbits is followed by their disappearance within a few hours or days, but here and there single bacilli or clusters could be found for a long time in the lungs and liver adhering to the vessel walls without any marked changes in the latter. But after a variable time, generally in the lung first and subsequently in the liver, a cell proliferation took place in the vicinity of the dead tubercle bacilli, which led to the development of small nodular new growths bearing a close morphological similarity to miliary tubercles. In structures of this nature, while there was often cell necrosis, no evidence of caseation could be found, and instead of any multiplication of the bacilli there was rather a steady diminution in their number. Finally Prudden and Hodenpyl concluded that the new structures originate in a proliferation of the endothelium of the blood-vessels under the stimulus of the dead and disintegrating bacilli. These formative tissue changes, they suggest, may be due to the action of the bacterioprotein of the tubercle bacillus, set free as the germs die and disintegrate in the tissues, while the equally important coagulation may be largely the result of those soluble, freed metabolic products of the life processes of the organism which are not present under the conditions of these experiments.

In a subsequent study of experimental pneumonitis in the rabbit induced by the intratracheal injection of dead bacilli, Prudden showed that when dead tubercle bacilli are introduced in small flocculi into the air spaces of the lung there occurs at their seat of lodgment a large accumulation of small spheroidal cells in the air spaces which is followed by a proliferation of epithelioid cells and the formation of giant cells in the contiguous vesicles. Eventually the small round-cell accumulation of the central parts disappears by necrosis, disintegration, and absorption, accompanied by a conversion of the peripheral portion into connective tissue, which contracts until the primary lesion is indicated only by a small mass of dense fibrous tissue. In short, then, the conclusions of these researches indicate that intravenous injection of dead tubercle bacilli killed by heat produce small nodules in which giant cells are occasionally present, but no caseation.

In the main these results have been confirmed by a number of investigators, among whom may be cited Straus and Gamaleïa, Vissman, Kostenich, Grancher, and Ledoux-Lebard, Abel, and Babes and Proca. However, Straus and Gamaleïa sometimes found traces of caseation. The bacilli could be well recognized in the tubercles by the ordinary staining-method. Similar lesions have been produced by intraperitoneal and intrapleural injection. The introduction of dead bacilli beneath the skin produces only a local abscess without secondary tubercles in the viscera. And not alone this, but Prudden, and Straus and Gamaleïa observed that a condition of marasmus may set in and sometimes gradually lead to a fatal termination. Frequently repeated inoculations in time will develop a greater or less immunity.

Auché and Hobbs investigated the effects of dead tubercle bacilli in frogs and produced by intraperitoneal inoculation lesions of the same character. Extending the study further Stockman induced identical lesions with dead tubercle bacilli in the horse, hog, and cat.

EXPERIMENTAL TUBERCULOSIS IN BIRDS.

Avian tuberculosis is easily induced in birds with tubercle bacilli from avian sources. Inoculations readily succeed whether the route be subcutaneous, intravenous, intraperitoneal, or by way of the digestive tract. Whatever the mode of infection the lesions are essentially abdominal in distribution. If the inoculation be subcutaneous the point of entrance will be the seat of a localized tuberculosis, quite firm and not caseous. The loss of weight is always considerable in this disease. The liver will be found greatly enlarged and completely studded with fine miliary tubercles. The spleen is similarly affected; tuberculosis of the lungs is less common. The bone marrow in birds seems to constitute a favorable soil for the development of the tubercle bacillus, for lesions of this tissue are very common.

In 1888 Hip. Martin published his results of unsuccessful attempts of inoculation of various birds with human tuberculosis. Although these results were confirmed by Straus and Wurtz, Rivolta, Marfucci, A. Gärtner, and a host of others, experiments of later date show that the establishment of certain conditions permits the reproduction of the disease in its typical form. Investigations by Cadiot, Gilbert, and Roger showed that rabbits are susceptible to inoculation with avian tuberculosis, but in guinea-pigs a local caseous abscess is at the most produced.

Like Rivolta, Marfucci, and Straus and Gamaleïa, the majority of experimenters have failed in their attempts to incite tuberculosis in birds with tubercle bacilli of mammalian origin. All have noted that the guinea-pig resists ordinary subcutaneous inoculation of avian tubercle bacilli, and that should it succumb to intraperitoneal inoculation the lesions produced are very different from those incited by the bacilli of human origin: the spleen is much augmented in size, red, and soft, and rarely contains visible tubercles, nor do the liver and lungs. Nevertheless the spleen and liver are riddled with microscopic tubercles containing many bacilli. Dogs resist even the intravenous inoculation of considerable quantities of culture of avian tubercle bacilli. On the other hand, Cadiot, Gilbert and Roger, Courmont and Dor, and Nocard state that inoculation of mammalian tubercle bacilli into fowls sometimes succeeds in establishing the lesions of tuberculosis. The rabbit, however, is receptive to both types of bacilli, and after two or three passages it is often impossible to differentiate the two forms from the lesions produced.

The Relationship Between the Tubercle Bacilli From Different Sources.

Now that the unity of the bacillus tuberculosis of mammals has been established, discussion has largely centred itself upon the relations of human tubercle bacillus (mammalian) to that of avian origin. Formerly regarded by Koch as identical they afterwards came to be considered as distinct varieties, the principal argument for this conception basing itself upon certain cultural differences and dissimilarities of pathogenic behavior in animals, the latter particularly explaining the varied opinions entertained by investigators.

The prominent differences are summed up thus: Cultures of human origin are dry, scaly, and cohesive, while those of avian derivation are more luxuriant, softer, and unctuous, and multiply at 43° C., a temperature at which tubercle bacilli of mammalian source cease to grow. As to the differences in pathogenic effects, advocates of the doctrine of dualism (Martin, Gärtner, Auclair, Straus, Wurtz), claim that ordinarily it is impossible to incite mammalian tuberculosis in fowls, whatever the mode of inoculation employed. And some mammals, notably the dog, are refractory to avian tuberculosis; but guinea-pigs which are not susceptible to subcutaneous inoculation of fowl tubercle bacilli, succumb to intraperitoneal infection with lesions totally unlike those provoked by the infecting agent of human tuberculosis.

Per contra the opponents of this view uphold, notwithstanding cultural and other differences, that human and avian tubercle bacilli are but variations of the same organism modified by circumstances of environment. Sometimes they find that it is possible to incite tuberculosis in fowls with bacilli of mammalian sources, and that this form is inoculable in series (Bollinger, Koch, Nocard, Cadiot, Gilbert and Roger, Courmont and Dor). Moreover, some animals are equally receptive to human and avian bacilli; and after a small number of transfers the lesions induced by one and the other become similar. This is especially so for rabbits, and Nocard has shown that the same thing is true for the horse. Commonly so resistant to experimental tuberculosis, this animal frequently becomes infected under natural conditions, the evolution of the infection being divisible into two distinct types. In the one the disease is essentially limited to the

abdominal viscera, invasion of the lungs occurring only in the latest
stages of the affection; the other type, on the other hand, is characterized by primary involvement of the lungs, extension to the abdominal
viscera taking place much later. Comparison of these two groups
permitted Nocard to show that in the same degree that the pathological presentation differed so were there evident distinctions in the tubercle bacilli found in both types of infection. While the pulmonary type
was incited by an organism identical with that of human tuberculosis,
the abdominal was excited by a bacillus similar to that of avian source,
except that it had been more or less modified by the condition in
which it subsisted. But the rabbit and horse are not the only mammals capable of contracting avian tuberculosis. The same observer
found that a tuberculous sputum, markedly pathogenic for rabbits,
was scarcely at all so for guinea-pigs; and the animals that died presented at the autopsy lesions closely simulating those of avian tuberculosis. Cultural comparison proved that the bacilli were identical
with those of known avian derivation. The important distinction
was noted, that inoculated hens almost all resisted, but those that
died showed lesions comparable to the findings of the natural disease
in this animal.   .

It has been shown by Kruse, Fischl, Pansini, and others that in
human beings one occasionally meets with tubercle bacilli which
grow like those of fowl tubercle; and which also resemble them in
their pathogenic effects on rodents. Then, again, there are on record
a certain number of observations which apparently have proven that
the ingestion of phthisical sputum by fowl was followed several
months afterwards by tuberculosis in the birds. The strongest argument brought forward for the view that human and avian tubercle
bacilli are identical is embodied in the experiment of Nocard, who
has been able apparently to transform bacilli of the first source into
those having all the characters of the second. But before him Fischl
obtained certain results, which at least suggested the possibiliy of
this demonstration. Cultivation of mammalian bacilli in eggs and
subsequent transplantation to boric acid or thymol glycerin agar resulted in the production of long threads and clubs, which when introduced into guinea-pigs and rabbits incited changes somewhat similar
to those produced by the organism of bird tuberculosis.

Utilization of the collodion sacs, which yielded such fertile results
in the hands of Metchnikoff, Roux, and Salimbeni in their studies
upon the toxin of the spirillum of Asiatic cholera, and Nocard and
Borrel in their work on pleuropneumonia of cattle, was extended to
the study of tuberculosis by Nocard. These sacs are small, thin,
collodion bags in which cultures are placed, and when the bags are

sealed they are introduced into the peritoneal cavity of the animal experimented with. Although permitting the passage of fluids in either direction, the bags do not allow the bacteria to escape. In this way free interchange occurs between the animal fluids without and the bacterial products within. Nocard introduced bags of this kind containing human tubercle bacilli into the peritoneal cavity of fowls. At the end of five to eight months the birds were killed and the sacs were removed from a mass of adhesions. It was found that the cultural characters had been so profoundly modified that instead of growing like human tubercle bacilli they possessed the characteristics of fowl tubercle bacilli. And this modification was not limited to the cultural side only, for pathogenic differences were now pronounced. Guinea-pigs resisted subcutaneous inoculation, although sometimes at the point of inoculation a small abscess would form which healed readily without any generalization of the process.

If the inoculations were intraperitoneal death followed in more than one-half of the cases, and at the autopsy tubercles were found on the peritoneum, omentum, and spleen, the lungs and liver usually escaping. The type form of experimental disease was not produced. Rabbits were very susceptible and after intravenous injection died in from six to ten weeks with lesions like those of avian tuberculosis. Fowls resisted inoculation except ultimately, when the bacillus was so altered that the disease could be reproduced in its typical form.

Investigations by Theobald Smith lead him to think that there are certain constant differences between human and bovine tubercle bacilli sufficient to make a race. He believes that bovine and other animal tubercle bacilli (except Nasua, which is regarded as coming from man) grow less vigorously than sputum bacilli; are much less influenced by certain modifications of the culture medium; and tend to remain short, the human bacilli being more slender from the start or becoming so during cultivation. Bovine bacilli produce more rapid death and more extensive lesions in pigs than human bacilli. These conclusions accord with those of Dinwiddie (1899).

Critical survey of the facts at hand bearing on this problem shows us that we are near the ultimate solution of this heretofore much vexed question. Now that the investigations of Bataillon, Terre, and Dubard on the tuberculosis of cold-blooded animals have been verified, it seems clear that the unity of all tubercle bacilli from whatever the source has been established. Variations observed are merely accidents of long habit in certain environments. The gradual and progressive introduction of conditions common to one or the other type will convert them at will to forms, realizing in time all the distinctive features which they did not previously exhibit. So Nocard

changed mammalian tubercle bacilli to those having characters of
bacilli of avian origin; and now Dubard, Kráhl, and others have shown
that with the establishment of adequate conditions human or avian
bacilli may induce tuberculous lesions in cold-blooded animals, such
as frogs, serpents, fish, lizards, etc.

TUBERCLE BACILLUS-LIKE ORGANISMS.

Apart from the smegma, lepra, and syphilis bacillus (?), other
organisms have been described within the last few years which possess similar tinctorial and other characters of the bacillus tuberculosis. The most important of this class are:

Moeller's Timothy-Grass Bacillus.—The organism was found by
Moeller in 1898 in infusions made from timothy grass (Phleum pratense). Since then it has also been obtained from other grasses, such
as *Bromus erectus* and *Alapecurus pratensis*—grasses which are common
in temperate climates and largely used for feeding cattle. According
to Moeller and Lubarsch it is difficult to differentiate this microorganism from the tubercle bacillus. It behaves like the tubercle bacillus to stains, and by means of pure cultures Moeller produced a disease in guinea-pigs resembling experimental tuberculosis. Culturally
the main difference seems to be its rapid growth as compared with
that of the tubercle bacillus.

Moeller's Grass Fungus II.—Closely resembling the timothy-grass
bacillus and the bacillus tuberculosis is the grass bacillus II., which
differs culturally from the preceding organism in its close resemblance
to the bacillus of avian tuberculosis. Inoculation with cultures of
this bacillus produces tubercle-like lesions.

Moeller's "Mistpilz" (Manure Fungus).—The manure bacillus was
obtained from cow dung, and like the other organisms just described
resembles the tubercle bacillus. Like the other organisms also it
often appears in the form of branching filaments with clubs.

Rabinowitsch's Butter Bacillus.—Rabinowitsch found in a certain
proportion of specimens of butter an organism which when inoculated
into guinea-pigs incites the development of lesions similar to tubercles. Doubtless this organism, like others mentioned, is closely related to the tubercle bacillus.

Concurrent Infections in Tuberculosis.

The question of concurrent infections in tuberculosis is one which
has come to the front within a comparatively recent date. The greater
part of the work relating to this problem is intimately associated

with the disease in its pulmonary form. Long ago Koch had pointed out the necessity of considering these associated infections in their relation to the course of the disease. The discovery of pyogenic bacteria in the expectoration of tuberculous patients along with the tubercle bacillus, and their frequent virulence, necessitated modification of the earlier views regarding the pathogenesis of tuberculosis. Some observers like Ortner, Weichselbaum, Strümpell, Roger, Dieulafoy, Mosny, and Marfan have laid much stress on the influence of secondary infection; they regard pulmonary tuberculosis as a mixed infection, the secondary invading microorganisms being wholly or in large part responsible for the toxic symptoms and cavity formation. Wolf, Osler, Spengler, Muhlmann, King, and Samter hold a more or less similar view. Indeed, recently some have gone further in attributing a more conspicuous part to these infections. *Per contra*, Straus, Leyden, Baumgarten, Fraenkel, and Troje have endeavored to minimize their importance.

Doubtless in some cases their action has been overestimated. The point generally lost sight of is that the mere presence of associated microorganisms with the tubercle bacillus by no means in itself furnishes sufficient evidence that they exercise any noteworthy action. In some cases the mixed infection may be considerable, and yet no special effects follow therefrom. Accessory processes probably are added in another category of cases; or old lesions may be accentuated by these bacterial invasions. It is still early to define with any certainty the precise relations of infections of this kind to the evolution of tuberculosis.

Suggestive experimental work has been done along these lines. In 1894 Prudden carried out a series of experiments to determine the part played by concurrent infections in the formation of cavities in pulmonary tuberculosis. Intratracheal inoculations were made into rabbits, some receiving pure cultures of the tubercle bacillus, others simultaneous inoculations of this organism and the streptococcus pyogenes; and finally a third series received only the streptococcus infection some time after having been inoculated with the tubercle bacillus. While the final significance of these experiments, as Prudden points out, will be clear only after a more extended study of the frequency and varying conditions of such concurrent infections in man, certain results were sufficiently suggestive to be emphasized in this place in view of their practical importance. The rabbits inoculated with the tubercle bacillus alone presented an acute tuberculosis similar to that in man, save that cavity formation was of exceptional occurrence. These studies further show that the introduction of cultures of the streptococcus pyogenes into rabbits' lungs, which are already the seat of extensive tuberculous consolidation and necrosis, is followed not by an increased amount of exudative pneumonia, but, in many cases, by the extensive development of cavities.

Passing over the earlier studies of Babes, Kitasato, Cornet, Pasquale, Patella, Ortner, and.Czaplewsky to more recent investigations, it is at once apparent that the results of later workers have been quite uniform, so far as the bacteriological findings in such cases are concerned. The bacteria most commonly met with in lung tuberculosis are the streptococcus pyogenes, staphylococci, diplococcus lanceolatus, and Friedländer's bacillus, sometimes associated singly with the tubercle bacillus or in other combinations. In addition to these microorganisms a host of others have been mentioned.

Invasion of the blood by secondary infecting organisms in the course of tuberculosis is uncommon. Associated infections in tuberculous disease of the serous membranes—meninges, peritoneum, pleura, and joints—are less frequent than those met with in pulmonary tuberculosis. Usually the streptococcus, staphylococci, and diplococcus pneumoniæ are the organisms isolated in these cases.

Artault recently studied the bacteriology of pulmonary cavities in 35 cases. In addition to the tubercle bacillus he found the streptococcus 20 times, staphylococci 12 times, the pneumococcus in 9 cases, the colon bacillus in 6, the bacillus pyocyaneus in 4, the micrococcus tetragenus in 3 instances, and the influenza bacillus in 1 case. In addition to these organisms he found the proteus vulgaris, bacillus prodigiosus, sarcinæ, saccharomyces, amœba pulmonalis, cercomonas, and trichomonas. Schütz also studied the mixed infections in pulmonary cavities. He frequently found in the sputum and lungs bacilli of greater or less similarity to the diphtheria bacillus in patients who had not had diphtheria.

The microbic associations in genitourinary tuberculosis have been studied by Albarran. He concludes that whatever the mode of commencement, urogenital tuberculosis does not evolve long before secondary infections occur. These invasions are frequently due to the colon bacillus, streptococcus, and staphylococci. The colon, either alone or associated with staphylococci, according to Albarran, is the most important of these secondary infecting organisms. From an anatomical standpoint, the author believes that the concomitant pyogenic infections quicken the progress of the tuberculosis and augment its destructive tendency.

Bacteriological Diagnosis.

Recourse to bacteriological examination always constitutes one of the important features in the diagnosis of any case of tuberculosis.

EXAMINATION OF THE SPUTUM.

The morning sputum is preferably collected in a clean bottle with a wide mouth provided with a tight stopper. Care should be exercised in the selection of the specimen. Frequently naso-pharyngeal mucus only is obtained, whilst the material should be coughed up from the lungs. Whenever the sputum is small in amount, it is advisable to collect the whole twenty-four hours' expectoration. In the examination of sputum for tubercle bacilli the fine cheesy particles should be carefully selected, as they are more apt to contain bacilli. For their detection portions of sputum are placed upon a plate of glass of suitable size, and this is then covered by a second similar plate, and by pressing the two together the sputum is thereby spread into a thin layer. The whole is placed on a black background, when the caseous particles will stand out more distinctly. Specimens are stained in the manner already indicated in the section dealing with tinctorial reactions.

When few bacilli are present, Simon recommends the following procedure: About 100 c.c. of sputum are boiled with double the amount of water, to which from six to eight drops of a ten-per-cent. solution of sodium hydrate have been added, until a homogeneous solution has been obtained, water being added from time to time to allow for evaporation. This is then set aside for twenty-four to forty-eight hours, and examined for tubercle bacilli and elastic tissue. The use of the centrifugal machine is of great assistance when the tubercle bacilli are few in number. Some have thought that placing sputum in a warm chamber for twenty-four hours or more facilitated their detection. This would result from the multiplication of the tubercle bacilli in the sputum, an occurrence which has been demonstrated by Nuttall. Simon urges the employment of this procedure. In infants and children it is often difficult to obtain expectoration for diagnostic purposes on account of the fact that they frequently swallow the sputum. Washing out the stomach, however, particularly in the morning, will often give the desired material.

When tubercle bacilli are found in sputum, this evidence is obviously demonstrative; but a negative result, even after a number of attempts, does not by any means necessarily bar out the existence of tuberculosis. Many examinations are often required before the tubercle bacilli are detected. Sometimes guinea-pig inoculations are required. In acute miliary tuberculosis the bacilli may not be found for a long time.

Pappenheim found in sputum smegma bacilli which he mistook for tubercle bacilli. Commenting on this case, Fraenkel states that he had had several cases of gangrene in which he made a similar mistake. He says that in ordinary mucopurulent sputum the smegma bacillus does not resist decolorization, but that in all cases of decomposing sputum rich in fatty acids and myelin the ordinary methods of staining the tubercle bacillus are unreliable as a means of differentiation of the two bacilli.

Some observers have thought that from the number of tubercle bacilli in the sputum certain conclusions might be formulated regarding the prognostic aspect of the case. More careful observations show that the number of bacilli found in a specimen possesses little prognostic value in itself. Comparative studies of the number in a single case would be more likely to give suggestive indications. Thus, if the specimens from a patient were examined from time to time and the bacilli were seen to become less and less numerous, this might be significant of amelioration. But on this point we would not care to insist too much, for we have seen cases in which the bacilli diminished in number with the increasing severity of the clinical course.

Examination of the Urine.

Frequently tubercle bacilli are present in the urine in tuberculosis of the urogenital system, but their detection here is often difficult and uncertain. For purposes of bacteriological examination the urine should be obtained through a catheter to avoid contamination with the smegma bacillus, which morphologically and tinctorially resembles the tubercle bacilli closely. It is advisable to collect the sediment by means of the centrifuge. Cover-glass preparations are then made and stained in the usual manner. Frequently they will not be found even when present, especially when in small numbers. The writer in his experience has found inoculation of the sediment into guinea-pigs the most reliable. Subcutaneous inoculation answers very well.

Cover-slip examinations for tubercle bacilli in the urine have another disadvantage. The smegma bacillus, which is present about the genitals, stains not unlike the bacillus tuberculosis, and unless special precautions be used, might easily be mistaken for it. The safest way out of the difficulty at the present time remains in the use of the animal inoculation. The smegma bacillus produces no lesions, of course, of tuberculosis.

Numerous special methods have been devised to differentiate the tubercle and smegma bacilli by tinctorial manipulations. The method of Giacomi, which is to heat the specimen in the solution of carbolic fuchsin to ebullition and then decolorize by perchloride of iron, has not proved very satisfactory. The method of Fraenkel—which consists in staining with carbolic-fuchsin solution and decolorizing by a mixture of nitric acid, alcohol, and methylene blue—stains the tubercle bacilli, but unfortunately they may also be decolorized by this method. A procedure devised by Weichselbaum gives better results. After staining in the ordinary way with the carbolic-fuchsin solution and washing, the specimen is treated with a concentrated alcoholic solution of methylene blue. The tubercle bacilli alone are supposed to remain in red. Grethe recommends the method devised by Czaplewski, who decolorizes the specimen, after staining with fuchsin, with an alcoholic solution of fluorescin and methylene blue.

Perhaps the best of the various methods is that of Bunge and Trantenroth, the steps of which are as follows: Let the preparation remain in absolute alcohol not less than three hours and then transfer for fifteen minutes to a five-per-cent. chromic-acid solution; stain with carbolic-fuchsin solution; decolorize with dilute sulphuric acid for two to three minutes; then pass into concentrated alcoholic solution of methylene blue for about five minutes.

Honsell recommends the use of hot carbolic-fuchsin solution followed by the action of three-per-cent. hydrochloric acid in absolute alcohol for not less than ten minutes, counterstaining with a solution of methylene blue in fifty-per-cent. alcohol. Pappenheim uses a solution of corallin in absolute alcohol.

The writer has not found any of these methods wholly satisfactory, hence generally relies on the inoculation test.

EXAMINATION OF SEROUS EXUDATES.

The search for tubercle bacilli in the exudates of tuberculous pleurisy, peritonitis, meningitis, or arthritis is often uncertain and tedious. The exudates are to be removed with bacteriological precautions and collected in sterile receptacles. Fluid may be obtained from cases of meningitis by lumbar puncture. For microscopical examination, it is important to centrifugate the fluid because tubercle bacilli are almost always few in number in such exudates. The crucial and most reliable method consists in introducing the centrifugated sediment beneath the skin of the thigh of a guinea-pig. If the specimen contains tubercle bacilli involvement of the glands will soon take place. Cover-slip preparations of the broken-down glands will show the tubercle bacilli, so that it is unnecessary to wait until the disease is widespread or the animal dies to make the diagnosis.

EXAMINATION OF THE INTESTINAL DISCHARGES.

The search for tubercle bacilli in the stools is generally difficult. Rosenblatt recommends giving laudanum until the stools become hard and sausage-like, and then examining the surface of the stool, particularly any mucopurulent areas. He states that when tubercle bacilli are present he usually finds them in the first preparation. In his opinion the hard scybala, in passing over the ulcerated surface, brush off bacilli and carry them along with them, while ordinary diarrhœal stools do not dislodge them.

AGGLUTINATION TEST.

The serum test so extensively used in the diagnosis of typhoid fever has been recently applied to tuberculosis with some modifications, particularly by French observers. The test was first applied in tuberculosis by Arloing and Courmont (1898). Upon the admixture of fluid cultures of tubercle bacilli and sera from rabbits or goats which had previously received several subcutaneous inoculations of tuberculin or tubercle bacilli, the bacilli became agglutinated.

Cultures of tubercle bacilli to be used in the test must be homogeneous emulsions of the microorganism. The best medium for cultivating them for this purpose is six per cent. glycerin bouillon containing one per cent. peptone. The agglutination capacity is said to be twice as great with six to eight per cent. glycerin as when only two per cent. is employed (Arloing and Courmont). Cultures eight to twelve days old are the best. Arloing and Courmont give the following directions for carrying out the test: The method which gives the most delicate results necessitates the employment of serum obtained from a venous puncture with aseptic precautions. However, blood secured by simple puncture of the skin gives good results. It is collected in small sterilized capillary tubes, and the serum (which must be utilized fresh) is used free from formed blood elements. With each serum prepare three dilutions: 1:5, 1:10, 1:20. Dilutions lower than 1:5 are of no value; with dilutions higher than 1:20 agglutination is rare. The diluted serum and culture, which are preferably placed in sterilized tubes of small diameter, are inclined to an angle of 45° to facilitate agglutination. The time in which the reaction is developed is variable with different sera; in some cases it is complete in two hours, while in others it may take twenty-four hours. Observations should be macroscopic and microscopic. A complete reaction consists in the deposition of a fine sand-like material along the side of the tube, while the control shows no similar deposit. Of course, microscopical examination must show clumping of the tubercle bacilli. The serum reaction may be considered positive when clumping is abundant, although clarification may not be complete.

Some clinical work has been done with this test. For instance, Arloing and Courmont, in 26 cases of pulmonary tuberculosis, obtained 24 positive results. Of the 24 positive reactions 18 were obtained with a dilution of 1:10 or 1:20. Of 22 cases of slight pulmonary or pleural tuberculosis examined by this method 95.5 per cent. gave positive results; of 12 surgical tuberculoses 50 per cent. gave distinct reactions, while the remaining cases gave only feeble reactions. Twenty-one diseases other than tuberculosis were tested, and 14 gave negative results, while positive reactions were noted in 7 cases; these included cases of appendicitis, hysteria, pneumonia, Bright's disease, rheumatism, erysipelas, cancer, chlorosis, etc. The test was also applied in 9 cases of typhoid fever with 4 negative results. In 16 apparently healthy people from eighteen to thirty years of age Arloing and Courmont got 5 positive results.

Micheleau obtained a positive result in a case of acute miliary tuberculosis, and Mongour and Buard tested the serum of many patients suffering from various diseases, and on the whole reached conclusions similar to those of Arloing and Courmont. Knopf tried pleuritic fluids from tuberculous guinea-pigs with positive results. In 10 cases of pulmonary tuberculosis he got 4 well-marked positive results, 2 slight reactions, 1 doubtful, and 3 negative. A case of miliary tuberculosis showed a slight reaction. On the whole Knopf questions the great value of this test. The writer tried it in 4 cases of pulmonary tuberculosis, with a marked reaction in but 1 case and a doubtful reaction in another; the remaining 2 were negative. It is yet too early to reach any definite conclusions regarding the value of the test. More extended studies alone can decide its practical value.

PATHOLOGICAL ANATOMY.*

The presence and growth of the bacillus tuberculosis in the tissues incite certain reactive phenomena on the part of the body cells, which under different conditions vary considerably in character. The nature and extent of the process depend on several factors— number and virulence of the infecting bacilli, susceptibility of the

---

* The limitations of this article restrict the discussion mainly to a consideration of the histogenesis of the tubercle and pathological anatomy of pulmonary tuberculosis. The pathology of the tuberculosis of other tissues has been treated of more or less exhaustively by those who have written on the diseases of special organs.

individual, and finally the nature of the tissue involved. As a sequence of infection with tubercle bacilli, the fixed tissue cells in their vicinity are stimulated to proliferation and an emigration of leucocytes from the blood-vessels occurs; or the poisonous products of the germs may cause death of the cells. Any tuberculous process is necessarily characterized by a productive, exudative, or necrotic inflammation. Sometimes the three are concomitant, but often two or only one of these phases will be present.

Certainly one of the most striking features of a tuberculous inflammation is the occurrence of a special type of necrosis which appears in the form of an opaque material of yellowish color. This has been likened in its appearance to cheese; hence the designation caseation, caseous or cheesy degeneration. Regarded as a phase of coagulation necrosis, changes of this kind are largely referable to the action of products given off by the bacillus tuberculosis.

Ordinarily tuberculosis is characterized by the development of small spheroidal nodules, varying from one millimetre in diameter to the size of a small pea. The latter are commonly caseous in the centre; the small tubercles usually have a gray, translucent appearance. To these nodular bodies has been given the name *miliary tubercles*. "The term miliary tubercle, which arose from the crude coincidence in size between small foci of tuberculous inflammation and some forms of millet seed, is now very liberally applied to tubercles which are very much larger as well as to those which are very much smaller than millet seeds" (Delafield and Prudden). Very frequently two or more tubercles are joined together to form greater or smaller tubercles—*conglomerate tubercles*.

Tubercles are not entirely distinctive of tuberculosis, for similar formations are met with in other diseases.

Morphologically contrasting with the tubercle is another type of process, which occurs in the form of diffuse tuberculous inflammation. Tissues affected in this manner often have a white or yellow color in the central portions; peripherally these areas are frequently surrounded by a zone of tubercle tissue or by a dense fibrous capsule. Diffuse tuberculous inflammation commonly occurs in the brain, serous membranes, lymph nodes, kidneys, testicle, etc. Tuberculous processes are not infrequently accompanied by the formation of inflammatory exudates—pus, fibrin, serum, etc. The intensity and rapidity of the local poisoning by the bacillus is sometimes so considerable as not to permit of the production of organized new tissue, but only of exudative products. A less severe degree of exudative inflammation may develop in the vicinity of miliary tubercles anywhere in the body, but more particularly in the lungs.

If caseous tuberculous tissue becomes disintegrated, cavities result which are filled with pus and débris of the broken-down caseous. mass. The cavity wall consists either of already caseous tissue in the process of breaking down or of granulation tissue containing tubercles.

Tuberculosis generally begins in the form of a local process in the lungs, intestinal tract, or skin—tissues more or less readily accessible from without. The frequency of involvement of these tissues varies. For instance, in children intestinal tuberculosis is more common; in adults the lungs are the seat of election for tuberculous disease. Retaining the features of a localized inflammation, the disease may run for years without extension of the process to neighboring or other organs. Lupus is a good example of this. Often local tuberculosis is followed by clinical evidences of systemic infection. If the process continues to advance in the interior of an organ, or if softening occurs in a tuberculous focus, a blood-vessel may become involved and tubercle bacilli thus be thrown into the blood stream; or the bacilli may gain the blood channels by way of the lymphatic vessels through the thoracic duct. By either of these routes metastatic foci may be established in succession, or at the same time in many parts of the body and so give rise to *general miliary tuberculosis.*

The number of tubercle bacilli which may be present in the lesions of tuberculosis differs considerably under different circumstances. Great numbers of them may be found in the walls and contents of tuberculous pulmonary cavities and in tissue which is undergoing caseation. Considerable numbers are often found in the cells, particularly the giant cells of the tubercle. They are usually to be found in tuberculous lesions in any part of the body, but under some conditions, especially in old processes, tubercle bacilli may not be demonstrable.

Whether or not it is possible for tubercle bacilli to enter the body through the uninjured mucosa has been much debated within the last few years. Surely in the light of recent knowledge such an occurrence is not wholly inconceivable. Indeed, experimental studies of Dobroklonski and Straus have shown the possibility of such a thing for the intestinal canal. Feeding animals with cultures of tubercle bacilli Dobroklonski was able to demonstrate bacilli in the walls of the intestine and in the mesenteric glands so soon as four or five days after their ingestion. The writer has been able to confirm this on a number of different occasions. Probably the same holds good for the respiratory system.

Distribution of Tuberculous Lesions in the Body.

Under different conditions the frequency of tuberculosis in the organs of the body varies within certain proportions. Thus the distribution of tuberculous lesions in early life is somewhat different from that observed in later years. Lymph-gland, bone, and joint tuberculosis constitute a high percentage of this disease in childhood. From a series of 123 autopsies in children Schwer gives the following figures:

Liver	104	Meninges	53
Respiratory organs	103	Thyroid gland	12
Kidneys	83	Striated muscle	2
Intestine	61		

Statistics by many others give higher figures for the respiratory organs.

In adults the lungs are certainly the most common seat of tuberculosis. Osler states that in 1,000 autopsies 275 cases presented tuberculosis; with but two or three exceptions the lungs were constantly involved. The distribution of the lesions in other tissues was as follows:

Intestine	65	Liver	12
Peritoneum	36	Generative organs	8
Kidneys	32	Pericardium	7
Brain	31	Heart	4
Spleen	23		

Warthin gives the relative per cent. of the distribution of the tuberculous lesions in 50 cases as follows:

Lung	100 per cent.	Fallopian tubes	7 per cent.
Pleura	100 "	Uterus	7 "
Bronchial glands	100 "	Tonsils	4 "
Liver	100 "	Duodenum	4
Spleen	100 "	Appendix	4
Kidneys	100 "	Retroperitoneal glands	4 "
Small intestine	95 "	Tongue, adrenals, bladder	2 "
Mesenteric glands	95 "	Nose, testes, seminal vesicles	2
Meninges	24 "	Cervical glands, prostate, stomach	2
Large intestine	17 "	Rectum, mamma, skin	2 "
Peritoneum	9 "		
Bone	9 "		
Brain	7 "		
Heart	7 "		

Figures from the clinic in Würzburg show that surgical tuberculosis has a very different distribution. Of 8,873 patients 1,287 were found to be tuberculous. The frequency of involvement of different tissues was as follows:

Bones and joints	1,037	Mucous membranes	10
Lymph glands	196	Urogenital organs	20
Skin and connective tissues	77		

Histogenesis of the Tubercle.

The history of the study of the histogenesis of the tubercle naturally falls into two distinct periods separated by the discovery of the bacillus tuberculosis. The prebacterial period was essentially one of a study of pathological histology in a restricted sense; the period that followed has attempted a solution on broader lines. Having no knowledge of the exciting factor of tuberculosis, the earlier investigators perforce directed their attention wholly to the morphological side of the study. Unable to correlate their findings with the bacteriological conception, insistence on many features of a purely secondary nature was often the result. Notwithstanding this the main morphological points had been well brought out by them.

Virchow, as has already been explained in the historical section, regarded tubercle as a special product made up of a mass of small round cells disposed in a stroma. The analogy of the appearance of the cells to those of lymphatic tissue was pointed out; and he classed these tuberculous neoplasms among the lymphomata. Investigations by Langhans (1868) established the frequent association with the tubercle of multinucleated cells, since known as the giant cells of Langhans. Before him Rokitansky (1855) and E. Wagner (1861) had observed similar cells; but to Langhans belongs the credit of having given a fuller significance to these elements.

In 1869 Koster returned to Virchow's conception of the tubercle; and E. Wagner (1870), carrying the similarity of the tubercle to a lymphoid production still further, found no other differences between the two sorts of tissue than the absence of blood-vessels in the former. A notable advance in this study was made by Schüppel the following year. He differentiated the tubercle from lymphoid tissue by the following characters: the latter is made up of a mass of uninuclear cells embedded in a fine reticulum; it contains capillaries, which are never found in the tubercle. Moreover, the tubercle contains giant and epithelioid cells, neither of which are found in the lymph nodes. To this day Schüppel's description of the tubercle has remained classical.

At this period the giant and epithelioid cells had come to be regarded as specific of tuberculosis. But Heidenhain, G. Weiss,

Baumgarten, and Ziegler shortly thereafter discredited this notion by experimentally proving the presence of giant cells in tissues following the introduction of foreign bodies beneath the skin or in the peritoneal cavity. Since then these cells have lost their original significance.

Widening the point of view inquiry was next directed to the determination of the cells giving rise to the elements making the tubercle. Among those earliest in the investigation of this side of the question were Lubimoff and Ziegler. With the discovery of the tubercle bacillus the scope of research assumed new and different proportions, and with this change in experimentation study of the genesis of the tubercle also underwent modifications.

As a derivative of experimental results secured within the last few years, two conceptions of the genetic history of the tubercle have been elaborated. According to the advocates of the one the migratory cells of the blood are the important factors in the production of this tuberculous neoformation—a view wholly dominated by the phagocytic theory of Metchnikoff. Others, including those of the German school, attribute to the fixed tissue cells the essential part. Still a third group conceive both factors as important elements in the production of this newly formed tissue.

THE TUBERCLE.

Histological and experimental investigations alike show that one of the first local effects of the presence and growth of the tubercle bacillus in tissues is to stimulate the fixed tissue cells to proliferation, and also to call forth an emigration of the leucocytes from the blood. Some of these cells become larger, of rather clear vesicular appearance, and from their resemblance to the epithelial cell type have received the name *epithelioid cells*. In the development of the tubercle giant cells may be formed. Concomitant with these processes a fine reticulum is developed. So, in a general way, the histological tubercle is made up of a peripheral zone of small, deeply staining round cells, with little protoplasm. Between them and in the central portions of the tubercle are disposed the epithelioid cells; finally the type tubercle also contains giant cells.

At this stage of development the tubercle is a grayish and translucent spheroidal body. It is a non-vascular formation which shows little tendency to the formation of new blood-vessels; old vessels are usually obliterated as the new growth takes place. After a time evidences of retrogressive changes appear in the new-formed tissue as well as in the old tissue of the infected area. These changes are referable to the action of poisons of the tubercle bacillus, and this degenerative change is in small part possibly also due to the non-vascularity of the tissue.

Retrogressive Changes in the Tubercle.—When the tubercle has reached a certain size retrogressive changes usually appear; they are usually classified under one of two headings: (1) caseation, and (2) sclerosis or fibrosis.

Caseation.—With the elaboration by the tubercle bacilli of certain products which act upon the cells, a process of coagulation necrosis

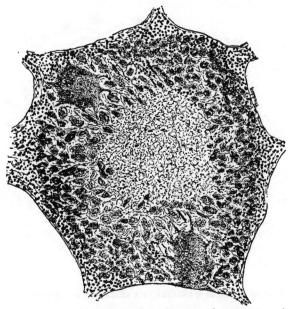

Fig. 6.—A Nodule of Tuberculous Inflammation (Miliary Tubercle) in the Lung. Showing polyhedral cells, small cells, giant cells, and coagulative necrosis at the centre. (Delafield and Prudden.)

is produced which first appears in the centre. Baumgarten states that the leucocytes are the earliest to die, then the epithelioid cells follow. At this stage a partial necrosis of the giant cells is also apparent. The process by extension from the centre outwards may convert the whole mass into a hyaline, structureless, or granular substance. Finally the mass may change to an opaque and yellowish-white appearance. This goes to make up what is spoken of as caseation. The cheesy masses may undergo softening, fibrosis, and calcification.

Fibrosis.—This is essentially a conservative process and is the result of secondary inflammatory reaction. So the whole tubercle

may be changed into a nodule of hard fibrous tissue. Such a conversion is common in chronic tuberculosis. Not infrequently, instead
of complete fibrous transformation, only the peripheral portion of the
tubercle is fibroid, while the central parts are caseous. This is often
spoken of as encapsulation.

Calcification.—The deposition of lime salts (chiefly phosphate of
lime) in the tubercle is observed in old tuberculous lesions in man and
some animals. Thus, while common enough in cattle and pigs, it is

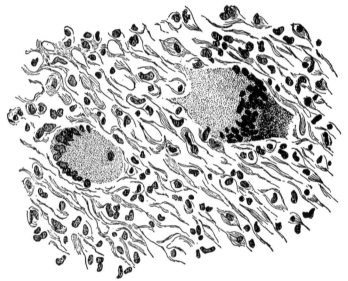

Fig. 7.—Giant Cells in Tubercle of a Rabbit's Lung After Injections of Dead Bacilli (Straus).

not met with in rabbits or guinea-pigs. Calcification of tubercle has
been noted as early as one hundred and six days after inoculation in
the pig.

The Fixed Tissue Cells.—Foremost among the champions of the
theory of a genesis of tubercle from fixed tissue cells is Baumgarten,
whose brilliant researches regarding the histogenesis of this neoformation have rallied many to his belief in the importance of the fixed tissue
cells in its development. This investigator made inoculations of tubercle bacilli into the anterior chamber of the rabbit's eye, and studying the development of the lesion from day to day was able to follow
the process step by step. Up to the fifth day Baumgarten was unable
to observe any appreciable changes except those related to the healing
of the inoculated wound. At this time he was able to detect a few

bacilli, some free, others in the fixed cells of the tissue around the inoculation point. The main reaction seemed to be limited to the production of isolated karyokinetic figures. On the sixth day there were noted, in places where the bacilli were more numerous, cells of new formation which had the character of epithelioid cells. By the seventh and eighth days the karyokinetic figures had become more abundant; in the neighborhood of the bacterial foci they could be observed in almost all the cells of the tissue of the iris—connective-tissue cells, endothelial cells of the blood-vessels, and epithelial

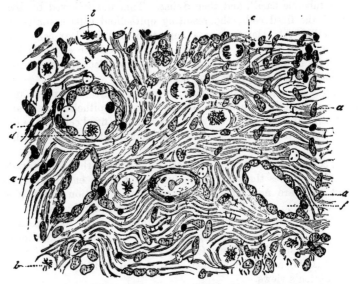

Fig. 8.—Schema of Development of the Tubercle, after Baumgarten. a, Epithelioid cell; b, karyokinetic figure; c, migratory cell; d, endothelial cell; f, capillary. (Straus)

cells covering the surfaces of the iris. Several days later in these portions an abundance of epithelioid cells were to be found. Step by step he was able to follow the transformation of the fixed tissue cells into cells of an epithelioid character. The dividing cells were generally free from bacilli (see Fig. 8).

At this period, according to Baumgarten, another phenomenon occurs in the form of an invasion of the parts concerned by migratory cells. These are small uninuclear and multinuclear leucocytes. Karyokinetic figures were never observed in the migratory cells by Baumgarten.

About the tenth or twelfth day it was noted that there appeared in the interior of the tubercle, between the epithelioid cells, a fine fibrillary reticulum. At the same time a sort of encapsulation of the nodule could be noticed. The leucocyte migration was observed to become greater and greater until the tubercle presented the appearance which Virchow had long before taken as the type form of tubercle.

Brissaud and Toupet and Pilliet are also partisans of Baumgarten's conception of the origin of the tubercle from the fixed tissue cells. Kostenich and Volkow (1892), repeating the studies upon the eye of the rabbit, concluded that soon after the inoculation there occurred a multinuclear leucocytosis, the leucocytes taking up the tubercle bacilli and then dying. This was followed by division of the fixed cells, the resulting epithelioid cells assimilating the bacilli. At a later stage a migration of uninuclear cells took place into the tubercle; finally, when all the cellular elements had undergone necrosis, a new influx of multinuclear leucocytes occurred and they in turn disappeared by necrosis.

Straus also accepts Baumgarten's explanation: "The primordial and characteristic elements of the tubercle, the epithelioid cells and giant cells, are derived by karyokinesis from the fixed cells of the tissues: connective-tissue cells, vascular endothelium, and epithelial cells. The migratory elements (multinuclear and uninuclear leucocytes) come from the inflamed vessels of the neighborhood and invade at different times the tubercle nodule. But these emigrated lymphoid cells are not capable of progressive evolution; they give birth neither to epithelioid nor to giant cells, but rapidly undergo nuclear fragmentation, chromatolysis, and other regressive modifications of cells in the process of disintegration." The researches of Nikiforoff (1890), Ziegler (1891), Klebs (1894), Thoma (1894), Schieck (1896), Kockel (1896), and Broden (1899), have contributed to the support of Baumgarten's views.

Phagocytes.—Although Koch, perhaps influenced by the investigations of Cohnheim and Ziegler on diapedesis, regarded the leucocytes as capable of entering into the production of the tubercle, it remained for Metchnikoff and his pupils to develop the conception that the tubercle was the result of phagocytic activity. So well known are the remarkable investigations of this savant regarding phagocytosis that the relation of his views of the production of the tubercle to this theory must appear obvious. Studying the action of avian tubercle bacilli upon a small rodent (spermophilus guttatus) Metchnikoff affirms that giant cells and epithelioid cells are not degeneration forms, but on the contrary, are endowed with abundant phagocytic properties. As proof he mentions the regressive forms of the tubercle bacillus which one finds in their protoplasm. Weigert strongly argues against this interpretation.

In a later study Metchnikoff returns to the same question and looks for new arguments in favor of his view in experiments by intravenous injection of avian tubercle bacilli in rabbits. In this investigation the liver was especially utilized. The epithelioid and giant cells, according to him, develop from phagocytes—large uninuclear leucocytes and endothelial cells of the capillaries; other phagocytic cells may become transformed into epithelioid cells. Hepatic or epithelial cells would take no part in the process.

Other investigations, by Yersin (1888), Stchastuy (1889), Gilbert and Girode (1891), Borrel (1894), Leredde (1895) and Peron (1895), have led these experimenters to similar conclusions.

Some, like Pilliet and Welcker, believe that the phagocytes and fixed tissue cells both play some part in the production of the tubercle. This seems to the author more nearly the truth than either of the conceptions of Baumgarten and Metchnikoff considered separately. But the limitations of the part of each in the process are still problems for future solution. Apparently, however, the fixed tissue cells assume the more important rôle.

ORIGIN OF THE GIANT CELL.

The manner of formation of the giant cell has been the subject of study at different times. Langhans long ago conceived two possible modes of origin. According to one view the giant cell originates from a single modified cell, or else is the result of the confluence of several cells. Ziegler fancied that they developed at the expense of the leucocytes; Schüppel also maintained a somewhat similar origin. At a later period Schüppel admits their endothelial origin, a view accepted by Cornil and others. Charcot and Gombault explained the formation of the giant cell by the massing and superimposition of many cells.

Two definite theories in time arose to explain the mode of formation of the giant cell—the unicellular and the pluricellular. Among the partisans of the first Koch may be mentioned. He assumed that the migratory cell containing the tubercle bacilli underwent nuclear multiplication and was thus transformed into a giant cell. Weigert also admits the unicellular origin of these cells, presumably due to feeble irritation capable of inciting nuclear division. Baumgarten likewise adopts this mode of development; Metchnikoff, on the other hand, believes that giant cells may have either a unicellular or a pluricellular origin.

Arnold and his pupils accept the pluricellular derivation of giant cells. These cells, in their opinion, originate from the confluence of several swollen epithelioid cells. Yersin also practically accepts this derivation, but thinks that the mechanism in their formation is somewhat different. According to him, from the necrotic action of the bacilli there are formed in places areas of granular detritus formed of destroyed cells. Leucocytes surround these areas in a semicircle, and finally penetrate them; and so the giant cell is developed. Borrel believes that the uninuclear leucocytes, after having sent prolongations around the tubercle bacilli, become fused and thus the giant cell is formed. According to Kostenich and Volkow a fusion of several cells and multiplication of the nuclei are both necessary factors.

Pathology of Pulmonary Tuberculosis.

Tuberculosis of the lungs usually begins as a local disease, but the tuberculous pulmonary inflammation may be only a part of a general process with similar lesions in other viscera. Infection of the lungs takes place most commonly by way of the respiratory tract (pneumatogenic tuberculosis), or the bacilli may reach these organs through the blood-vessels (hæmatogenic tuberculosis); finally in another set of cases the infection occurs by means of the lymphatics (lymphogenic tuberculosis). When the infection is hæmatogenic or lymphogenic the lesion is usually secondary to tuberculosis elsewhere, the tubercle bacilli entering the circulation from some other point, often a caseous lymph node. Occasionally the process is limited to the lungs and may be secondary to an older tuberculous lesion of the lung itself.

Pulmonary tuberculosis may present itself under so many different guises that any classification based on sharp distinctions must necessarily not include a large series of intermediate forms, in which often are seen the characteristics of several types. Anatomical variations largely depend on the channel by which the tubercle bacillus gains access to the lungs; also on features peculiar to the individual himself and the tissue involved. And not alone this, but the number of bacilli introduced constitutes a most important factor in the determination of the character of the inflammatory process incited. Other less related processes, such as those induced by concomitant bacterial infections, and preëxisting lesions, add to the multiplicity of postmortem pictures observed in lung tuberculosis.

The presence of tubercle bacilli in the lungs incites tissue reactions, giving rise to exudative and productive inflammation, the variety produced depending on a whole series of more or less complex conditions. To these phenomena may be added necrosis of the exudate, newly formed tissue and portions of the lung parenchyma.

When the number of bacilli inhaled is considerable, both varieties of inflammation are produced, frequently with preponderance of the exudative variety. Should, on the other hand, the number be small, then focal areas of productive inflammation are generally observed. Many of the changes incited in the lungs by the tubercle bacillus may be reproduced and well studied experimentally in animals. Prudden, by the injection of tubercle bacilli, alone and associated with streptococci, into the air passages of rabbits has been able to reproduce closely in many respects the lesions of phthisis. "If a small quantity of the culture be used and distributed in very minute flocculi through a considerable quantity of salt solution, so that the emulsion has a faint milky appearance and a large amount, say from two to three cubic centimetres of the material, be introduced into the lungs through the trachea, the animal being held on its back with the head and shoulders high and turned from side to side, one can usually so distribute the germs in the lungs that small discrete areas of consolidation result, having the gross appearance of miliary tuberculosis. If, on the other hand, larger quantities of the tubercle bacillus are used, so that from three to five cubic centimetres of a deep milky emulsion are introduced, no special pains being taken to distribute it in the lungs, large areas of consolidation may be induced involving whole lobes or whole lungs. Under these circumstances the right upper lobe and the posterior parts of both lower lobes of the lungs are most apt to be consolidated and to present a gross appearance similar to that of many phases of solid lungs in acute phthisis or cheesy pneumonia. In regard to the experimental control of the quality of the lesion, it may be said, in general, that when very large amounts of the tubercle bacillus are introduced, the early phases of the resulting lesion are apt to be dominated by the occurrence, in addition to the local cell proliferation and productive inflammation and cheesy degeneration, of an exudative inflammation especially characterized by the accumulation in the air spaces of fibrin and leucocytes or lymphocytes" (Prudden).

For the sake of simplicity and clearness we shall consider tuberculous inflammations of the lungs under two main headings: miliary tuberculosis and tuberculous pneumonia or phthisis. Such a classification seems best for the purposes of this article.

MILIARY TUBERCULOSIS.

This form is characterized by an eruption of tubercles in one or both lungs, usually on both sides. The development of miliary tubercles in the lungs is usually only part of a generalized tuberculosis, although these organs are often the seat of most prominent involvement. In generalized miliary tuberculosis the organs, besides the lungs, most conspicuously involved are the kidneys, spleen, liver, and meninges. Sometimes the apex of one or the other lung contains a tuberculous focus which occasionally is the starting-point of the miliary tuberculosis. More commonly tubercles are scattered through the lungs; at other times they are aggregated in irregular fashion or localized in certain parts. Although ordinarily discrete in distribution, the tubercles may be so close together as almost to render the lung solid.

In very acute tuberculosis the tubercles may be so small and transparent as almost wholly to escape macroscopic detection; with oblique light, however, they are more readily perceptible. In the hæmatogenous miliary tuberculosis the characteristic cellular aggregations are first seen around and implicating the arterioles and capillaries in the intraalveolar septa. When the infection, on the other hand, takes place through the lymphatics the tubercles are seen distributed along the lymph vessels coursing in the interlobular septa, or around blood-vessels and bronchi.

With the development of the tubercles, the alveoli and smaller bronchioles in relation with the bacterial foci become filled with cells. The anatomical forms of miliary tubercles in acute miliary tuberculosis are divisible into three groups: 1. Miliary tubercles embracing a group of alveoli filled with granular material, a few shrunken cells, and a peripheral zone of pus cells. The alveolar walls may be still visible and infiltrated with exudate or they may be necrotic. 2. Miliary tubercles formed by the infiltration of the wall of the bronchiole or air passage with tubercle or granulation tissue. It may extend to the walls of adjacent vesicles, the vesicles themselves often containing tubercle tissue or epithelium, fibrin, and pus. 3. Miliary tubercles made up of a group of alveoli, of which the walls are infiltrated and the cavities filled with granulation or tubercle tissue. The alveolar spaces are filled with tissue or exudate as in the second form (Delafield and Prudden).

Other forms of miliary tuberculosis, more chronic in their evolution, instead of having a more or less simultaneous development in all parts, frequently begin at the apex of one lung with subsequent extension of the process until a large part of the organ is involved. The areas of involvement are generally more considerable than in acute miliary tuberculosis, and the tubercles are harder and denser. With chronic miliary tuberculosis there commonly exist catarrhal bronchitis and bronchiectasiæ; interstitial pneumonia is sometimes present and pleural thickening is common enough.

Certain authors hold that chronic miliary tuberculosis is produced by infection through the blood or lymph channels; presumably in these instances small numbers of bacilli enter the thoracic duct, possibly from infected and broken-down lymph nodes, in a gradual manner. Such an explanation answers for many of these cases, but others are not explicable in this way.

The various tissues of the body are apt to undergo parenchymatous degeneration in miliary tuberculosis, especially in the acute forms; fatty degeneration is also observed. The heart, liver, and kidneys are very prone to changes of this kind. No striking changes can be observed in the morphology of the blood.

TUBERCULOUS PNEUMONIA.

Under the general term *tuberculous pneumonia* or *phthisis* we shall include practically all of the forms of pneumatogenous tuberculosis. Any form of phthisis may evolve clinically as an acute or chronic process. Anatomically, it may in a general way conform to a bronchopneumonic or lobar distribution; either may develop with or without cavity formation. These two types are modified by a whole series of tributary and secondary processes—concomitant bacterial infections, preëxisting or newly formed anatomical lesions such as emphysema, interstitial pneumonia, bronchiectatic cavities, etc.— which give rise to a diversity of post-mortem appearances.

Infection by way of the air passages is the most common mode of invasion in pulmonary tuberculosis. The tubercle bacilli are inhaled and are arrested in the terminal bronchioles or alveoli, in parts where the epithelium is not ciliated. Very rarely do they become fixed in the larger bronchi on account of active ciliated movement. After a variable period tissue changes are incited by the bacilli, most marked in the peribronchial connective tissues and alveolar cavities. Thus an area of peribronchitis and bronchopneumonia is produced. Tubercle bacilli may penetrate the bronchial mucous membrane and pass to the bronchial lymph nodes without leaving any trace of their passage.

Although any part of the lung may become involved, topographical studies show that some portions are implicated with much greater frequency than others. Indeed, the frequency with which the apex of the lung, especially the right, is the seat of tuberculosis has been universally appreciated since the time of Louis. Much less often are other parts the seat of the primary lesion. The frequency of localization of the lung lesion differs considerably according to the age. For instance, in children a primary basic origin is considerably more common; the posterior border of the lung, especially perhaps the upper portion of the lower lobe, is more often the point of early implication. In the case of children bronchial gland disease seems almost without exception to be coexistent.

Explanations of the common apical distribution of lung tuberculosis have not been wanting, but it must be confessed that no attempt of this kind has been wholly satisfactory. Some have insisted upon

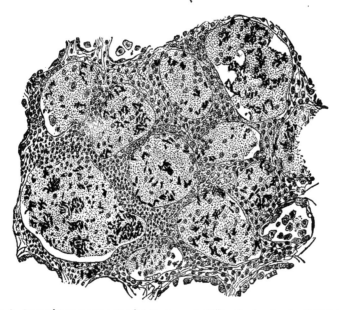

Fig. 9.—Tuberculous Pneumonia (Focal) in the Lung of a Child. Showing the alveoli filled with necrotic exudate. (Delafield and Prudden.)

and, in this relation, said much of the restricted movement of this part of the organ, owing to a comparative rigidity of the ribs in the upper chest. Others, assuming that the circulation of this portion of the lung is less active than elsewhere, seem to think this sufficient to explain the local susceptibility.

Whenever the tubercle bacilli are present in great numbers and other conditions are favorable, caseous pneumonia is more likely to be produced than tuberculous nodules; if the bacilli are few in number the condition is usually reversed. But both processes develop concomitantly. Hand-in-hand with the development of these processes there are taking place changes of a destructive and reparative nature. On the one hand, caseation affects large portions of the tubercle tissue and lung tissue; reparative processes in the form of small round-cell infiltration and cell proliferation in the tissue surrounding the affected parts is also noticed. The portion of lung between the nodular areas of tuberculosis may remain unaltered for a long time; or circulatory and other disturbances are produced with consolidation of the alveoli from inflammatory exudate. Like the tissue around it the consolidated areas are apt to undergo caseation.

Acute Pneumonic Tuberculosis (Acute Pneumonic Phthisis; Tuberculous Infiltration, Laennec; Caseous Pneumonia).—From the rapidity of the clinical course acute pneumonic tuberculosis has often been designated *galloping consumption*. It is observed in both adults and children, but much more frequently in the latter, in whom it is often mistaken for simple bronchopneumonia. It is not infrequently secondary to a preëxisting tuberculous focus in the lung itself, either an apical cavity or a softened bronchial gland which has ruptured into a bronchus.

Fraenkel and Troje have shown that in this form of disease, in which the exudative is apt to dominate so largely over the productive lesion, the tubercle bacillus alone was present in the lung in eleven out of twelve cases; in the remaining case the lung contained large numbers of streptococci. According to these investigators the morphological difference between caseous pneumonia and tubercles is due to the fact that while the tubercles are developed in the interalveolar structures of the lungs to which bacilli are brought by way of the lymphatics and blood-vessels, largely free from poisonous substances, the infection by aspiration is mainly intraalveolar and the bacilli are accompanied by greater or less quantities of diffusible poisonous material developed at the original seat. Prudden has likewise shown this.

Lobar Pneumonic Tuberculosis.—The amount of involvement is always considerable; one lobe or in some instances an entire lung may be affected. The implicated portions do not collapse but are firmly consolidated and airless, and on section present somewhat varying appearances. Sometimes the appearance is that which is seen in red hepatization; more often the cut surface resembles that seen in the intermediate stages of red and gray hepatization or in that of gray hepatization itself. In the later phases of the process the appearance has very fittingly been likened to that of Roquefort cheese, a background of yellowish-white irregularly streaked with lines of black. Naturally, the yellowish-white portions are the caseous material, while the deeply pigmented parts correspond to the areas of anthracosis. The *gelatinous pneumonia* of Laennec is much less commonly observed involving large areas of lung tissue; but associated with the form mentioned it is not uncommon to observe small gelatinous infiltrations here and there. Areas of this kind are recognized by their œdematous, more or less colorless appearance in parts.

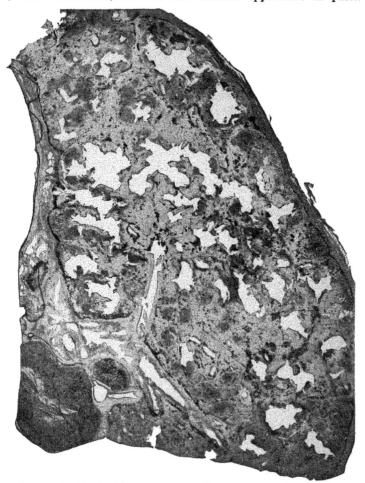

Fig. 10.—Acute Phthisis. Condition formed by softening of the areas of coagulated necrosis. (Delafield and Prudden.)

Microscopically it is seen that such parts contain serum and desquamated cells from the walls of the alveoli.

The consolidation sometimes presents a few discrete foci of older tuberculosis; a cavity at the apex or in some other portion of the lung is commonly enough seen. Miliary tubercles may occasionally be detected elsewhere in the pulmonary tissue. Probably when cavity formation is present the resulting lobar infection is an aspiration process.

The upper lobe is oftenest affected in the lobar pneumonic form of phthisis. Pleural inflammation is a constant association; sometimes it is a dry pleurisy, and when not dry the overlying pleura is found covered with exudate, either fibrinous or caseous. The bronchi also present evidences of active inflammation.

The microscopical characters of the exudate vary within wide limits, but the elements present are always essentially the same, notwithstanding differences of appearance—red blood corpuscles, leucocytes, serum, fibrin, and desquamated epithelial cells from the alveolar lining.

Bronchopneumonic Tuberculosis.—The occurrence of this form is much more frequent, particularly in children, and it constitutes the majority of cases of *phthisis florida,* or galloping consumption. Anatomically, it consists of disseminated foci of bronchopneumonia commencing in the smaller bronchi. The consolidated areas are of different size; they may be soft and cheesy. The tubes are blocked with caseous material, and the surrounding air spaces contain products of exudative inflammation, much of which undergoes caseation. By confluence of contiguous foci large areas of lung tissue, indeed a whole lobe, may thus become consolidated, but between the bronchopneumonic patches areas of crepitant tissue are generally observed. Miliary tubercles are not abundant. Softening is a usual occurrence in the nodules of tuberculous involvement, resulting in cavity formation. As in the lobar pneumonic phthisis, pleurisy is also a frequent accompaniment of the disease in this form.

Chronic Tuberculous Pneumonia (Chronic Ulcerative Phthisis). —By this term is designated a tuberculosis of the lungs, in which exudation and productive inflammation are common features. Beginning purely as a tuberculous inflammation it becomes after a variable time a greatly complicated process, many of the complicating features being more or less directly the result of secondary bacterial infections (see Concurrent Infections). By far the largest number of cases of pulmonary tuberculosis naturally fall in this class. Like the preceding forms chronic phthisis is most often an apical lesion at the start. Of 427 successive cases Osler found that in 172 the right apex was involved; in 130 it was the left apex, and both apices in 111. The proportion of basic lesions to those of the summit of the lung is about 1 to 500 (Percy Kidd). In the majority of cases the apex lesion is not located at the extreme tip, but from one inch to one inch and a half from the summit and nearer the posterior and external margin.

The changes in the lungs in chronic phthisis are essentially those of the acute disease, but more or less modified by the chronicity of the inflammation. Productive inflammation is more accentuated than in the acute lesions. In all specimens of chronic phthisis patches of pneumonia may be seen distributed through the organ, usually bronchopneumonic in character.

The tubercle bacilli lodge in the terminal bronchioles and give rise to bronchopneumonic areas of consolidation; and from these foci other portions of the lung are infected. The affected portions of the lung are solid, of grayish-white or yellow color. The bronchi are usually filled with mucopurulent exudate. Destructive and reparative processes will be noted side by side in the affected tissues. Miliary tubercles may not be present or a few discrete ones are detected here and there—the "secondary crop" of Laennec—about the caseous portions.

The exudate of the consolidated areas in chronic tuberculosis is very similar to that in acute phthisis. The consolidation of the alveoli may extend for some distance from the foci of tuberculosis, and the inflammatory process may be either specific or of other nature. Areas of gelatinous pneumonia are not uncommon.

One of the most characteristic features of chronic tuberculosis of the lungs is the tendency of the products of inflammation to degenerative and necrotic processes, which lead to cavity formation. The cavity or vomica usually contains a variable quantity of ill-smelling material, consisting for the most part of detritus in which bits of elastic tissue are often recognizable. Moreover, tubercle bacilli, pyogenic bacteria, and other microorganisms are usually present. The number and dimensions of the cavities vary very widely in different cases; sometimes only a single vomica, scarcely over 1 or 2 cm. in diameter, is present at the apex; at other times a whole lobe or more may be almost completely excavated. Multiple discrete cavities are not uncommon; larger cavities are frequently formed by the coalescence of smaller ones. The cavity wall is uneven and ragged or covered with granulation tissue.

A remarkable series of investigations by Prudden (1894) showed the relation of secondary infection of the lung with the streptococcus pyogenes to the experimental formation of cavities in pneumonic tuberculosis. "On the other hand, a large proportion of these lungs which had been the seat of concurrent infection with the tubercle bacillus and the streptococcus showed, in addition to the lesions of a tuberculous bronchopneumonia, a most remarkable formation of cavities. Nine lungs out of the thirteen were, as has been stated, considerably consolidated, and eight out of these consolidated lungs showed cavities in various phases of development. . . .

"These cavities are due to the softening and absorption of the necrotic small cell masses or the cheesy centres of the areas of tubercular consolidation artificially induced. They run in size from that of a pin head to those involving nearly a whole lobe. In some cases there is one cavity; in others a series of communicating chambers, crossed by cords and bands of old lung structures. They all communicate with the bronchi, and can be filled with fluids through the trachea. A few are lined with remnants of bronchial epithelium. They may be surrounded with little or much consolidated lung tissue, or, in fact, closely resemble the cavities which are prone to form in human beings in acute phthisis. The softening of the consolidated lung may begin as early as twenty-four hours after the introduction of the streptococcus. It may involve tubercular foci as small as two millimetres in diameter, or those which occupy a whole lobe. The cords and bands stretching across these cavities usually contain a bronchus and its surrounding connective tissue.

"The necrotic centres of the consolidated areas may within twenty-four hours begin to become friable and loose in texture, or the central portion of the necrotic mass, retaining its coherency, may become sequestrated and loosened from the surrounding solid lung tissue. Then disintegration of the necrotic mass proceeds rapidly with disappearance of the detritus, apparently by absorption, leaving a cavity bounded by whatever form of tissue composed the outer zone of the consolidated area involved. If the tubercular lesion were advanced so that the outer zones were fibrous, as in the rabbit may happen within two or three weeks, then the walls of the cavity may be fibrous and lined with an irregular layer of cell detritus. If, on the other hand, the particular tuberculous mass were composed in its outer zones of densely packed epithelial cells, or of these with more or less new-formed stroma, or of a zone of dense living tissue infiltrated with spheroidal cells, then the wall of the new-formed cavity has one or other of these structural characters. Cavities forming close beneath the pleura may have dense fibrous walls containing many old and new-formed, often dilated blood-vessels" (Prudden).

Cavities are formed in one of two ways: either through dilatation of the weakened walls of ulcerated bronchioles or through disintegration of the caseous masses. Extension occurs by breaking down of the caseous walls or by actual ulceration; both processes are often active. In acute phthisis the fresh ulcerative cavities contain no lining membrane, but the walls are made up of softened and caseous masses. When located just beneath the pleura cavities of this sort may rupture and give rise to pneumothorax. The walls are frequently lined with a pyogenic membrane. Projecting bands of lung tissue crossing the cavity may subdivide the interior into a series of sinuses. The rough inner surface of a cavity is often ribbed by projecting bands which represent the trabeculæ and blood-vessels which have resisted the necrotic process more persistently than the immediately surrounding tissue. Blood-vessels may resist until the entire tissue around them has disappeared and they are left coursing across the centre of a cavity. When this occurs thrombosis ordinarily takes place. On the other hand, such blood-vessels or those in the walls often enough show aneurismal dilatations. And from just such dilatations the fatal hemorrhages in the later phases of tuberculosis often take place. The hemorrhages observed in the early stages of the disease are more often due to erosion of the smaller vessels of the bronchial tubes or to capillary rupture, the result of congestion.

The bronchial tubes are the seat of inflammatory changes, incited either by the tubercle bacillus or by other microorganisms. Ulceration of the mucous membrane is by no means uncommon. The bronchial lymph nodes likewise generally show tuberculous changes.

In almost every case of chronic tuberculosis the pleura will be found involved, not always, however, in a specific inflammation. The adhesions are generally old fibrous ones, sometimes thin, in other cases dense and firm. Serous, purulent, or sanguineous fluid may be present in the pleural cavity. Extension of the disease to other viscera is common, particularly to the intestine which becomes infected largely by swallowed sputum.

Amyloid degeneration is often observed in these cases in the liver, spleen, kidneys, etc. Fatty changes are also frequent enough, particularly in the liver. The endocarditic lesions in tuberculosis have been well studied by Teissier (1894). Endocarditis was present in twelve of Osler's cases and in twenty-seven of Percy Kidd's five hundred cases. Laryngeal tuberculosis is frequent in chronic phthisis.

FIBROID PHTHISIS.

Under the heading of fibroid phthisis very widely different processes have been described. Hadley and Chaplin divide it into three groups: 1. Pure fibroid; fibroid phthisis, an interstitial pneumonitis without tuberculosis. 2. Tuberculofibroid disease—a process tuberculous from the start but running a fibroid course. 3. Fibrotuberculous disease—a process primarily fibroid, which has subsequently been tuberculous in character.

The second type is usually seen following a chronic tuberculous bronchopneumonia or chronic pleuritis incited by the bacillus tuberculosis. At times a similar process is going on hand-in-hand in chronic ulcerative tuberculosis. Finally the picture of tuberculous fibroid phthisis assumes the character of ordinary chronic interstitial pneumonia, a description of which may be found in Vol. VI. of this series.

Zoological Distribution.

Tuberculosis in natural conditions is very common in some species of animals and in others is wholly unknown. Undoubtedly some animals, such as the goat, possess a marked immunity against the disease. Although unknown in wild animals, the disease affects a large proportion in captivity.

MAMMALS.

Discussion of tuberculosis among mammalians will be limited to the more important species.

Cattle.—Bovine tuberculosis has been known to stock-breeders for many centuries, but the knowledge of its nature was so vague that no efforts were made to prevent or cure the disease. By reason of its frequency and the relations of the bovidæ to man, much interest has naturally been aroused in this phase of the subject. Long since known among the English as " pearl disease," as " Perlsucht " to the Germans, and in France as " pommelière," tuberculosis has been known to affect cattle more than any other domesticated animal. The proportion affected varies largely according to the regions considered. In some localities ten, fifteen, or twenty-five per cent. or more are estimated to be diseased; in other places the disease is practically absent. The Danish herds which were said to be sound until after the importation of Schesing and short-horn cattle in 1840 and 1850 are now generally infected, seventeen per cent. of the cattle slaughtered showing tubercles, while over sixty per cent. of the dairy herds showed disease under the tuberculin test. Statistics from German abattoirs give 6.9 per cent. of tuberculosis for cows, for oxen 3.6 per cent., for bulls 2.6 per cent., and for yearlings and calves 1 per cent. In Saxony, for example, official statistics of the abattoirs show that in 1891, 17.4 per cent. were affected; in 1892, 17.79 per cent.; in 1893, 18.26 per cent.; in some cities this percentage approaches 30. According to the returns of the Leipsic abattoirs for 1897, 36.4 per cent. of the 27,191 cattle slaughtered were tuberculous. Nearly one-half (48.09 per cent.) of the cows were affected, while only one-fifth (20.49 per cent.) of the bullocks and heifers showed disease. Notwithstanding this only 2.08 per cent. were totally condemned as food.

In Copenhagen 16.6 per cent. of the cattle were diseased in 1891, according to abattoir returns. In other countries statistics show about the same figures. Doubtless if more careful examination of the slaughtered cattle were made, much higher returns would be given. A careful inspection of 43 well-nourished cattle revealed the fact that 21 had bronchial gland tuberculosis. Law states that by the tuberculin test of New York State herds (2,417 head) in 1894, 16.75 per cent. were proved to be infected. Estimations by Cassidy and Smith would give something like 75,000 tuberculous cows in the State of New York alone. In other States the disease is also very high. Much has been done to determine the frequency of the disease, especially in Massachusetts and Pennsylvania, where it is stated the affection is on the decrease.

A marked characteristic of the disease in the bovidæ is its frequent localization in the serous membranes, especially the pericardium and pleura. Here it forms the well-known grape-like masses of dense fibrous tissue, occasionally containing thick pus in their interior. These masses cover the whole surface of the membrane, and their appearances have given the name to the disease, "the grapes." Many of the lesions elsewhere appear to have this tendency to surround themselves with dense fibrous tissue. Broadly stated it may be said that purulent softening is rarer than in man. It may be generally calculated that in one hundred cases of tuberculosis the pleura and lung will be involved forty times, from twenty to twenty-five times the lung alone, and from fifteen to twenty the pleura and peritoneum alone. Sometimes the animals may present a form of disease largely limited to the lymphatic glands.

Horses do not readily contract the disease under ordinary circumstances, but this cannot be attributed mainly to insusceptibility, since they take it easily when inoculated. The relative immunity is probably in part due to absence of frequent exposure, and in some degree also to the outdoor life and well-developed state of the system. Occasionally infection occurs under ordinary conditions; and it seems that in this animal the disease progresses more rapidly and generalizes itself more easily than in cattle. The abdominal viscera are points of election for infection; less often the thoracic viscera are implicated from the beginning. Although it is known that the inoculation takes place by way of the digestive apparatus, nothing is known of the source of the infection. Lehnert in 1888 published the interesting observation of a pony that became tuberculous following a long stay in a stable containing tuberculous cattle.

Swine.—This animal is also subject to tuberculosis, especially through the consumption of·uncooked offal of slaughter-houses and the milk of tuberculous cattle. While much rarer than in cattle, tuberculosis is much more frequent in hogs than in the horse, sheep, or goat. According to Johne, of 230,808 killed in Saxony in 1891, 2,477 (1.07 per cent.) were affected; in 1892 out of a total of 276,851 killed 3,804 (1.37 per cent.) showed the disease; in 1893 the percentage reached 1.64. For Amsterdam the proportion is somewhat less (Thomasset). Contrasting with these figures are those of Bang, who states that 11.38 per cent. of swine killed at Copenhagen were tuberculous. Scharenberger states that at the abattoir of Dantzig, out of 40,000 hogs slaughtered 11 per cent. were affected, and among those fed in certain dairies this proportion reached 60 and 70 per cent. In contrast to the infrequency of tuberculosis in calves is its prevalence in young swine. Contamination by way of the respiratory organs is infrequent. Nine times out of ten the infection is an ingestion tuberculosis. Chronic glandular lesions were for a long time and are still spoken of as scrofula of swine; this form is often accompanied with disease of the gut. Bone lesions are not uncommon. Experimentation shows the possibility of contamination by sputum.

Goats and Sheep.—In their natural environment infection of goats or sheep is rare. In Saxony, where bovine tuberculosis is very frequent (18.26 per cent.), 85,701 sheep were killed in 1891, and of this number only 30 were found infected with tubercle (.035 per cent.); in 1892 the figures remained the same—39 out of 104,987. In 1893 the percentage was slightly higher. Figures from Prussia are about the same (.09 per cent.). From the fact that verminous bronchopneumonia closely simulates caseous pneumonia in man, Nocard believes that perhaps only one-half of this number were really tuberculous.

There have been reported a few isolated examples of sporadic tuberculosis in goats. Carstens, Harms, Gerlach, Lydtin, and Detroye have contributed a few cases. Those of Matz, van der Huys, and Korevaar relate to goats in the same immediate environment as tuberculous cows. Thomassen reported an interesting case of infection of a goat probably from the ingestion of the milk of a diseased cow. Finally Alston, König, Moulé, and Siegen have added other reports of non-experimental tubercle in goats.

Dogs and Cats.—The carnivora, the dog more especially than the cat, were a long time regarded as immune. Experimentally they resist ordinary subcutaneous inoculation, but intravenous inoculation of a small quantity incites tuberculous lesions. The dog, however, resists inoculation even of large quantities of avian tubercle bacilli. Outside of experimental conditions tubercle is occasionally met with in dogs. Since attention has been directed to its occurrence, examples are now not uncommon, and veterinary literature at the present time contains several hundred observations (Bang, Jensen, Cadiot, Chantemesse and Le Dentec, Ebers). Cadiot in an important monograph upon tuberculosis of the dog relates 40 such examples among 9,000 dogs brought to the Alford Clinique in two years (1891–93), a proportion of 1 to 125. The dog, like man, infects himself largely through the respiratory tract, as shown by the frequency with which the lungs are the seat of tubercle; in 28 cases Jensen found the lungs affected in 19, Eber 9 times out of 11, and Cadiot 33 times out of 40. The pleura and peritoneum are likewise frequently involved; intestinal lesions are unusual. Experimental evidence bears out this fact also, for the inhalation type is comparatively easily reproduced, whereas ingestion tuberculosis is successful only when the infected material is repeatedly given.

Tuberculosis in dogs would seem to be the result largely of association with individuals suffering from phthisis. In half the collected cases of Cadiot this mode of infection seems evident; for the remaining cases the etiology is less clear.

Jensen has cited twenty-five cases of spontaneous tuberculosis in cats. As in the dog, the lungs are greatly involved, and contrary to what occurs in dogs the pleura and peritoneum are rarely affected, but the digestive organs are frequently the seat of tubercle. Ingestion tuberculosis apparently is more common than infection by way of the lungs.

Monkeys.—To the author's knowledge no observation has been made of tuberculosis of monkeys in their native condition. But in captivity it is common enough, chiefly affecting the pulmonary organs. While the larynx and pleura are infrequently affected, the lesions are commonly seen in the liver, spleen, and intestine. The tubercles are characterized by a tendency to undergo a form of puriform softening, so much so that Koch likened them to multiple abscesses. In the Zoological Garden of London Forbes states that forty-three per cent. of the monkeys die of tuberculosis; Saint-Yves Ménard estimates this mortality in the Jardin d'Acclimatation in Paris at twenty per cent.

The experimental side has been fully studied by Dieulafoy and Krishaber, who found that this mortality of the animals in captivity was largely due to the fact that cages were imperfectly cleansed or healthy animals were placed in cages with affected ones.

Other Mammalians.—Domestic animals are by no means the only animals in which tuberculosis has been observed. In Egypt it has been noted among camels. Giraffes, antelopes, gazelles, and zebus are also known to become victims when captive, but fuller reports exist of its occurrence in the lion, tiger, jackal, panther, kangaroo, fox, llama, etc., under this condition.

BIRDS.

In its epidemic form tuberculosis in birds is fairly well known. As a natural disease it affects fowls, pigeons, pheasants, turkeys, and other birds which are in captivity.

Parrots are frequently affected. Fröhner out of one hundred and fifty-four parrots treated from 1886 to 1893 found thirty-six per cent. tuberculous. In these animals the disease is characterized by affections of the skin which are absent in fowls and pheasants. The lesions consist of grayish tumors, often of a horny appearance and located on the lids, conjunctiva, beak, pharynx, tongue, skin of the wings, articulations, etc. The skin of the head is the seat of election for these tumors. The internal organs are occasionally invaded, the lungs more frequently than the liver or intestine.

Owing to the investigations of Johne, Nocard, Nevers, Mollereau, de Lamellerée, and several others it is now known that fowls not uncommonly become infected by the ingestion of tuberculous material, but more especially tuberculous sputum. However, this is by no means the habitual manner of inoculation. In the great majority of cases tuberculosis appears after the importation of new birds and so the disease may rapidly spread.

The distribution of the lesions in birds is strikingly different from that in mammals. Instead of the lungs being the commonest site of the lesions they are the rarest among the great viscera to become diseased. The chief seat is in the abdominal viscera; the liver first, then in order the spleen, the wall of the intestine, and the mesenteric glands. Nodules when in the lung are small, round, and firm, and shell out from the lung parenchyma in removing the organs from the chest. These are of brownish color, firm consistence, and often contain deposits of urates. The cause of death in the birds is generally diarrhœa.

Tuberculosis of bones and joints seems to be more common in birds than in mammals. Pus is practically unknown in birds.

COLD-BLOODED ANIMALS.

The study of tuberculosis in cold-blooded animals is yet too recent to formulate any very definite opinion as to its occurrence under natural conditions. Sibley, of London, had the opportunity to examine a case of tubercle in a snake (trepidonatus natrix) which died in captivity. Later his observations included other instances of this. In 1897 Bataillon, Dubard, and Terre communicated a most interesting note apropos of tuberculosis in carp in waters contaminated by sputum and intestinal discharges from a case of tuberculosis. Our knowledge of the disease has been largely extended in this sphere by further studies of these and other investigators.

ETIOLOGY.

Frequency in Man.

Taking the mean death-rate of the whole population to be 22 per 1,000, and the average of death from phthisis of the lungs to be 3 per 1,000, we find that the deaths from consumption are nearly one-seventh of the entire mortality (Hirsch). This mortality exceeds the combined deaths from war, famine, plague, cholera, yellow fever, and smallpox. In former times fully 80 per cent. of all deaths were attributable to maladies at the present time considered preventable, yet now with a reduction to one-quarter of what the mortality formerly was, one-fourth of all deaths among the adult populations is due to this scourge. Estimating the total yearly mortality of the world to be 35,000,000, we find that about 5,000,000 deaths are referable to this cause, being the greatest number reported by reliable observers as due to any single disease (Evans). Ransome, in his Milroy Lectures on the etiology and prevention of phthisis, delivered before the Royal College of Physicians of London in 1890, says: "Tubercle in its various forms at the present day carries off annually nearly 70,000 persons (in England). In the form of phthisis, at ages between fifteen and forty-five—the most useful stages of human existence—it kills one-third of the people who die at those ages, and nearly half between fifteen and thirty-five. . . ."

According to the official returns for Germany (1893), out of a total of 268,500 persons dying between the ages of fifteen and sixty, of whom the cause of death was reported, 88,654 died from tuberculosis—a mortality of 33 per cent. for these ages. Leyden estimates the annual death rate from phthisis in that country to be 170,000, and the total of living tuberculous patients to be 1,300,000. Statistics show that of a mortality of 850,000 in France, fully 150,000 deaths are due to tuberculosis. Allowing 15 deaths per 1,000 on our 70,000,000 population, this would furnish us 150,000 deaths from tuberculosis in the United States. The United States Census Report for 1890 gives 102,188 deaths due to consumption. Basing his estimation on the Census Report, Vaughan concludes that the total number of persons suffering from tuberculosis is 1,050,000, or 1 in every 60 of the population. In New York State more than 13,000 deaths annually occur from pulmonary consumption, while in Paris alone it is estimated that there are over 11,000 deaths each year from it; in London in 1897, they were 80,943 deaths, 10,984 of which were from tuberculosis; in New York City considerably over 8,000 deaths a year are attributed to this cause. The same proportion holds good for most of the other large American cities. Thus Dr. Max C. Starkloff, in the Annual Report of the City of St. Louis for 1898, writes: "The present population of the City of St. Louis, calculated from the returns of the election commissioner, is 635,000; of this number it is lamentable to have to say, but it is nevertheless the fact, that 90,700 will die of tuberculosis."

Such figures would become still higher were we to add those from other forms of tuberculosis—intestinal, urogenital, osseous, meningeal, etc. Moreover, the evidence derived from post-mortem examinations of persons who have died of other diseases than phthisis would swell this number still further. For instance, in Cruveilhier's, Roger's, and Dejerine's researches on this point 50 per cent. of their patients, who did not die of tuberculosis, showed signs of caseous and calcareous formations. Bollinger in 256 similar cases found 27 per cent. with indications of healed tuberculosis; Standacher 26 per cent.; Massini 30 per cent.; and Harris estimated that in at least 39 per cent. of the necropsies at the Manchester Royal Infirmary there were evidences of healed phthisis. Fürbringer, of the Berlin General Hospital, says 10 per cent. show healed tuberculosis; Renvers, of the Moabit Hospital, Berlin, 30 per cent. An inquiry into this subject by H. P. Loomis demonstrated 8 times out of 30 invasion of the bronchial glands with tubercle bacilli without any demonstrable past or recent lesions elsewhere.

The following statistical compilation, which appeared in the *Münchener medicinische Wochenschrift* for 1896, gives sufficiently approximate figures of the mortality from consumption, for each one thousand population, in various large cities for purposes of comparison:

FRANCE.

Cities.	Population.	1894.	Cities	Population.	1894.
Havre	116,000	50.0	Roubaix....	115,000	29.7
Rouen...........	111,000	45.0	Lille	700,000	28.2
Paris	2,424,000	41.6	Bordeaux.......	252,000	25.5
Nancy	86,000	33.7	Sainte-Etienne...	133,000	23.5
Lyons	431,000	33.6	Marseilles	406,000	21.8
Rheims..........	105,000	32.6	Toulouse	148,000	17.7
Nantes	122,000	30.1	Algiers	83,000	16.5

GERMANY.

Cities.	Population	1892–93.	1894.	Cities.	Population.	1892–93.	1894.
Würzburg ...	65,000	41.6	52.4	Dresden	316,000	28.1	26.0
Nuremberg ..	161,000	41.7	39.3	Altona......	149,000	28.5	24.7
Breslau	361,000	40.1	34.9	Leipsic	404,000	25.8	24.3
Augsburg....	81,000	33.4	33.5	Gorlitz	67,000	24.8	24.3
Munich	393,000	30.8	30.8	Chemnitz ...	150,000	23.6	22.7
Cologne	309,000	30.8	28.2	Berlin......	1,703,000	25.7	22.3
Frankfort....	201,000	29.1	27.8	Hamburg ...	604,000	25 2	21.1
Elberfeld....	138,000	28.1	26 6	Lubeck	69,000	16.5	16.1

OTHER COUNTRIES.

Cities	Population.	1894.	Cities.	Population.	1894.
Budapest	552,000	49 3	Glasgow	686,000	22.6
Vienna	1,465,000	45.4	Naples	535,000	21.1
St. Petersburg ...	954,000	44.3	Buenos Ayres....	580,000	20.7
Moscow	753,000	42 9	Manchester.......	522,000	19.6
Warsaw	500,000	25.7	London	5,300,000	17.3
New York.......	1,925,000	24.1	Chicago	1,600,000	13.4
Philadelphia	1,115,000	23.7			

The following table, taken from A. Newsholme's "Elements of Vital Statistics," 1899, gives the chief figures as to the mortality from tuberculous diseases in England and Wales. The facts as to phthisis are classified according to age and sex.

MORTALITY FROM PHTHISIS IN GROUPS OF YEARS, 1861–96, PER MILLION OF EACH SEX LIVING AT EACH GROUP OF AGES.

Males.

Periods	All ages	Under 5.	5–10.	10–15.	15–20.	20–25.	25–35.	35–45.	45–55.	55–65.	65–75.	75 and upwards.
1851–60............	2,579	1 3.9	525	763	2,399	4,052	4,081	4,004	3,830	3,331	2,389	928
1861–70.	2,467	990	431	605	2,190	3,883	4,094	4,166	3,861	3,297	2,024	659
1871–80... ...	2,209	783	340	481	1,675	3,092	3,699	4,120	3,860	3,195	1,924	603
1881–90	1,847	553	253	342	1,287	2,353	3,024	3,562	3 488	2,916	1,816	688
1891–95. .	1,633	467	197	260	1,076	2 036	2,548	3,268	3,205	2,687	1,572	563
1896................	1,485	392	150	203	913	1,848	2,285	3,029	3,042	2,599	1,329	512

Females.

	All ages.	Under 5.	5-10.	10-15.	15-20.	20-25.	25-35.	35-45.	45-55.	55-65.	65-75.	75 and upwards.
1851-60.........	2,774	1,281	620	1,293	3 516	4,288	4,575	4,178	3,121	2,383	1,685	716
1861-70.........	2,483	947	477	1,045	3,112	3,967	4,378	3,900	3,850	2,065	1,239	447
1871-80.........	2,028	750	375	846	2,397	3,140	3,543	3,401	2,464	1,777	1,093	467
1881-90.........	1,609	518	327	699	1,800	2,315	2,787	2,730	2,053	1,512	974	397
1891-95......	1,303	421	260	561	1,428	1,740	2,155	2,305	1,742	1,294	800	350
1896.............	1,139	349	204	454	1,183	1,562	1,874	2,090	1,543	1,170	676	375

The following table is taken from Polk's "Medical and Surgical Register" for 1898 :

State.	Total number of deaths from consumption during 8.	Death rate from consumption per 1,000 of capita ion.	Deaths from consumption per 1,00 of total deaths.	State.	Total number of deaths from consumption during 1896.	Death rate from consumption per 1,000 of population.	Deaths from consumption per 1,000 of total deaths.
Alabama.....	2,163	1.43	103.50	Missouri	3,559	1.32	109.72
Alaska	....	....	...	Montana	55	0.42	54.34
Arizona......	68	1.14	118.67	Nebraska....	604	0.57	71.52
Arkansas	1,219	1.07	84.01	Nevada......	35	0.77	80.65
California....	2,889	2.39	163.19	New Hampshire	729	1.93	103.05
Colorado.....	489	1.18	89.68	New Jersey..	3,388	2.34	112.65
Connecticut..	1,743	2.34	120.46	New York...	14.854	2.47	120.65
Delaware	476	2.83	153.20	N. Carolina..	2,212	1.37	112.00
District of Columbia..	827	3.59	138.87	N. Dakota ..	167	0.91	97.32
Florida......	377	0.96	90.95	Ohio	6,393	1.74	128.26
Georgia......	2,155	1.17	101.77	Oklahoma...	21	0.34	59.66
Idaho........	36	0.43	46.69	Oregon......	305	0.97	118.45
Illinois......	5,698	1.49	107.26	Pennsylvania	7,689	1.46	104.57
Indian Territory.......	....	....	....	Rhode Island	921	2.67	121.84
				S. Carolina..	2,112	1.83	136.30
Indiana......	3,504	1.60	144.91	S. Dakota...	208	0.63	76.89
Iowa........	1,832	0.96	104.56	Tennessee ..	3,637	2.06	152.47
Kansas	1,368	0.96	113.83	Texas	2,059	0.92	77.93
Kentucky....	3,538	1.90	148.18	Utah	62	0.30	29.26
Louisiana....	1,516	1.35	92.70	Vermont....	661	1.99	121.84
Maine	1,477	2.23	147.05	Virginia	3,050	1.84	131.28
Maryland....	2,315	2.22	128.61	Washington.	278	0.79	103.15
Massachusetts	5,981	2.67	132.58	W. Virginia.	1,143	1.50	138.15
Michigan	2,747	1.31	109.81	Wisconsin ..	2,015	1.19	107.97
Minnesota....	1,532	1.17	98.92	Wyoming...	18	0.30	43.48
Mississippi...	1,433	1.11	96.18				

From the following table of mortality in 662 cities in France in 1891 (Lagneau), it will be seen that the number of deaths from tuberculosis diminishes both relatively and absolutely in the different groups of cities with the diminution of the population, having its maximum in Paris, where the proportion reaches 4.90, while in the towns of less than 5,000 the mortality is only 1.81 per 1,000 inhabitants.

	Pop- ulation.	TUBERCULOSIS.			PROPORTION PER 1,000 POPULATION.		
		From phthisis.	From other tuberculous affections.	Total mor- tality from tuberculosis.	From phthisis.	From other tuberculous affections.	Total mor- tality from tuberculosis.
Paris	2,424,705	10,287	1,608	11,895	4.24	0.66	4.90
11 cities. Population from 430,000 to 100,000...	2,143,380	6,262	1,535	7,798	2.92	0.71	3.63
46 cities. Population from 100,000 to 30,000 ...	2,361,244	5,474	1,764	7,238	2.31	0.74	3.05
50 cities. Population from 30,000 to 20,000	1,220,019	2,595	935	3,530	2.12	0.76	2.88
127 cities. Population 20,000 to 10,000	1,799,443	3,682	1,219	4,701	2.04	0.67	2.71
332 cities Population 10,000 to 5,000............	2,274,757	3,773	1,164	4,937	1.65	0.51	2.16
95 towns (chef. lieu) less than 5,000.......	330,802	493	107	500	1.49	0.32	1.81

The Decrease of Tuberculosis.—It is a matter of frequent observation that the aggregate death rate from tuberculosis has been decreasing in many countries for a number of years. Italy by methods of prevention reduced mortality from this disease in less than a century from that of a most virulent epidemic to a comparatively rare disease. Cornet finds that in Prussia the general mortality from tuberculosis for the period 1875–86 was 30 per 10,000 inhabitants; since the application of prophylactic measures it has fallen to figures below 25, a diminution from which Cornet estimates a saving of 70,000 persons who would else have died from tuberculosis between 1889 and 1893. Other German states show a similar favorable decrease; in Saxony since 1892 the mortality rate has fallen from 25 to 21; in Baden from 30 to 26, etc.

In 1896 E. F. Wells published a paper in which he indicated by statistics that pulmonary tuberculosis is diminishing in prevalence in some parts of the United States. While the last decennial census in this country does not show any such diminution, nevertheless in many of the large cities the decrease has been considerable. Wells states that in New York in 1805 there were 5.72 deaths per 1,000 of tuberculosis, which ratio had decreased in 1894 to 3.29. In Baltimore in 1815 the figures were 4.10, and in 1894 the decrease was down to 2.71. In Philadelphia in 1835 it was 3.52; in 1894, 2.65. In Massachusetts the decrease has been considerable also, the mortality rate having fallen from about 42 per 10,000 population in 1853 to 21.8 per 10,000 in 1895.

Investigating the same question in England the Royal Commission on Tuberculosis wrote in 1897: "We note, therefore, with satisfaction that death from tuberculous disease in all its forms and at all ages has steadily fallen from 3,483 per million during 1851–60 to 2,122 during 1891–95, a reduction of 39.1 per cent.; and also that at every age period for which statistics are available there has likewise been a decrease, sometimes of a very substantial character."

Since 1884 the decrease in the number of deaths from tuberculosis in Berlin has been progressive. In 1883 it was 3.42 per cent., and in 1896 only 1.26 per cent. Large cities elsewhere reveal varying figures of diminution also.

Geographical Distribution.

The widespread prevalence of tuberculosis is shown by the universality of its geographical distribution over all parts of the inhabited globe. Close critical study of the relations of tuberculosis to the geographical conditions must appreciate the independence of the existence and frequency of the disease to climate, latitude, and altitude. If we take the map of almost any country in the world and shade its several provinces so as to denote the varying prevalence of tuberculosis, we shall discover not only that a great variety of tint has to be used, but also that the dark places alternate with the light without any reference to geographical position, north or south, east or west. In Scotland consumption is almost unknown in the Western Hebrides, but in towns on the west of the mainland with a similar climate and race of people it is very common. Writers frequently cite the Scottish Hebrides, Iceland, Newfoundland, coasts of Hudson Bay, northern parts of Norway and Sweden, Lapland, Finland, etc., as localities free from tuberculosis. F. A. Cook, who accompanied Lieutenant Peary's Arctic expedition, says that the Esquimos of South Greenland are commonly subject to the disease, and estimates that two-thirds of the inhabitants suffer from it. In the Arctic highlands, however, he found no cases of it. It is common on both the east and west coast of Mexico, in the seacoast towns of Yucatan, the Isthmus of Panama, and Nicaragua; in the highlands in the interior of these countries *per contra* phthisis is almost unknown. Ransome states that the disease is common and pernicious on the coasts and plains of Guinea, while it is almost unknown among the native inhabitants of the mountainous parts of the country. It is also very frequent in all the islands of the West Indies, in Ceylon, and in the warmer regions of the Pacific. Recent years show an increase in the prevalence of tuberculosis in the maritime districts of Peru, Ecuador, and Chili. It is not infrequently seen in the valleys of the Andes, and in the forest regions of Peru, at so high an altitude as 500 metres (1,625 ft.); the higher plateau regions, on the other hand, are very free from it. It is said that persons living in very dry climates are comparatively immune. Common reports have it that the interior regions of lower Egypt and the Nile valley are uncommonly free from phthisis; and in India sections of country with a dry climate are also said to be singularly free from tuberculous disease.

But it must be remembered that there is, comparatively speaking, in just such regions—deserts, northern regions, and mountain plateaux—a sparse population free from the many stimulating factors to disease which become inherent conditions of large and close aggregations of human beings. In Christiania and Stockholm, where the social and economic conditions are more or less similar to those of other large European cities, the death rate from this disease is practically the same as that of cities in more temperate latitudes. The same holds good for St. Petersburg and Moscow.

A shaded map, indicating the variations in prevalence of tuberculosis in a general way, also denotes the relative density of the population in different parts of the world. In other words, the mortality rate from tuberculosis is directly proportionate to the number of individuals aggregated on a given space of ground; and any differences in the death rate in various large cities throughout Europe, Asia, Africa, and America are obviously referable to other causes than climate.

Altitude.—Inasmuch as altitude has been commonly looked upon as bearing a certain relation to the prevalence of the disease, and especially in view of its practical and therapeutical application, this subject merits some special consideration. Gastaldi, who was among the first to refer to the immunity of elevated regions, thought that at a height of 200 metres or over this influence became apparent, while in situations below this the disease was quite as common as on the plains. Smith and Tschudi believed in a similar rarity of phthisis on the plateaux of the Peruvian Andes, and Bowdin made the same observation for those of Mexico. That these elevated localities are comparatively free from the disease cannot be doubted, but it should also be remembered that the population is less than that on the plains, the mode of life less confined, and the air much less polluted with organic matter. That the immunity is not simply due to the rarity of the air is completely proved by E. Müller, who has shown that there is no complete immunity from the disease in Alpine Switzerland. A certain number of the inhabitants of this section die of tuberculosis, the rate depending not upon the elevation above the sea, but upon the nature of their occupation. Industrial indoor pursuits give a rate varying from 6.5 to 10.2 per cent., and one of the highest of these rates (9.8) is at an elevation of 3,400 to 4,400 feet; above this to 5,000 feet the rate is 7.7 per cent. for mixed labor.

More especially since the investigations of Bowditch in America and Buchanan in England the relations of *moisture of soil* and consumption have received a good deal of attention by some writers. These two writers believed that it prevails much more in places situated upon a damp, impenetrable subsoil than in those upon a porous soil. Additional evidence has shown that observations of this kind, while true for some sections of country, cannot hold for other districts. Furthermore, there are in some parts of the world extensive tracts of country that are very damp, many the seat of much malaria, and yet are so free from tuberculosis that a few writers have thought that malaria is antagonistic to phthisis—a view wholly unwarranted by facts.

Facts necessitate our falling back upon the conditions of social and economic life as more potent factors than the influence of either climate or altitude.

Briefly then it must appear evident that the number of cases of tuberculosis is proportionate to the aggregation of human beings, indoor life, malnutrition, and unhygienic surroundings—conditions all of which favor the element of infection. Create an *ensemble* of the kind existing in most large cities and tuberculosis will be found as fatal among populations living on the highest plateaux as it is in cities of the plains at the present day.

Predisposing Conditions.

Most certainly any condition which tends to diminish the vitality of an individual necessarily increases his susceptibility to tuberculosis. Clinical evidence sustains this view in a most emphatic manner.

ENVIRONMENT.

There is a general agreement that under certain circumstances calculated to establish extreme impurity of the air, tuberculosis becomes much more frequent. Environment becomes a factor which cannot too strongly be insisted upon in an estimate of predisposing conditions. Absence of sunlight and ventilation are important tributary causes of predisposition.

Experimentally it is known that animals in these conditions die more readily than others placed in more favorable surroundings. Trudeau inoculated a number of rabbits with the same quantity of tubercle bacilli. One-half of the animals were allowed to run free in the open air and the remainder were placed in a dark damp hole under ground, deprived of sunlight. The animals in both series were killed at the same time; those which had been permitted to run wild had either recovered or showed only slight lesions. The confined animals presented extensive tuberculosis.

The increase of phthisis in the majority of civilized countries co-incides with the irresistible tendency which more and more takes the population of the country to cities, from which it results that sedentary occupations are substituted for an active open-air life. Statistics show that the ratio of tuberculosis diminishes, within certain limits, in proportion to the density of the population, the country districts showing a less mortality rate from tuberculosis than the cities.

Those belonging to the poorer classes and surrounded by unhygienic conditions of existence naturally give the greatest number of victims to this scourge. According to Holti, the death rate from phthisis for males of over fifteen years of the upper class in Helsingfors is 27.7 per cent. of the general mortality, while it is 44.6 per cent. for those of the necessitous classes.

INHERITED VULNERABILITY.

Knowledge of inherited susceptibility dates back to the earliest writers and has ever since been the subject of study and interest. Formerly accorded a most important rôle, inherited predisposition has been much less insisted upon since the discoveries of the inoculability and the inciting factor of tuberculosis. Indeed Villemin and some others went so far as to consider it as a negligible quantity. Doubtless it has been much exaggerated, but to discard its influence in any consideration of tributary causes in the face of recent statistical knowledge would be inconsistent with the facts.

The chief argument in favor of vulnerability by inheritance lies primarily in the fact that tuberculosis is very commonly met with in the ascendants of those affected. It is commonly stated that an hereditary influence may be found in from twenty-five to thirty per cent. of all cases of consumption if inheritance from parents alone is taken into consideration, and in about sixty per cent. when phthisical grandparents also are concerned. How much of this comparatively greater excess of tuberculosis in the offspring of consumptives can properly be put down to heredity is still an unsolved problem. Assuming that one death occurs from tuberculous disease in every five individuals above one year of age or that number for every three between fifteen and sixteen years, it would not be strange to find one or more deaths attributable to this cause in average-sized families. Extending the study to cousins, how few families there would be without tuberculous taint!

Perhaps one of the most careful investigations bearing on this question is that of Leudet, which included 143 families, comprising

1,485 persons, of which 312 were tuberculous. Some families could be followed for four, five, and six generations. These are the figures of Leudet's analysis:

55 families included	415 persons	presenting per family	1 tuberculous subject.
43 " "	373 "	" "	2 " subjects.
25 " "	320 "	" "	3 " "
13 " "	253 "	" "	4 " "
4 " "	48 "	" "	5 " "
1 family ".	19 "	" "	6 " "
1 " "	17 "	" "	7 " "
1 " "	40 "	" "	11 " "
143 families "	1,485 "	" a total of	312 " "

It will be seen that out of 55 families, comprising 415 persons, tuberculosis presented itself only once in each family; in 88 families, making 1,070 persons, the number varied from 2 to 11 per family. Taking those 143 families, which comprised three or four generations, he subdivided them in 214 families of less number.

Heredity from mother to children,	existed in	57 families.
" " father to children,	"	21 "
" " mother and father together,	"	4 "
" " grandmother to grandchildren,	"	4 "
" " grandfather "	"	1 "
" " aunt to nephews and nieces,	"	14 "
" " uncle " " "	"	7 "
		108

In the 106 remaining families no heredity existed from father, mother, grandmother, aunt, or uncle.

Vallin, who also made a collective investigation of this question, concludes his report as follows: "One cannot deny that heredity plays an important rôle in the development of tuberculosis; but by reason of the great frequency of this affection it is difficult to exactly define the limits of this influence; it does not seem to manifest itself in more than one-half the cases. Moreover, a certain number of cases may be the effect of family contagion. The chances are greater that the child will become tuberculous when the mother at the time of conception was tuberculous; when the father alone is phthisical the children often remain free." A statistical examination of 432 cases of tuberculosis by Kuthy (1894) showed that in 23.8 per cent. one or both parents were tuberculous; in 11.5 per cent. the father had the disease; the mother in 9.9 per cent. Both parents were affected in only 2.4 per cent. of the cases. Rilliet and Barthez give the following figures: Of 24 children with tuberculous fathers 20 died of the disease; of 32 with phthisical mothers 22 were affected and died. Finally 4 children out of 6 died when both parents were affected.

More recently Squire has published some statistics which minimize the influence of heredity. In 275 families in which there was no phthisis in the parents, comprising a total of 1,745 children, 24.87 per cent. of these became phthisical; while in 199 families of consumptive parents, with a total of 1,182 children, 33.71 per cent. of the chlidren became phthisical. This shows a difference of only nine per cent., a comparatively small excess in the incidence. of phthisis on the offspring of tuberculous parents, which might well be accounted for in Squire's mind by the greater exposure to infection of those whose parents were already infected. Out of 12,509 cases of consumption the parents were phthisical in 3,101 cases (24.79 per cent.); in 12,146 consumptives there was a history of phthisis in 7,563 cases (parents, grandparents, uncles, or aunts) or a percentage of 63.34. Impressed with the fallacy of results in this kind of investigation from a study of ancestors, he noted how many of the children of a consumptive became tuberculous. Starting with the diseased individual, the offspring instead of the ancestors were traced, with the result that, the same method of analysis being applied to the non-phthisical, there was a difference of only a little over nine per cent., from which Squire concludes that the influence is considerably less than has been generally believed.

Other statistics give variable figures. Thus Williams found in 1,000 cases that there were 48.4 per cent. with family predisposition, 12 per cent. with parental, 1 per cent. grandparental, and 34.4 per cent. with collateral heredity. Of 250 cases investigated by Solly 28.8 per cent. showed parental taint, 7.6 per cent. grandparental, and 19.2 per cent. collateral heredity. Osler states that of 427 cases at the Johns Hopkins Hospital there were 53 in which the mother had had tuberculosis, 52 in which the father had been tuberculous, and 105 in which a brother or sister had suffered from the disease. Of 13,000 cases at the Görbersdorf Institute Brehmer says that in 36 per cent. there was hereditary influence; Detweiler, of Falkenstein, states that about 33 per cent. show it.

Interesting physiological differences were studied in the offspring of tuberculous parents. In an investigation of this character Riche and Charrin have shown that in infants born of tuberculous mothers, contrasted with infants born of healthy parents, the urine had a higher degree of toxicity, intense myosis was often present, and sometimes the reflexes were considerably exaggerated. Salivation was also occasionally observed.

Constitutional Peculiarities.

The association of a certain habit of body and physiognomy—*habitus phthisicus*—had been pointed out by medical writers of antiquity. "The form of body peculiarly subject to phthisical complaints was the smooth, the whitish, that resembling the lentil; the reddish, the blue-eyed, the leucophlegmatic, and that with the scapulæ having the appearance of wings" (Hippocrates). Similarly Galen and Aretæus noticed that there is often a peculiar shape of the thorax in phthisical persons. The most casual observations show the frequency with which the long, flat chest is met with in tuberculous patients. The significance is merely that of an imperfect, fragile constitution. The writer certainly can see no specific significance in this condition.

This type of thorax has been attributed to smallness of the lungs and to undue rigidity of the bony framework. The important characteristic lies in "the straightening of the upper ribs, with widening of the intercostal spaces, and undue obliquity of the lower rib, whose intercostal spaces are narrowed. The thorax is thus flattened in its anteroposterior diameter, as well as being long and narrow, and the respiratory movements are diminished in extent, owing to the modification in the curvature of the ribs. The increased obliquity of the lower ribs and the falling of the shoulders also cause prominence of the scapulæ, giving rise to the 'alar' or 'pterygoid' chest of Galen and Aretæus. Other forms of the phthinoid thorax are also described, and in many cases there are other characteristics, such as delicacy of skin, fairness of hair, length of eyelashes, early development of teeth which have thin enamel and often decay early, transparency and bluish tint of conjunctivæ, large pupils, rigidity of the bones, with insufficient growth of their cartilages, in consequence of which they are long and slender; precocity of intellect" (Sir W. Jenner).

These manifestations are often accompanied by weakness of resisting-power and susceptibility to catarrhal inflammations—all indications of perverted physiological functions. Beneke believes that one-third of this class show imperfect development of the heart and hypertrophy of the whole arterial system, the pulmonary artery being relatively wider than the aorta, a condition favoring intrapulmonary blood pressure, which explains the liability to catarrhal processes.

AGE.

Estimating the number of deaths from tuberculosis at various ages per 10,000 population, Würzburg shows that the mortality is highest with the advance of age as follows:

From 60 to 70 years	.... 93.18	From 0 to 1 year	.... 23.45
" 50 to 60 "	.... 67.94	" 1 to 2 years	.... 20.41
" 70 to 80 "	.... 61.72	" 15 to 20 "	.... 18.87
" 40 to 50 "	.... 48.42	" 2 to 3 "	.... 12.51
" 30 to 40 "	.... 41.12	" 3 to 5 "	.... 6.23
" 25 to 30 "	.... 36.73	" 10 to 15 "	.... 5.86
Beyond 80	.... 25.80	" 5 to 10 "	.... 4.68

For Brussels (1885-86-87) Destrée and Galemaertz found that the death rate from divers tuberculous affections, making comparisons in the same manner, was greatest in children from 0 to 12 months of age in which period the mortality reached the astounding figures of 168 per 10,000 living at the same age. The minimum mortality was observed from 6 to 15 years, at which period it was only 15 per 10,000 living. In adult Age the number reached 89 per 10,-000 for men at 40 years and 21 for women at the same age. From 60 to 70 the mortality was only 49.8 for men and 15.9 for women per 10,000. The diminution was then progressive. Holsti gives the greatest mortality during the first two years of life; the least between the ages of 5 and 15.

According to the following figures, taken from Newsholme, the ages of maximum phthisis mortality have been postponed in both sexes. This may be ascribed to a greater saving of life at those ages formerly most liable to death from phthisis or to a postponement of death in those who are attacked by the disease. Probably both factors are important.

AGES OF MAXIMUM MORTALITY FROM PHTHISIS (ENGLAND).

(The Age Groups in heavy type have the maximum rates, the others being approximate.)

Periods.	Males.	Females.
1851-60	20-25, 25-35, 35-45	25-35
1861-70	25-35, 35-45	25-35
1871-80	35-45	25-35
1881-85	35-45	25-35
1886-90	35-45, 45-55	25-35, 35-45
1891-96	35-45, 45-55	35-45

"We must accept as conclusive the evidence that with the advent of adolescence a very decided increase in the susceptibility of the lungs to the development of tubercle takes place, and that the development of the disease may be in most cases quite independent of any existing lesion. But it is quite otherwise when the other forms of tubercular disease are considered. Tabes mesenterica, which is most closely related to food infection, and has its chief incidence in the early periods of life—almost three-fourths of its deaths occurring between the age 0–5 years—is no doubt frequently confused both in practice and in the registrar's returns with other forms of chronic diarrhœa which are not tubercular; but quite as great a statistical difficulty arises because of what may be called the clinically interchangeable character of the various forms of tubercular disease which are not phthisis" (Chambers).

It is generally agreed that tuberculosis is rare during the first months of life. The observations of West, Henoch, Bouchut, Barthez, Sanné Schwer, and others have thrown a flood of light upon tuberculosis in the young. Froebelius found in infants from one to four months only 416 affected with tuberculosis out of a total of 18,569 deaths. The statistics of Schwer show that although very rare during the first few weeks of life it becomes frequent with advance of age. Thus Landouzy found tuberculosis in one-third of the children who died under two years. Queyrat, Aviragnet, and Boltz give practically similar figures.

Authors are far from being in accord upon the frequency of tuberculosis in old age. Notwithstanding divergence of opinion on many points the studies of Ruelle, Gilbert, and Michel tend to show that senile phthisis is much less uncommon than was formerly supposed. Laennec made an autopsy on a woman who died at the age of ninety-nine years from tuberculosis.

OCCUPATION.

The influence of some occupations in so modifying the tissues as to make them more vulnerable to infection with the bacillus tuberculosis is not without much practical interest. Statistics show that those following some occupations become more often victims of tuberculosis than others. Observations of this kind have, however, as Straus has pointed out, certain limitations of interpretation: it is certainly eminently improper, for instance, to assume that because tailors furnish a large number of patients this occupation necessarily predisposes to phthisis, for it should be remembered that it is chosen by preference often by weak persons incapable of much muscular effort. Inversely some occupations necessitate vigorous individuals, and if the death rate is low from tuberculosis this should not be interpreted as indicating a healthful calling; often it simply signifies greater resistance by those engaged in the work.

Notwithstanding these restrictions tuberculosis is much more frequent among persons following one occupation than among those following another, other things being equal.   Italian statistics show that in 1890 the greatest mortality from tuberculosis was among students; for every 1,000 general deaths among them 459 were referable to this disease. Typographers and lithographers came next with 347.6; then clerks with 248 per 1,000.   In England, according to the figures of Farr and Ogle, among printers the rate was 430.1 per 1,000 deaths; among workers in cloth in Manchester, 340; knife workers, 283.5; shoemakers and tailors, ·274.7 to 259.6 per 1,000.   In Brussels the highest tribute is paid by waiters—666 per 1,000 general deaths.   Otis, in an analysis of a series of 232 cases of pulmonary tuberculosis, found that 91 followed indoor occupations and 53 outdoor.   Moreover, those following dusty occupations gave a very high number as compared with the others.

Sex.

From 1851–65 the death rate in England was greater among females, the differences between the two gradually diminishing. Since 1866 the rate of mortality from phthisis has been greater among males, and increasingly so. Statistical investigations by Würzburg and Lehmann also show the greater prevalence of tuberculosis among males.

Studying the mortality statistics of Bavaria for the years 1888–89 Zwickle shows that the death rate increases with age, and is higher in males. For 100,000 population the figures are approximately as follows:

Years.	Males.	Females.	Years.	Males.	Females.
6 to 15	100	100	41 to 50	530	350
16 to 22	180	250	51 to 60	640	400
21 to 30	425	375	61 to 70	690	460
31 to 40	490	475			

Statistics by Holti and Benny Frank indicate the same differences. At the Brompton Hospital C. T. Williams records that out of 1,000 cases 625 were male and 375 female; this accords with J. Pollack's experience, which indicates that 60.75 per cent. of males were affected, and 39.25 per cent. of females.

Race.

Differences of prevalence among various races depend to a very small extent on inherent peculiarities of a race. Marked differences of this·kind are referable to other factors. In this country it is stated that the Irish and Negroes are especially prone to the disease. The annual death rate from consumption per 100,000 of population in New York City for the six years ending the 31st of May, 1890, was: for the Irish, 645.73; colored, 531.35; Germans, 328.80; American whites, 205.14; Russian and Polish Jews, 76.72 (J. S. Billings).

THE RELATION OF TRAUMA TO TUBERCULOSIS.

It is generally admitted, notably since the experimental investigations of Max Schüller, that an intimate association exists in many cases between trauma and the subsequent development of a tuberculous lesion in or about the injured parts. Results recently brought forward by Lannelongue and Achard, however, would tend to minimize the importance heretofore given to this belief. Friedrich's experiments apparently confirm the conclusions of these French investigators.

Considered in its relation to accidental injuries of various parts of the body this question becomes of considerable interest to the physician and surgeon. Experience shows that some parts are much more prone than others to the development of tuberculosis after lesions of this kind. Thus the joints, lungs, and meninges are particularly vulnerable under these circumstances. Convincing cases of pleural or pulmonary tuberculosis following injury are limited to a very small number of reports. Chauffard in 1896 published three cases of traumatic pleurisy which argue strongly for the influence of such injuries in the development of the subsequent process. For example, the first case was in a healthy individual sixty-two years of age, with an alcoholic history, who injured his side, fracturing the seventh rib; eight days later he had repeated chills and dyspnœa and from this time the formation of a pleural effusion was noted. One month later tapping was used to remove two litres of blood-stained fluid. No lung lesions were apparent. The following month thoracentesis on two separate occasions removed 1,500 and 1,200 c.c. respectively. During all this time there were no fever, loss of flesh, or general symptoms. Another case, of a still more convincing nature, was that of a middle-aged man who fell, striking the right side, particularly the chest wall. Ten days later he was taken with chill, pain in the injured side, fever, and dyspnœa. On examination he presented signs of a right-sided pleurisy with effusion, and on aspiration 1,500 c.c. of fluid was withdrawn. There was no return of the effusion and the patient recovered. Inoculation experiments with the pleuritic fluid produced tuberculosis in a guinea-pig. The last case was that of a healthy old woman who fell, fracturing the seventh and eighth ribs. The subsequent history was essentially the same as in the second case. The animal experiment was equally positive.

Stern, in his monograph on the traumatic causation of internal diseases, recognizes only two authentic cases, though some have been reported since. Schrader in 1897 reported the case of a young man, twenty-nine years old, previously perfectly healthy. The day following an injury to the right chest he had fever, headache, dyspnœa, and cyanosis. Physical examination at this time showed dulness over both lower lobes on the right side, and the diagnosis of pneumonia was made. Later there developed an irregular fever, and tubercle bacilli were found in the sputum. In time he recovered. Harris added another interesting case the following year. Following an injury to the chest a pneumonia developed, the patient dying about eleven weeks after the accident. The autopsy showed very recent cavities and several old latent foci of tuberculosis.

Considering the frequency of latent tuberculous foci in the body it seems probable that in cases like Schrader's the infecting bacilli came from the old lesions; in the case of Harris this is evident. Examples like those of Chauffard may have a similar origin, but to the writer, in the light of Hodenpyl's observations of miliary tuberculosis of the pleura without other tuberculous involvement of the lung, cases of this kind are more readily explicable from the view point of previous miliary tuberculosis of the pleura. Hodenpyl showed that in fully fifty per cent. of all cases without tuberculosis of the lungs the surface of the pulmonary pleura showed minute miliary tubercles, the morphological peculiarity of these tubercles being a tendency to fibrous tissue metamorphosis.

Tuberculous meningitis following injury to the head is a striking occurrence. Reports by Buol and Paulus, Schilling, Potain, and others contain a few interesting observations of this nature. The case of Schilling was that of a boy who injured his head and was unconscious for two days. Eleven days after the accident he developed marked meningeal symptoms and died in ten weeks after the injury. The autopsy showed the presence of tuberculous meningitis and caseated tracheal lymph glands. No other tuberculosis was discovered. Other cases present in a general way a similar history, and the autopsy usually shows some old tuberculous lesion elsewhere. The case of Buol and Paulus, on the other hand, presented no old focus, but the patient had a history of having had left-sided apex disease some time before.

Traumatic joint tuberculosis is such a well-recognized condition that little need be said beyond referring to the subject. The researches of Cheyne in England, Gibney in America, and Koenig, Verneuil, and others on the continent have done much to put this subject in a practical light. The relation of surgical trauma in local tuberculosis to the generalization of the disease has been fully studied by Koenig, Verneuil, Prengrueber, Kirmisson, Poncet, and Lucas-Championnière. Studies of this kind include cases in which an operation caused the sudden appearance of local lesions where none previously existed, in which the local lesion has been much aggravated, and in which an operation was followed by general miliary tuberculosis. Eilers, Demars, Poncet, and Szuman have reported tuberculous meningitis after surgical operation, sometimes about the head, often in parts quite remote from it. Generalization of the process is explained by assuming that during the operation tubercle bacilli are freed and escape into the general circulation. The more curetting is done the greater is the danger of such an accident supposed to be.

OTHER PREDISPOSING CAUSES.

Some of the acute infectious diseases, notably influenza, whooping-cough and measles, are commonly followed by tuberculosis. According to Landouzy this is also true of variola. Barthez and Rilliet state that almost ten per cent. of all those having measles in hospitals die of tuberculosis. How often this is attributable to a recent infection with tubercle bacilli is obviously still an open question; nevertheless, when we consider the frequency of latent tuberculosis, as shown by post-mortem investigations, it seems that the disease must often be referable to a revivescent focus. In the same way that other disturbances increase the vulnerability to tuberculosis so may syphilis. In children gastroenteritis and enterocolitis sometimes create in the subject a favorable soil for the development of tuberculosis. From the earliest times the influence of diseases of the respiratory system has often been mentioned. Catarrhal affections evidently play the most important part. Occasionally one sees tuberculosis after pneumonia.

Innumerable other conditions occupying varying positions as predisposing factors have been specifically mentioned, among the principal of which are alcoholism, chronic nervous and mental disorders, pregnancy, chronic diseases of the kidneys, liver, and heart, arteriosclerosis, etc. The relation of diabetes to tuberculosis has been fully studied by Bertail, Leyden, and Bayou. In the same way syphilis has been studied by Guidone, Potain, and Jacquinet. In hospital practice a large proportion of individuals, the subjects of chronic disease, present lesions of tuberculosis, Osler believes frequently of the serous membranes.

Regarding typhoid fever there has been considerable discussion; some authors like Thirial, Barthez, Revilliod, and Paul have thought that a certain antagonism existed between this disease and tuberculosis. Others like Laennec and Monneret have contended that no such relation was evident. Experimental evidence certainly in no measure sustains the contention of the first-named observers. Last year Arloing and Dumarest undertook some experiments in this direction, from which they conclude that a belief in such an antagonism is unwarranted. A considerable number of cases are now on record of the coexistence of both infections; Guinon and Meunnier, Chantemesse and Raymond, and others have observed cases of this kind.

Impressed with the great rarity of tuberculosis and cancer in the same individual Rokitansky taught that a certain antagonism must exist between the two conditions; Dittrich modified this opinion by saying that the two affections were never seen in the same organ. Both these opinions have been discredited by the numerous observations of Lebert, Virchow, E. Wagner, Friedrich, and O. Weber. Loeb in 495 cases of tuberculosis and 111 of cancer found the two associated in 31 patients; Lubarsch out of 2,668 tuberculous cases found 117 with carcinoma also. Instances in which both processes were found associated in the same organ have been studied in detail. C. Friedländer, Zenker, Cordua, Crone, and Baumgarten have contributed many such examples.

The Infectious Character of Tuberculosis.

The contagion idea of phthisis dates back to the time of Galen, who included it among those diseases which could be communicated from one subject to another. Some others who followed taught the same thing. Ballonius, a physician of large practice in Paris in the fifteenth century, had noted the frequent occurrence of the disease in those who tended consumptive patients. Two centuries later Paolo Zacchia discussed the interesting problem, whether if one of a married couple was the subject of phthisis the other was bound to pay the "conjugal debt." Nicholas Chesneau (1672), of Marseilles, held that the wife was more liable to contract phthisis from the husband than he from her, because she was busier ministering to his needs. The idea of contagion was strongly impressed in Morgagni's mind: "Ego vero illa [sc. cadavera phthisicorum] fugi de industria adolescens, et fugio vel senex."

Jeannet des Longrois in his "Traité de la Pulmonie" (1781) re-**lates** that at Nancy in 1750 the magistrates had burned in the great place of the city the furniture of a phthisical woman, who, although well before, became infected by having often slept in the same bed with a consumptive patient. A little later similar regulations came into vogue in Languedoc. In the latter half of the eighteenth century this belief must have occupied a prominent position in the minds of many in some parts of Italy. Already in 1754 the members of the College of Physicians of Florence pronounced themselves, on the whole, in the affirmative on this most important question of the communicability of the disease. In 1767 the Republic of Lucca recognized the contagious character of tuberculosis by passing certain regulations. At Naples a royal edict of September 20th, 1782, prescribed the sequestration of consumptives. The disease had become almost epidemic and the death rate reached ten per thousand. Stringent laws were enacted which ordered in addition to isolation of the patient the disinfection of the locality, effects, furniture, books, etc., with vinegar, eau-de-vie, lemon juice, sea water, fumigations, etc., under a penalty of three years in prison; for the nobles violation of this order was punished by three years' confinement in a chateau and a fine of 300 ducats ($684). The physician who failed to make known a phthisical case was subject to a fine of 300 ducats for the first offence, and upon repetition, banishment for ten years.

So definite had the conception of the contagiousness become in some that Baumes of Montpellier went so far as to designate the contagious element as a virus, and in 1807 Vienholdt wrote a book wholly devoted to the contagiousness of phthisis.

The fear of contagion from phthisis was so deeply implanted among the inhabitants of Spain and Portugal that in 1839 Georges Sand, travelling in Spain with Chopin who was consumptive, writes: "At the end of a month poor Chopin, who, since he left Paris has continued to cough, became very ill. I called in a physician, two physicians, three physicians, each one a greater ass than the other, who spread out the tale that our patient was in the last stages of phthisis. There was an immense excitement; phthisis is seldom seen in these climates, and is classed as a contagious disease. We were regarded as pest-breeders. . . . The proprietor of the small house we had rented put us out of doors and threatened us with prosecution for infecting his house. We were plucked by the law like chickens." At Barcelona they had more or less similar experiences.

The work of Villemin did much to popularize the idea that tuberculosis was an infectious disease. In 1874 H. Weber communicated to the Clinical Society of London a report "On the Communicability of Consumption from Husband to Wife," which aided in extending this belief. Laveran about the same time pointed out its frequency in military nurses; in 1875 the mortality rate was 4.40 per 1,000 men, while that for the entire army was only 2.27. Since the discovery of the tubercle bacillus the infectious character of tuberculosis has become common knowledge.

The Collective Investigation Committee of the British Medical Association was able in 1883 to collect 158 cases in which tuberculosis was apparently transmitted from husband to wife, or *vice versa*. The following year the Berlin Medical Society collected 40 similar cases. In 1884 Vallin reported for the Medical Society of the Paris Hospitals 107 instances of this kind, of which 64 were from husband to wife and 43 from wife to husband. The reports of Leudet, Dubousquet-Laborderie, and others contributed numberless cases of this nature. Among members of religious orders the mortality from tuberculosis is often two-thirds of the entire death-rate; in prisons the high prevalence of former times as compared with recent figures is also suggestive. Since the establishment of prophylactic measures in 1887 Cornet states that statistics indicate a diminution of mortality in Prussian prisons. During the period 1875–76 the average mortality from tuberculosis per 10,000 prisoners living was 118.9; from 1878 to 1884 it increased to 140.8, while in 1887 it reached 174.7. From 1887 to 1890 under improved conditions it fell to 101; in 1890–92 to 89.4; 1892–94 to 81.2. Prisons in other States show similar results. Baer states that in a general way tuberculosis is four times more prevalent in prisons than outside. Figures of this kind are glaring demonstrations of its infectious character. Among nurses the mortality from tuberculosis sometimes reaches sixty-three per cent. In Paris they are decimated by the disease. In many other places, however, particularly where considerable care is exercised in the disposition of infected material, tuberculosis is uncommon among the attendants.

In a large business house in the centre of Paris twenty-two persons were employed about eight hours a day; one of them, aged forty, had been phthisical about three years and did not leave his work until three months before his death. Within the ten years following, of twenty employed fifteen had died, fourteen of them from phthisis. Another citation equally illustrative is that of Napias. A large manufacturer, several years ago, impressed with the great number of his employees who became victims of tuberculosis, ordered a medical inspection, from which it was found that the diseased individuals would expectorate on the floor and that the healthy ones became infected from the contaminated dust. Improvement of existing conditions was quickly followed by the disappearance of the epidemic.

Bec has reported several very interesting rural epidemics, in villages previously free from tuberculosis, which followed the appearance of a case of which the infection had occurred elsewhere. To Praeynes, a hamlet of 46 inhabitants, a young girl comes back from the city with acute miliary tuberculosis; in less than one year 4 other young girls, her companions, succumb to the disease. At Majastres, a village of 202 inhabitants, 12 persons died of tuberculosis within three years after the arrival of a victim of the disease. In Brunet, with 418 inhabitants, 18 deaths followed under similar circumstances; within seven days 3 became infected.

The researches of Flick regarding infected houses are interesting in connection with the subject of the infectious character of tuberculosis. In studying the distribution of tuberculosis in a single ward in Philadelphia he showed that only ten per cent. of the houses in which this disease occurred were in an isolated position. Furthermore in a number of years more than one and frequently three or four cases had occurred in thirty-three per cent. of the infected houses. Moreover, the distribution of tuberculosis corresponded almost exactly with that of the more acute diseases.

In the same way the Board of Health of New York City has shown that in one ward there were 28.2 per cent. of infected houses which contained 55.8 per cent. of the cases of tuberculosis, and these occurred in only 10.5 per cent. of all the houses in the ward. In another ward 44.3 per cent. of the cases occurred in 18.9 per cent. of the infected houses, and these constituted only 7.1 per cent. of all the houses in that ward.

In visiting many of the so-called health resorts especially frequented by pulmonary tuberculosis invalids in all stages of the malady, one cannot fail to become impressed with the danger arising from the indiscriminate spitting everywhere. So much is this so that in some places tuberculosis has materially increased in regions previously almost free from the disease. The chief health officer of Nice, Dr. Balestre, in a communication to Dr. S. A. Knopf, writes: "It is a well-known fact that Nice, and especially Menton, have seen the number of their consumptives increased in an enormous proportion since phthisical patients have frequented these resorts." The secretary of the New Mexico Territorial Board of Health, Dr. F. H. Atkins, writing to the same gentleman, says: "Like other communities much resorted to by consumptives, we are year after year discovering cases of phthisis occurring in New Mexico among people born here, or quite recently come here and healthy, and in many of them there has been a definite exposure to the infection of the tubercle bacillus." On the other hand, Gardinier states that at Colorado Springs, in which for twenty years tuberculous patients have been living, the number of cases of tuberculosis originating in the city is very small. W. Æbi makes a similar statement for Davos, notwithstanding the fact that a large sanatorium is located there.

Distribution of the Bacillus Tuberculosis.

That the tubercle bacillus is abundantly distributed should be the cause of little surprise when one considers the indifferent attitude and ignorance of patients regarding the disposition of infected material. By far the most fertile source of dissemination is to be found in the sputum. Remembering the estimate of Nuttall that the twenty-four hours' sputum of a consumptive patient may contain between 300,000,-000 and 4,000,000,000 tubercle bacilli, or that of Bollinger, that 1 c.c. of sputum may contain from 810,000 to 960,000 bacilli, it becomes evident with what ease this ubiquity is maintained. Cadéac and Bournay have shown that the fecal discharges of cattle contain virulent tubercle bacilli. In its moist state sputum is devoid of great danger, risk occurring chiefly when drying takes place which reduces the infected material to a fine powder that is spread in all directions. Perhaps nothing more forcibly emphasizes the importance of the danger of infection from such sources than the investigations of Straus, who demonstrated the presence of the bacillus tuberculosis in the nasal cavities of various healthy individuals frequenting the wards of the Charité and Laennec Hospitals in Paris. Of the twenty-nine attachés, nurses, and patients examined, nine gave positive results when tested by guinea-pig inoculations. From the nasal mucus of six machinists and the orchestral leader of the Opera the results were negative in all instances save that from the leader of the orchestra. Kelsch, Boisson, and Braun obtained one positive result from the nasal mucus of a series of soldiers examined.

Dust.—One of the best known studies relating to the existence of tubercle bacilli in dust is that of Cornet, who published the results of his work bearing on this question in 1888. He experimented with the dust obtained from the walls and floors of various dwellings in which tuberculous patients had been by inoculating guinea-pigs and carefully excluding all possibility of infection from outside sources. In this way twenty-one rooms of seven Berlin hospitals were examined, and bacilli were found present in most of them. Positive results were similarly obtained with the dust from asylums and prisons. In the same manner the apartments of a considerable number of consumptive patients were investigated and the dust in many of them was found to be virulent. The dust was regularly virulent when the patient had been in the habit of spitting on the floor or in a hand-kerchief; when the spit-cup had been used the results were negative. In a room which had been occupied by a tuberculous patient the dust was shown to contain virulent tubercle bacilli six weeks after her death.   These experiments showed that while quite commonly present in the neighborhood of consumptive patients, tubercle bacilli are infrequently found elsewhere.

Repeating the investigation in the hospital at Bonn, Krüger took sixteen specimens of dust from medical wards in which phthisical patients had been for some weeks and obtained two positive results; with eight specimens of dust from other localities in which no such patients had been, the results were all negative.   Bollinger's pupil, Kaster, got similar results with dust from the Munich clinic. At the instigation of Bollinger this subject was again taken up by Kustermann, with dust from the penitentiary at Munich, where for two years disinfection of the floor and walls had been rigorously carried out.   In no instance was he able to demonstrate any tubercle bacilli.   However, similar results were obtained from a public waiting-room in which no such precautions were used; this led Kustermann to conclude that the propagation of tuberculosis (in prisons and similar institutions) must depend on other conditions than the spreading of dried expectorations and the presence of bacilli in the dust of floors and walls.   Such an interpretation of this observation is discredited by the investigations of more recent experimenters.   Related to the same problem, the researches of Kirchner in 1896 established the presence of tubercle bacilli in the dust of the trousers and other clothes of soldiers in three of six specimens examined.

The dust in railway cars is often particularly infectious.   Petri (1893) demonstrated tubercle bacilli in the dust of the pillow, railing, and ceiling of a berth occupied by a traveller.   Similarly Prausnitz two years before him had also found them in railway coaches. Hance examined the dust from street cars; one in five cars was shown to contain dust contaminated with tubercle bacilli.   Since then a considerable number of studies have demonstrated the not unusual contamination of such localities.

Meat.—It is natural to suppose, from the frequency with which domestic animals, particularly cattle, are affected with tuberculosis, that the meat distributed for public consumption must often contain more or less virulent tubercle bacilli.   Knowledge of tuberculosis in meat dates back a considerable time, but appreciation of the frequency with which it is affected is of comparatively recent date and largely based upon systematic inspection of the abattoirs.   Dominated by the ideas of Toussaint, Bouley regarded all meat from a tuberculous animal, howsoever slightly affected, as unfit for use. This conception was again embodied in the resolutions of the fifth International Congress of Veterinary Medicine held at Paris in 1889. The relative immunity of the muscles to infection was, however, demonstrated very clearly by Nocard in 1888. Perroncito four years later carried out another series of extensive experiments related to the same theme. Of more than four hundred guinea-pigs and rabbits inoculated with meat extract obtained from the flesh of tuberculous ànimals none was infected.

More recently still Reismann in an article of high practical interest arrives at certain conclusions which embody the opinion of the time and recognize the occasional danger of meat from infected animals. Perhaps the most extensive and thorough investigation of the whole subject was undertaken by the Royal Commission on Tuberculosis and carried out by Sydney Martin. Throughout the experiments muscle substance only was used; fat, tendons, and lymph glands in the intermuscular spaces were removed and no obvious focus of tuberculosis was allowed to remain. Of 48 animals inoculated with meat or meat-juice 10 developed tuberculosis; of 102 animals (guinea-pigs, rabbits, pigs) fed with the meat 6 developed the disease. The positive results were obtained from the meat of 8 of the cows—viz., of 1 cow with mild, of 3 with moderate, and of 4 with advanced and generalized tuberculosis. In experiments with the meat of 16 cows (no advanced or generalized tuberculosis) 35 animals were inoculated and 5 developed tuberculosis; of 81 animals fed with the meat not one showed any sign of the disease. The meat or meat-juice of 4 cows affected with generalized disease was inoculated into 13 animals; of these 5 became affected. In another series of 4 cows 21 animals were fed, but only 6 developed lesions.

Many points of considerable interest were brought out by this investigation. The meat of no one carcass was sufficiently infectious to produce tuberculosis in all the inoculated animals; and of those fed the number of positive results was still less. It was additionally shown that while the meat of one carcass might be uniformly infective by inoculation and yet produce no constant results when fed to animals, other meats produced a reverse order of conditions. Martin advances a consideration which explains some of the anomalies he met with. In preparing the meat for sale the butcher uses the same knife with which he has already cut infected tissues, and so the surface of meat is irregularly contaminated with tuberculous material.

Two years ago Lignières reported that a piece of cooked sausage was brought to him which had been served in a restaurant. It contained gray areas which were seen under the microscope to be lymph nodes containing tubercle bacilli. Fortunately inoculation experiments proved that the tubercle bacilli were dead. Examination of the meats served by the same butcher revealed other infected material.

Milk.—The frequency with which milk is contaminated has been variously estimated by different experimenters. Impressed with the frequency of tuberculosis of the udder in cows Van Hersten was among the first adequately to appreciate the danger which might arise from the use of milk of such derivation. Another important step in this direction was made by Bollinger (1879) in showing that not only was the use of milk from animals with such disease fraught with peril, but that milk from tuberculous cows without tuberculous lesions of the udder occasionally contained virulent tubercle bacilli. However, more especially the work of May, Stein, Galtier, Bang, Hirschberger, Gebhardt, Gaffky, Ernst, and still more recently the investigations of Obermüller, Zacharberkoff, Fiorentini, Sydney Martin, Buege, Petri, Massone, Kanthack and Sladen, Allan Macfadyen, and Woodhead and Wood have done much to define the danger and limitations of the infectious character of milk of this kind. In 1892 Gaffky also pointed out the possibility of milk contamination with tubercle bacilli from fecal dejections of cattle. In highly centrifugated specimens of infected milk Bang demonstrated tubercle bacilli in great numbers; and further experiments by Scheurlen showed that it was impossible to remove all the tubercle bacilli by the use of the centrifuge.

The infectious character of milk has been shown to vary considerably in different places. In the Bulletin Municipal Officiel de la Ville de Paris of November 23d, 1896, it is stated that of ten samples of milk collected so many as four contained tubercle bacilli. And it must not be thought that this danger is wholly limited to the milk of animals with marked tuberculosis, for a report by Rabinowitsch and Kempner and another by Ostertag have shown that at times the milk of cows even apparently healthy but reacting to the tuberculin test contains virulent tubercle bacilli. The first two observers found 66.6 per cent. of such milk virulent; Ostertag, on the other hand, concludes that the milk of cows clinically presenting no indications of tuberculosis may be regarded as free from danger. Other evidence certainly points to such an interpretation.

In samples obtained from 36 different cows, all of them presenting more or less distinct signs of tuberculosis of the lungs or elsewhere, but none of them having marked signs of disease of the udder of any kind, Ernst showed a percentage of detected infectiousness of 27.7 per cent. By centrifugation and inoculation Obermüller, out of 40 specimens of milk, demonstrated tubercle bacilli in some; using the cream and sediment, he obtained 10 positive results out of 26. Zacharberkoff obtained 4 positive results out of 80 specimens examined in St. Petersburg. Of 50 specimens of milk collected in Milan Fiorentini detected tubercle bacilli in 4. Petri found 14 per cent. of the examined samples of milk infected; Massone 9 per cent.; Thomassen 25 per cent.; Delepine in one series found only 5.55 per cent., in another 17.6 per cent.; Kanthack and Sladen found that the specimens of 9 dairies were infected out of 16 examined, and the results of Woodhead and Wood showed that 5 specimens out of 50 contained virulent tubercle bacilli. Also Rabinowitsch and Kempner found that 7, or 28 per cent. of 25 samples of Berlin milk contained tubercle bacilli. The studies of Kanthack and Sladen proved the cream infective 9 times, while the sediment from the specimens was so only 6 times. An explanation of this is readily found in the interesting observations of Freeman, who found that as the cream rises to the surface it carries with it more than 90 per cent. of all the bacteria, leaving the milk relatively free from microorganisms. The experimental researches of the Royal Commission on Tuberculosis tend to show that tuberculous disease of the udder must be established before the milk becomes infective. Sydney Martin tested 10 cows, all tuberculous to a greater or less degree, but without udder disease, and obtained negative results in all instances.

Butter and Margarin.—A considerable number of investigations have shown that butter made from tuberculous milk is often infective, and the experiments of Heim and Gasperini demonstrated that tubercle bacilli may live and retain their virulence in butter for a period of one hundred and twenty days. In thirty days, however, Gasperini found that the virulence began to diminish. Brusaferro tested 9 samples of butter, using 22 guinea-pigs, with 1 positive result; by intraperitoneal inoculations Roth succeeded in establishing the infective character of the butter in 2 samples out of 20 examined. Schuchardt took 42 samples and inoculated with them 28 animals; one became tuberculous. Groening got 47 per cent. of positive results.

The researches of Rabinowitsch in 1897 threw much new light upon this whole question. In the light of her experimental results former investigations lose much of their scientific value. Of 80 samples of butter collected in Berlin and Philadelphia she was unable to demonstrate tubercle bacilli in any, but in 23 samples (28.7 per cent.) she found organisms producing lesions simulating those of tuberculosis; by closer study they could be distinguished, however, without any difficulty. Others have since described similar microorganisms: Petri in milk, Moëller in infusions of timothy grass (Phleum pratense), dust of grasses, cow-dung, and milk. The bacillus isolated by Rabinowitsch is *säurefest*, and grows on all ordinary media with the production of an ammoniacal, unpleasant odor. Spores are not formed; and animals infected with it do not react to tuberculin. The tinctorial reactions of this organism are essentially the same as those of the tubercle bacillus. With pathogenic and tinctorial reactions to some extent simulating those of the tubercle bacillus, it is obvious that earlier investigators might well have confounded the two organisms. Hence the hesitancy in accepting *in toto* results anterior to 1897.

Similar inquiries by Hormann and Morgenroth showed that in a series of experiments tubercle bacilli were present in 6 samples of the 13 examined; and of 15 samples of cheese tested positive results were obtained in 3 cases. In a second research Rabinowitsch determined the presence of pseudo-tubercle bacilli in 13 specimens and tubercle bacilli in 2 out of a total of 15 examined. A careful bacteriological examination of 10 samples of butter bought in 10 different markets in Berlin by Obermüller demonstrated the existence of tubercle bacilli in 7; Petri found that 32.3 per cent. of a large number of specimens contained the same organism, whereas Goggi obtained only 2 positive results in 95 specimens submitted to tests.

But few examinations of margarin have been reported with a view to determine the presence of tubercle bacilli. Morgenroth last year communicated the results of the examination of 20 specimens, 9 of which gave positive results (45 per cent.). Working on the same subject, Annett produced tuberculosis but once with a series of 28 samples of margarin collected in Berlin and Liverpool.

Hands.—Scarcely any mention has hitherto been made of soiled hands as carriers of tubercle bacilli. Not long ago this was made the subject of an interesting investigation by Baldwin, of Saranac Lake. The hands of 15 patients were examined and of this number 10 were contaminated with the specific organism. From these experiments he concludes that living tubercle bacilli are not infrequently present on the hands of patients who are not careful in the use of handkerchiefs, clothing, or cuspidors.

Other Possible Sources of Infection.—Observations of recent years have shown that tubercle bacilli are commonly present in the saliva of individuals suffering from phthisis, and so this is recognized as a means of spreading these organisms in many directions. Petit a few years ago undertook some experiments, the results of which are of practical interest. Confirming the frequent presence of tubercle bacilli in the saliva, as pointed out by Freudenthal and Kerez, he established the fact that from this source considerable danger exists in the practice of kissing, and in eating and drinking from utensils used by consumptive patients. My confrère Hiss found tubercle bacilli on the mouth of a medicine bottle, and I have demonstrated them on a spoon used by a consumptive patient.

There seems to be a certain element of danger in cigars and cigarettes made by hand. The saliva which the tuberculous laborer uses to fasten the wrapper of the cigar or cigarette may convey the tubercle bacilli to the smoker. Petit points out that in some places it is customary for individuals to collect cigar stumps to utilize the tobacco in the manufacture of new ones, and it is probable that such tobacco is often contaminated. Kerez had already emphasized such a mode of infection from tobacco, and Spenser has actually demonstrated the presence of tubercle bacilli in various specimens of cigars submitted to him for examination.

A propos of this subject the report of the United States Commissioner at Constantinople additionally emphasizes this risk. He says that the sanitary officer at Cavalla had been impressed by the spread of tuberculosis among the workmen in the tobacco factories there, and on investigation found that, in order that the special qualities for which it is so highly prized may not be lost, Turkish tobacco is exposed to the air as little as possible; consequently, in the course of its manufacture into cigars, no circulation of air is allowed in the workrooms. These rooms, besides being ill-ventilated, are damp; the workmen are crowded in them and inhale all the dust caused by the manipulation of the herb. They sleep in the rooms, bronchitis is universal, pulmonary tuberculosis is common among them, and they spit all about the rooms.

Midwives and at times physicians apply the mouth to that of an asphyxiated infant and inflate the child's lungs in order to bring its respiratory organs into play. If the operator is a consumptive the danger of imparting the disease is considerable. The habit some midwives have of sucking the mucus from the child's throat by direct application of the mouth is equally hazardous. Reich two years ago reported ten cases of tuberculosis caused by this practice. A midwife in the village of Neuenberg became phthisical in 1874 and died of the disease in the middle of the summer of 1876. Ten children without hereditary taint attended by this woman in the months of April and May, just preceding her death, died before reaching the age of one year and one-half. This midwife was in the habit of sucking the mucus from the mouths of the newborn children and blowing air into their lungs.

A suggestive case of infection by means of a penholder was also reported by Petit. A strong, healthy woman, who was in the habit of placing a penholder in her mouth when writing in the evening, after the same thing had been done by a phthisical individual more or less during the whole day, developed tuberculosis after a time.

In the act of circumcision the Mosaic law prescribes that the final act of the operation, hæmostasis, be performed by the operator suck. ing the wounded surface. Such an act performed by a phthisical subject naturally then becomes of considerable danger, as the obser. vations of Lindemann, Lehmann, Hofmokl, Elsenberg, W. Meyer, Karewski, Ware, Pott, Moskowitch and others attest. This subject will receive more detailed consideration in the section on inoculation tuberculosis.

So this question of infection of the saliva has a far-reaching im. portance in more than one direction. Public drinking-cups, the communion cup, as used in Protestant churches, bible-kissing, etc., must often likewise be sources of some danger.

Innumerable other lurking-places for the tubercle bacilli present themselves, such as money, notes, and books. Bissel has proven the existence of tubercle bacilli in second-hand clothing; and recently Abba, of Turin, has found tubercle bacilli in holy water.

The inhumation of either expectorated or fecal matter from tuberculous patients without its having been previously treated by disinfectants might not under all circumstances be perfectly safe. Lortet and Despeignes presented to the Académie des Sciences of Paris, January 25th and July 4th, 1892, a report of some experiments by which they showed that the earth worm may be instrumental in bringing to the surface again the bacilli from interred tuberculous material. The belief that flies which have fed on tuberculous sputum may serve as carriers and disseminators of this microorganism has furnished a theme for investigation to Spillman and Haushalter (1886), who have demonstrated by extensive experiments that the fly may become the propagator of the tuberculous virus. The abdominal cavities of flies caught in the rooms of consumptives were found to contain living bacilli, so also the fly specks scraped from the walls and windows of hospital wards and rooms where consumptives habitually sojourned. E. Hoffmann (1888), wishing to control these results, investigated the intestinal contents of flies obtained in an apartment recently occupied by a subject of pulmonary tuberculosis. Tubercle bacilli were found in four flies out of six examined, and also in the excreta. Flies fed with tuberculous sputum died in a few days, and after twenty-four hours bacilli could be demonstrated in their excreta. Similar observations have been made by Alessi. Larkin, and the writer. Dewèvre (1892) collected many bedbugs from the bed of a consumptive patient and found that they contained tubercle bacilli.

Modes of Infection.

Natural tuberculosis in man in many respects is not unlike that of some animals. So also as in experimental tuberculosis certain well-defined forms are recognized, depending on the point of entrance of the infecting agent, the disease in man conforms to the same divisions according to the channel of infection. Of these the most frequent is tuberculosis by inhalation; infection by way of the intestinal tract is less common; and transmission by heredity and inoculation is the less important from a practical point of view by reason of its greater infrequency.

Congenital Tuberculosis.

Still one of the most vexed and unsettled problems in the pathology of tuberculosis, the influence of heredity has been the theme of a rich and abundant literature. Since Baumgarten formulated the doctrine of bacterial transmission from parent to offspring much activity has been shown in this department of scientific thought. Even before the discovery of the tubercle bacillus Baumgarten conceived that heredity of tuberculous disease was rather a transmission of the bacterial inciting factor than the inheritance of simple susceptibility of the tissues. Such a conception must assume in a large proportion of cases a latency of bacterial manifestations—a potential stimulus which under little understood conditions is capable of remaining in abeyance for long periods. Baumgarten holds that such heredity is analogous to what may occur in syphilis or variola.

So actively and with so much energy has Baumgarten developed this view that opinion is divided at the present time between those accepting this interpretation, and others, the larger number, who would see such a conception applicable only in rare instances, and regard inheritance of soil as the preëminent factor. The great rarity of congenital tuberculosis in man and animals must remain a forceful argument against this doctrine of bacterial inheritance. Furthermore, the belief in a particular resistance of embryonic tissues, which presumably explains so much in the conception, is based on insufficient evidence to be taken at all seriously. In the first place the frequency of tuberculosis in early age is in itself a serious obstacle to such an hypothesis; moreover, experiments of Sanchez-Toledo, Straus, and Kockel and Lungwitz discredit this assumption.

The inheritance of the bacilli themselves is, however, supported by a number of facts; and recent investigations tend to show that congenital tuberculosis is considerably more common than was admitted by Virchow and Cohnheim. Certain writers, like Cnopf and Goldschmidt, have endeavored to support Baumgarten's views by statistical evidence, showing the great frequency of tuberculosis in the first periods of life. Imbued with the same idea Aviragnet investigated this question, but found that in many instances it was possible to establish postnatal infection. Furthermore, the observations of Demme, Straus, Wassermann, and others invalidate the contention of those who would prove congenital transmission by the arguments of Cnopf and Goldschmidt. And then a host of observers have shown that tuberculosis is often found in the early life of children free from any possible influence of inheritance. Another argument advanced in support of congenital infection, and which has met with some favor, is the existence not only in infancy but also in adult life of primary tuberculous foci in lymphatic glands, bones, articulations, etc., without any associated lesions of the respiratory system. But at the present time it is universally admitted that infection can well occur through other channels — tonsils, intestines, etc.—without necessarily any apparent lesions at the point of entrance.

To sum up, then, Baumgarten's conception is that tuberculosis, and not alone hereditary disease so called, but tuberculosis in general, in the majority of cases is the pathological sequence of an infection which may occur through the sperm or the ovum, or by way of the placenta. In all cases the bacilli would be very few in number, so that at birth lesions would be uncommon; occasionally their number would be sufficient to cause lesions, as shown by the few cases of congenital tuberculosis reported. To explain the long period of latency, resistance of embryonic tissue is invoked. The bacilli present in small numbers become lodged in organs where solid particles are most apt to be arrested—lymph nodes and marrow of bones, and there they remain for long periods of time, months, often years, without any manifestation of pathogenic activity.

Transmission by Sperm.—The belief in this mode of infection is based on analogy, experimental demonstration being wholly lacking. From the fact that seminal infection causes such hereditary infectious diseases as syphilis, it has been assumed that the same mode of infection holds good for tuberculosis. The investigation of the infectious character of sperm in tuberculosis was undertaken by Landouzy and Martin, Gärtner, Baumgarten, and Marfucci with affirmative results in some instances. The experiments of the last-named observer are not without interest in this connection. He inoculated rabbits with mam-

malian tuberculosis and examined the sperm at the end of forty-eight
hours and at different intervals for three months. Only about the
twenty-fifth day were the bacilli abundant in the sperm. From the
fact that few of the offspring of the animals experimented with showed
tuberculosis, presumably by sperm transmission, no definite conclusion can be reached. More recently Binghi (1898) introduced tubercle
bacilli into the testicles of guinea-pigs, but their offspring did not
develop the disease. Experimentation is obviously not conclusive
in this respect, and further and fuller investigations are necessary to
permit any dogmatic utterance. Benda contends that the spermatozoa
are incapable of transporting immotile bacilli, an objection, however,
which has little weight.

If the sperm of animals suffering from tuberculosis not infrequently
contains tubercle bacilli, the same cannot be said from the evidence at
hand of that of human beings. The work of Westermeyer, Walter,
Dabroklowski, Albrecht, and Jaeck certainly seems to indicate that
the seminal fluid of ordinary subjects of phthisis without miliary,
genital, or pelvic tuberculosis is not infective. Nakarai has again
(1898) gone over the same ground with results essentially similar to
those of previous investigators. The comparative infrequency of
genital tuberculosis in the female genital organs—vagina, uterus—
argues against the infective character of the semen under ordinary
conditions of tuberculous pulmonary disease.

Turning to the side of clinical medicine, we find that the literature of congenital infection of paternal origin is limited to the reports
of Zippelius, Landouzy, Bang, and Sansom, in all of which it is
possible there was heredity of predisposition with subsequent bacterial infection. Thus at the present time there does not exist a
single case which leads us to think that inheritance of a germ infection from the father occurs in tuberculosis.

Maternal Transmission.—This may take place through the ovum
or by way of the placenta. Some have contended that heredity from
the ovum is impossible, believing that an infected ovary is incapable
of development. Such a view does not appear to be substantiated by
observation. In the strictest sense infection in this way is the only
true form of hereditary maternal infection—tuberculosis of placental
origin being merely a congenital tuberculosis. However, separate
consideration of the two forms is impracticable.

Closer study in the domain of animal and human pathology has
permitted the publication of a moderate number of cases of congenital tuberculosis. Clinical knowledge of this condition is based on
some forty cases in the human subject, and more than sixty-five examples in calves. Thus Johne, Malvoz and Brouwier, Misselwitz,

Walter, Csoker, Bang, Ruser, and Macfadyen have contributed some studies of congenital tuberculosis in calves; Landouzy and Martin, and Cavagnis in guinea-pigs; Sibley in fowls, etc. Probably Charrin (1873) was the first to report an authentic case of this nature in human beings born of a tuberculous mother. Merkel observed an infant born with a caseous focus in the palate, and another in the neighborhood of the thigh. This child died shortly afterwards of glandular tuberculosis. Baumgarten and Roloff, Berti, Jacobi, Demme, Rindfleisch, Sarwey, Sabouraud, Lehmann, Schmorl, and Kockell have added to the list.

Congenital tuberculosis without lesions, but in which the tubercle bacillus was demonstrated, has been observed a number of times by Landouzy and Martin, Armanni, Schmorl and Birch-Hirschfeld, and Thiercelin and Londe.

INHALATION TUBERCULOSIS.

The common primary localization of tubercle in the lungs indicates that in a large proportion of cases infection takes place by inhalation. Pizzini inoculated lymph glands from forty people, who died of accident or acute disease, into guinea-pigs. From the results of the inoculation experiments he concluded that forty-two per cent. of healthy people have tubercle bacilli in their glands, mostly in the bronchial. Statistics of the Paris morgue show that a considerable proportion of all who die of accident or suicide have evidences of some tuberculous disease in connection with the respiratory system.

Villemin was among the first experimentally to demonstrate this mode of infection. Dried tuberculous sputum insufflated into the trachea of rabbits through an opening into this organ produced the disease in its characteristic form. In his paper lies the whole anticipation of the experiments of Cornet, to which we have already referred. To Tappeiner, however, belongs the credit of having first firmly established the experimental production of the disease by inhalation. His experiments were carried on with dogs. By throwing a fine spray of diluted sputum into closed cages in which the animals were placed, he succeeded in infecting the dogs. The spraying was repeated for one hour twice daily for from twenty-five to fifty days. At the autopsies all the animals showed lung tuberculosis with frequent extension to other organs. Repetition of more or less similar experiments by Bertheau, Veraguth, Koch, de Toma, and Thaon confirmed these results.

The best conceived experiments on the relation of dust to inhala-

tion tuberculosis are those of Cornet, who established the frequent
infectivity of the dust collected from localities in proximity to
phthisical patients. Flügge, looking at the question in another
light, argues that the propagation of phthisis by dried tubercle bacilli, which has been so largely admitted since the researches of
Cornet, is far from being demonstrated. Indeed, he says that the
majority of experiments in which animals were made to respire dust
containing dried tuberculous sputum have given negative results.
Cornet himself, he says, succeeded in infecting animals only by injection into the peritoneal cavity of dust collected in the vicinity of
consumptive patients. Juxtaposition of these facts permits Flügge to
believe that the danger from inhalation of such dust is at a minimum,
and at all events that it is not the principal mode of propagation of
pulmonary tuberculosis. On the other hand, he thinks that infection must commonly occur from the fine moist particles thrown off
by consumptive patients. This view is supported, Flügge believes,
by the fact that it is much easier to infect animals by the vaporiza-
tion of infected fluids than with dust.

With these ideas in mind he undertook some experimental studies in this direction. Consumptives were placed in spacious boxes,
in which plates of agar-agar were disposed at variable distances.
Once in the box the patient was requested to talk, cough, and sneeze.
In another series of tests the patient was made to do the same thing
outside of the box through an orifice, after which the air in the case
was aspirated and passed through a solution of sodium chloride. In
a third series culture media were placed at variable distances from
the mouths of the patients who were lying down and who were made
to talk, cough, etc. All these tests were positive in showing that
when a phthisical subject talks there is formed around him a humid
atmosphere, imperceptible to the naked eye and containing tubercle
bacilli. More recently Flügge has repeated his experiments with con-
firmative results. Other observers—Engelmann, Weismayr, B. Fraenkel—have obtained like results. Heymann measured the tiny drops
after they had fallen on the slides. Their average diameter was
about 35 μ, and microscopically they consisted of mucus, pus cells,
epithelial cells, and many tubercle bacilli.

Weismayr caused a number of persons to rinse their mouths
with fluid cultures of the bacillus prodigiosus, and then to cough.
Under such conditions he found that bacilli were projected in the quiet
air of a closed room for a distance of 4 metres, while if a door were
opened and shut they spread 2 metres behind and to the side of the
person coughing. Spitting also spread the bacteria for some distance.
Experimenting along similar lines Hubener ascertained that loud

talking, sneezing, and coughing would project microorganisms; sometimes five hundred were found in plates 5 metres from the patient.

Very recently Moeller, of Goerbersdorf, went over some of the work of Flügge and his pupils. He moistened glass slips with glycerin or gelatin and suspended them over the beds of consumptives in all stages, at different hours of the day, for various intervals of time, and at all distances up to a metre. About one-half of all the phthisical patients whose sputum contained tubercle bacilli were able to project the infected particles of spray upon the glass slips. The morning and evening hours appeared to give the most marked results. In some cases even a few acts of coughing were sufficient to contaminate the slips, while in other cases an exposure of hours was necessary. Furthermore, those with watery sputum projected the most particles into the air. The reading-room of the Goerbersdorf Sanatorium was often used for theatrical performances; naturally there was here much laughing, followed often by paroxysms of coughing. After the close of a performance lasting from two and one-half to three hours the air from the room was pumped through a sand filter; then the sand was washed in bouillon and the liquid tested for tubercle bacilli. The result was negative. On the other hand, positive results were obtained with the dust collected from the walls, ornamental plants, etc.

Mozza argues against Flügge's conclusions. But Cornet's work is the most important in support of the opposite view. In admitting the negative attempts of Sirena, Pirence, Toma, Celli and Guarnieri, Cadéac and Molet, and himself, to infect animals regularly with dried sputum dust by inhalation, he explains this by the fact that in conditions of experimentation the bacilli, by virtue of hygroscopic properties, take up moisture from the expired air of the animals and become agglutinated into too voluminous particles to be inhaled. This would explain the failure of many previous experiments.

Other experiments conducted by Cornet were carried out under the most natural conditions. Tuberculous sputum was spread on the carpet of a room, mixed with dust, and allowed to dry for two days. Animals were placed in the room in different groups, some were placed on the floor, and others upon stages at various heights: 7, 40, and 120 cm. Then the floor was swept in the usual way with a stiff broom, a cloud of dust being raised. A second group of animals were submitted to direct inhalation of infected dust. Sputum was dried and finely pulverized and held a distance of 20 cm. from the animals. Of forty-eight guinea-pigs used forty-six became infected. Cornet protected himself by wearing an overall coat reaching to the feet, and by covering his head with a hood containing an opening filled with glass to see and to breathe through. Despite all precautions he was able to infect an animal with mucus from his nasal cavity.

Neisser carried out other experiments which tend to emphasize the danger of infected dust. He proved that dried tubercle bacilli can be transported from place to place in mild currents of air. By mixing tubercle bacilli with fine dust, and then directing a gentle current of air upon the mixture, the bacteria were carried to distant points. Moreover, he found that dried tubercle bacilli can be held for some time in the suspended dust of ordinary rooms.

INGESTION TUBERCULOSIS.

In the observation of Malin (1839) we have, perhaps, the earliest expression in literature of any definite recognition of ingestion tuberculosis. He relates the case of a consumptive woman who had a pet dog which swallowed during a year. the expectorations of the patient. At the end of six months it became sick, emaciated, and finally died. Another dog took its place, and like its predecessor swallowed the sputum and died at the end of five months. On opening the thorax both lungs were found almost entirely destroyed by "suppuration."

Chauveau, Villemin, Parrot, and Klebs were among the first to undertake systematic study of this form of infection. Their results were sufficiently constant to demonstrate the possibility of ingestion tuberculosis under experimental conditions. Since then Gerlach, Bollinger, Orth, Toussaint, and Peuch have successively taken up the subject. At the present time few doubt its occurrence under natural conditions in man and animals.

In 1882 a Commission of the Dresden Veterinary School was appointed to investigate the danger from the use of infected meat or milk. The experiments which were published by Siedamgrotsky were in the main affirmative. Baumgarten caused rabbits to swallow infected milk with uniformly positive results. Wesener in 1885 published an important memoir upon ingestion tuberculosis in which were recorded a large number of experiments essentially confirmatory of anterior conclusions.

Examples of primary intestinal tuberculosis are not very common. Stang observed one case of this kind. The case was one of a finely developed five-year-old boy, the son of healthy parents without any hereditary taint. The child died from miliary tuberculosis of the lungs with enormously enlarged tuberculous mesenteric glands. At the autopsy it was learned that the boy had habitually drunk the milk of a cow which had been killed shortly before he died and which had tuberculosis. Ollivier and Bouley have reported six cases which developed in an institution where was used the milk from a tuberculous cow. Bang has also reported similar instances. Demme has put on record a most interesting observation. Three infants, the offspring of sound parents and without any hereditary taint, were placed in the care of a nurse with tuberculosis of the jaw, with a fistula communicating with the buccal cavity. The infants died during the first year of life from primary intestinal tuberculosis. A fourth child, placed in the care of the same nurse under similar conditions, also died of intestinal tuberculosis. Inquiry revealed the fact that this woman was in the habit of first placing the food, which she prepared, in her mouth and then giving it to the children. Infection probably occurred from the infected saliva.

A complication of phthisis in the form of ingestion tuberculosis is often produced by the patient swallowing the infected sputum. Apart from its association with lung disease and its mode of origin its points of interest are those of ordinary intestinal tuberculosis.

Inoculation Tuberculosis.

Tuberculosis by accidental inoculation has been sufficiently well studied to be mentioned under a separate head. This form of the disease is more apt to be met with in those working with the infected tissues, such as pathologists, butchers, handlers of hides, etc.

Tschering, of Copenhagen, in 1888 reported a case of this nature. The sufferer was a veterinary surgeon who wounded his finger while making an autopsy on a tuberculous cow. Three weeks after the accident the wound had healed, but the adjoining parts became swollen and later suppuration occurred. Despite treatment the process advanced, and the diseased portion was removed. Microscopical examination of the tissues demonstrated tubercle bacilli. In 1885, another veterinarian of Weimar cut his thumb under similar conditions. The wound healed, but six months later Pfeiffer, who reported the case, detected cutaneous tuberculosis about the cicatrized wound. In the fall of 1886 the patient presented symptoms of pulmonary tuberculosis. He died, and at the autopsy tuberculous arthritis was found at the site of the original wound. Jadassohn has reported a case of inoculation infection from tattooing.

In 1894 Rémy related a case of inoculation tuberculosis produced by a tuberculous mother sucking the child's wound, and Kelsh three years later reported two cases of tuberculosis following infection of wounds of the foot with dust containing tubercle bacilli. Cases of infection of washerwomen from washing linen soiled by consumptive patients are reported by Eiselberg and White. Fischer reports infection in a nurse as a result of a cut from a spit-cup. Lefévre has collected a moderate number of these cases, and Martin du Magny, Law, and others have added to the list. Other modes of inoculation have been mentioned, such as the bite of a tuberculous subject, and the transplantation of skin (Czerny). White, of Boston, has reported a case in which piercing the ears was followed by a local tuberculosis of the ear lobes.

Of the large number of cases of inoculation tuberculosis reported, a considerable proportion have followed the ritual circumcision of infants as practised by orthodox Hebrews. The Mosaic law prescribes that the final act of the operation be carried out by the operator sucking the wounded surface. Naturally, if the operator be the subject of tuberculosis and his saliva contain tubercle bacilli, the chances for infection must often be great. Lindemann, Lehmann, Hofmokl, Elsenberg, Willy Meyer, Karewski, Ware, Moschkowitz, and others have contributed instructive cases of this nature. Small epidemics, the result of such practice, have been reported, particularly in Russia. Thus, Eiselberg reported four and Lubliner five such cases, and in Eiselberg's cases the tubercle bacilli were found not only in the diseased skin but also in the sputum of the operator.

Primary infection of the genitourinary tract may occur by direct infection during coitus. It is probably less frequent than some authors will admit; and the probability of the occurrence of infection by direct contagion is lessened by the fact that this localization is commonly met with before the period of sexual activity. Experimentally Dabroklowsky established the possibility of inoculation of these parts. Clinically this mode of infection has been known for a long time. Cohnheim recognized that it was possible for the urethra of man to be contaminated by the secretions of a tuberculous uterus, and that the sperm of a tuberculous patient might be the cause of infection in women. Verneuil, Verchère, Fernet, and Bonis have published histories of presumably such inoculations.

Bibliography. *

Herard, Cornil, et Hanot: La Phtisie Pulmonaire, Paris, 1888.
Damaschino: Leçons sur la Tuberculose, Paris, 1891.
Arloing: Leçons sur la Tuberculose et certaines Septicémies, Paris, 1892.
Klebs: Die causale Behandlung der Tuberculose, Leipsic, 1894.
Straus: La Tuberculose et son Bacille, Paris, 1895.

---

* The references given are not intended to be a complete bibliographical list of subjects treated in the article; the citations cover only some of the more important literature. Many of the references given have been specially selected on account of their bibliographical value.

Cornet: Die Tuberculose, Vienna, 1895.

Dürck: Ergebnisse der allgemeinen Pathologie und pathologischen Anatomie des Menschen und der Tiere   Lubarsch und Ostertag, Wiesbaden, 1897.

Important literature may also be found in the numbers of the *Revue de la Tuberculose*, Paris, and in the *Études expérimentales et cliniques sur la Tuberculose*, published in Paris under the direction of Verneuil. The transactions of the Congrès pour l'Étude de la Tuberculose, Paris, contain many interesting reports.

History.—Young: Practical and Historical Treatise on the Consumptive Diseases, etc., London, 1815.

Waldenburg: Die Tuberculose, etc., Berlin, 1869.

Spina: A History of Tuberculosis (Translation), Cincinnati, 1888.

BACTERIOLOGY.

Tinctorial Reactions.—Ehrlich: Deutsche medicinische Wochenschrift, 1882, p. 269; Charité Annalen, 1886, pp. 123–138.

Ziehl: Deutsche medicinische Wochenschrift, 1882, p. 451.

Neelsen: Fortschritte der Medicin, 1885, p 200.

B. Fraenkel: Berliner klinische Wochenschrift, 1884, pp. 193–214.

Gabbet: Lancet, 1887, p. 757.

Hauser: Comptes rendus de la Société de Biologie, 1898, p. 1003.

Kühne-Borrel: Annales de l'Institut Pasteur, 1893, p. 602.

Bienstock: Fortschritte der Medicin, 1886, p. 193.

Gottstein. Ibidem, 1886, p. 252.

Hammerschlag: Sitzungsberichte der kk. Academie der Wissenschaften, Wien, December 13, 1888; Centralblatt für klinische Medicin, 1891, p. 1.

Weyl: Deutsche medicinische Wochenschrift, 1891, p. 256.

Aronson: Berliner klinische Wochenschrift, 1894, p 484

Morphology.—Koch: Mittheilungen aus dem Kaiserlichen Gesundheitsamte, 1884, Bd. 2, p. 22.

Ehrlich: Charité-Annalen, 1886, p. 124.

Nocard et Roux: Annales de l'Institut Pasteur, 1887, p. 28.

Metchnikoff: Virchow's Archiv, 1888, Bd. cxiii., pp. 63, 70.

Czaplewski: Die Untersuchung des Auswurfs auf Tuberkelbacillen, Jena, 1891.

Bruns: Ein Beitrag zur Pleomorphie der Tuberkelbacillen. Inaugural Dissertation, Strassburg, 1895.

Coppen Jones: Centralblatt für Bakteriologie und Parasitenkunde, 1895, Bd. xvii., pp. 1 and 70.

Craig: Journal of Experimental Medicine, 1898, p 363.

Babes et Levaditi: Archives de Médecine expérimentale et d'Anatomie pathologique, 1897, p. 1041.

Schultze: Zeitschrift für Hygiene, 1899, Bd. xxxi., p. 153.

Friedrich: Deutsche medicinische Wochenschrift, 1897, p 653.

Friedrich und Nösske: Ziegler's Beiträge, 1899, Bd xxvi., p 470.

Biology.—Lubinski: Centralblatt für Bakteriologie und Parasitenkunde, 1895, Bd. xviii, p. 125.

Schneiderlin: Ueber die Biologie des Tuberculoserregers (Tuberkelbacillus). Inaugural Dissertation, Freiburg, 1897.

Schottelius: Centralblatt für Bakteriologie und Parasitenkunde, 1890, Bd. vii., p. 265.

Straus et Dubarry: Archives de Médecine expérimentale et d'Anatomie patho logique, 1889, p. 7.

Heiman: New York Medical Journal, 1892, vol. lv., p. 287.

Schumowski: Centralblatt für Bakteriologie und Parasitenkunde, 1898, Bd. xxiii., p. 828.

Germicidal Action of Various Substances.—Woodhead: Lancet, 1896, vol. i., p. 945.

Schill und Fischer: Mittheilungen aus dem Kaiserlichen Gesundheitsamte, 1884, Bd. ii.

Voelsch: Ziegler's Beiträge zur pathologischen Anatomie, 1888, Bd. ii., p. 239.

Yersin: Annales de l'Institut Pasteur, 1888, p. 60.

Grancher et Ledoux: Archives de Médecine expérimentale et d'Anatomie pathologique, 1892, p. 1.

Forster: Hygienische Rundschau, 1892, p. 869.

Bonhoff: Ibidem, p. 1009.

De Man: Archiv für Hygiene, 1893, Bd. 18, p. 133.

Smith: Journal of Experimental Medicine, 1899, p. 217.

Malassez et Vignal: Comptes rendus de la Société de Biologie, 1883, p. 366.

De Toma: Annali universali di Medicina, July, 1886.

Sawizky: Centralblatt für Bakteriologie und Parasitenkunde, 1892, Bd. 11, p. 153.

Mitchell and Crouch: Journal of Pathology and Bacteriology, 1899, p. 14.

Ausset: Journal de Clinique et de Thérapeutique infantiles, February 11, 1897.

Blaikie: Scottish Medical and Surgical Journal, 1897.

Pott: Lancet, 1897, p. 1314.

Thoinot: Annales de l'Institut Pasteur, 1890, p. 500.

Parrot et Martin: Revue de Médecine, 1893, p. 809.

Rovsing: Fortschritte der Medicin, 1897, p. 257.

Baumgarten: Berliner klinische Wochenschrift, 1887, p. 20.

Murray: British Medical Journal, 1899, vol i , p. 202.

Falk: Virchow's Archiv, 1883, Bd 93, p. 144.

Wesener: Beiträge zur Lehre von der Fütterungstuberculose, Freiburg, 1885, p. 55.

Straus et Wurtz: Archives de Médecine expérimentale et d'Anatomie pathologique, 1889, p. 370.

Chemistry.—Hammerschlag: Sitzungsberichte der kk. Academie der Wissenschaften, Wien, December 13, 1888; Centralblatt für klinische Medicin, 1891, p. 1.

Weyl: Deutsche medicinische Wochenschrift, 1891, p. 256.

De Schweinitz und Dorset: Journal of the American Chemical Society, August, 1895; Centralblatt für Bakteriologie und Parasitenkunde, Bd. 19. p. 707.

Ruppel: Zeitschrift für physiologische Chemie, vol. xxvi.

Aronson: Berliner klinische Wochenschrift, 1898, p. 484.

Behring: Ibidem, 1899, p. 537.

Auclair: Bulletin de l'Académie de Médecine, November 20, 1898.

Koch: Deutsche medicinische Wochenschrift, 1890, p. 1029; Ibidem, 1891, p. 101; Ibidem, 1189.

Hueppe und Scholl: Berliner klinische Wochenschrift, 1891, pp. 88, 193.

Hueppe: Ibidem, 1891, p. 1121.

Hunter: British Medical Journal, 1891, vol. ii., p. 164.

Kühne: Zeitschrift für Biologie, 1893, Bd. 29, p. 26; Bd. 30, p. 221.

Hoffman: Wiener medizinische Wochenschrift, 1894, p. 712.

Matthes: Deutsches Archiv für klinische Medicin, 1894.

De Schweinitz: Journal of the American Medical Association, 1897.

Stroebe: Ueber die Wirkung des neuen Tuberkulins, T. R., etc., Jena, 1898.

Engelking: Zur Behandlung der Tuberulose mit Tuberkulin R. Inaugural Dissertation, Marburg, 1898.

Bezançon et Gouget: Comptes rendus de la Société de Biologie, 1899, p. 525.

Stockman: British Medical Journal, 1898, vol. ii., p. 601.

Goldschmidt: Berliner klinische Wochenschrift, 1891, p. 28.

Babes und Kalendero: Deutsche medicinische Wochenschrift, 1891, p. 115.

Straus et Tissier: Semaine médicale, 1893, p. 364.

Cultural Characters.—Kitasato: Zeitschrift für Hygiene, 1892, Bd. xi., p. 441.

Czaplewski und Hensel: Centralblatt für Bakteriologie und Parasitenkunde, 1897, Bd. xxii., p. 643.

Hesse: Zeitschrift für Hygiene, 1899, Bd. xxxi., p. 502.

Ledoux-Lebard: Archives de Médecine expérimentale et d'Anatomie pathologique, 1898, p. 362.

Hip. Martin: Ibidem, 1889, p. 77.

Powlowsky: Annales de l'Institut Pasteur, 1888, p. 303.

Tomasczewski: Ueber das Wachstum der Tuberkelbacillen auf Kartoffelhaltigen Nährboden. Inaugural Dissertation, Halle, 1898.

Sander: Archiv für Hygiene, 1893, Bd. xvi., p. 238.

De Schweinitz and Dorset: Tuberculosis Investigations. United States Department of Agriculture, Bulletin 13, 1896.

Marfucci: Giornale di Anatomia et Fisiologia, 1889, fasc i ; Riforma Medica, May, 1890; Zeitschrift für Hygiene, 1892, Bd. v., p. 445.

Bataillon, Dubard, et Terre: Comptes rendus de la Société de Biologie, 1897.

Bruns: Ein Beitrag zur Pleomorphie der Tuberkelbacillen. Inaugural Dissertation, Strassburg, 1895.

Craig: Journal of Experimental Medicine, 1898, p. 363.

Experimental Tuberculosis.—Smith Journal of the Boston Society of Medical Science, November, 1898; Boston Medical and Surgical Journal, 1899, p. 31.

Moore: Journal of Pathology and Bacteriology, 1899, p. 94.

Dinwiddie: Arkansas Agricultural Station Bulletin No. 57, 1899.

Armanni: Movimento medico-chirurgico, Naples, 1872.

Salomonsen: Nordisk medicinsk Archiv, 1879, No. 19.

Tappeiner: Virchow's Archiv, 1878, Bd. 74, p. 393.

Chauveau: Bulletin de l'Académie de Médecine, 1868, p. 1007; Association française pour l'avancement des sciences, 1873, p. 717; Ibidem, 1874, p. 943.

Klebs: Virchow's Archiv, 1870, Bd. xix., p. 291.

Orth: Ibidem, 1880, Bd. lxxvi., p. 217.

Wesener: Kritische und experimentelle Beiträge zur Lehre von der Fütterungstuberculose, Freiburg, 1885.

Dobroklowski: Archives de Médecine expérimentale et d'Anatomie pathologique, 1890, p. 253.

Action of Dead Tubercle Bacilli.—Prudden and Hodenpyl: New York Medical Journal, June 6 and 20, 1891.

Grancher et Ledoux-Lebard: Archives de Médecine expérimentale. 1892, p. 1.

Auche et Hobbs: Comptes rendus de la Société de Biologie, 1898, p. 13.

Leroy: Le Bacille tuberculeux chez l'Homme et dans la série animale, Paris, 1897, p. 83.

Lannelongue et Achard: Académie des Sciences, April 26, 1897.

Relationship between Bacilli from Different Sources. —Nocard: Annales de l'Institut Pasteur, 1898, p. 561.

Bataillon et Terre: Comptes rendus de la Société de Biologie, 1899, p. 608.

Nicolas: Ibidem, 1899, p. 617.

Moeller: Deutsche medicinische Wochenschrift, 1898, p. 876.

Lubarsch: Zeitschrift für Hygiene, 1899, Bd. xxxi., p. 187; Centralblatt für Bakteriologie und Parasitenkunde, 1899, Bd. xxv., p. 369.

Concurrent Infections.—Prudden: New York Medical Journal, 1894, vol. lx., p. 1.

Gruber und Bernheim: Ergebnisse der allgemeinen Pathologie, etc. (Lubarsch und Ostertag), 1897, pp. 1–67.

Spengler: Zeitschrift für Hygiene, 1894, Bd. xviii., p. 342.

Ehrhardt: Ueber die Mischinfektion bei Lungentuberkulose. Inaugural Dissertation, Königsberg, 1897.

Albarran: Annales des Maladies des Organes génito-urinaires, 1897, p. 1.

Schröder und Mennes: Ueber die Mischinfektion bei der chronischen Lungentuberkulose, Bonn, 1898.

Schütz: Berliner klinische Wochenschrift, 1898, p. 297.

Bacteriological Diagnosis.—Wurtz: Bacteriologie clinique, Paris, 1898.

Pappenheim: Berliner klinische Wochenschrift, 1898, p. 809.

Fraenkel: Ibidem, 1898, p. 880.

Grethe: Fortschritte der Medicin, 1896, Bd. xiv.

Bunge und Trautenroth: Ibidem.

Rosenblatt: Centralblatt für innere Medicin, 1899, p. 755.

Micheleau: Journal de Médecine de Bordeaux, July 21, 1898.

Knopf: Journal of the American Medical Association, 1899, p. 1445.

PATHOLOGY.

Schwer: Ein Beitrag zur Statistik und Anatomie der Tuberculose im Kindesalter. Allgemeine medicinische Central-Zeitung, No. 6, 1886.

Osler: Practice of Medicine, 3d edition, p. 270.

Warthin: Medical News, 1899, vol. lxxiv., p. 455.

Histogenesis of Tubercle.—Virchow: Die Cellular-Pathologie, 1858.

Langhans: Virchow's Archiv, 1868, p. 286.

Koster: *Ibid.*, 1869, vol. xlix., p. 114.

Wagner: Archiv für Heilkunde, 1870, vol. ii., p. 497; 1871, vol. xii., p. 1.

Schüppel: Lymphdrüsen-Tuberculose. Inaugural Dissertation, Tübingen, 1871.

Baumgarten: Zeitschrift für klinische Medicin, 1885, Bd. ix., pp. 93, 245; Bd. x., p. 24; Lehrbuch der pathologischen Mykologie, 1890, Bd. ii., pp. 555–600.

Metchnikoff: Virchow's Archiv, 1888, vol. cxiii., p. 63.

Weigert: Fortschritte der Medicin, 1888, p. 809.

Arnold: Virchow's Archiv, vol. lxxxii., lxxxiii.

Josué: Histogénèse du Tubercle. Thèse de Paris, 1898.

Welcker: Ueber die phagocytäre Rolle der Riesenzellen bei Tuberculose. Inaugural Dissertation, Jena, 1895.

Broden: Archives de Médecine expérimentale et d'Anatomie pathologique, 1899, p. 1.

Pulmonary Tuberculosis.—Prudden: New York Medical Journal, 1894, vol. lx., p. 1.

Fraenkel und Troje: Zeitschrift für klinische Medicin, xxiv., 30, 1894.

Baumgarten: *Ibid.*, 1885, Bd. ix. and x.
Borrel: Annales de l'Institut Pasteur, 1893.
Letulle: Anatomie pathologique, Paris, 1897.
Teissier: Thèse de Paris, 1894.

ZOOLOGICAL DISTRIBUTION.

Nocard: Les Tuberculoses Animales, Paris, 1895.
Eber: Die Tuberkulose der Thiere. Ergebnisse der allgemeinen Pathologie, etc. (Lubarsch und Ostertag), Wiesbaden, 1899, p. 859.

ETIOLOGY.

Hirsch: Handbook of Geographical and Historical Pathology, New Sydenham Society translation, London, 1885.
Evans: Handbook of Historical and Geographical Phthisiology, New York, 1888.
Ransome: British Medical Journal, 1890, vol. i., p. 523; Researches on Tuberculosis, London, 1897; Practitioner, 1898, p. 575.
May: Münchener medicinische Wochenschrift, 1897, p. 253.
Wick: Wiener klinische Wochenschrift, 1895, p. 525.
Otis: American Journal of the Medical Sciences, 1898, vol. cxvi., p. 532.
Hodenpyl: Medical Record, 1899, vol. lv , p. 903.
Holsti: Zeitschrift für klinische Medicin, 1893, Bd. xxii., p. 317.
Bang: Presse médicale, 1898, p. 70.
Beevor: Lancet, 1899, vol. i., p. 1005.
Leudet: Bulletin de l'Académie de Médecine, 1885, p. 532.
Thompson: Family Phthisis, 1884, p 45; British Medical Journal, 1894, p. 1364.
Squire: British Medical Journal, 1896, p. 459; American Journal of the Medical Sciences, 1897, vol. cxiv., p. 537.
Riche et Charrin: Comptes rendus de la Société de Biologie, 1897, p. 355.
Kurlow: Archiv für klinische Medicin, 1889, p. 436.
Solly: American Journal of the Medical Sciences, 1895, vol cx., p. 133.
Jenner: Medical Times and Gazette, 1860, vol. i., p. 259; Ibidem, 1861, vol. ii., p. 2.
Schmidt: Ueber die Heredität der Tuberculose nach statischen Untersuchungen an der medizinischen Poliklinik. Inaugural Dissertation, Erlangen, 1897.
Zander: Charité Annalen, 1899, p. 391.
Destrée et Gallemaertz: La Tuberculose en Belgique, Brussels, 1889, p. 95.
Aviragnet: De la Tuberculose chez les Enfants, Paris, 1892.
Michel: Étude sur la Tuberculose chez les vieillards. Thèse de Paris, 1894.
Frank: Statistik des Lungenschwindsucht. Inaugural Dissertation, Freiburg, 1895.
Kocks: Ueber die Sterblichkeit an Tuberkulose in der Rheinprovinz bezüglich ihrer Abhängigkeit von industrieller Beschäftigung. Inaugural Dissertation, Bonn, 1890.
Bertillon: Annuaire statistique de la Ville de Paris, 1891, p. 130.
Bagou: La Tuberculose pulmonaire dans le Diabète sucré. Thèse de Paris, 1888.

Jacquinet: Contribution à l'Étude de la Tuberculose chez les Syphilitiques. Thèse de Paris, 1895.

Claude: Cancer et Tuberculose   Paris, 1900.

Baldwin and Wilder: American Journal of the Medical Sciences, June, 1899.

Schrader: Berliner klinische Wochenschrift, 1897, p 1001.

Harris: Lancet, 1898, vol. ii , p. 1045.

· Wiener: Beitrag zur Statistik tuberculöser Knochen- und Gelenkleiden nach Trauma. Inaugural Dissertation, Breslau, 1897.

Reichel: Ueber die wesentliche Beziehung zwischen Trauma und Tuberculosis Inaugural Dissertation, Breslau, 1898.

Erster: Zeitschrift für klinische Medicin, 1884, Bd. viii , p. 572.

Vallin: Bulletin de la Société des Hôpitaux de Paris, 1886.

Leudet: Union médicale, 1891.

Knopf: Prophylaxis and Treatment of Pulmonary Tuberculosis, Philadelphia, 1899, p. 37.

Flick: The Contagiousness of Phthisis, 1888.

Wise: Lancet, 1899, vol. i., p. 1359.

Römpler: Deutsche Medicinal-Zeitung, 1890, No. 31.

Distribution of the Tubercle Bacillus —Cornet: Zeitschrift für Hygiene, 1888, Bd. v., pp. 191–332; Ueber Tuberculose, Leipsic, 1890.

Krüger: Einige Untersuchungen des Staubniederschlages der Luft in Bezug auf Tuberkelbacillen. Inaugural Dissertation, Bonn, 1889.

Kirchner: Zeitschrift für Hygiene, 1896, Bd xxi., p. 493.

Petri: Arbeiten aus dem Kaiserlichen Gesundheitsamte, 1893, Bd ix., p. 111.

Prausnitz: Centralblatt für Bakteriologie und Parasitenkunde, 1891, p. 320.

Perroncito: Centralblatt für Bakteriologie und Parasitenkunde, 1892, p. 429.

Reismann: Hygienische Rundschau, 1896, p. 856.

Royal Commission on Tuberculosis, Lancet, 1896, vol. i., p. 575.

Lignières: Recueil de Médecine vétérinaire, 1898, p. 71.

Ernst: American Journal of the Medical Sciences, 1889, p. 439.

Martin: Lancet, 1896, vol. i., p. 945.

Kanthack and Sladen: Lancet, 1899, vol. i., p. 74.

Macfadyen: Lancet, 1899, vol. ii., p. 849.

Woodhead and Wood: Lancet, 1899, vol. i., p. 537.

Freeman: Archives of Pediatrics, 1899.

Annett: Lancet, 1900, vol. i., p. 159.

Schuchardt: Inaugural Dissertation, Marburg, 1896.

Rabinowitsch: Zeitschrift für Hygiene, 1897, p. 90; Deutsche medicinische Wochenschrift, 1899, p. 1.

Hormann und Morgenroth: Centralblatt für Bakteriologie und Parasitenkunde, 1899, p. 84.

Morgenroth: Hygienische Rundschau, 1899, p. 1121.

Annett· Lancet, 1900, vol. i , p. 159.

Baldwin· Philadelphia Medical Journal, 1898, p. 1198.

Freudenthal. Archiv für Laryngologie, Bd. v.

Reich: Berliner klinische Wochenschrift, 1878, No. 37.

Spenser: Medical News, 1897, p. 639.

Bissel: Ibidem, 1899, p. 156.

Alba: Lancet, 1899, vol. ii., p. 1782.

Spillmann et Haushalter: Comptes rendus de la Société de Biologie, 1887, p. 352.

Celli: Bolletino della Società Lancisiana degli Ospedali di Roma, 1888, fasc. i., p. 1.

Dewèvre: Comptes rendus de la Société de Biologie, 1892, p. 232.

Congenital Tuberculosis.—Baumgarten. Zeitschrift für klinische Medicin, 1883, p 61 Lehrbuch der pathologischen Mykologie, 1890, p. 628; Arbeiten aus dem Institut zu Tübingen, 1892, p. 322.

Bolognesi Recherches cliniques, bactériologiques, histologiques, et expérimen. tales, pour servir à l'histoire de l'hérédité de la tuberculose humaine. Thèse de Paris, 1895.

Hauser: Deutsches Archiv für klinische Medicin, 1898, p. 221.

Kuss. De l'Hérédité parasitaire de la Tuberculose humaine, Paris, 1898.

Inhalation Tuberculosis.—Göbell Ueber die Infection der Lungen von den Luftwegen aus. Inaugural Dissertation, Marburg, 1897.

Baer: Ueber die primären Lokalisationen der Inhalationstuberkulose. Inaugural Dissertation, Erlangen, 1896.

Pizzini. Centralblatt für Bakteriologie und Parasitenkunde, 1892, p. 872.

Tappeiner. Virchow's Archiv, 1878, Bd lxxiv, p. 393.

Bertheau. Deutsches Archiv für klinische Medicin, 1880, Bd. xxvi, p 523.

Veraguth: Archiv für experimentelle Pathologie, 1883, Bd. ii., p 261.

De Toma: Annali universali di medicina, June, 1886

Thaon: Comptes rendus de la Société de Biologie, 1885, p. 582.

Preyss· Münchener medicinische Wochenschrift, 1891, p. 421.

Cornet: Zeitschrift für Hygiene, 1888, Bd. v., p. 191; Berliner klinische Wochenschrift, 1898, p. 317.

Flügge: Deutsche medicinische Wochenschrift, 1897, p. 665; Zeitschrift für Hygiene, 1899, Bd. xxx., p. 179.

Engelmann Inaugural Dissertation, Berlin, 1898.

Heymann: Zeitschrift für Hygiene, 1899, Bd. xxx., p. 139.

Hubener: Ibidem, 1898, Bd xxviii., p 348.

Moeller: Ibidem, 1899, Bd xxxii., p 205.

Mazza: Rivista d'Hygiene e Sanità pubblica, 1897, p 809.

Neisser: Ueber Luftstaubinfektion, ein Beitrag zum Studium der Infektionswege, Leipsic, 1898.

Ingestion Tuberculosis.—Lydtin: Report of the Veterinary Congress of Brussels, 1883, p. 288.

Lyon: Gazette des Hôpitaux, 1891.

Gebhardt. Münchener medicinische Wochenschrift, 1889, p. 731.

Law: Proceedings of the United States Veterinary Medical Association, 1898, p. 84.

Inoculation Tuberculosis.—Lefèvre. Sur la Tuberculose par inoculation cutanée chez l'Homme, Paris, 1888.

Nocard: Les Tuberculoses animales, Paris, p. 121.

Tardivel· Contribution à l'Étude de la Tuberculose d'Origine cutanée. Thèse de Paris, 1890.

Rémy: Journal de Clinique et de Thérapeutique infantiles, March 14, 1894.

Kelsch: Revue d'Hygiène, 1897, p. 868.

Ware: New York Medical Journal, 1898, vol 67, p. 287.

TUBERCULOSIS.
(SYMPTOMATOLOGY.)

BY

HENRY W. BERG,
NEW YORK.

TUBERCULOSIS.

(SYMPTOMATOLOGY.)

TUBERCULOSIS, although an infectious disease, and having many of the characteristics of other infectious diseases, with regard to its propagation is almost unique in that, while it is a constitutional disease originating in a local infection, its characteristic lesions are not limited to the site of the local infection. On the contrary, the infection, at first local, almost invariably extends until it involves other organs and tissues of the body. This extension is limited either by spontaneous cure, after the disease has made a limited progress, or by the death of the patient. It follows then that a clinical description of tuberculosis involves a discussion of the tuberculous process affecting all of the organs of the body. In the case of each organ, while the pathological development of the tubercle is very much alike, allowances being made for difference due to the individual anatomy of the different organs, the resulting symptomatology and clinical history, both subjective and objective, will vary with the organs and tissues involved. Thus the characteristic cough, sputum, hemorrhage, etc., which reveal tuberculosis of the lungs, will be entirely absent in primary tuberculosis of the cornea, provided the lungs in the latter instance are not involved. It is, therefore, necessary to discuss the clinical history and symptomatology of tuberculosis of the different organs and tissues separately, and consider each as an entity.

Furthermore, there are practically two ways in which the tubercle bacillus is disseminated throughout the system—by the lymphatic channels, and by the blood-vessels. The mode of dissemination through the blood stream, while fortunately by far·less frequent than that through the lymphatic vessels and glands, is much more rapid and causes the involvement of all the organs and tissues of the body in a very short space of time. Not only does the latter mode of dissemination differ in rapidity and virulence from the more common mode of spreading by means of the lymphatics and secondary infection, but it gives rise to a distinct difference in the clinical course. In the miliary tuberculosis, which is the result of infection carried by the blood-vessels, the disease is eminently of the acute type and rapidly fatal; while in the cases in which the virus is disseminated by the lymphatic system, the disease progresses with varying degrees of slowness to other organs than those originally the seat of infection, and which are involved only after longer periods of time, while frequently the process remains limited to the organs first infected. We shall, therefore, consider acute disseminated or miliary tuberculosis separately, as a distinctive condition, after we have discussed the ordinary and comparatively chronic form of pulmonary tuberculous disease.

As to the relative frequency with which various organs and tissues are affected by tuberculosis, there is no question that certain structures, notably the lungs, are affected much more frequently than others. It is not here intended to discuss the comparative frequency with which the disease occurs in the various tissues. But this variable liability to the disease is not due, as has been claimed by, the older writers, to an excessive predisposition for the disease on the part of individual organs, but to the fact that certain organs, such as the lungs, for instance, are anatomically so situated that they are pre-eminently subject to contact with the outer world, by which they may become infected with live tubercle bacilli; when the organ in question is so constituted anatomically as to form a favorable nidus for the growth and development of the tubercle bacilli and the tubercles which they cause, the conditions necessary to favor the frequent occurrence of tuberculosis in such organs are fulfilled. The lungs answer both of these conditions, and accordingly it is found that the lungs are most frequently affected by tuberculosis. The skin, on the other hand, answers the first condition better even than the lungs, but is so well guarded against ordinary infection by contact, from the nature of its anatomical structure, that tuberculosis of the skin is rare, and occurs only when the skin has first become the seat of a lesion in continuity.

Occasionally even here, however, tuberculosis occurs as a secondary manifestation of the disease primarily located in some other organ. The lungs are most frequently primarily infected through contact with inspired air, which carries tuberculous matter and bacilli. But pulmonary tuberculosis also occurs secondarily to tuberculosis of other structures in the human body. In such cases the clinical manifestations, due to the presence of the disease in the lungs, are added to the symptomatology of the primary affection. Here, as in other forms of tuberculosis, whether surgical or medical, the consideration of the disease as a primary affection does not imply that any of the organs cannot become secondarily affected, without regard to the original source of infection. Thus tuberculous meningitis, complicating Pott's disease of the spine, is either an extension

of the primary tuberculous process from the bones ,o the nerve structures, or an instance of secondary involvement of the nerve structures
in a general tuberculosis of which tuberculous disease of the vertebræ
was the primary disease. So, also, the lungs may be the primary
seat of the disease, or they may become affected by juxtaposition
with some neighboring tissues, the seat of primary tuberculosis, or
as part of a general tuberculosis affecting the whole body.

In the present article the symptomatology of pulmonary tuberculosis only will be considered, that of the other localizations of the
disease (which do not come in the domain of the surgeon), having
been treated of elsewhere in this work.

PULMONARY TUBERCULOSIS.

When tubercle bacilli have gained lodgment in the lungs, either
through the inspired air or through the lymphatics, and have begun
their malign existence at the expense of the pulmonary tissues and
nutritive fluids of the body, no local symptoms will be perceived for
several weeks in any case, and in some cases for several months, or
even years. Not even constitutional symptoms will appear until the
tubercle begins to undergo disintegration. Then the soluble proteins
set free in the disintegration process are absorbed into the lymph
channels and blood-vessels, and carried to distant organs and centres,
where their toxic activity gives rise to the early constitutional symptoms. Those portions of the broken-down tubercle or tuberculous
focus which do not admit of absorption, sooner or later infect and
destroy the healthy pulmonary tissue which separates them from a
terminal bronchus or air cell, and thus gain access to a channel communicating with the open air, whence and through which they can be
expelled from the lungs, chiefly by means of and through the expul-
sive power of cough. So that this destruction and breaking down
of healthy lung tissue, separating a primary tuberculous focus from
the air cells and terminal bronchus, although pathological, is in one
sense a conservative effort, the object being to afford egress from the
system of the broken-down tuberculous tissue. Nevertheless, it is
this process which first gives rise to such local symptoms as cough
and expectoration. Indeed, the process, if conservative at first, soon
ceases to be such, for it is in this way that the extension of the tuberculous focus occurs in the early stages of the disease. Nevertheless,
sputum, cough, and expectoration begin only when the disintegration
products of tubercle reach the air cell or bronchus, and this is the
reason why general constitutional symptoms precede the occurrence
of local manifestation in pulmonary tuberculosis.

Constitutional Symptoms.

These constitutional symptoms vary in kind and in degree. One of the earliest is *anæmia*. The patient is objectively pale. The conjunctivæ are not so red as usual, the cheeks are of an ash color. Very rarely, even in this early stage, an examination of the blood shows changes characteristic of simple anæmia, in respect to the relative number of the red blood corpuscles and leucocytes, and a diminution in the percentage of the hæmoglobin. These changes, exceptional in the early stage, become more marked as the disease progresses. Very rarely, indeed, however, does pulmonary tuberculosis cause more than a slight diminution in the number of red blood globules, and a slight reduction in the percentage of hæmoglobin. It is very difficult to distinguish these cases of anæmia and chlorosis due to early tuberculous infection from simple anæmia and chlorosis, although it is characteristic of these patients that the ashy gray color of the skin, almost like that of pernicious anæmia, is not accompanied by such invariable reduction in the number of the red blood globules and in the percentage of hæmoglobin as one would expect. Even those cases which show a decided diminution in this respect in the early stage, frequently reveal an improvement in these factors as the disease progresses. This is probably due to the fact that the excessive perspiration of the second stage of phthisis improves the hydræmia by diminishing the watery constitutents of the blood, thus restoring to the normal the relative number of the red blood globules and the percentage of the hæmoglobin. It may be proper here to state, however, that all authorities are practically agreed that, when cases of phthisis have reached the stage of mixed infection with its sepsis and high fever, there is generally found a more or less considerable leucocytosis. V. Limbeck, however, states that miliary tuberculosis is never accompanied by leucocytosis. Many authorities report a marked leucocytosis, and the appearance of large uninuclear leucocytes and eosinophiles after injections of tuberculin. The anæmia of the early stage of phthisis is accompanied by loss of appetite and loss of flesh. These symptoms are frequently the result of another symptom of far more importance, namely, fever.

As to how early a *febrile movement* occurs in this affection, various cases differ. Some chronic cases of phthisis run their course with but little rise of temperature, while others of the more acute variety have a high temperature curve early in the disease; and this factor, owing to the ravages which it causes in the strength and vitality of the patient, becomes the most important symptom of the disease. The causation of the fever in pulmonary tuberculosis is various: 1. The fever following injection of Koch's tuberculin into the blood proves that the absorption of the ptomains and products of decomposition of the tubercle bacillus by the lymphatics and blood-vessels from the tuberculous focus is capable of causing fever in phthisical patients from the earliest stage to the latest. 2. Mixed infection by the germs that cause suppuration, such as the staphylo-coccus, streptococcus, etc., is one of the causes of the fever in cases in which the process has gone on to purulent destruction of tissue. 3. The spread of the inflammatory process in the lungs around the tuber-culous foci as new areas of tissue become involved, either by direct ex-tension or by other means of infection, is a constant factor in the pro-duction of the fever, in both acute and chronic pulmonary tuberculosis.

There is no characteristic temperature curve in any stage of pul-monary phthisis. The well-known fact that a large proportion of phthisical patients who have so-called hectic fever have a remission in the early morning hours, and a gradual rise in temperature until late in the afternoon and evening, when the temperature reaches its height, again to decline after midnight, has popularly given rise to the impression that the febrile movement of phthisis has this charac-ter in every case. But an observation of large numbers of patients will show that fever is not present in every case of pulmonary tuber-culosis, even when large cavities have been formed; that the extent and duration of the fever are not always a measure of the gravity of the disease; and that even in an individual case the temperature varies from day to day, and in different stages of the disease. In some cases, complete remissions occur; in others, there is constant fever. A high temperature occurring daily, and unaffected by treatment, is an element of extreme gravity in the prognosis. In the early stages as well as in later stages of the disease, chills and rigors followed by exacerbations of fever, and later on by a drop of temperature to nor-mal, or, in advanced cases, to even below the normal, occur very frequently in this disease. These chills are probably synchronous with the absorption of ptomains into the blood or mark the begin-ning of new areas of infection. Frequently the fever of pulmonary phthisis, together with the chill which precedes it, resembles the fever of malaria, and can be differentiated only by an examination of the blood during the rigor for the plasmodia malariæ. Very seldom, however, does the fever of pulmonary tuberculosis show any such regular remissions and intermissions as malaria. It must not be forgotten, however, that the two diseases may affect the patient simultaneously.

It will be instructive to illustrate graphically the temperature·
curve of various cases of phthisis. The accompanying charts repre﹕

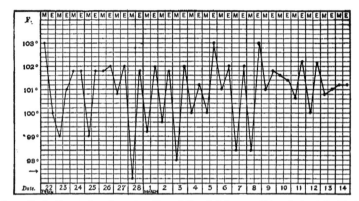

CHART No. 1.—Temperature Curve in a Case of Chronic Pulmonary Tuberculosis at the Monte-
fiore Home.

sent average temperature curves in cases of incipient, chronic, ard
advanced pulmonary tuberculosis.

Upon the severity and permanence of the fever will depend, to a
great extent, the severity of another important symptom which also
occurs very early in the disease, frequently even before the fever is
well marked, and that is excessive *perspiration*. Even the patient
learns to fear this symptom. Although it represents only a hyperactivity of a normal function of the skin, it has much influence in

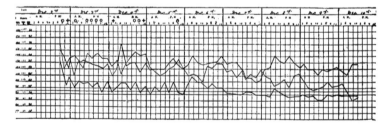

CHART No. 2.—Chronic Phthisis with advanced Pulmonary Changes.

weakening the physical energies of the sufferer. In the early stages
of the disease it generally occurs toward early morning, at two or
three o'clock. The amount of the sweating varies in different cases,
some patients finding the skin only slightly moistened on awakening,

others finding themselves bathed in perspiration, so that they are compelled to change their underclothing as well as the bed clothes. The symptom is most troublesome at night, although some patients perspire more or less constantly. In some, one part of the skin is more affected; in others, other portions. The severity of the symptoms bears a direct proportion to the acuteness of the disease. Patients suffering from advanced tuberculosis with a constant high fever sometimes cease to perspire, the skin on the contrary being dry and hot to the touch. It would appear that the sweating is chiefly dependent upon the fever, being a conservative process for the reduction of the high temperature. It furthermore appears to me that it may well be the result of an attempt on the part of the consti-

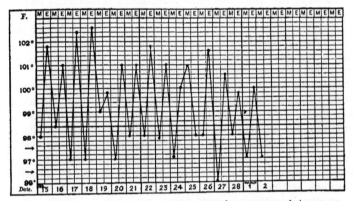

CHART No. 3.—Temperature Curve in a Case of Advanced Pulmonary Tuberculosis at the Monte-fiore Home for Chronic Invalids. The subnormal morning temperature is marked.

tution to get rid, by the skin acting as an emunctory, of the ptomains and poisonous products absorbed into the circulation from the tuberculous focus. In this way one could account for the rashes and sudamina which occur as a result of the hyperidrosis on various portions of the cutaneous surface, regarding them as the irritation of the sweat glands and the surrounding elements of the skin by the tuberculous ptomains contained in the sweat. It is well known that rashes of various types, chiefly erythema, multiform in character, follow the injection of tuberculin in quite a percentage of the cases.

Another very early symptom of this disease, and one which frequently is present even before there is any fever, is *excessive rapidity of the pulse*, tachycardia. At first, this excessive rapidity, 90, 100, or even more in adults, is noticed only on exertion. Later on it becomes constant, and even in fever patients is disproportionate to the temperature. The pulse is usually regular, but thin and fluttering, and is accompanied by the subjective sensation of palpitation of the heart. Various explanations of the causation of this symptom have been given. By some authorities it is supposed to be due to irritation or pressure upon the vagus or phrenic nerves by the tuberculous lymphatic glands in the posterior mediastinum or neck. In advanced cases the symptom has been ascribed to tuberculous disease of the pericardium. In the last stages of pulmonary phthisis, the resistance to the passage of the blood in the diseased lung tissue results in hypertrophy followed by dilatation of the right venticle which would manifest itself by a fluttering rapid pulse. This is not the place to speak of tuberculous disease of the muscles or valves of the heart, although tuberculous myocarditis and endocarditis are not so very rare. I have myself seen a case in which a loud systolic mitral murmur developed as a complication of pulmonary tuberculosis of an extremely chronic type three weeks before death. In this case the development of the murmur was preceded by a chill, followed by high temperature and a convulsion. Unfortunately an autopsy was not allowed, although clinically the diagnosis of ulcerative endocarditis, possibly due to secondary infection, was highly probable. It is proper, however, to refer here to the fact that the general loss in adipose tissue throughout the body would presuppose a similar loss in the fat cushion around the heart of a stout patient. Thus the emaciation, by removing what is practically a support of the heart, becomes a factor in the causation of the weak and rapid pulse in advanced cases of phthisis. The wasting of the heart muscle must be expected to go on *pari passu* with the wasting of the muscular tissue throughout the body. All of these causes which might account for the rapid and fluttering pulse of cases of marked phthisis, can hardly be considered as explaining the rapid and fluttering pulse as a symptom of the prodromal stage. This latter appears to me to be the result of a deleterious action on the nervous mechanism of the heart, which is caused by the absorbed ptomains formed as a result of the activity of the tubercle bacillus.

The above symptoms occur in the prodromal and early stage of pulmonary tuberculosis, although they continue and progress through the later stages of the disease. Blueness of the lips, rapid heart action and pulse, slight rise of temperature, especially toward night, and night sweats are almost entitled to be considered as placing upon the physician the burden of proving the non-existence of tuberculosis. At least, they must awaken the attention to the importance of repeated physical examinations and examinations of the sputum.

Local Symptoms.

We now come to consider symptoms of tuberculosis of a more local character, which do not occur until physical changes, even if slight in degree, begin to take place in the lungs. Frequently even when there is considerable cough, which is the first of these symptoms to which I shall devote my attention, and characteristic expectoration, the most careful physical examination will fail to reveal any organic changes in the lungs, recognizable by either percussion or auscultation. But fortunately at this stage the broken-down disorganized tubercles and lung tissue begin to appear in the sputum, these elements having gained access to air cells or terminal bronchi, and being thence expelled to the outer air. The most important finding in the sputum in such cases is the tubercle bacillus. Its presence in the expectoration shows the existence of the bacillus in the deeper air passages. Its absence in the sputum does not equally imply its absence from the lungs; hence the importance of repeated examinations of the sputum when constitutional symptoms of the character I have described point to the suspicion of pulmonary tuberculosis.

Cough being a reflex manifestation of an irritation of the mucous membrane of the respiratory tract, presupposes the presence of irritating material, such as sputum or other foreign substance, in some portion of this tract. Thus it will be seen that a cough can be the result of an irritation by a neoplasm, an enlarged bronchial gland, or inflammatory conditions of the mucous membrane of the larynx, trachea, bronchi, air cells, or even pleura. It may also be a reflex manifestation as a result of an irritation of nerve branches distinct from those of the air passages, as, for example, the cough which accompanies nausea, hysterical cough, etc. A cough thus in itself does not even indicate disease of the respiratory tract, and yet cough is so frequent in pulmonary diseases that it is considered the most common symptom of pulmonary tuberculosis. With relation to cough we have to consider its character and its frequency. A loud cough of barking character indicates disease of the larynx and irritation of the vocal cords. This does not always signify that the original cause of the cough is disease of the larynx, for frequently a cough of a softer character, due to tracheal or bronchial lesions, so irritates the glottis as to cause a secondary hyperæmia of the vocal cords, which results in giving a barking character to the cough. This irritation of the glottis necessarily results from the fact that cough is mechanically produced by the forced expulsion of air through a closed glottis by the action of the expiratory muscles. A cough due to a bronchial or tracheal irritation is softer in character. It is harsh, however, if there be expelled but little sputum, glairy and white and of extreme consistency, while it is much softer if the sputum which causes the irritation is more plentiful in quantity and non-tenacious in quality. A cough in the early stages of tuberculosis is generally only a slight hack, occurring at any time during the waking hours, and followed by the expulsion of scarcely any sputum. It is probably the manifestation of the irritation of a tuberculous focus upon the mucous membrane of a terminal bronchus. As the disease progresses the cough becomes longer in duration, and has for its object the expulsion of a white, glairy, tenacious mucus, which is the cause of the irritation in the deeper bronchi. This mucus is so sticky and has such a tendency to adhere to the walls of the air passages in its progress upwards, that spasmodic attacks of coughing, long in duration, sometimes terminating in vomiting, are required for its expulsion. Later on the secondary bronchitis which complicates the formation of tubercle results in the effusion into the bronchus of large quantities of mucus, the sputum material becomes more plentiful and fluid in character, and the cough, although more frequent, becomes correspondingly easy and soft, the expectoration being raised with no difficulty.

The frequency of the cough in cases of tuberculosis of the lungs varies with the amount and character of the sputum. The latter, as we shall presently see, varies under different conditions, and its quantity is not always a measure of the gravity and extent of the disease. Many patients go through pulmonary tuberculosis of long. duration with comparatively little cough, while others suffer more inconvenience from the cough than from all the symptoms of their malady combined. Some patients cough more at night than in the day. The majority of patients cough most in the morning, owing to the fact that the sputum which has collected during sleep exerts its reflex irritation immediately on waking, which does not cease until the patient has expelled all of the sputum. Some patients cough more on lying down even in the waking hours, others more in the erect posture. In some cases lying on the diseased side gives rise to cough, while in others lying on the healthy side causes an excess of coughing. Many of these apparent inconsistencies could be explained by the fact that these various positions in individual cases are favorable to the action of gravity acting upon the sputum in such a manner as to bring it in contact with the bronchial mucous membrane.

A peculiar cough occurs in some cases, when the patient has been asleep for a time. He suddenly wakes with a spasmodic cough of the most violent character, which causes him to jump up from bed, and cough somewhat like patients with pertussis, until vomiting relieves the attack. The cough is probably due to a small amount of mucus having gained access to the larynx, either from the mouth or from the trachea. This variety of cough seriously disturbs the rest of the patient. The passage of small particles of food into the larynx during swallowing, owing to functional weakness of the epiglottis, is occasionally seen as a cause of violent cough in advanced cases of pulmonary tuberculosis. In such cases the patient is so distressed by this cough as to dread the necessity of eating or drinking, and the appetite is accordingly seriously disturbed.

In the cases in which the attacks of coughing are long continued and severe, hoarseness frequently occurs, sometimes temporary in duration, and sometimes lasting throughout the disease. Hoarseness in pulmonary phthisis, however, apart from those cases in which irritation of the vocal cords by the cough is the cause, may be due to laryngeal tuberculosis, catarrh of the larynx and vocal cords, owing to the irritative action of the sputum, or, finally, to paralysis of one or both vocal cords. Either of these will cause a serious diminution in the intensity and quality of the voice. In almost all cases of pulmonary phthisis the voice is lower in pitch and diminished in power. In many cases, however, of very severe pulmonary disease, the voice remains clear and ringing even to an abnormal extent. Many professional singers, suffering from tuberculosis of the lungs, retain the full sweetness and power of the voice. This, however, is the exception, while a gradually increasing aphonia is the rule. At the final stages of the disease some patients suffer from such absolute aphonia as to be inaudible in speaking.

In every case, cough, as a symptom, should be carefully investigated, not only on the theory that it is caused by pulmonary diseases, but with a view to the possible exclusion of tuberculosis, by finding other causes for its occurrence.

Closely connected with and standing in a causative relation to the cough is the *sputum*. This varies in its gross appearance, such as color, consistence, quantity, and component elements. I have already spoken of the fact that the cough in its earliest stages is followed by very little expectoration; later on the expectoration consists of a whitish, glairy mucus, rather transparent and viscid in character. In the further stages of the disease this sputum becomes more opaque and yellowish in color; it is apt to be streaked with reddish and rust brown spots, due to blood, and in advanced cases, especially those in which cavities and dilated bronchi have been formed, to be intermingled with pus. Different observers have also found the color vary with the presence of various chromogenic bacteria. The quantity of the sputum varies. In some patients the quantity is small, in others so great that large receptacles are filled within the course of twenty-four hours. The expulsion of such large masses of sputum constitutes a serious drain upon the vitality of the patient, on account of the physical effort required to expel it. When cavities are present the sputum is especially plentiful, of a foul, disgusting odor like that from gangrene of the lungs, and of a sweetish taste. The same is true in cases in which bronchiectasis is present.

The composition of the sputum is important, chiefly because here the presence of tubercle bacilli gives indisputable evidence of tuberculosis, even if the physical examination fails to reveal any changes. It must not be forgotten, however, that in tuberculosis which is propagated through the blood-vessels, and when a tuberculous focus has not yet opened communication with a bronchus, tubercle bacilli would not be present in the sputum, so that their absence does not exclude tuberculosis. It is not the function of the writer of a clinical article on tuberculosis to speak of the bacteriological technique necessary to reveal the presence of tubercle bacilli and other bacteria in the expectoration, but it is proper to indicate in brief the component elements of tuberculous sputum. In addition to tubercle bacilli various observers have found numerous other forms of bacteria, whose chief importance lies in the causation of the "mixed infection," which so modifies pulmonary tuberculosis, adding to the baneful nature of the disease and lending it its multifarious aspects. These bacteria are all the forms of the septic bacteria, such as streptococcus pyogenes, staphylococcus pyogenes aureus and albus, the bacillus pyocyaneus which imparts a bluish color to the sputum, the pneumococcus, the tetragonus, and numerous other bacteria. None of these, however, is as constant as the tubercle bacillus.

When the sputum is examined microscopically for elements other than bacteria, it is found to contain pus corpuscles, epithelium of the mucous membrane of the larynx, trachea, and bronchi, pavement and cylindrical epithelium, and granular cells, leucocytes, red blood corpuscles and detritus, and broken-down lung-tissue elements. Among the latter the most important are elastic fibres; they occur whenever lung tissue has undergone destruction by a pathological process. They are the most resistant anatomical elements of lung tissue, and before the discovery of the tubercle bacillus were considered the most characteristic element of the sputum (see Fig. 11).

These elastic fibres are easily found in fresh thin layers of unstained specimens of tuberculous sputum, and occur as frequently as in ninety per cent. of the cases of pulmonary tuberculosis. Although, as I have said, these elastic fibres in the sputum are the result of destruction of lung tissue by the tuberculous process, and would, therefore, appear in the sputum chiefly during the third stage of the disease, when the consolidated tuberculous areas are breaking down, resulting in the formation of cavities, yet they are seen frequently in the sputum of even the early stage of the disease, when the destructive process is not yet sufficiently extensive to give rise to physical changes in the lungs more grave than localized catarrhal bronchitis. The chemical components of the sputum, found mostly in sputum which has remained in the body for a length of time, and thus undergone changes of decomposition, have been extensively studied, and

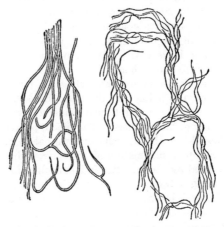

Fig. 11.—Elastic Fibres from Tuberculous Sputum (Bizzozero)

are of interest chiefly in regard to the albuminoid bodies which they contain. Several investigators have even isolated from the sputum a digestive ferment.

Hæmoptysis.—The consideration of the blood so frequently expectorated in phthisis is of much greater importance. Indeed, it is of the greatest importance when the quantity of blood expectorated is sufficient to endanger the life of the patient. This symptom, which logically is properly considered in connection with the sputum, although not uniform in pulmonary tuberculosis, is considered by the patient as of the gravest import. Authorities differ as to the frequency with which it occurs in the course of pulmonary tuberculosis. Some statisticians affirm that it occurs in fully two-thirds of all cases of the disease, others have found it less frequent. There is reason to believe that climate, that is to say increased atmospheric pressure, has much to do with the liability to hemorrhage, and increase in the general humidity of the atmosphere predisposes to hemorrhage in a tuberculous patient. Thus, it will be observed that cases of pulmonary hemorrhage occur in groups about at the same time, and generally in humid weather. In my own practice I have long noted that, when one of my tuberculous patients has a severe hemorrhage, other cases are quite sure to come under my care at about the same time. It does not appear that age and sex are predisposing factors to hemorrhage from the lungs, except in so far as they are predisposing factors to the contraction of pulmonary tuberculosis.

Hemorrhage from the lungs may occur during any stage of the disease, from the earliest period when there is only the localized bronchitis with slight surrounding dulness, in the second stage of peribronchitis and extensive consolidation of lung tissue, and with greatest frequency in the cavernous stage, when the friable walls of vessels surrounding large cavities break under slight provocation, and give rise to severe hemorrhages.

In the earliest stages severe hemorrhage is frequently the first intimation that there is pulmonary disease. Indeed, in these cases, the hemorrhages were for a long time considered the etiological factor in the causation of the phthisis. The blood, poured out from the broken blood-vessel into the air cells or terminal bronchi, was supposed to give rise to inflammation of the surrounding lung tissue, resulting in a localized bronchitis and consolidation. That such blood clots, forming a favorable nidus for the development of tubercle bacilli, could explain cases of active pulmonary tuberculosis, in which, before the initial hemorrhage, there was only a quiescent tuberculous focus, giving no symptoms, is possible. But the fact that tubercle bacilli are discovered in the expectorated blood in these cases, even if no physical signs of pulmonary disease are present, is sufficient proof that the tuberculosis precedes the hemorrhage. As to the pathological process which results in the hemorrhage in these early cases, views differ. What probably occurs is that a tuberculous focus so weakens the walls of a terminal blood-vessel that the ordinary blood pressure results in a minute aneurysmal dilatation. This miliary aneurysm, if it may be so called, bursts and pours out its blood, small in quantity, as a rule, into the air cell. This hemorrhage is checked spontaneously by the formation of a thrombus and the influence of the pressure of the surrounding healthy lung elements. When such miliary aneurysms, either single or multiple, communicate with a terminal bronchus, so situated that the blood poured into it is readily evacuated, then the hemorrhage is checked only by a blood clot, which forms more slowly owing to the fact that the blood is coughed up as fast as it flows out. In such a case the hemorrhage may be quite severe.

Hemorrhages in pulmonary tuberculosis occur with by far the greatest frequency during the third stage of the disease, when cavities are being formed. Here the hemorrhage may be due to an eroded blood-vessel, which, if large, may cause a fatal loss of blood. Or again it may be due to the bursting of vessels, the seat of the aneurysmal process, above described, and either located in the wall of a cavity or even passing across a cavity. The hemorrhage may also arise from the bursting of blood-vessels in congested areas of lung surrounding a cavity, dilated tuberculous bronchus, or other tuberculous area. The amount of blood poured out varies from enough to cause a mere tinge of red in a few mouthfuls of sputum up to a quart or more. The danger in the severe cases lies not only in the amount of blood lost, but also in the more important consideration as to whether the patient can get rid of the blood from the trachea and larynx as rapidly as it is poured into them from the bleeding bronchus. If not, death by suffocation is the result. Frequently the small hemorrhages are preceded by the appearance of a few slight streaks of blood in the sputum for some time before the real bleeding occurs. At other times there is little warning before a severe hemorrhage sets in. It rarely happens that a hemorrhage ends fatally in a few minutes, although this does occur occasionally. The prognosis of a hemorrhage in a case of pulmonary tuberculosis with cavities is more serious than in incipient cases.

These hemorrhages are brought on by various causes, such as excessive coughing, physical exertions, violent exercise, increased humidity of the atmosphere, the inhalation of irritating gases and vapors, anger, excitement, and any condition that augments the blood pressure. In a given case of pulmonary hemorrhage it is of great importance to recognize the lungs as the source of the hemorrhage. The color of the blood in these cases is bright red. As the hemorrhage subsides it grows lighter in color, until, finally, only a foamy sputum is expectorated. After a day or two small, black clots are generally brought up, intermingled with the ordinary elements of the sputum. In cases of even moderate severity it can generally be determined that the blood is coming from the lungs by hearing bronchial râles over the affected side of the chest. If the hemorrhage be severe these râles can be heard in the larger bronchi and trachea even by the bystanders. In cases of even small pulmonary hemorrhages careful auscultation will localize bronchial râles over a limited area of the chest, either in front or at the back. Having heard these râles, one can affirm the pulmonary character of the hemorrhage, but it must not be forgotten that even in the absence of these râles the bleeding may still be pulmonary in origin. Not all pulmonary hemorrhage, however, is caused by tuberculosis. It may be due to aortic aneurysm, certain organic lesions of the heart valves or muscle, pneumonia, gangrene of the lung, pernicious anæmia, hæmophilia, pulmonary infections, tumors of the lung causing congestions of a limited lung area, etc., etc. Vicarious menstruation through hæmoptysis has been occasionally reported. All of these instances of hemorrhage should be carefully and frequently investigated as to the presence of tubercle bacilli in the sputum before the case is negatived as to the existence of pulmonary tuberculosis. The vomiting of blood (hæmatemesis) may be mistaken for pulmonary hemorrhage and *vice versa*. The vomited blood from hemorrhage into the stomach is generally blackish and clotted, except when poured out in very large quantities. The points already mentioned as characteristic of pulmonary hemorrhage will help to differentiate these cases. Blood from the posterior nares, nasopharynx, mouth, and gums will sometimes be mistaken as of pulmonary origin. A careful investigation is necessary to clear up doubtful cases.

The symptoms I have hitherto described have been those which may be present in the incipient stage of pulmonary tuberculosis. I have discussed their manifestations in the later and final stages of the disease, to avoid the repetition of again enumerating these symptoms in describing clinical manifestations in the advanced stages of the malady. The local symptoms I have detailed are uniformly present in every instance of tuberculosis, although cases vary as to which of these manifestations is prominent, and which is subordinate.

There are other local symptoms, however, not uniformly present, although occurring to a greater or less extent in the large majority of the cases. Of these local symptoms, pain and dyspnœa are the most prominent, although by no means general in tuberculosis of the lungs.

Pain is not usually a troublesome symptom in pulmonary tuberculosis. It is generally localized over the diseased area of the lung, and most perceptible to the patient when taking a deep inspiration or when, on coughing, sneezing, or any other more or less violent exertion, the movements of the lungs are brought into play. Occasionally there is pain on pressure over the diseased area of the lung. Even the percussion on the part of the examiner causes the patient uneasiness. The degree of pain varies. Sometimes it is sharp and lancinating, the patient feeling as though cut with a knife on taking deep inspiration. Sometimes he complains of being unable to take a full breath, on account of the sharp pain. Occasionally the pain is localized over the terminations of the intercostal nerves. It is necessary also to mention that the general constitutional condition of the patient causes a hyperæsthesia of the muscles and skin of the whole body, which results in pains in the limbs and muscles analogous to a feeling of weariness rather than of pain. The cause of the pains over the diseased area of lung is manifestly the pleurisy which almost always affects the pleura at the location of the pulmonary disease. This pain is the result also of the stretching of the pleuritic adhesions with every movement of the lung. Destruction of lung tissue itself, unless the pleura be involved, gives rise to no pain. Nerve trunks involved and pressed upon by tuberculous glands, either in the mediastinal spaces or in the pleural cavities, will give rise to neuralgia in the course of the distribution of such nerves. Abdominal pain may be the result of a diaphragmatic pleurisy. Tuberculous neuritis, complicating pulmonary tuberculosis, is not to be considered under this head.

Dyspnœa is a rather interesting symptom in this connection, not on account of its frequency, for it is not by any means frequent, but on the contrary because it is absent in so many cases in which the extent of the lesion would lead one to expect its presence. When the progress of the disease is slow, dyspnœa rarely supervenes except, perhaps, in the very last few days or even hours. Enormous and numerous cavities and large areas of consolidation may be present, and yet the patient suffer only very slightly from dyspnœa, and then only upon extreme exertion or excitement. Even then the dyspnœa is rather the result of the increased rapidity of the heart's action, than of the diminished breathing surface. Cases are not infrequent, however, in which dyspnœa occurs in spasmodic attacks, closely resembling those of asthma. Such attacks occur more or less frequently, and can with difficulty be differentiated from spasmodic asthma. The difficulty is all the greater owing to the presence of the whistling and sibilant râles which mask all other auscultatory symptoms. In these cases careful percussion and examination of the sputum, together with a subjective history of tuberculous symptoms, will enable one to arrive at a diagnosis. In the interval, too, of the spasmodic asthmatic attacks the physical signs pointing to pulmonary tuberculosis can be elicited.

Although, as I have said, dyspnœa is rare except in the last stages of pulmonary tuberculosis, irrespective of the extent of lung surface involved in the disease, a striking exception to this general rule occurs in cases in which a sudden involvement of large, fresh areas of pulmonary surface by inflammatory disturbance takes place.

Thus a pneumonia involving hitherto healthy areas of lung tissue, or the sudden occurrence of pleuritic effusion, will give rise to dyspnœa, frequently of a very severe type. We must not forget, too, that the involvement of the vagus, recurrent laryngeal, or phrenic nerves, either from pressure by enlarged or cheesy lymphatic glands or through tuberculous neuritis, may cause a dyspnœa owing to the disturbance of the respiratory function controlled by these nerves. It may be proper here also to mention that paralysis or irritation of the nerves supplying the muscles of the larynx, owing either to these causes or to local laryngeal tuberculosis, may cause most frightful laryngeal dyspnœa. Dyspnœa due to the latter cause, together with difficulty in deglutition (dysphagia), should properly be considered in connection with laryngeal tuberculosis.

Symptoms in Other Organs than the Lungs.

I have already discussed certain early constitutional symptoms of pulmonary tuberculosis, both in their early manifestation and in their development throughout the course of the disease. Such symptoms were fever, rapid pulse, changes in the constitution of the blood, and the excessive perspiration. There are other constitutional disturbances which come on generally when the disease is fully developed. I have preferred to discuss these after the essentially local symptoms. Among these constitutional effects the most important, because the most frequent, are disturbances of the digestive tract, the stomach and bowels.

The *stomach* is frequently disturbed as regards its function in pulmonary phthisis, although it cannot be said that the character of these altered gastric manifestations is at all characteristic, either of the disease in general or of any stage of the disease. For while some patients have normal appetite and normal digestive power, others suffer from almost complete anorexia, and the little food they take is vomited. There is also a third class of patients whose appetite is excessive, while the functional activity of the stomach is so increased that the abnormal quantity of the food is properly digested. Such patients are very apt to increase in weight, while all the physical signs show a constant progress in the tuberculous disease. The factors which determine the appearance of gastric symptoms in cases of phthisis are the fever and the cough. Patients suffering from fever more or less constant are very apt to have loss of appetite, while the presence of free HCl in non-febrile phthisical patients is replaced by the lack of free acid in the stomach contents of patients suffering from fever. This latter condition is very apt to be present in the second and third stages of the disease. The motor power of the stomach in fever patients also suffers, especially in advanced cases, so that frequently these patients suffer from the symptoms of dilatation of the stomach in addition to the more essential symptoms of their disease. In some cases of phthisis, dyspepsia is frequently the causative element in the lowering of the vitality of the patient, which enables the tubercle bacillus to find a nidus in the lungs, and in such cases the gastric symptoms for a long time monopolize the attention of the patient and even of the physician, until a hemorrhage or persistent cough calls attention to the lungs, and an examination discloses marked physical changes. The cough also frequently influences the digestive functions by causing vomiting, owing to spasmodic contraction of the diaphragm. In these cases the thick viscid sputum is expelled only after violent spasm, which is relieved by vomiting the contents of the stomach. After such vomiting some patients refill their stomachs with food, while others are so exhausted that they have no desire to eat, and a serious disturbance of the appetite results. Catarrhal gastritis in phthisis is frequently the result of injudicious medicinal and dietetic treatment of the disease, thus adding the horrors of dyspepsia to the emaciating effect of the tuberculosis. The swallowing of masses of foul sputum, and the constant odor of disorganized and decaying animal matter which is always present with the patient, have no slight influence in the production of the catarrhal gastritis and the anorexia. The typhoid condition which marks the closing stage in many cases of phthisis has its characteristic gastric and intestinal disturbances.

The *bowels* are frequently absolutely normal in cases of pulmonary tuberculosis. In other cases, however, especially in the early stages, there is sometimes constipation. The latter symptoms generally occur in patients in whom there is increased appetite with good digestion. In many cases of phthisis, however, particularly in the more advanced stages of the disease, diarrhœa is a troublesome symptom. This diarrhœa may be due to a catarrhal inflammation of the mucous membrane of the small intestines, or more frequently to a colitis of the catarrhal or ulcerative type. These ulcers are not necessarily of a tuberculous character, but are simply erosions, the results of advanced catarrhal lesions of the bowel. Etiologically they may be due to irritative action of the chemical constituents of the sputum swallowed by the patients, which is so frequently the cause of the gastric catarrh. The diarrhœa resulting from these ulcers is extremely difficult to treat and control. It is frequently temporary, stopping as the inflammation or ulcerative conditions heal, and returning when they again irritate the bowel by their presence. These patients frequently suffer form colic in connection with their diarrhœa. In addition to these cases diarrhœa frequently occurs in phthisical patients as a result of inflammatory or tuberculous changes in the follicles of Lieberkühn, and the lymphatic vessels and glands. Tuberculous disease of the bowels also causes diarrhœa. Occasionally blood appears in the stools, owing to hemorrhages from the ulcers above described or from tuberculous ulcers. In this connection we must not forget to allude to the frequency of hemorrhoids in these patients, owing to the enlargement of the superficial hemorrhoidal veins. This is probably the result of the venous engorgement which is the effect of the slowness of the portal circulation accompanying the general asthenia characteristic of the disease. Owing to the weak condition of the patient, both the organic and functional diarrhœas are of the utmost gravity. Their importance is increased by the fact that most of these diarrhœas are extremely difficult to check.

Partly in consequence of the fever, the sleeplessness, the loss of appetite, vomiting, cough, and diarrhœa, and partly in consequence of the toxæmia which affects secondarily all of the vital functions, there results one of the most characteristic symptoms of the disease, namely,

Emaciation.—This consists of a loss of all the fatty tissues of the body and an atrophy and wasting of even the muscular tissue. The amount of emaciation varies greatly, being less in patients in good circumstances who have good care, and in whom the disease progresses slowly and is not accompanied by stomach disturbances, while it is more marked in those in whom the disease progresses more rapidly, and in whom the vital disturbances are more serious. The fat disappears first from those portions of the body in which its deposit is most marked, as on the abdomen, and an important symptom which early attracts the attention of the patient is the fact that his clothes are growing too large for him. Of all the causes of this loss of flesh, the fever is pre-eminently the first, but all of the factors I have enumerated are distinctly important in this connection as causative agents. Here it is interesting to call attention to a peculiar fibrillary contraction of the muscles which is seen in patients who are very much emaciated. This fibrillary twitching, involuntary in character, is most frequently seen on the chest. It is elicited by sharply stroking the pectoralis muscles with the edge of the finger. It is best seen in muscles that lie close to bones; thus the deltoid, the triceps, and the pectoralis, will show this symptom in advanced cases of tuberculosis. It is a symptom due to the general muscular atrophy which is present in all wasting diseases.

Integuments.—The facies of the phthisical is so characteristic that it is not astonishing to find that the integument of such patients undergoes constant changes. We have already spoken of the pale color of such patients. Some are not only pale, but the skin has a gray tint; the veins shine through a transparent integument and some patients are even livid and cyanotic. The skin is readily sunburnt, contrasting forcibly with parts of the body that have been protected from the sun. The extreme softness of the surface of the skin in patients suffering from phthisis is of common observation. The terminal phalanges of the fingers and toes are clubbed and thickened. The fingers are darker in color than the rest of the hand, owing to the slowness of the capillary circulation. The nails take on a curved contour transversely and longitudinally, and are apt to become roughened and scaly. The hair falls out, and becomes less glistening, and is apt to turn gray early. The hyperidrosis is very apt to cause chromophytosis or pityriasis versicolor, especially on the chest and back. In the last stages of the disease a pityriasis somewhat resembling pityriasis rubra is occasionally seen. Chloasma chiefly marked upon the forehead and cheeks is frequently observed. In the last stages of the disease there is very apt to be in phthisical patients œdema, particularly of the feet and legs, even in cases in whom there is no tubercular lesion of the heart or kidneys, or disturbance of the portal circulation. This is due to the intense anæmia and slowness of the venous return.

Urine.—In the earlier stages of tuberculosis of the lungs the urine shows, as a rule, no changes from the normal, either quantitatively or qualitatively. Later on, as the hyperidrosis increases, the quantity of urine is apt to be diminished. When amyloid degeneration of the kidneys occurs, there is generally albumin present, occasionally granular and hyaline casts and pus globules. The presence of tubercle bacilli in the urine signifies tuberculous degeneration somewhere in the genitourinary tract. Indican is occasionally found, according to some authorities, especially in children. Ehrlich's diazo reaction is present in advanced cases of phthisis quite frequently, but does not always indicate an acute exacerbation of the symptoms, nor has it any diagnostic value.

I must not neglect here to call attention to the frequency with which pulmonary tuberculosis complicates diabetes mellitus. So frequent is this condition that in every case of pulmonary tuberculosis the urine should be carefully and repeatedly examined for sugar.

On the part of the *nervous system* we have symptoms referable to the peripheral nerves and symptoms due to disturbances of the brain and spinal cord. A multiple neuritis, slow in progress and gradual

in development, is occasionally seen. This causes paralysis or pare-
sis of various nerves, atrophy of muscles supplied by them, and various anæsthesias, hyperæsthesias, and paræsthesias. We do not
here include cases due to real tuberculous degeneration of nerve
trunks, but rather such as are due to pressure of tuberculous lymphatic glands upon nerve trunks or to a toxic neuritis. We must not
forget to mention the comparatively frequent occurrence of herpes
zoster, particularly over the areas supplied by the intercostal nerves.
In these cases the affection runs its usual course, accompanied by
intense pain, and followed by attacks in other neighboring areas.

On the part of the *brain*, motor disturbances, such as convulsions
and paralyses, are rare except in cases in which there is ground for
assuming a tuberculous meningitis or cerebritis. Mono- or hemi-
plegias certainly indicate a grave lesion of the brain structures.
Phthisical patients in the later stages of the disease, however, suffer
from. visual troubles due to a disturbance of the circulation and
atrophies in the optic nerve and other structures of the eye. Distant
vision, I have observed, becomes more difficult as the disease advances. Convulsions, however, do occur as a result of the high temperature, which follows a chill, especially in young patients. Such
chills, for instance, are observed some days after a severe hemorrhage, owing to septic absorption from decomposing blood clots.
Headaches occur frequently in phthisis, as in other febrile and
wasting diseases. They have no diagnostic importance.

The *mental condition* of phthisical patients is peculiar. Every
one is familiar with the tendency which is marked in these sufferers
to minimize the gravity of the disease with which they are affected.
They readily believe the physician who speaks of their condition as
a "cold" or a "bronchitis," even when they sojourn in an institution
devoted to the treatment of pulmonary tuberculosis, and are surrounded with patients suffering from this disease. Thus a physician
who was under my care in the last stages of pulmonary tuberculosis,
finding much relief from an occasional injection of morphine given to
quiet excessive pleuritic pains, whispered to me one morning that he
felt certain that he would recover soon, if I would consent to let him
have his morphine several times a day, instead of occasionally as the
pain indicated. Other patients are very much depressed and worry
over their condition, notwithstanding earnest assurances of their recovery. Such patients are apt to pass sleepless nights in thinking
over their "hopeless state," the digestion becomes disturbed, and not
only do they materially imperil their chances of recovery by their
gloomy forebodings, but occasionally develop real melancholia. I
have seen several cases of melancholia complicating phthisis. Occa-

sionally the melancholia gets well, but sometimes it persists to the end.   In such cases illusions, delusions, and hallucinations, not connected with the disease, develop and the insanity becomes a prominent factor in the patient's death.   The melancholia may be complicated by violent attacks of mania.   A patient who was under my care for pulmonary tuberculosis for years, suddenly developed a melancholia with delusions of persecution based upon fancied criminal acts in early life.   Within a few days after the melancholia set in, a violent mania supervened, in which she almost succeeded in cutting her throat with a broken window pane.   This mania persisted until her death within two weeks.

The mental ability of patients suffering from pulmonary tuberculosis is generally not affected, although the mental processes are frequently slower, and memory is no longer so acute.   The energy of the patient is generally diminished, owing to the weakness following the fever and emaciation.   Many patients, however, keep at their work, dying almost in harness.   Thus a clerk under my care died of hemorrhage at his desk at the counting-house.   Another young man, although suffering from advanced phthisis with high fever in the afternoon, kept at his work up to three days before death, contrary to all advice.   The absorption of the tubercle proteins into the circulation, the fever, and the sweating are the chief causes of the loss of strength.   The patient is frequently unable, owing to the loss in strength, to work at his occupation, although he earnestly desires to do so; nevertheless, the working ability of the patient is interfered with, as a rule, only in the advanced stages of the disease.   Especially is this true of patients who follow a sedentary occupation.

The *sexual power* of phthisical male patients is not altered in any way in the early period of the disease.   In the later stages of the malady, however, many of these patients have no erection under any circumstances, and have no desire for sexual gratification.   This is true even of those patients who, in health, ran to excess in the gratification of the sexual passion.   To this general rule there are, however, many exceptions, and patients have been reported who had sexual intercourse almost up to the day of their death.   In women, as a rule, also, advanced tuberculosis is accompanied by a loss of sexual desire.   This does not preclude, however, many consumptive women, who suffer the embraces of their husbands, from becoming pregnant.   A more pitiable picture than that of a patient in the final stages of pulmonary phthisis undergoing the torments and pains of labor can hardly be imagined.   It is very common, however, for women suffering from the later stages of pulmonary tuberculosis to lose their menses.   This is probably due to the intense anæmia, and may be an etiological factor in the fortunate rarity with which women suffering from advanced phthisis become pregnant. Many patients, however, ascribe all of their symptoms, *post hoc, propter hoc,* to the cessation of the menses.

Physical Signs.

The physical examination of a patient with pulmonary tuberculosis has for its object the eliciting of symptoms by means of, first, general inspection of the patient, especially of the conformation, measurements, and movements of the thorax; second, percussion of the chest walls; third, auscultation; fourth, palpation. While the aggregate of symptoms thus obtained will yield a very fair conception of the physical condition of the lungs and the changes they have undergone, it cannot be said that any of them are pathognomonic of pulmonary tuberculosis. They simply indicate a physical condition of the lung tissue and the chest walls which can then be considered positively due to tuberculosis only when the presence of tubercle bacilli in the sputum has been demonstrated. It is evident, too, that, since pulmonary tuberculosis is a generally chronic and progressive affection, the physical changes in the lungs, as they progress, give rise to changes in the physical symptoms elicited by inspection, auscultation, and percussion. It is only by a careful study of the relations between the pathological changes and the physical signs which accompany them, especially from an etiological standpoint, that we can gain from a physical examination of the thorax a knowledge of the condition of the lungs.

INSPECTION.

Inspection of the patient generally reveals a thorax of the form known as the paralytic thorax; that is to say, a thorax in which the longitudinal diameter is increased, and the horizontal, particularly the anteroposterior diameter is diminished. The scapulæ are found to stand away from the ribs, the angles being prominent, the intercostal spaces are deeply placed and appear wider than usual, the muscles of the chest are atrophied, and the vertebral column is more deeply buried between the scapulæ than normal. This kind of chest is considered characteristic of phthisis. It is the so-called phthisical chest. It is supposed that individuals with such chests are more liable to contract tuberculosis than others. As a rule, however, it simply indicates that the patient is weak, being lean and emaciated, and not necessarily that the emaciation is the result of a predisposition to tuberculosis; nor does it indicate that the patient is emaciated as a result of an existing pulmonary tuberculosis. Weak patients do, when subjected to infection by the tubercle bacilli, contract the disease more readily than stronger people. That the latter do contract tuberculosis quite frequently, however, is shown by the numerous cases in which a strong, muscular physique and well-shaped chest have not prevented the patient from acquiring tuberculosis. Localized irregularities in the thoracic wall or in its circumference during rest, inspiration, and expiration furnish important data as to the condition of the lungs and pleura. Such changes in action and diameters of the chest wall are present only when the tuberculous process has so far progressed as to cause marked lesions in the lungs. Thus consolidation of lung tissue, if extensive, will cause a diminished respiratory movement in the corresponding portion of the chest. The formation of a cavity and shrinking of lung tissue that has undergone fibroid changes will show a corresponding falling in of the chest wall over the seat of lesion.

The most frequent falling in of the chest wall is seen over the left apex, and next in frequency over the right apex underneath the clavicles, because it is these portions of the lung which most frequently are primarily affected. Much of the apparent retraction in this region is due to wasting of the chest muscles, owing especially to the diminished amount of labor which the phthisical patient naturally exerts.

Palpation.

Palpation offers but few indications of tuberculous pulmonary disease in the earlier stages. Later on, however, we can gain some confirmatory knowledge of changes, the existence of which have been revealed by auscultation and percussion. Thus with the palmar surface of the examiner's hand pressed against corresponding portions of two sides of the chest it becomes easy to recognize increased or diminished amplitude of the expansion and recession of the chest walls with the inspiratory and expiratory movements. A diminution in the extent of these movements occurs over portions of the lungs which have suffered consolidation or infiltration, or fibroid changes. Increased resistance is felt over extensively diseased areas. By palpation the vocal fremitus, normally existing, is felt to be increased or diminished over the diseased areas of the lungs. Especially is this true when the diseased areas are bound by pleuritic adhesion of the chest wall. Thus increased vocal fremitus would indicate tuberculous cheesy degeneration, fibroid degeneration, or pneumonic infiltration of the portions of the lung over which the symptom was appreciable. Diminished or absent vocal fremitus would indicate a tuberculous pleurisy with effusion localized over the affected area, or a pneumothorax with no patent communication into the bronchi. A cavity separated from the surface of the lung by consolidated pulmonary tissue will also cause increased vocal fremitus, especially if the cavity be near the surface. Absence of any change in vocal fremitus of the two sides is neither a positive nor a negative indication of disease. In tuberculous, as in other empyemas palpation of the intercostal spaces over the pus-containing pleural cavity will detect a feeling of fluctuation if a sharp blow be given on the same half of the chest at a point distant from the palpating hand.

PERCUSSION.

Percussion furnishes valuable indication of pulmonary disease, when the percussion note produced by the pleximeter or the fingers of the examiner differs from the normal note of the corresponding healthy portion of lung either in quality, pitch, intensity, or duration. Here, again, corresponding portions of the chest walls must be examined to differentiate between the normal and the abnormal, making proper allowances for areas of dulness or flatness due to underlying solid viscera, especially the heart on the left side and the liver on the right. It must not be forgotten that changes in the lungs can cause corresponding changes in the percussion note only when they have advanced to a considerable size. Thus diminished resonance on percussion will not show itself unless the consolidated area on the surface of the lung has a circumference of 4 to 6 cm. and a thickness of 2 cm., while dulness will not appear unless the area is at least 5 cm. thick. It follows, therefore, that the percussion note will not be much altered when the patient suffers only from isolated tuberculous masses, or even in cases of advanced miliary tuberculosis. In the latter case, indeed, there may be even increased pulmonary resonance or even tympanitic resonance owing to the secondary emphysema, which results from the overdistention of the alveoli remaining healthy. It follows, therefore, that percussion is of very little value as an early diagnostic agent.

On the other hand, diminished resonance or dulness on percussion heard over either apex is of extreme value as a symptom of pulmonary tuberculosis, for the reason that here the earliest changes of a tuberculous character in the lungs so frequently occur. It must be remembered, however, that tuberculosis frequently begins at other portions of the lungs, as, for instance, low down posteriorly on the right side. Ordinary pulmonary resonance over the apices of the lungs should normally be obtained from 3 to 5 cm. above the clavicles. Any diminution in the percussion note below this point, as compared with normal pulmonary resonance obtained by percussing over healthy lung, is an important symptom of pulmonary tuberculosis, especially when taken in connection with other symptoms. When both sides show such diminished pulmonary resonance, it becomes necessary to compare the note repeatedly with that of normal pulmonary resonance before a decision can be arrived at. Such dulness, however, may be the result of a thickened pleura over the apex. While a secondary emphysema following tuberculous consolidation may serve to substitute a tympanitic percussion for diminished resonance over consolidated areas, mediastinal tumors, aneurysms, etc., also may cause the changed percussion note in patients with healthy lungs. Dulness over tuberculous areas is rarely so extremely flat as over areas of lung consolidation in pneumonia. It must be remembered, however, that frequently the latter disease complicates pulmonary tuberculosis, so that when long-standing dulness over limited portions of the chest suddenly and largely increases in extent the probability of a complicating pneumonia may be suspected. The sudden advent of a tuberculous pleurisy with effusion will give rise to flatness over the fluid in addition to or in place of the dulness due to the tuberculous consolidation of the lung. On the other hand, a pneumothorax due to the entrance of air into the chest cavity will cause a tympanitic resonance to replace the dulness due to the phthisis. So manifold, therefore, are the variations that it is never advisable to depend upon the results of percussion alone for an absolute diagnosis.

Flatness, as I have stated, rarely is present over phthisical lungs. It does occur over tuberculous as well as other pleuritic effusions. A dull percussion note, varying in degree, is obtained over those portions of phthisical lungs in which the alveoli or bronchi are more or less filled with cheesy or fibrinous material or fluid, such as blood or serum. A more marked dulness verging on flatness is obtained over tuberculous pleuritic exudations.

A slighter degree of dulness with a ringing echo is obtained over areas of pneumothorax, with no communication with a bronchus, and where the air is under pressure.

A non-tympanitic, yet ringing percussion note indicates emphysema of the underlying portion of lung.

A clear tympanitic note is obtained over cavities in the lung, such cavities indicating a breaking down of tuberculous foci in the lungs, bronchiectasis, gangrene, or pulmonary abscess. Should such cavities, however, be full of fluid, such as blood, pus, etc., then a tympanitic area will be found to have become dull on percussion.

A tympanitic percussion note of a duller character may be obtained over completely infiltrated tuberculous areas of lung, when such consolidated areas carry the vibration of the column of air in the trachea or a large bronchus to the surface. Compressed areas of lung over pleuritic exudations may cause a similar transmission of vibration from a large bronchus.

A clear tympanitic percussion note is obtained through a pneumothorax, connecting with a bronchus through an opening formed by a breaking down of lung tissue.

Metallic or amphoric resonance is obtained over cavities with smooth walls, or those surrounded by homogeneously infiltrated and consolidated lung tissue, provided they are quite near the surface and not covered by normal healthy lung tissue, and at least 6 cm. in diameter, and in pneumothorax in which the air is not compressed.

Cracked-pot resonance, *bruit de pot fêlé*, is heard over cavities communicating with an open bronchus through a narrow opening and superficially placed. It is frequently heard over cavities in the upper portions of the lungs, and in pneumothorax communicating with a bronchus or external air.

Alteration in the position of patients suffering from cavities in the lungs gives rise to peculiar variation in the tympanic resonance obtained by percussion over these cavities. This resonance varies as we lengthen or shorten the vibrating column of air communicating with the cavity, by changing the position of the patient, or by causing the latter to open his mouth. Alterations so obtained over cavities are described under various names. Thus a raising of the pitch of the tympanitic percussion note by percussing when the patient's mouth is open, and a lowering of it when the patient's mouth is closed, is known as Wintrich's modified tympanitic resonance. Elevating the pitch of the tympanitic note by causing the patient to lie down, and lowering it by having him sit up, was a procedure of Gerhardt's, and is known under his name.

That deep inspiration sometimes raises the tympanitic pitch over cavities was first spoken of by Friedreich, and the phenomenon is known under his name. Tuberculous pleurisies with effusion of serum or pus, and the extension of tuberculous areas by a complicating acute pneumonia will be shown by the characteristic increase in the latter case of the dulness, and in the former case of the flatness. I have already spoken of the importance of looking for some such complication as a causation for a sudden marked increase in the area of dulness or flatness.

AUSCULTATION.

We now come to consider the auscultatory phenomena of pulmonary tuberculosis which certainly·outrank in importance any other signs to be obtained by the physical examination of the patient as indicating the character and extent of the disease. While not so infallible as to the nature of the disease as the finding of the tubercle bacillus in the sputum, the symptoms to be obtained by auscultation of the chest of a phthisical patient give far more information of the physical conditions of the lungs under examination than any other method of investigation to which the living patient can be subjected. Furthermore, auscultation enables us to detect pulmonary changes in their very early stages—as soon, indeed, as the primary tuberculous focus has established a communication with a terminal bronchus or alveolus, thus enabling the ear of the examiner to hear the earliest râles. In cases in which the individual tubercles are sufficiently superficial to cause pleurisy, we shall hear pleuritic râles even before the tubercle begins to break down.

The auscultatory phenomena in pulmonary tuberculosis depend upon the changes in the normal respiratory murmur owing to the presence of individual tuberculous areas, of broken down, consolidated, or indurated lung tissue, and of pleuritic changes. As is the case with the symptoms obtained by percussion, the earliest manifestations in cases of pulmonary tuberculosis are heard in the apex of either lung. Such auscultatory changes, when compared with the normal respiratory murmur of the other apex, and found constant, will give very early knowledge of tuberculous disease. One of the earliest symptoms thus heard is a prolonged, louder, and rougher expiratory murmur as compared with the inspiratory murmur. Normally the latter is longer and louder than the former. The prolongation of the expiration is explained by the obstacle to the exit of air from the alveoli and finer bronchi, owing to the tuberculous deposits, and the bronchial character of the expiration is explained by the fact that the bronchial breathing is better transmitted through consolidated lung tissues than through normal lung. In advanced tuberculous pulmonary consolidation we get almost pure bronchial or tubular respiration instead of the normal respiratory murmur. A breaking up of the inspiratory murmur into two or more "sections" or murmurs, instead of one continuous sound, until inspiration is completed, with a similar modification in the expiratory movement, indicates a pleurisy over a superficial tuberculous focus under the surface where it is heard, and is generally an early manifestation of pulmonary disease.

Rhonchi or *râles*, coarse and fine, crepitant and subcrepitant, dry and moist, are heard in the early stages of pulmonary disease, and indicate the presence of the local bronchitis which is an **early**

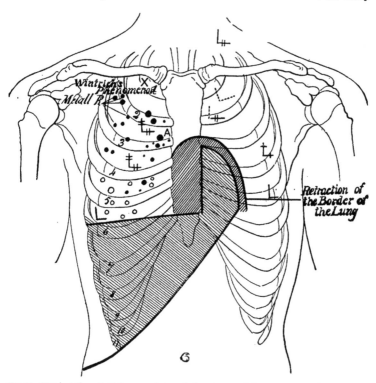

FIG. 12.—Physical Signs in Pulmonary Tuberculosis On the right are advanced lesions, while the changes are beginning only on the left side. (After Sahli.)

L, Weak vesicular respiration;	○, coarse
L, sharp vesicular respiration;	○, medium } moist râles;
ᴸ₊, mixed breathing;	○, fine
ᵗ₊, bronchial breathing;	●, coarse
Lᴴ, bronchial expiration;	●, medium } sonorous râles;
ᴸᴴ, irregular breathing with bronchial expira-	●, fine
tion;	**A**, amphoric breathing;
Lᵤ, irregular respiration;	**X**, tympanic resonance.

sign of tubercles which have caused bronchial involvement. These râles, when local, are a very important symptom, at first heard only occasionally with forced and prolonged respiratory effort, and after the patient is asked to cough; but later on they are heard almost constantly. When heard over a limited area of the lung they are a very suspicious symptom, and a thorough examination of the affected area of lung by all the means at our command should be made. Amphoric breathing, like amphoric resonance, metallic tinkling, and bronchophony are heard in cavities under certain conditions—*e.g.*, that the cavity be 5 or 6 cm. in diameter, and that the walls be smooth and enclose only air. Increased voice and increased breathing, like increased respiratory and vocal fremitus, indicate consolidation of lung. Ægophony is heard over small cavities surrounded by consolidated lung tissue, as well as at the level of the fluid in tuberculous pleural. effusions. In patients suffering from general bronchitis with dilated bronchi, such as chronic asthmatics, the general distribution of coarse râles over the chest and back may conceal the presence of tuberculous foci, which should be sought for by other than auscultatory means if the bronchitis is long persistent.

The auscultatory symptoms obtainable in pulmonary tuberculosis are as follows: Diminished respiratory murmur with prolonged and louder and rougher expiratory as compared with the inspiratory murmur indicates an obstruction in the smaller bronchi, at the spot over which the sounds are heard, due to a localized tuberculous bronchitis. Broken inspiration and expiration indicate a localized pleurisy.

Bronchial breathing is heard over tuberculous consolidated or even indurated pulmonary areas, enclosing or near a large bronchus, over areas of lung compressed by tuberculous pleural effusions, and over dry cavities communicating with a large bronchus. There is diminished or absent respiratory murmur when the bronchus is plugged with secretions or swollen mucous membrane.

Sibilant, sonorous, moist râles, coarse and fine, crepitant and subcrepitant, as I have already stated, indicate the presence of secretion, large or small in quantity, viscid or fluid, in the bronchi of the affected area, in cavities formed in the lung tissue, or in bronchiectasis. Amphoric breathing and metallic tinkling indicate large cavities, and pneumothorax and pyopneumothorax communicating with a bronchus. Ægophomy I have already described. Pleuritic friction sounds indicate tuberculous pleurisy.

Absence of voice and breathing, coming on suddenly in pulmonary tuberculosis, may indicate a sudden effusion into the pleura, but it is to be confirmed by other signs. At no time is it wise to form an opinion concerning the symptoms of a given case before a thorough and conclusive examination has been made by inspection, palpation, percussion, and auscultation. I am accustomed to auscultate first, and confirm these findings by percussion.

MENSURATION.

. The measurement of the circumference of the chest during maximum inspiration and maximum expiration enables us to estimate the expansive power of the lung. Such measurement is best taken by passing the tape over the two nipples and under the angles of the

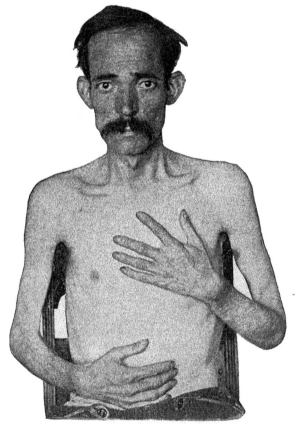

FIG. 13 —Facies of Incipient Pulmonary Tuberculosis.

scapulæ. Normally it is found that there is a difference in adult, healthy males of 7 cm. between the maximum expiration and maximum inspiration. This difference is markedly diminished in phthisis, the measurement of maximum inspiration being diminished and that of maximum expiration increased. The increase in the latter is more marked than the diminution in the former.

In phthisis the vital capacity of the lung, that is to say, the amount of air which the patient can expire from the lungs, beginning with a maximum inspiration and ending with a maximum (forced) expiration, is very much diminished. Even in the incipient stages it is about one-tenth less than normal, while in the advanced stages of phthisis, when the patient has become very weak, the vital capacity is diminished to less than one-half of the normal, in both the male and female.

GENERAL APPEARANCE.

The facies of a pronounced case of pulmonary tuberculosis is very characteristic, and is well shown in the accompanying illustration. Fig. 13 is from a photograph of a man with incipient pulmonary tuberculosis. The patient is tall and thin, the neck is long, the bones are slender, the muscular system is badly developed. The forehead is high, the hair is thin, the eyes are abnormally bright, and the cheek bones are prominent. The chest is flat and long, the hollows under the clavicles are abnormally deep, the scapulæ stand away from the ribs at their ver-

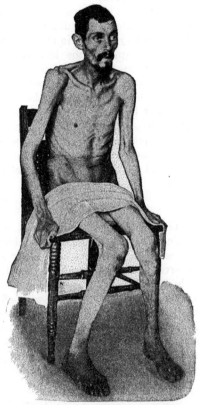

Fig. 14.—Facies of Advanced Pulmonary Tuberculosis.

tebral border (winged scapulæ). This form of chest, known as the paralytic thorax, is supposed to be due to weakness of the muscles which retain the scapula against the chest wall. The tendency to clubbed finger ends and the claw-like curving of the nails are also shown in the illustration. The extreme pallor, amounting almost to blueness and cyanosis, is, of course, not shown in the picture, but was present in the subject.

In Fig. 14, from a case of advanced pulmonary tuberculosis, are shown admirably the extreme atrophy and emaciation which have given this condition the name of consumption. I wish to call especial attention to the sinking in of the chest above and below the clavicles, owing to consolidation and retraction of the apices of the lungs. The marked prominence of the extrinsic respiratory muscles, both in the neck and in the abdomen, and the drawing in of the costal wall at the line of insertion of the diaphragm, all indicate the hyperactivity of the respiratory muscles in the attempt to obtain sufficient air for oxygenation in spite of the incapacitated pulmonary tissue. This is further shown by the position of the patient, the chest and neck curved forward, the chin raised in the effort to obtain air, while the whole attitude is eloquent of the lack of sufficient muscular strength to support the weight of the body. We see in this patient also the dull, apathetic, yet emaciated countenance. The strained look of the eyes in viewing distant objects, so characteristic of extremely advanced cases of consumption, was well marked in this case. The rapid and short respiration was also a marked and obvious clinical feature.

SKIAGRAPHY.

The Roentgen or x-ray has not as yet given us any valuable diagnostic points in the symptomatology of phthisis, although tuberculous lungs have been extensively studied by the x-ray by many observers. Normal lungs are not indicated in the x-ray picture of a healthy chest. Tuberculous consolidations, tuberculous pneumonias, tuberculous pleurisy with effusion give rise to a shadow in the picture, not so marked, however, as that of the bones. A shadow at the apex of the lungs appears, according to many authorities, as soon as there is consolidation at this point. At best, this method of examination is still in the beginning, and requires much labor before positive symptomatic indications will have been attained.

TUBERCULIN.

Injections of tuberculin for the purpose of ascertaining the presence of tuberculous foci of which a physical examination elicits no symptom, and when an examination of the sputum is negative, have been practised with some results in the human subject. Very properly the diagnosis of tuberculosis in human beings by this means is not popular, although the method is an extremely valuable aid in the recognition of tuberculosis in the lower animals, particularly cattle. The procedure depends upon the well-ascertained fact that such injections are followed within eight or ten hours or even sooner after the injection by a rise of body temperature, accompanied by a local reaction at the seat of the tuberculous focus in the lungs, giving rise to local symptoms which had been previously in abeyance. These local manifestations and the fever gradually subside, and in a few days the patient returns to his ordinary condition. Should no febrile movement occur, the temperature having been carefully observed every few hours for several days, a second injection may be made, and even a third, until, these repeated injections being followed by no reaction, the test may be set down as negative in result. The tuberculin generally employed is the old tuberculin of Koch, the quantity used is 1 mgm. for the first injection, 2 mgm. for the second, and 4 mgm. for the third. It does not appear, even to the most enthusiastic observers, that this method of examination for diagnostic purposes is to be recommended in human beings, not so much because of any positively ascertained injurious effect from the tuberculin injections, but rather from the dread that an agent capable of increasing the local symptoms in the tuberculous focus, and of producing sufficient disturbances to cause the appearance of symptoms in portions of lung tissue previously apparently healthy, may cause more than a mere temporary reaction, and even prevent a regression of the symptoms to the *statu quo* before the injection was made; this, notwithstanding the enthusiastic employment of very much smaller doses of modified tuberculin (T R) in the treatment of phthisis by many very able therapeutists. For this purpose the dose is much smaller than when the injection is made for diagnostic purposes.

Modes of Onset.

This account of the symptomatology of pulmonary phthisis which I have given, while it aims to consider each of the individual symptoms, will be recognized by those who are accustomed to see much of pulmonary tuberculosis as still leaving out an important factor, which is necessary to complete a clinical picture applicable to most cases of the disease. This factor has to do with questions as to whether a given case is of the acute or chronic type. For there are clinically considered two classes of cases of pulmonary phthisis: one group in which the pathological changes are rapidly progressive and the symptoms eminently acute in character; and another group in which the disease is but slowly progressive and chronic in character, lasting frequently many years, or even terminating in an apparent cure. The acute cases must not be classed with acute miliary tuberculosis, although both diseases progress rapidly to a fatal termination. It is to be understood that there are many cases which, at one period of their course, will seem to belong to the acute type, and later the disease process becomes less rapid, the symptoms regress, and the patient improves, still continuing, however, to suffer from the chronic type of pulmonary phthisis.

In the *acute cases* the very inception is generally marked by serious symptoms. The disease at the outset may be a pneumonia, or a hemorrhage from the lungs, or a severe bronchitis. Or the patient may suddenly develop a hectic fever after recovery from typhoid fever or malaria or any weakening disease. Whatever the inception may be, very soon changes in the lungs manifest themselves, accompanied by cough, by the presence of tubercle bacilli in the characteristic sputum, high fever, loss of appetite, loss of strength, anæmia, night sweats, and great emaciation. The symptoms progress rapidly, the physical changes of destructive character progress correspondingly, and within three or four months the most frightful destruction of lung tissue has taken place, and the patient dies. These cases rarely, yet occasionally, progress rapidly for a month or two, then suddenly improvement sets in, and the disease follows a slower and more chronic type.

In the *chronic cases* the patient for a long time suffers from no apparent lung symptoms. There may be a slight dry cough, which the patient ascribes to a cold or catarrh of the pharynx, or there may be dyspeptic symptoms or general anæmia and chlorosis. There is at the beginning little or no fever. The patient at intervals feels perfectly well; a careful general examination may reveal some of the earlier symptoms of disease at the apex, although frequently the lesions are so slight that a physical examination will show nothing positively. An examination of the sputum generally reveals tubercle bacilli, although the absence of these does not positively indicate that no pulmonary disease exists. When changes begin to appear in the lungs they progress very slowly, the patient frequently being able to continue at his employment and remaining in the enjoyment of comparatively fair health for many years. These cases,-too, frequently undergo fibroid degeneration of the affected area of lung tissue, and sometimes the symptoms regress, and the patient considers himself and appears, indeed, to be cured. Others go on gradually to the stage of the breaking down of the consolidated areas of the lung, cavities are formed, and the various manifestations due to mixed infection cause a rapid progress of the patient towards death. In the later stages of the disease the progress may be extremely rapid. In these cases, moreover, the disease may, at any period, suddenly assume the acute type, and progress to a rapidly fatal termination. Many author-

ities have described the symptoms and pathology of pulmonary tuberculosis by dividing these chronic types of the disease into three
stages: the inception stage, the stage of consolidation, and stage of
the breaking down of the tuberculous areas, with the formation of cavities.   While for descriptive purposes this division may be useful, it
must be understood that the clinical picture does not admit of such
decided differentiation of the symptoms into these different stages.
The term hasty consumption, or galloping consumption, is frequently
applied to the cases belonging to the acute type.

MILIARY TUBERCULOSIS.

The symptomatology of general miliary tuberculosis differs so
materially from that of chronic or even acute tuberculosis of the various organs that a description of the symptomatology of the latter
does not give in any way the clinical story of the former.   General
miliary tuberculosis is more than a general distribution of tubercle
bacilli, and the formation of tubercles throughout the organs and tissues of the body.   It is an infectious constitutional disease in which
the tubercle bacilli have been disseminated throughout the body by
way of the blood-vessels and lymphatics.   As a result the organs and
tissues affected have scattered through them innumerable tubercles.
Even in the most acute cases of chronic tuberculosis the affected tissues only gradually become invaded by a comparatively slowly spreading pathological process which gradually destroys more and more of
the organ, but in general miliary tuberculosis all parts of the affected organs become invaded at one time by the tuberculous disease,
giving the clinical picture of tuberculosis of multiple organs.   In addition to this we have general septicæmic and pyæmic symptoms,
which are the result of embolism of the minute capillaries, depending
upon the part which the blood-vessels play in the dissemination of
the pathological factors of the disease.   Although it is not the function of this section to treat of the etiology of miliary tuberculosis, it
is an important fact in connection with the symptoms of the disease
that in many cases general miliary tuberculosis occurs as a secondary
disease and not as a primary affection.   In other words, it becomes
important in making the diagnosis of acute miliary tuberculosis to be
able to find a primary focus of tuberculous disease in some portion of
the body, generally in the lungs; and even more frequently tuberculous
lymphatic glands can be demonstrated, some of which have undergone cheesy degeneration, and the tuberculous material thus set free
has gained access to the circulation.   In other cases general miliary
tuberculosis has been preceded by the tuberculous abscesses which

occur as a result of tuberculous joint disease or osteomyelitis. Again, tuberculous nephritis complicating these latter conditions may in turn be complicated by general miliary tuberculosis. Tuberculosis of the serous membranes frequently forms the connecting-link between chronic tuberculosis of the lungs and general miliary tuberculosis. Whatever the primary seat of the tuberculosis may be, the diagnosis of general miliary tuberculosis presupposes the presence of some primary tuberculous focus.

Symptoms.

The symptoms of this condition are constitutional and local. The constitutional symptoms are the manifestation of the general infection, while the local symptoms depend upon the individual organs which are involved in the general infection, and upon the local seat of the distribution of the bacilli and of the miliary tubercles.

Of the *constitutional symptoms* which mark the general infection of the system by the tubercle bacillus and its products, the most important and perhaps the most constant is the fever. This fever is continuous in character, now rising, now falling without any special, absolutely characteristic temperature curve. Sometimes, however, the temperature resembles very closely that of typhoid fever, and it becomes important to distinguish between the two maladies. For this purpose the absence of the Widal reaction, the frequent occurrence of brain symptoms early in the disease, the presence of tubercles on ophthalmoscopic examination of the choroid, the symptoms of general capillary bronchitis and pneumonia complicating phthisis, and, above all, the isolation of the tubercle bacillus from the blood, especially that withdrawn from the spleen, all speak in favor of a general tuberculous infection. Very frequently, however, the temperature curve is not that of typhoid fever, but on the contrary the highest rise is in the morning and a decline occurs in the evening. Occasionally the fever is like that of malaria of the quotidian or tertian type. These cases can be differentiated from malaria by the absence of the malarial organisms on repeated examination. Occasionally, too, cases of general miliary tuberculosis run an apyretic course. In such cases as a rule the diagnosis is made at the autopsy, the chief symptoms having been of a cerebral character, and the patient having been supposed to suffer from mania. In contradistinction from typhoid fever the fever of acute miliary tuberculosis is generally accompanied by an extremely rapid pulse. The pulse may reach 150, with a temperature of 104°. When the fever declines there is a corresponding diminution in the rapidity of the pulse, but even when the patient has normal temperature the pulse is extremely rapid. This rapidity of the pulse is important because it enables one to differentiate cases of this disease from meningitis, in which the pulse has a tendency to be slow.

The fever and the rapid pulse are almost necessarily accompanied by constant and excessive perspiration; and owing to this as much as to the fever and the loss of appetite there is rapid emaciation with loss of strength. When the fever and wasting are accompanied by mania and delirium, the case resembles on superficial examination one of advanced typhoid fever. Ehrlich's diazo reaction occurs frequently early in the disease. Albuminuria is very often present, and occasionally also peptonuria and propeptonuria, which serve to raise the suspicion of concealed sepsis.

Further constitutional symptoms are intense anæmia, deep cyanosis, and dyspnœa. These two latter symptoms are of especial interest from the fact that they are entirely independent of extensive pulmonary disease, whether of a chronic or acute character. Their value as diagnostic symptoms lies in the fact that with no or only slight physical changes in the respiratory organs and passages and no recognizable vascular or cardiac lesions, deep cyanosis and dyspnœa exist. The respiration in these cases is very rapid, and the patient maintains his body in the erect or sitting posture with the shoulders well forward, gasping for air. This dyspnœa is possibly due to irritation of branches of the vagus nerves by miliary tubercles. Whatever its cause, it forms in conjunction with the absence of respiratory and vascular changes a very characteristic symptom group.

Although in chronic tuberculosis of the various organs tubercle bacilli are as a rule entirely absent, yet, when they can be found in the blood, they become an important corroborative evidence of acute miliary tuberculosis. Frequent examinations of the blood of suspected cases must be made, for the bacilli when present are few in number. They are especially apt to be found in blood withdrawn from the spleen. These bacilli thus carried in the circulating blood and lymphatics are generally carried, as I have already said, from some chronic tuberculous focus and deposited in the various organs, where they form tubercles in vast numbers which cause by their presence inflammatory irritation.

Local Symptoms.—Owing to these local inflammatory disturbances, together with the general sepsis, death is so rapidly produced that the tubercles thus formed do not have time to break down and go through their usual degenerative changes. It follows, therefore, that the symptoms of acute miliary tuberculosis of the various organs are radically different from those of chronic tuberculosis of the same organs. The most generally and commonly affected organs in acute

miliary tuberculosis are naturally the lungs, for here generally is the
primary focus of chronic tuberculosis; from this acute tuberculous
infection of the blood originates.   The local symptoms of such an
acute miliary tuberculosis of the lungs are the same as those of acute
bronchitis, or more rarely bronchopneumonia.   These are cough, spu-

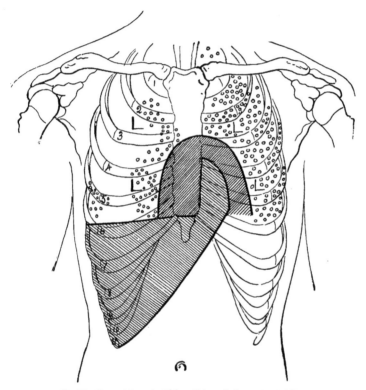

Fig. 15.—Physical Signs in Miliary Tuberculosis   (After Sahli.)

L, Weak vesicular respiration;   O, coarse
L, sharp vesicular respiration;   o, medium } moist râles.
                                           o , fine

tum frequently of the rust-brown character, rapid respiration and
dyspnœa, and occasionally hemorrhage.   On physical examination
there are coarse and fine râles, dry and moist, whistling, crepitant, and
subcrepitant.   If the miliary tubercles have caused isolated patches
of pulmonary inflammation, we will obtain over these areas the physical signs of localized pneumonia, on both auscultation and percus-

sion; otherwise the percussion note will be normal over areas where auscultation shows a bronchitis. Occasionally, however, we obtain, especially near the clavicles, tympanitic and cracked-pot resonance. When, however, the primary pulmonary chronic tuberculosis is far advanced and extensive physical changes are present, the signs of the deposit of miliary tubercles are apt to be mistaken for the manifestations of the primary disease, and even symptoms caused by tuberculosis of other organs than the lungs are apt to be ascribed to the tuberculous phthisis. In such cases the diagnosis will depend upon a careful examination of the blood and the presence of tubercles in the choroid. Although tubercle bacilli are present in the sputum of many cases of acute miliary tuberculosis, this must not be ascribed to the miliary tubercles present in the lungs, but rather to the fact that so large a proportion of miliary tuberculous cases are secondary to pulmonary tuberculosis. The presence of bacilli in the sputum depends upon the breaking down of tubercles, and since in acute miliary tuberculosis death results before the tubercles have time to break down, it is evident that bacilli will not appear in the sputum if the lungs are the seat only of an acute miliary tuberculosis secondary to tuberculosis in some other organ; so also the appearance of tubercle bacilli in the urine would indicate chronic tuberculous disease of the genitourinary organs or tract rather than acute miliary tuberculosis of these tissues. In the latter case, again, we would have the local symptoms due to inflammation of the kidneys, bladder, etc., following the general distribution of the miliary tubercles in these organs. The patient generally would die of the constitutional manifestations long before the tubercles had broken down sufficiently to give rise to bacilli in the urine. When a pleurisy, peritonitis, or pericarditis results from the deposit of miliary tubercles over these serous membranes, in the course of acute miliary tuberculosis, the resulting local symptoms of these inflammations are very similar to those characteristic of the same affections when due to other causes.

In the pleurisy of acute miliary tuberculosis the exudation may be serous or hemorrhagic.

Tuberculous peritonitis when it occurs is general, and depends for its diagnosis upon the constitutional symptoms, examination of the blood and retina, etc., rather than upon any individuality in the local symptoms of the peritonitis. Frequently a cardiac lesion is shown by the presence of murmurs, which develop suddenly and increase rapidly. These murmurs are generally due to a tuberculous endocarditis. If the patient suffering from such a lesion complicating acute miliary tuberculosis lives until the tubercles break down, he is liable to suffer from infarctions of the various organs and tissues, together with all other clinical manifestations of septic endocarditis.

When miliary tubercles affect the kidneys they give rise to an acute or subacute parenchymatous nephritis, and all of the progressive symptoms characteristic of such inflammations of the kidneys will gradually develop. The urine will show the presence of albumin and the customary microscopic changes. It must be noted, however, that the presence of albumin in the urine is not always caused

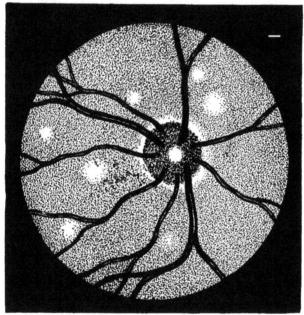

Fig. 16.—Tubercles of the Choroid. (After Sahli.)

by the deposit of miliary tubercles in the kidneys, but may occur in acute miliary tuberculosis even if there are no miliary tubercles in these organs. In other words, the albuminuria may be the result of the general infection which accompanies acute miliary tuberculosis, or it may be the result of a tuberculous endocarditis or some other tuberculous complication competent to cause albumin to appear in the urine. It must not be forgotten also that acute miliary tuberculosis of the kidneys does not imply that tubercle bacilli will be found in the urine of such patients, for the reason that as a rule the patients do not live long enough for the tubercles to break down and set free the tubercle bacilli to be voided with the urine. When such bacilli occur in the urine it speaks rather for the presence of a primary or secondary tuberculosis of the kidney in which the tuberculous masses have reached the stage of disruption.   In acute miliary tuberculosis of the kidney the patient is apt to pass a largely diminished quantity of urine.   I have already mentioned that the diazo reaction of Ehrlich is found in the urine in most cases of miliary tuberculosis.   In chronic tuberculosis the diazo reaction in the urine indicates an increased gravity of the prognosis.   Most of the cases in which such reaction occurs end in death.   In miliary tuberculosis, however, the prognosis being fatal in any case, the Ehrlich diazo reaction in the urine simply helps to confirm the diagnosis, and does not in any way affect the prognosis.

One of the most characteristic symptoms of miliary tuberculosis, and one to which great diagnostic importance should be attached, is the observation of miliary tubercles over the choroid in the fundus of the eye.   These tubercles can be seen in the living patient by the use of the ophthalmoscope.   They appear as slightly yellowish, irregular, circular spots or bodies, having a bright centre and rather dark outline, and resembling the optic papilla in size and general contour.   They may be only one or two in number, or there may be large numbers of them.   They do not seem to disturb the vision, although they are more apt to be present in cases in which the meninges are the seat of miliary tubercles.   They should be sought for in every case of suspected acute miliary tuberculosis.   In a large majority of the cases of acute miliary tuberculosis the delirium and stupor which are present would indicate involvement of the brain and the meninges in the disease.   It must not be forgotten, however, that delirium and stupor are symptoms frequently present in all infectious febrile diseases of a severe type.   Autopsies, however, as well as symptoms during life very frequently indicate the involvement of the meninges of the brain and spinal cord in acute miliary tuberculosis. In these cases they will be present in addition to the subjective symptoms of cerebral disease, such as headache, delirium, stupor, and coma, and to the usual objective symptoms of the involvement of the meninges, such as the pupillary disturbances, opisthotonos, convulsions, paralyses, vomiting, etc.   In these cases, as I have already stated, repeated examinations should show the presence of miliary tubercles in the fundus of the eye.   It is needless to say that the tubercle bacilli are carried by the circulation to practically all the other tissues and organs of the body.   The spleen especially has been found to be the seat of numerous miliary tubercles, and the bacilli can be most readily found in the blood drawn from the spleen.   Ulcerating tuberculous lesions are found quite frequently in this disease in the lymphatic glands, throat, larynx, tongue, and mucous membranes. The presence of all such lesions strengthens the diagnosis.

It is sometimes very difficult to differentiate acute miliary tuberculosis from other diseases. The pathognomonic symptoms are the presence of tubercle bacilli in the blood and the finding of miliary tubercles in the optic fundus. When these symptoms are absent the diagnosis cannot positively be made.

The disease is apt to be confounded with typhoid and typhus fevers, malarial fever, cancer of the lung, bronchitis, sepsis, meningitis, nephritis and uræmia, septic endocarditis, and even poisoning by some narcotic drug. In all of these diseases the two absolutely characteristic symptoms which I have described above are absent.

The duration of the disease may be from a week to six weeks or more; generally, however, three or four weeks. The prognosis is generally fatal, although some authorities consider that recovery is a possibility. In such cases chronic tuberculosis of a more general type is apt to result. Occasionally, too, the affection shows signs of apparent improvement, only to be followed by exacerbation of the symptoms and death.

It gives me pleasure to express my obligations to Dr. Joseph Fraenkel and Dr. Wolf, of the Montefiore Home for Chronic Invalids, for their courtesy in connection with the clinical material under their charge.

TUBERCULOSIS.

(DIAGNOSIS, PROGNOSIS, PROPHYLAXIS, AND TREATMENT.)

BY

S. A. KNOPF,

NEW YORK.

TUBERCULOSIS.

(DIAGNOSIS, PROGNOSIS, PROPHYLAXIS, AND TREATMENT.)

Introduction.

THE word tuberculosis probably has its origin in the writings of Baillie,[1] who was certainly the first (1793) to describe the tubercle as a special pathological production in phthisis pulmonalis. The pathological unity of all tuberculous diseases was discovered by Laennec[2] at the beginning of the nineteenth century. In 1865 Villemin[3] demonstrated the inoculability of tuberculosis and the necessity of classifying this affection under virulent diseases. Lastly, Koch's great discovery in 1882[4] gave us the absolute proof of the specificity of tuberculosis by demonstrating the presence of a distinct microorganism. All doubts as to the truth of Laennec's teachings were thus dispelled. It is now known that there is but one tuberculosis, though it may manifest itself in various forms, attacking the visceral, bony, muscular, or cutaneous structure; but its specific pathological factor is always the bacillus tuberculosis. In the present article, dealing with the methods now in vogue to combat tuberculosis successfully, the subject will be discussed under the following heads: 1, Sources of infection and individual prophylaxis; 2, general public prophylaxis; 3, special prophylaxis of tuberculosis in childhood; 4, prevention of tuberculosis in cattle and other domestic animals; 5, predisposition and preventive treatment; 6, early diagnosis of tuberculous diseases; 7, the hygienic treatment in sanatoria, special hospitals, and at home (with a description of a model sanatorium); 8, aërotherapy and the pneumatic cabinet; 9, solar theraphy; 10, dress and personal hygiene; 11, hydrotherapy; 12, dietetic treatment; 13, medicinal and symptomatic treatment; 14, the treatment of complications in phthisis and other forms of tuberculosis; 15, education, discipline, and marriage relations; 16, hypurgy; 17, culture products in the treatment of tuberculosis; 18, climatotherapy, health resorts, and sports; 19, pathological and clinical proofs of the curability of pulmonary tuberculosis; 20, prognosis; 21, public care of the consumptive poor and the social aspect of tuberculosis; conclusions.

PROPHYLAXIS.

Sources of Infection and Individual Prophylaxis.

For a tuberculous disease to manifest itself in a living organism two things are necessary, viz., the presence of the bacillus and the condition suitable to its development. In order to understand its presence we will consider the various ways in which the infection may be transmitted from one individual to another.

An individual suffering from pulmonary tuberculosis is estimated to expectorate as many as seven billions of bacilli in twenty-four hours. This patient may not be sick enough to be in bed; in fact, the patient in bed is perhaps less a danger to his fellow-men, for, if he is careless, he must confine his unsanitary habits to one room, while the unscrupulous or ignorant consumptive still able to be about disseminates the germs of his disease wherever he goes. As long as the sputum remains in the liquid state there is less danger from it, but matter expectorated on the floor, in the street, or in a handkerchief usually dries very rapidly, and, becoming pulverized, finds its way into the respiratory tract of any one who chances to inhale the air in which is floating this dust from expectorations, laden with many kinds of bacteria. The most dangerous is the tubercle bacillus, which retains its virulence in the dried state for several months.[1]

If an individual is perfectly well, the inhalation of the bacilli will not hurt him. In health not only does the nasal mucous secretion possess bactericidal properties,[2] but the nasal mucous membrane is endowed, more than any other similar structure in the human body, with a marked reflex action to mechanical and chemical irritants. But if any one with a weakened constitution, or suffering from chronic catarrh of the nasopharyngeal or laryngeal tract should be exposed to the frequent inhalation of particles of dried and pulverized tuberculous expectoration, he would certainly be in danger of thus contracting pulmonary tuberculosis. Countless are the cases reported which prove beyond a doubt this mode of propagation of the disease. In addition, tuberculosis has been produced by this method experimentally in the lower animals. The writings and experimental work of Villemin,[7] Weber,[8] Tappeiner,[9] Cornet,[10] Krüger,[11] Straus,[12] Hance,[13] Murrell,[14] etc., all confirm what has just been said on the danger from the careless and promiscuous expectorating of tuberculous individuals. Personal investigations in this respect have shown that what is proved experimentally and clinically to be possible, does occur on a large scale.

Some years ago, when visiting many of the European and American health resorts much frequented by consumptives, and watching the careless method pursued by them in disposing of their sputa, I became convinced that these unconscientious and ignorant tuberculous visitors constituted a menace to the permanent population. Inquiries addressed to the proper authorities confirmed my suspicions, and the recently proposed restrictions on the immigration of consumptives into California, Colorado, etc., give additional evidence of the truth of my observations.

To stop the spread of tuberculosis by the careless or ignorant consumptive we must begin by convincing him of the wrong he is doing to himself and others by the manner in which he disposes of his infectious expectoration. The danger of his becoming continually reinfected must be particularly impressed upon him. Such a patient should be taught never to expectorate except in a proper receptacle. The habit of expectorating in a handkerchief should be considered as dangerous as expectorating on the ground, for the frequent unfolding of a handkerchief containing the dried sputum is a most common way of disseminating the bacilli, and, besides, not infrequently the patient reinfects thus his upper air passages. The frequent coexistence of pharyngeal and laryngeal tuberculosis with relatively little advanced pulmonary lesions may well be explained by this mode of secondary infection, especially when there has been a denudation of epithelium through catarrhal conditions.

In all places where there are likely to be tuberculous patients able to be about, whether in private residences, workshops, offices, hospitals, or sanatoria, there should be the proper kind of spittoons, and a sufficient number of them, properly placed and kept. Cuspidors placed on the ground should be done away with, for while a fair number of male patients may possess a certain dexterity in disposing of their sputum, it is usually more difficult for a woman to hit the spittoon. Where much expectoration is going on, one usually finds the brims of the cuspidors that are placed on the floor covered with dried sputa, and even the piece of oilcloth sometimes placed underneath as a precautionary measure often shows signs of the inexperienced spitter. To obviate these difficulties, and also to make the presence of numerous cuspidors in either private dwelling, hospital, or sanatorium as little objectionable as possible, the following arrangement of elevated spittoons, visible only when in use, is to be recommended. In the walls of parlors, halls, galleries, etc., at appropriate distances, are constructed small niches or cupboards three or three and a half feet from the floor. They are large enough to hold a spittoon eight inches high and about the same diameter. Not to expose the persons entrusted with cleaning these vessels to the possible danger of inoculation by breakage of porcelain, metal spittoons should be used. Blue enamelled iron seems to be the most practical of all. The dark blue color makes the contents less visible. The cuspidor is supported by a metal ring attached to the door of the cupboard. The patient desiring to expectorate opens the little door, thus bringing the spittoon within his reach, and closes it again when he gets through. In the grounds surrounding the hospital or sanatorium the niches may be replaced by boxes mounted on stands or attached to the trunks of trees. The drawing will more fully explain the construction and the working of this arrangement. The cuspidor of metal, elevated and covered, has additional advantages over the usual uncovered vessel of porcelain or earthenware. Animals, such as cats, dogs, etc., will not be able to reach the contents of the cuspidor; and there is less danger of its bursting when placed outdoors at freezing temperature if enclosed in a box. In the grounds of institutions where porcelain vessels have been placed it has happened that the frost cracked the spittoons and caused their contents to be spread over the ground. Now, it is well known that the tubercle bacillus does not die at the freezing

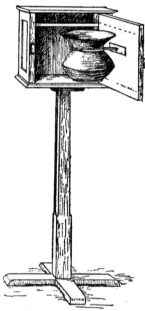

Fig. 17 —Elevated Spittoon for Home or Institutions.

temperature, and hence there is danger in the use of porcelain vessels. Galtier,[13] and later Cadéac and Malet, exposed the tuberculous expectoration to repeated freezing and thawing, and a temperature of −8° C. did not destroy the virulence of these tuberculous products.

For factory and workshop use, Predoehl's enamelled iron spittoon, of which a drawing is also given, seems to answer all practical purposes. The cover is essential to prevent the entrance of flies—not an unimportant item in the prophylaxis of tuberculosis. Spillmann and Haushalter,[14] of Nancy, have demonstrated by extensive experiments that the fly may become the propagator of tuberculosis. The abdominal cavities of flies caught in the rooms of consumptives were found to contain the living bacilli, so also did the fly specks scraped from the walls and windows of hospital wards and rooms where consumptives habitually sojourned. The same experiments were repeated and verified by Hoffmann." Now, the danger from

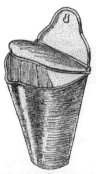

FIG. 18 —Predoehl's Spittoon for Factories and Workshops.

FIG. 19.—Spit-Cup for Use on the veranda and at the Bedside.

these infected insects is twofold. They die and crumble to dust which contains the bacilli, and the microorganisms may thus enter the system through the respiratory tract. Or the fly which may have partaken of the tuberculous expectoration deposits its excrements at the next opportunity upon some article of food, whence the

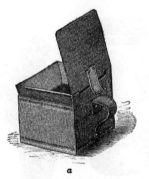
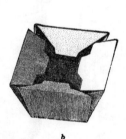

a   b

FIG. 20.—Seabury and Johnson's Spitting-Cup. a, Frame; b, folded cardboard.

bacilli contained in the deposit find their way into the alimentary tract of man or beast.

Predoehl's cuspidor—which is about nine inches high, eight inches at its largest, and three inches at its smallest diameter—may be suspended at any height, and can be very easily cleaned and disinfected.

A third kind of spittoon is the small mug, which should also be of some unbreakable material—enamelled iron, tin, or aluminum—and, of course, with a tightly closing cover.   On account of its light-

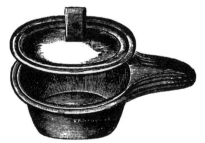

FIG. 21.—Sanitary Spittoon-Cup Made of Pressed Paper.

ness, the last-mentioned metal is preferable.   The drawing shows the form which seems to me most convenient.   Another kind of spittoon of practical use, at home or in institutions, is the Seabury & Johnson spitting-cup, made of impermeable pasteboard, to fit in a metallic frame with handle and cover.   When the cup is filled, the pasteboard is taken out and burned, with its contents.   These are

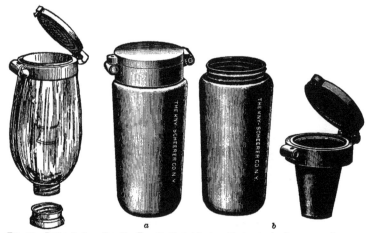

FIG. 22.—Dettweiler's   FIG. 23.—Knopf's Pocket Sputum Flask of Aluminum.   a, Closed; b,
"Hustenfläschchen"   taken apart for cleaning.

the cuspidors for patients in bed or for those who are taking the rest cure on the veranda.

There exists also a sanitary sputum cup, manufactured by the Kny-Scheerer Company, which may serve as a receptacle for the sputum at the bedside or when the patients are outdoors on reclining chairs. It is made of heavy pressed paper, has a convenient handle and a closely fitting cover. Its cheapness and easy destruction by fire (cup and contents together) make this cup a useful article in the prevention of the spread of tuberculosis through expectoration.

Patients who are too weak to make use of even this light paper cup should have (placed within easy reach) a number of rags, kept moist, wherein they may expectorate. These rags should be burned before they have a chance to dry.

We come now to the fourth kind of spittoons—the pocket flask which, when properly and faithfully used by the pulmonary invalid, will prove one of the most important factors in the prevention of tuberculosis. It should be carried by the tuberculous individual all the time, and used whenever he cannot conveniently get at the stationary cuspidors. The first pocket spittoon was Dr. Dettweiler's "Hustenfläschchen." It is a flask of blue glass, about four inches long and six inches in its largest circumference, provided with a hermetically closing top and bottom, of white metal, and so constructed that it can easily be cleaned. The lid flies open at a slight

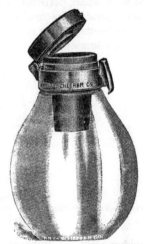

FIG. 24.—Knopf's Sputum Flask of Glass. The funnel is longer than it appears in the drawing.

pressure on the spring, and after use is closed by pushing the top down again. Since the appearance of this flask, many similar utensils have been devised, partly with a view of simplifying the mechanism and also of producing an article cheap enough to be within the reach of every one. In the endeavor to attain these ends I have designed two models. The better of these is, perhaps, an aluminum flask constructed like Dettweiler's, but without the extra opening at the bottom. It is lighter, less bulky, and unbreakable. It is easy to disinfect as it may be boiled without injury. It possesses every advantage except that of cheapness. The other is a strong glass flask modelled like the aluminum flask just described. The funnel is of vulcanized rubber and the cover of white metal. The cleaning and disinfection are simple, and its cost is only about one-third of that of the aluminum flask. It is made in various sizes so that smaller hands (ladies' and children's) can manipulate the flask with ease. All of these flasks are so constructed that the contents cannot be spilled if tipped over, even when the cover is open.

There is one precaution to be observed in connection with the use of the pocket flask and the cuspidor in general.   The same handkerchief should never be used for wiping the nose that is used to wipe the mouth after having expectorated.   Patients should have two handkerchiefs with them, and always hold one before the mouth during an attack of coughing or sneezing, to guard against the expulsion of small particles of sputum.   Flügge and Latschenko[18] have demonstrated the need of such precaution by careful and extensive experiments.   They requested some consumptives to cough (but not to expectorate) in a large glass box.   The patients had to put on new

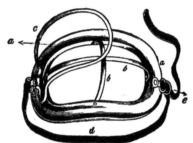

FIG. 25.—Fraenkel's Mouth Mask. (⅓ natural size.) a, Metal ring; b, supporter; c, saddle; d, elastic band: e, rings for fastening.

rubber coats and rubber shoes, to make the detaching of particles of dried sputum, which might have been on their clothes, impossible. Sterilized glass plates, somewhat moistened, had been previously placed in the upper portion of the big box.   Animals inoculated with the substance scraped off these plates were rendered tuberculous. These experiments have since been verified by Goldie[19] and others.

In special institutions—sanatoria and hospitals—prophylactic measures to guard against the expulsion of particles of sputum can be carried out which would be much less practicable for patients outside of such establishments.   At the Berlin Charité Prof. B. Fraenkel insists that all the tuberculous inmates must wear masks to catch the germs they expel in speaking and coughing when they are in the common room, and remove them only while eating or expectorating. The patients soon become accustomed to the mask, as by impregnating the gauze, which is held in place by a metallic frame, with some medicinal substance they suppose it is to be worn for their own personal benefit, instead of for the protection of others.   Bacilli are frequently found in the gauze.   It is, of course, understood that the gauze, lint, or cotton removed from these respiratory masks is to be burned immediately, and the masks disinfected at regular intervals.

Fraenkel's mouth mask is, however, most important perhaps in the prevention of mixed infections. Where there are many consumptives in the advanced stages there will always be a smaller or greater number suffering from a mixed infection, therefore the expulsion of countless pus-creating microorganisms, such as the streptococci and the staphylococci, into an atmosphere which is breathed by consumptives can be prevented by the wearing of such a mask.

That an expulsion of particles of infectious sputum is possible during the act of speaking cannot be denied. The experiments of Latschenko and Heymann in the laboratory of Professor Flugge have, however, demonstrated that for the infection to take place through the expulsion of particles of sputum a close proximity to the invalid is essential. At a distance of over four feet from the patient this mode of infection is no longer possible. Again, this danger is still more reduced by the fact that not all individuals afflicted with pulmonary tuberculosis have bacilli in their saliva; also the time the physician, nurse, or friend need be in close proximity to the patient is rarely longer than a few moments.

A patient should have two pocket flasks, so as never to be without while one is being cleaned. In hospitals and sanatoria the same rule should hold good for the fixed cuspidors. In such institutions the person who attends to the cleaning of these vessels should, during his work, be provided with rubber gloves, so as to remove all possible danger of inoculation through an abrasion of which he might not be aware.

The most thorough method of cleaning any cuspidor filled with tuberculous sputum is certainly the one recommended by Prof. Grancher of Paris.[20] It consists in placing the spittoons—contents and all—in boiling water, where they are left for five or ten minutes; by the addition of some bicarbonate of soda the boiling-point will be raised to 102° or 103° C., which will destroy the tubercle bacilli most certainly. The next best, and perhaps the most convenient method, is to mix the tuberculous expectoration freely with a five-per-cent. solution of carbolic acid. After this in order of efficacy comes the bichloride solution of 1:1,000. This should always be used in combination with tartaric acid, citric acid, or some other preparation that will prevent the coagulation of albumen. According to the experiments of Yersin,[20 a] it takes thirty seconds to kill the tuberculous germs immersed in a five-per-cent. solution of carbolic acid, while it takes ten minutes before all the germs are killed when immersed in a bichloride solution of 1:1,000. Every stationary cuspidor, and also the hand-cup in the sick-room or on the little table next to the steamer-chair where the patient takes his rest cure, should be filled every morning about one-fifth with a five-per-cent. carbolic-acid solution. Of late, wood vinegar (acidum pyrolignosum) has proved to be an excellent disinfectant for tuberculous secretions. It kills the bacilli after six hours, and takes away the unpleasant aspect of the expectorated matter.

To encourage the use of the pocket flask, one must make its manipulation, and especially the process of cleaning, as simple as possible. Thus the directions which accompany the aluminum pocket flask above referred to are as follows: To empty the flask, unscrew the top and pour the contents into the water-closet; or fold a newspaper into several layers, pour the contents on to this, and throw the whole at once into the fire, being careful not to spill any. Rinse the flask in hot water and wash the hands immediately afterwards.

Some consumptive individuals will not use the pocket flask, in spite of all persuasion, fearing to attract attention to their malady. For these there is but one thing to do—to use squares of soft muslin, cheap handkerchiefs, or Japanese paper handkerchiefs specially manufactured for that purpose,[21] which can be burned after use. But they should place in their pockets a removable lining of rubber or other impermeable substance which can be thoroughly cleaned. This additional pocket could be fastened to the inside of the ordinary pocket by clamps, and thus be of no inconvenience to the patient. Of course, all invalids using handkerchiefs as receptacles for expectorations take their chances of infecting their hands, and should always wash them thoroughly before touching any food.

There is no doubt that a frequent cause of infection by ingestion is the use of tuberculous milk or meat as nutriment. In children especially the delicate intestinal epithelium offers to the bacilli contained in tuberculous milk a most favorable abiding-place. The reason we so rarely find primary intestinal tuberculosis in adults, in spite of the frequent ingestion of tuberculous substances, may perhaps be explained by the fact that with them the epithelial lining of the intestines is stronger and resists the colonization of cultures. If the individual is in poor health, and the phagocytic power of the blood is enfeebled, the bacilli ingested by a grown person usually find the apices of the lungs to be the *locus minoris resistentiæ*, which they reach through the medium of the circulation of the lymph or the blood. The individual can protect himself against the ingestion of tuberculous substances only by boiling or sterilizing all milk and thoroughly cooking all meat of doubtful origin.

The saliva of consumptives not infrequently contains tubercle bacilli. Petit,[21] Cornet,[22] and many others have reported their clinical experience in this respect, which shows that there is real danger in kissing tuberculous patients on the mouth. The napkins used by consumptives should be boiled after each meal. If, for economic reasons, a freshly washed napkin cannot always be had, Japanese paper napkins, which are burned after use, may be substituted. Knives, forks, spoons, glasses, etc., should be thoroughly boiled or sterilized after each use.

Consumptive men should either wear no beard at all or keep the mustache and beard closely cut, so that they may be easily kept clean and not become the cause of infection or reinfection.

It is of great importance to tell the patients never, out of false modesty or for any other reason, to swallow their expectoration. There is always danger of an intestinal infection. Among insane tuberculous patients, secondary intestinal tuberculosis is of most frequent occurrence.[24]

There seems to reside a certain danger in the cigars and cigarettes that are made by hand. If the cigarmaker happens to be tuberculous, the saliva which he uses to fasten the wrapper may convey the tubercle bacillus to the smoker. Dr. J. C. Spencer, of the San Francisco Board of Health, has actually demonstrated the presence of these bacilli in various specimens of cigars submitted to him for examination. Now, although the nicotine may kill the bacillus, it does not render it thereby inoffensive, for Prudden and Hodenpyl[25] have shown by their very interesting experiments that the dead tubercle bacilli still contain a specific protein capable of doing harm in the living tissue. Grancher and Ledoux-Lebard,[26] who carried on similar experiments, called the cellular reaction produced by the dead bacillus "necrotuberculosis." In view of the possible danger of this mode of infection, it would, of course, be well to advise all persons predisposed to consumption not to smoke at all, and the same rule may hold good for all individuals whose constitution is weakened from any cause.

Infection from the ingestion of tubercle bacilli is also made possible by the patient soiling his hands with the expectoration directly or, as has been stated above, through the medium of a soiled handkerchief, and then touching his food, thus conveying the bacilli to the digestive tract. That such infection from the hands in pulmonary phthisis is possible has been very clearly demonstrated by Dr. E. R. Baldwin, of Saranac Lake.

The soiled linen of consumptive patients should be placed in water immediately after the removal from bed or body, and be washed separately, or at least boiled before it is given to the general laundry.

Just as it must be considered unhygienic and a probable cause of the propagation of diseases to besprinkle one's self with holy water which has been standing for days in churches, and in which the multitudes have dipped their fingers, so does it seem unwise to use a common communion cup in the Protestant churches. The individual communion cup is certainly to be preferred. On the same principle we should also condemn the custom still frequent in this country of kissing the Bible when being sworn before court.

Midwives and also physicians will often, in the presence of an asphyxiated newborn child, apply the mouth to that of the infant and inflate the child's chest in order to bring its respiratory organs into play. If the operator is consumptive, the danger of imparting his or her disease to the infant is evident. To avoid such possibility, the mouth-to-mouth respiration should be replaced by the safer method of using the catheter, as recommended by Tarnier and Lusk. Laborde's method of rhythmical traction of the tongue will also often suffice to cause the child to breathe. The habit some midwives have, of sucking the mucus from the child's throat by direct application of the mouth, is equally to be condemned. Reich has reported ten cases of tuberculous infection through this method. A midwife in the village of Neuenberg became consumptive in 1874, and died of this disease in July, 1876. Ten children, without hereditary predisposition, attended by this midwife between April, 1875, and May, 1876, died before reaching the age of seventeen months. This consumptive midwife was in the habit of sucking the mucus from the mouths of newborn children, and blowing air into their mouths when there was the slightest sign of asphyxia.

The remnants of food left by tuberculous invalids should not be eaten by others.

The physician who is attending a consumptive engaged in such an occupation as that of dairyman, baker, confectioner, cook, or butcher should be particular to instruct his patient concerning the danger to himself and others of being careless with his expectoration or other secretions. If the patient is refractory, the physician's duty would be to report him to the authorities as a menace to public health.

We have already referred to the unsanitary habit of kissing. Probably consumption has often been transmitted in this way from one member of a family to another; but the habit of kissing domestic pet animals is equally dangerous. The parrot and the canary-bird, when domesticated, take tuberculosis most easily, and then constitute a real danger in the household.[27] Dogs and cats come next in the frequency of tuberculous infection. Kissing and caressing all such domestic pets, especially by children, should be strictly forbidden. The authorities should have a right to destroy small domestic animals if they are afflicted with tuberculosis.

In localities where there is not perfect sewerage it is always advisable to disinfect the stools from a patient suffering from intestinal tuberculosis. While it is true that the excreta coming from a healthy person contain saprophytic organisms which combat the tubercle bacilli, it is not unlikely that the stools of a phthisical patient are materially altered and permit a longer existence of pathological organisms. We know that the fecal matter coming from typhoid-fever patients does not lose its infectious qualities after having been ejected for some time or even thrown in the common cesspool.

In out-of-town institutions for consumptives, where a complete sewer system is often not easily installed, an oven for the burning of all fecal and expectorated matter is a prophylactic measure to be recommended. The superficial burying of tuberculous excreta (fecal matter or expectoration) should not be allowed unless it has been previously treated with a five-per-cent. carbolic-acid solution or a corrosive-sublimate solution of 1:1,000. Lortet and Despeignes reported to the Paris Academy of Science, on January 25th and July 4th, 1892, their experiments with the earth-worm, which show that it may be instrumental in bringing to the surface again the bacilli from buried tuberculous substances. Animals which might chance to pasture in the vicinity of spots where such substances have been buried are certainly in great danger of ingesting the tubercle bacilli. All persons handling vessels containing tuberculous substances should be very careful, for, while not having the disease themselves, they may unconsciously transmit it to others.

Consumptives who attend to the cleaning of their spittoons themselves must be especially prudent. . If they have anywhere a cutaneous abrasion, they must be careful not to soil it with saliva or expectoration. Surgeons and nurses should be particularly careful when attending surgical cases of tuberculosis. I have had occasion to observe such an inoculation in the service of a colleague. The unfortunate nurse came wellnigh losing his whole hand from dressing a tuberculous wound. The seat of entrance of the tuberculous infection was a slight abrasion of the skin which had passed unobserved.

Equally dangerous are the handling and washing of handkerchiefs and other linen used by consumptives. The slightest skin wound on the hands of the washer may be the cause of an inoculation which by friction is often rubbed into the deeper tissues. Steinthal,[28] Dubreuilh and Auché,[29] and von Eiselsberg[30] have reported cases demonstrating this source of infection. If the contact of the tuberculous material is in the region of the face, or near the genital region, it is not infrequent to see the development of typical lupus from the inoculation. Leloir[31] and Baginsky described a case in which a healthy girl contracted a lupus of the nose in consequence of frequent use of the soiled handkerchief of her tuberculous sister. A medical student in Germany, who was intrusted with the examination of tuberculous sputum, removed the scab from a recent duel wound with his infected finger-nails, which carelessness resulted in a facial lupus (Wolters[32]).

The most frequent mode of tuberculous inoculation is, of course, autoinoculation. I recall a case in which a tuberculous patient inserted an injured finger into his mouth and contracted tuberculosis of that member. Lipp[33] cites a case of lupus of the face, the anus, and the vulva in a consumptive as a consequence of perpetual scratching, the patient being infested with lice. Education and extreme care alone will be able to prevent such accidents.

Pathologists handling fresh tuberculous specimens, physicians performing autopsies, and students dissecting tuberculous subjects, are also greatly exposed to the danger of becoming inoculated with tuberculosis. The "piqûre anatomique" has, alas, too often developed into a serious tuberculous infection. To incise freely with an aseptic instrument at the seat of inoculation and apply a dressing of bichloride, 1:3,000, seems the best immediate step to take in case such an accident happens.

Infection from wet-nurse to child, and *vice versa*, is possible. Happily the cases in which a tuberculous mother nurses a child are now exceedingly rare. Unless a most thorough examination of the infant reveals no sign or symptom of tuberculous infection, or if there is the slightest doubt, a wet-nurse should not be exposed to the possibility of becoming infected by the child. Weber's case, cited in his Croonian lectures of 1885, gives a very striking example of the possibility of a tuberculous child communicating the disease to a healthy wet-nurse who had no hereditary predisposition.

The possibility of transmitting tuberculosis to a child through vaccination cannot be denied,[34] especially when one considers that the vaccine is now almost exclusively obtained from young bovine animals. Although Villain's statistics show a comparative rarity of tuberculosis in calves between the ages of four to six months, it seems to me good practice to follow Brouardel's suggestion[35] that, in order to obtain absolute security, the best thing would be to slaughter the animals immediately after they have served as vaccinifers, and not to use the vaccine until the examination of the slaughtered animals had shown that there was no trace of tuberculosis in their organs.

It is possible for tuberculous infection to take place through sexual relations. All phthisiotherapeutists have occasionally met with such cases. I need only to refer to the works of Reclus,[36] Schuchardt,[37] Carrera,[38] Cornet,[39] and Petit.[40] Education in private by the family physicians, and in some cases, perhaps, the sanitary police intervention, can alone do the necessary prophylactic work.

The ritual act of circumcision, practised according to Jewish rites, has, in numerous instances, been the occasion of transmitting to an innocent, healthy child the disease in question. The tuberculous inoculation manifests itself first as a local disease of the genital organs, from whence, in a large number of cases, it becomes generalized. Cases have been reported by Lindemann,[41] Jacobi,[42] Maas,[43] Meyer,[44] and others. The operation of circumcision, when skilfully and rapidly performed, is in itself trifling, but the sucking of the prepuce afterwards makes it dangerous. Since it will be difficult to stop this practice by a simple protest on the part of physicians, and as the law cannot interfere with the free exercise of a religious rite, I should suggest as a remedy that only such persons should be allowed to perform circumcision as have shown the necessary skill before a medical board of examiners, and that every time they are called upon to perform the rite they should submit themselves to a medical examination. Only when bearing a certificate from a regular physician, stating the absolute freedom from specific diseases, should they be allowed to perform ritual circumcision.

As another reliable prophylactic measure against the possibility of inoculating the child, when the parents insist upon the orthodox method of circumcision, is the suction by the aid of a glass tube, as practised in France and Germany.

Whenever a tuberculous secretion (saliva or sputum) enters an open wound, inoculation is possible. Thus, tattooing[45] or the simple procedure of piercing the ear lobe has given rise to local tuberculosis owing to the ignorance or carelessness of the operator when the latter happened to be consumptive.

General Public Prophylaxis.

In speaking of the communication of tuberculosis we have shown the individual and private means to prevent it. We now come to the duties of the sanitary authorities and of the general government in the prevention of tuberculosis in general, considered as what the Germans justly call a "Volkskrankheit" (disease of all classes).

We will first treat of the duties of the sanitary authorities in regard to the prevention of the propagation of the disease as it takes place from man to man.

The question of compulsory registration, or reporting cases of tuberculosis, is far from being settled. The vast majority of the profession is opposed to it. In an important meeting of the State and Provincial Boards of Health of North America, held at Detroit, Mich., in August, 1898, this matter was discussed. I quote the views I expressed at that time on the inadvisability of making the reporting of consumptive cases compulsory. My conviction in this matter has not changed since, but on the contrary has been strengthened by additional experience.

1. Pulmonary tuberculosis is not a contagious disease, but only communicable; the contact *per se* of a consumptive individual does not transmit the disease.

2. The scrupulous destruction of tuberculous expectoration and other secretions suffices to do away with all danger of infection and transmission.

3. Pulmonary tuberculosis is a chronic disease, lasting often for years, and once reporting it at a given time, and even the one and usually only visit on the part of a sanitary inspector, can have no lasting effect in the prevention of the disease.

4. The tuberculous patient who is likely to propagate his disease in the most extensive and dangerous way is not the consumptive unable to move about, and confined to one or a few rooms, but the relatively well tuberculous individual who, though expectorating daily millions of bacilli, is still able to attend to his occupations. Such a person, even when his case has been reported to the Board of Health, and when he has been visited once by the sanitary inspector, can change his residence, and his neighbors will have no idea of the danger they are in if the newcomer is unscrupulous with his expectoration.

5. While some boards of health refrain from sending a sanitary inspector when this is expressly stated as undesired in the family physician's report, other boards maintain that it should be done in all cases. Only the physician, who in many cases is not alone the medical adviser but also the counsellor and intimate friend of the family, will know that circumstances may arise in which making public the existence of a tuberculous disease in a family would mean disaster.

From the controversy going on in many parts of the world between boards of health and the medical profession at large, it is evident that the time for classifying tuberculosis with acute infectious and contagious diseases has not yet come.

What, then, remains to be done by the sanitary authorities in regard to this matter?

In the interest of demographical science, and in the hope of discovery of some of the underlying causes when the disease is seemingly confined to certain districts, all cases of tuberculosis should be reported. The reporting physician should receive printed measures how to insure a thorough prophylaxis, and also an offer that, if desirable, the sanitary inspector would visit the patient to give verbal instructions. It should be left to the discretion of the physician when and how often a disinfection of the patient's apartments during the course of his disease should take place. The disinfection of an apartment in which a consumptive person has died must, however, be enforced by law, and the physician should be held responsible that the authorities are notified of such a death. Disinfection should also be obligatory in case a room is vacated by a consumptive person; this should be especially enforced in hotels, boardinghouses, and health resorts. There should be no charge for disinfecting for the poor.

Formaldehyde gas, according to the experiments made by the Department of Health of the City of New York, is the best disinfectant known at present for use in infected dwellings. Its power of penetration is, however, inferior to that of steam or a dry heat of 230° F.; but for the disinfection of fine wearing apparel, furs, leather, upholstery, books, and the like, which are injured by great heat, it is better than any other means. I recommend the method indicated by Novy and Waite,[a] which is as follows: 1. All cracks or openings in the plaster or in the floor, or about the door and windows, should be caulked tight with cotton or with strips of cloth. 2. The linen, quilts, blankets, carpets, etc., should be stretched out on a line in order to expose as much surface to the disinfectant as possible. They should not be thrown into a heap. Books should be suspended by their covers, so that the pages will fall open and be freely exposed. 3. The walls and the floor of the room, and the articles contained in it, should be thoroughly sprayed with water. If masses of matter or sputum are dried down on the floor, they should be soaked with water and loosened. No vessel of water should, however, be allowed to remain in the room. 4. One hundred and fifty cubic centimetres (five ounces) of the commercial forty-percent. solution of formalin for each one thousand cubic feet of space should be placed in the distilling apparatus and be distilled as rapidly as possible. The keyhole and spaces about the door should then be packed with cotton or cloth. 5. The room thus treated should remain closed at least ten hours. If there is much leakage of gas into the surrounding rooms, a second or third distillation of formaldehyde should be made at intervals of two or three hours.

Each community should have health ordinances suitable to its own conditions. A place which is a favorite resort for pulmonary invalids will require much more stringent rules in regard to board-ing-houses and hotels than the average place. Wherever it is practi-cable the sanitary authorities should place spittoons containing dis-infectants in gardens, parks, public stations, etc. There should be a sufficient number and they should be kept clean. Elevated spittoons would be preferable. To put notices in public conveyances, halls, theatres, churches, etc., making spitting on the floor a punishable offence will prove a good thing everywhere. If it does not deter all the spitters from expectorating wherever they please, it will deter some.

It is also of importance that the floors of all public conveyances, instead of being covered with carpets or rope mats, which are often veritable filth and microbe collectors, should be simply left plain wood or covered with oilcloth which can be easily cleaned and washed off, as frequently as convenient and necessary. The removable slats used in street cars should be taken up at stated intervals and replaced by clean ones after the floor of the car has been thoroughly cleaned with disinfectant fluid. The disinfection of railway passenger cars, and especially sleeping-cars, should also be made obligatory, as well as all buildings in which large gatherings are held, such as theatres, churches, music halls, libraries, asylums, barracks, waiting-rooms, stores, pawnshops, etc. That such places need a regular and thor-ough disinfection has become evident by the interesting experiments of the late Professor Straus, of Paris. He took the nasal mucus of six employees and that of the leader of the orchestra of the Parisian opera, and also the nasal secretions of nine employees of the library of the medical faculty. He inoculated a guinea-pig with the mucus of each of these sixteen persons, and the result was that seven of the animals died soon very much emaciated, the autopsy showing typical tuberculous lesions. All the sixteen persons above mentioned had been previously examined by competent clinicians and pronounced free from any disease.

The disinfection of libraries, books, and documents seems quite important. Aside from the habit many people have of moistening the fingers with saliva to turn the leaves, the infection of the pages of books and documents may take place perhaps more frequently when a consumptive person is bending over a book for the purpose of reading or writing and is attacked by a coughing-spell. Small particles of bacilliferous saliva are thus thrown upon the pages. In the *Presse Médicale* of November 22d, 1899, a case was reported which illustrates this mode of infection. In Kharkov (Russia) twenty employees of the municipality became tuberculous successively. They all had worked over certain records of the city, which had previously been much handled by a consumptive. The bacteriologist of that city took scrapings from the various documents, and the examination showed the frequent presence of tubercle bacilli. Ledgers, or other large valuable books, are, however, rather difficult to disinfect thoroughly. The accompanying illustration (Fig. 26) will show a device

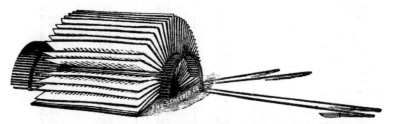

Fig. 26.—Apparatus for Separating the Leaves of Books to be Disinfected.

for making the process more easy and thorough. The book and the leaf separator are placed in an hermetically closing box into which the formaldehyde gas penetrates. To increase the efficacy of the disinfectant the box should have an arrangement which will permit the creation of a vacuum previous to the entrance of the gas.

For ordinary library books the use of this leaf-separating instrument is not necessary and Immerwahr's method suffices for all practical purposes. He advises placing the books, backs up with the covers so separated as to admit of some looseness of the leaves, in the upper part of an incubator heated from 86° to 95° F., with a formalin solution in shallow capsules at the bottom, and keeping them there for five or six hours.

A sanitary supervision of factories, workshops, and stores, with a view of securing hygienically constructed and managed places where the workers have to toil, is, of course, essential. In all industries where the inhalation of organic or metallic dust seems to be inevitable, the workers should be provided with respiratory masks, such as are in use in some of the factories in Europe.

The regulation of working-hours, especially for women and children, will also lead to a reduction of the mortality from tuberculosis.

No one is more prone to become consumptive than the overworked individual whose environments are the reverse of sanitary.

The following table, compiled by Archibald Kerr Chalmers, M.D., D.P.H.,'' showing the comparative mortality of individuals occupied in the various pursuits of life, will be the best guide to the sanitary authorities as to where intervention is most needed:

	Phthisis.	Other diseases of respiration.	Both together.	Per cent of phthisis to all diseases of respiration.
Agriculturist...............	106	115	221	48.0
Engraver (artist class).......	146	133	279	52.3
Storekeeper.................	172	178	350	49.1
Butcher....................	195	209	404	48.3
Commercial clerk...........	218	172	390	55.9
Watchmaker.................	243	193	427	54.8
Saddler	248	169	417	59.5
Shoemaker	256	181	437	58.6
Draper.....................	260	181	441	59.0
Tailor.....................	271	195	446	58.2
Hairdresser.................	276	213	489	56.4
Tobacconist, tobacco manufacturer	280	181	461	60.7
Hatter.....................	301	210	511	58.9
Musician	322	200	522	61.7
Bookbinder.................	325	218	543	59.9
Printer....................	326	214	540	60.4

This list relating to the frequency of tuberculosis among the various occupations coincides probably with the average experience of most physicians. It does not include the scientists nor the professions in general among which, nevertheless, a large number of deaths from phthisis occur. According to Raseri's statistics there are 13 cases of phthisis in each 100 deaths in Italy. Of these the "lazzaroni," or street-loungers, offer only 2.4 per cent., the scientists no less than 48 per cent. There are, however, in my experience also two classes of manual laborers which are frequently attacked by tuberculosis and which are not mentioned in any recently published statistics. These are, first, the employees in laundries entrusted with the task of assorting and marking the dirty clothing brought in by the collectors; secondly, and perhaps more frequently, I have found consumption prevailing among rag sorters. This occupation in most of our American cities is followed by poor Italians, who live, as a rule, in badly ventilated and most unhygienic basement rooms. It seems to me that some provision compelling laundry establishments to subject all the incoming pieces to a thorough disinfection by formaldehyde gas, steam, or boiling before they are given to the assorters might stop this mode of propagating the disease. Another means would probably be the recommendation of respiratory masks, through which the inspired air might be filtered. This latter precaution and additional hygienic instruction are probably also the only means to prevent the spread of tuberculosis among the Italian rag sorters.

The tailors, whom Dr. Chalmers places only as the seventh in the list, come in our great American cities pretty close to the printers in their mortality from tuberculosis, owing to the existence of the sweat-shop system. The terrible mortality among these laborers and their families, not only from tuberculosis but also from other infectious diseases in the city of New York, has been so great that a special law for the protection of these men, women, and, alas, children too, had to be enacted. The unhygienic mode of life and unsanitary homes in which these families live are, no doubt, additional factors in the propagation of tuberculosis. Here education must come to the help of legislation.

Cigarmakers, whom I presume Dr. Chalmers includes among tobacconists, are in my experience also a class particularly prone to consumption. There seem to be several reasons for this. First, it must be said that this occupation is not usually chosen by very robust people, and that many predisposed to tuberculosis join the ranks of the cigarmakers; a second cause is probably to be found in the irritating particles of tobacco dust; third, the presence of consumptive laborers who take no care of their expectoration; and finally, the close proximity in which these people work, which makes infection through the expulsion of small particles of saliva possible even during dry cough. A medical examination of the laborer who desires to enter a cigar factory is in my opinion a very rational prophylactic means to combat this source of infection. Of course, proper ventilation, the distribution of such spittoons as Predöhl's (Fig. 18), described on page 192, and the placing of the laborers in not too close proximity to each other should be made obligatory in all such factories.

In printing-offices good ventilation, more cleanliness, better hygiene, the wearing of respirators, and the better division of the time of labor, so as to enable the printers to spend more time in the open air, will certainly help to reduce the fearful mortality among this class of laborers. A periodical examination of the employees in printing-offices and the recommendation of a change of occupation in case the disease has been discovered will be helpful in promoting prophylaxis. Lastly, no one should be allowed to become an apprentice in a printing-office unless a physical examination has shown him to be in good health. Similar rules and regulations may be advantageously adopted for all those professions and trades which are notoriously dangerous in the propagation of pulmonary tuberculosis. Nurses and maids who have to clean the rooms of consumptives should wear a mask over mouth and nose during this work, to prevent the inhalation of dust which might be infected. All laborers who are exposed to the inhalation of dust from whatever source should be taught the importance of habitual nose breathing, to prevent diseases of the respiratory organs.

In some cities rigorous measures against the production of quantities of coal smoke would doubtless render the atmosphere purer and diseases of the respiratory organs rarer. In England there exists a Coal-smoke Abatement Society, the object of which is to combat the smoke nuisance and to enforce existing laws against black smoke. They are trying now to have a law passed making it illegal for any house to be built without being fitted with proper smoke-consuming appliances.

Damp, badly ventilated, and dark habitations seem to favor the development of tuberculous diseases. So long as the poor are housed by hundreds in dark, filthy, and badly ventilated buildings, so long will it be impossible to stamp out consumption. The hygienic condition of the poorer classes must be improved, but especially of those families wherein one or several members have already contracted tuberculosis.

That alcoholism is one of the greatest direct and indirect causes that prepare the field for the tubercle bacilli, is now generally conceded, not only by physicians and sanitarians, but also by all sociologists who have studied the question. It is not only a phthisiogenetic disease *par excellence* in adult life, but, according to statistics carefully kept in some of the European hospitals for scrofulous children, in more than fifty per cent. of the cases either the father or the mother, or both, were found to be, or to have been, alcoholics. Legislation alone will do little against the evil of alcoholism so long as there is no substitute for the liquor saloon. The establishment of places for healthy amusement where men, women, and children can go and obtain non-alcoholic drinks at reasonable prices should be encouraged by the authorities. In public thoroughfares there should be stands where in summer refreshing, non-alcoholic drinks, and in winter tea and coffee could be had at low prices. To combat alcoholism must be the work of the statesman and the sanitarian. With the diminution of the consumption of alcohol there will be a corresponding reduction in the mortality from pulmonary tuberculosis.

Syphilis is not infrequently a predisposing cause of pulmonary tuberculosis. To regulate prostitution, and thus diminish the danger of venereal infection, by humane but strict laws must, of necessity, become a portion of the public prophylaxis of consumption.

Of the importance of sanatoria, special hospitals, and dispensaries in the prevention of tuberculosis, we shall speak more in detail under a separate heading. Here I wish only to insist upon the necessity of a more general distribution of the pocket flask as a means of preventing expectoration in public. Dispensaries should distribute suitable pocket spittoons gratuitously to their very poor tuberculous patients. Those able to pay for them should be treated only under the condition that they provide themselves with such pocket flasks. I should like to go even further in this respect and insist upon the use of pocket flasks by all patients who expectorate, whether suffering from grippe, bronchitis, etc., or from typical pulmonary or laryngeal tuberculosis.

The strictest supervision on the part of the board of health in regard to tuberculosis should be exercised over insane asylums, prisons, convents, large boarding-schools, and all places where many people are constantly confined in a relatively small space. Statistics from all over the world show that the mortality from pulmonary tuberculosis in these places is higher than anywhere else.[48] My personal visits to some otherwise well-regulated prisons and similar institutions have convinced me of the need of more serious attention to this matter. A most commendable innovation in this respect is the projected convict camp of tuberculous prisoners of the State of Alabama.

In many cities tuberculosis seems to cling to certain localities and houses owing to the nature of their construction. The disease appears in a veritable endemic form, either from the fact that careless tuberculous patients have lived for years in these houses or from the equally important fact that the soil on which they are built, or the manner in which they have been constructed, is such as to favor the retention of the tuberculous infection indefinitely. That this is so has been shown by the report of Dr. Biggs,[49] of the Health Board of New York, and the interesting work on this subject by Dr. Flick, of Philadelphia.[50] When a thorough sanitary overhauling does not suffice to stamp out these centres of infection, the destruction of such dwellings seems the only remedy.

The published report of Dr. Gaston in the *Dietetic and Hygienic Gazette*, is a good example of such a case, and shows that a law should be enacted giving power to the sanitary authorities to enforce the destruction of such infected dwellings. The following is the history of the home of the S—— family: "The house was constructed at Mineral Ridge about 1830, and was occupied by a family of the name of F——. It is related that a young man who lived with the family was 'always ailing and in delicate health,' but the only death was that of a baby with bowel trouble. They resided in the premises until about 1846, when the house was occupied by a family named S——. They were an unusually strong and healthy family when they first came to this place, with no previous tuberculous history. The first one connected with this family to pass away was a lady boarder, but information does not reveal the cause of her death. It was quickly followed, however, by the death of two sons, two daughters, father and mother, from tuberculosis, leaving only one son, who had previously gone to Illinois on account of his health, and who still survives. From 1879 until now the house has been held by the present occupants. There was no history whatever of consumption in the family prior to their coming to this house. The daughter who died recently was born there. Her death was the seventh in the family in as many years from pulmonary tuberculosis. A sister, two brothers, and a mother survive, but the characteristic traces of the disease are plainly visible in the faces of one brother and the surviving sister. The building is a story and a half high, and is surrounded by dense foliage."

The circulars issued by a board of health in regard to any disease, but especially in regard to consumption, should be framed in clear, precise, untechnical, and comprehensive language. They should call attention to the danger from an unclean, unscrupulous consumptive, and explain wherein this danger lies and how to avoid it. But the circular should explain also that, if proper precautions are taken, there is no danger in associating with such a patient. Not to frighten very impressionable natures, the circular should state that pulmonary tuberculosis is one of the most curable and frequently cured diseases, for this has been amply proved; and the earlier the patient puts himself under the doctor's care the more chance has he of an early and complete recovery. Such circulars should be freely distributed, and especially in the densely crowded districts of large cities.

An excellent method of educating the public in regard to the necessity of preventive measures to stop the spread of tuberculosis is the formation of societies for this purpose. They exist now in nearly all civilized countries, and have done some very good work already. These societies are composed of laymen and medical men, and their purpose is usually twofold. The medical members deliver public lectures or compose tracts for distribution. The Pennsylvania Society for the Prevention of Tuberculosis, for example, distributed during one year fifty thousand tracts entitled "How to Avoid Contracting Tuberculosis," forty thousand tracts entitled "How Persons Suffering from Tuberculosis Can Avoid Giving the Disease to Others," and ten thousand tracts entitled "How Hotel-keepers Can Aid in Preventing the Spread of Tuberculosis," also an equal number on the "Predisposing Causes of Tuberculosis and How to Avoid or Overcome Them." The second very laudable purpose of some of these societies is the endeavor to establish sanatoria for the treatment of the tuberculous poor.

Streets should never be swept without having been previously thoroughly sprinkled. Professor von Schrötter calls the sweeping of unsprinkled streets and its accompanying raising of clouds of dust a crime towards one's fellow-men.

But, to my mind, equally dangerous is Dame Fashion, when she decrees that our ladies shall wear long street-dresses. To walk and breathe behind a lady dragging her dress over dusty, dirty sidewalks, often dotted with deposits of buccal, bronchial, and pulmonary secretions, sometimes containing the various pathogenic microbes, at others mixed with tobacco juice, must be dangerous to the health of every one. The poor woman who is afterwards obliged to clean these skirts, soiled with an accumulation of filth, dust, and too often disease-producing germs, is indeed to be pitied. If our ladies will not soon realize the danger of this mode of dress, I should certainly favor city ordinances prohibiting the wearing of trailing dresses in public streets.

Another means of preventing the possible dissemination of disease through dust might be an ordinance compelling all dealers in articles of food which have no natural covering or which are usually eaten uncooked and just as they are exhibited, to keep their display under a cover, preferably of glass. This ordinance should not only be enforced with the poor street vender, but also with the great department stores where candies and often other eatables are, perhaps, covered with far more dangerous dust than that of the street.

A very commendable precaution was recently instituted in some of the large bakeries of Germany, in connection with the handling and transportation of bread. The moment the bread comes out of the oven, while it is still too hot to be handled, it is placed, by the aid of a shovel, upon a piece of wrapping-paper large enough to envelop the whole loaf. By twisting the two ends of the wrapper the bread is completely enclosed. This is certainly a more hygienic way than the one now in vogue in nearly all countries. A loaf of bread coming from one of the public bakeries, and especially in the districts of the poor, usually passes through any number of hands. Sometimes it may be handled by those afflicted with disease, but nearly always passes through hands of doubtful cleanliness before it reaches the consumer's mouth. No one would think of washing the crust of bread which has been exposed to all sorts of contaminating influences in the bakeshop, bakery wagon, grocery store, etc.; but we would not think of eating any other article of food treated in the same way without submitting it to a thorough cleansing. I believe it would be a veritable protection to the people if the sanitary authorities would compel all public bakers and bread dealers to institute some such cleanly method of handling the bread as I have described.

A chapter on the prophylaxis of tuberculosis would not be complete without mentioning the danger arising from the present almost universal mode of the disposal of the dead. In connection with the disposal of the sputum and excretion I have already referred to the experiments of Lortet and Despeignes, whereby it was demonstrated that earthworms are capable of ingesting and ejecting the tubercle bacilli without the microorganisms losing their virulence. Other experimenters, such as Galtier,[51] of Lyons, showed that the bacillus of tuberculosis resisted putrefaction for several months. Gartner[52] buried the bacillus for one year, and it retained its infectious property, and Schottelius even claims that it resisted putrefaction for two years. In view of these and numerous other proofs of the danger of burying those who have died from tuberculous diseases, the Third Congress for the Study of Tuberculosis, held in Paris in 1894, adopted resolutions asking for obligatory disinfection of the bodies of diseased tuberculous individuals. A motion for recommending obligatory cremation of such bodies was not carried. Leaving the religious objection to cremation out of consideration, it seems to me that the objection raised from a medico-legal standpoint (inability to discover poison after cremation) can hardly have any weight in a case of death from a chronic tuberculous disease. As one of the means of stamping out tuberculosis in the human race, I would certainly favor the cremation of all bodies of individuals having died of a tuberculous disease. Thalassic submersion as a means for the disposal of the dead seems also preferable to the methods now so universally in vogue.[53]

It has been proposed by some authors that efforts should be made by the state to prevent the marriage of unduly youthful persons whose appearance indicates the possibility of tuberculosis, and that persons whose sputum contains tubercle bacilli should be absolutely forbidden marriage. In our present state of society this question must be left to the family physician, who alone can assert his influence in preventing a union, the result of which might be the propagation of a tuberculous disease.

In Germany a periodical physical examination of all people has been proposed as the best means to control tuberculosis among man. This stupendous task would, to my mind, be equally impossible to carry out without the cooperation of the general and family practitioner. In a well-regulated state, obligatory periodical examination is possible, but the selection of the physician for that purpose should be optional. But until the time when there will be ample provision for all the tuberculous poor, the obligatory physical examination will be of little avail in solving the tuberculosis problem.

Special Prophylaxis of Tuberculosis in Childhood.

Of the importance of this portion of our subject it is hardly necessary to speak, for the prophylaxis of tuberculosis in the child often means the protection of the individual from the disease throughout life. The prevention of tuberculosis in childhood must begin with the child *in utero*. We will outline the duties of the mother here, but under the heading of preventive treatment we shall speak especially of the woman who has reason to fear that a tuberculous tendency might be transmitted to her child.

Whenever the birth of a child is reported, there should be sent from the Board of Health to the mother, through the intermediary of the physician or midwife, printed directions in plain, comprehensible language as to her duties and the care to be exercised in order to prevent the child from contracting tuberculosis. These directions should treat of cleanliness, of ventilation, of nutrition, etc.; the danger of having the child sleep with the mother in the same bed, and the possibility of the transmission of a disease, if one exists, by kissing the child on the mouth. The various other modes whereby tuberculosis may be transmitted should be explained and the means of preventing them indicated. Instructions should be given in regard to the handling of milk, its sterilization, the cleaning of bottles, nipples, etc. Especial importance should be attached to the fact that the infection of children is very frequent during the age when they creep and play on the floor, touching everything with their little hands. The frequent existence of tuberculosis of the respiratory tract or the tuberculous invasion of the glandular system (scrofulosis) in children may thus be accounted for. Not only may these little ones inhale infected dust as well as grown persons, their frequent nasal catarrhs facilitating the entrance of the bacilli, but they will often, in addition to this, bring the infected fingers in direct contact with their nasal or buccal mucous membranes. A local tuberculosis by inoculation is also made possible by the often untrimmed nails.

Thus, through the above-mentioned circulars mothers should learn to let their babies play only on scrupulously clean floors (and be it said right here that a floor with a fixed carpet can never be clean). It would be better yet, if children could have their special clean mats to play on. Mothers and nurses should see that the children's fingers are kept as clean as possible and their nails cut. As long as the child is too small to clean its nose, regular nasal toilets with some mild borated solution or warm water should be instituted. Eczematous and other skin eruption should receive immediate medical attention; left to themselves they may give entrance to tuberculous infection.

Public nurseries, that is to say places where laboring-women may leave their children during working-hours, kindergartens, etc., should be under sanitary supervision. Expectorating on or near playgrounds for children should be considered a misdemeanor and punished accordingly. Playgrounds should be set apart for children in all communities. They should be kept especially clean and from time to time be strewn with clean gravel.

Concerning the hygiene of public schools, Emmet " justly says that many of them, as now conducted, are veritable "black holes," where the children are dying of autointoxication, and that there could not be found a better culture bed for the tuberculous germs than in these children, debilitated and with tissues starved through breathing devitalized and vitiated air. Public as well as private schools and colleges should be model houses in regard to cleanliness, hygiene, light, and constant ventilation—ventilation not only after the children have left, but all the time. Since windows and doors alone do not suffice properly to ventilate rooms when occupied by a mass of human beings, mechanical devices should be resorted to to secure always a plentiful supply of fresh air. Obligatory periodical disinfection by formaldehyde gas may also be advantageously instituted. To make the disinfecting and cleansing of the schoolroom as thorough as possible, I would suggest that desks and chairs be so constructed that they can easily be folded together after school hours. This innovation in school hygiene was first inaugurated by School Superintendent Akbroit, of Odessa, with most satisfactory results.

We should be anxious to give our children, during their school life, just as much opportunity of developing a sound vigorous body as of obtaining-culture and knowledge. Overcrowding of schoolrooms should not be tolerated. There should be a sufficient cubic air-space for each child; benches and desks should be constructed so as to make a faulty position of the body, or eye-strain, impossible.

The public school should be the place where the coming generation receives most of its hygienic education. There the children should be taught all that is conducive to health, and also how to avoid all that is unsanitary. The intelligent boy or girl will comprehend as well as the grown person why one should not expectorate except in a proper receptacle. Each child should have a cupboard where he should keep his own towel and drinking-cup. I have no doubt that thereby not only the frequency of tuberculosis, but also that of other infectious diseases would be greatly reduced among school children. Overwork during school life is an indirect cause of furthering a tuberculous tendency in many children, and indeed it is injurious even to a healthy child. The school physician (and every school should have one), charged with inspecting the children every morning for contagious diseases, should, on discovering a child developing tuberculosis, insist upon the exclusion of this pupil from the public school. Besides being a menace to the other pupils, the child will have no chance of getting well while daily attending school in a crowded classroom. Teachers suffering from tuberculosis should not be allowed to teach in public schools. Such regulation would be in their own interest as well as in that of the children.

There should be many small parks and playgrounds and public baths for old and young in the densely crowded districts of our large cities. City parks have justly been called the lungs of great centres of population. Here mothers and children of the poor can breathe purer and fresher air, which is one of the best means of preventing tuberculosis.

The Prevention of Tuberculosis in Cattle and Other Domestic Animals.

The prevention of tuberculosis in domestic animals is perhaps half the task in our combat against the "great white plague" in man. At the recent Congress of Tuberculosis in Berlin, no less a man than Virchow was selected to treat this important subject. The class of animals which requires our greatest attention in this matter is, of course, the bovine race. Dr. F. W. Smith, of the Tuberculosis Committee of the State Board of Health of New York, said to me: "The first great step towards the prophylaxis of tuberculosis in man is to stamp out the disease in cattle." Dr. Martin, of the Royal Commission of England, says: "The milk from cows with tuberculous udders possesses a virulence which can only be described as extraordinary."

Even the geographical distribution seems to point to the fact that the bovine race is in a large measure responsible for the prevalence of tuberculosis in man. In a very able paper, read before the American Health Association, at the twenty-fifth annual meeting, held at Philadelphia on October 26th to 29th, 1897, Dr. M. P. Ravenel,[55] of the Veterinary Department of the University of Pennsylvania, showed that in Northern Norway, Sweden, Lapland, and Finland, where reindeer constitute the bulk of farm animals; about Hudson Bay and in the islands of the Pacific, where no cattle exist; in the Scottish Hebrides, Iceland, and Newfoundland, where there are but few cattle, tuberculosis is far less prevalent in man. Particularly dangerous, on the contrary, seem to be the regions where cattle are housed in close proximity to the dwellings of the people as, for example, in Italy. This condition caused Perroncito to call tuberculosis " the scourge of man and beast."

The danger from tuberculous meat and milk should not be underestimated. It is well known that the bactericidal quality of the gastric secretions is rather insufficient in regard to the germ of tuberculosis. The only absolute defence against this mode of invasion seems to lie in the good phagocytic power of the blood of the healthy individual. Now, when we consider that milk, butter,[56] and the meat of cattle constitute most important and most universally used articles of food for man, and how relatively recently laws in regard to tuberculosis have been enacted at all, and in·how many States such laws do not exist or are but feebly enforced, I think it is not surprising when, in looking into the exact etiology of many cases of pulmonary tuberculosis, we find that a large number must have been caused by the ingestion and not by the inhalation of the bacillus.

What is now the present state of existing laws, for example, in the United States, to prevent the spread of bovine tuberculosis?

Some States have fairly good bovine laws and regulations and enforce them; others have good laws but cannot enforce them for lack of funds; again, some have regulations only concerning tuberculous milk, but none concerning tuberculous meat; and some have no laws or regulations concerning tuberculosis either in man or beast. It seems thus evident that, to combat effectually tuberculosis in cattle or other domestic animals, the central government alone is capable of doing the work. Much in the educational line of preventing bovine tuberculosis in the United States has been done by the Bureau of Animal Industry at Washington.

While each country and State may have to frame its bovine laws and regulations in accordance with the demands of its geographical, climatic, and perhaps also its political situation, there are some laws which should be common to all. As the result of a careful perusal of extensive literature on the subject, and an effort to make myself acquainted with the practical workings of the many different laws, regulations, and recommendations concerning the restriction of tuberculosis in cattle, I may suggest a few points which should form part of the rules essential to the prophylactic work instituted by any government in this respect:

1. There should be a central bureau, whence the work of the sanitary inspectors, especially educated for their duties, may be directed.

2. There should be an inspection of all cattle at regular intervals besides, of course, always upon the demand of the owner. Regarding the manner in which the inspection should be carried on, I have not found in all the literature on the subject anything more practical and more thorough than the directions given by Prof. Leonard Pearson,[7] the distinguished State veterinarian of the State of Pennsylvania, and I take great pleasure in reproducing them *in extenso:*

"*Directions for Inspecting Herds for Tuberculosis.*

"Inspection should be carried on while the herd is stabled. If it is necessary to stable animals under unusual conditions or among unusual surroundings that make them uneasy and excited, the tuberculin test should be postponed until the cattle have become accustomed to the conditions they are subjected to, and then begin with a careful physical examination of each animal. This is essential because in some severe cases of tuberculosis no reaction follows the injection of tuberculin, but experience has shown that these cases can be discovered by physical examination. This examination should be complete and include a careful examination of the udder and of the superficial lymphatic glands and auscultation of the lungs.

"Each animal should be numbered or described in such a way that it can be recognized without difficulty. It is well to number the stalls with chalk and transfer these numbers to the temperature sheet, so that the temperature of each animal can be recorded in its appropriate place without danger of confusion. The following procedure has been used extensively and has given excellent results:

"(a) Take the temperature of each animal to be tested at least twice, at intervals of three hours, before tuberculin is injected.

"(b) Inject the tuberculin* in the evening, preferably between the

---

* Average dose, 0.30 c.c. In diluting for an injection a ten-per-cent. solution of tuberculin is made by adding nine parts of a one-per-cent. solution of carbolic acid.

hours of six and nine. The injection should be made with a carefully sterilized hypodermic syringe. The most convenient point for injection is back of the left scapula.

"Prior to the injection the skin should be washed carefully with a five-per-cent. solution of creolin or other antiseptic.

" (c) The temperature should be taken nine hours after the injection, and temperature measurements repeated at regular intervals of two or three hours until the sixteenth hour after the injection.

" (d) When there is no elevation of temperature at this time (sixteen hours after injection) the examination may be discontinued; but if the temperature shows an upward tendency, measurements must be continued until a distinct reaction is recognized, or until the temperature begins to fall.

" (e) If a reaction is detected prior to the sixteenth hour, the measurements of temperature should be continued until the expiration of this period.

" (f) The thermometers used for this work should be accurate, and if several are used they should be compared before the examination is commenced.

" (g) If there is an unusual change of temperature of the stable, or a sudden change of weather, this fact should be recorded on the report blank.

" (h) If a cow is in a febrile condition when the initial temperatures are taken, tuberculin should not be used on her, because in this case the temperature curve is irregular and the result of the test uncertain.

" (i) Cows should not be tested within a few days before or after calving, for experience has shown that the result at these times may be misleading.

" (j) The tuberculin test is not recommended for calves under three months old.

" (k) In old, emaciated animals and in retests use twice the usual dose of tuberculin.

"In reporting upon the examination of the herd, the large temperature sheets should be filled out and returned, together with a more detailed record for each animal that proves to be tuberculous. This detailed report should be made out on the individual report blanks provided for this purpose.

"Condemned cattle must be removed from the herd and kept away from those that are healthy.

"In special cases inspectors may be directed to destroy and make post-mortem examinations upon the condemned animals as soon as they are recognized, but this must be done only when directions to this effect are given in the original letter of advice.

"In making post-mortems the carcasses should be thoroughly inspected, and all of the organs mentioned on the blank for reporting this work should be examined."

3. There should be thorough destruction of all tuberculous meat, etc., and a most careful disinfection and cleansing of the stables and all utensils which may have come in contact with the tuberculous animals. If the udders are the exclusive seat of the tuberculous lesion, and upon examination of the carcass·the other portions are found to be healthy, the meat can doubtless be used with safety. The owner of the cattle should be instructed in regard to the sanitary arrangements to prevent, as far as possible, a new outbreak of the disease. He should be especially instructed as to the precaution to be taken before introducing new animals into the herd.

4. There should be a just compensation for his loss according to the actual value and condition of the animals at the time of appraisement.

5. There should be a careful examination of all imported cattle and the strict exclusion of all tuberculous animals.

6. While several authors caution against the employment of a consumptive to help about cattle or in the dairy, I have failed to discover anything in the literature on the subject calling attention to the fact that the presence of any disease such as diarrhœa in children or adults, persistent cough, bronchitis, pleurisy, local badly healing sores in any one on or about the premises, might lead to the detection of bovine tuberculosis among the cattle of which they had charge, or of which they received milk. I would thus make it compulsory to notify the nearest sanitary authority of the occurrence of any of the above-named diseases, in addition to typhoid fever, scarlatina, diphtheria, etc., on the premises in the vicinity of where milch cows are kept.

7. A thorough supervision of all the slaughter-houses, milk depots, butcher shops, and retail milk stores is, of course, also one of the vital points to be considered in our strife against tuberculosis in man and beast.

8. The local boards of health of cities, towns, and villages should be in communication so as to be able to notify each other within a certain radius of the outbreak of any infectious disease in man or beast.

According to E. F. Brush,[8] a doctor of medicine and of veterinary surgery who has had vast experience in bovine tuberculosis, the frequency of this disease in cattle in civilized countries is to be explained by the method of inbreeding now almost universally in vogue, and the prolonged lactation. There seems to be no doubt that a cow, which from the time she is two years old or under, is milked continuously with the exception of a few weeks before her parturition, and which is pregnant during the greater part of the time that she is yielding her milk, must suffer from an impaired constitution and become an easy prey to the tubercle bacillus. A better education of our dairymen on the vital points of breeding cattle and the care of milch cows will doubtlessly lead to a reduction of bovine tuberculosis and be thus indirectly of vast prophylactic benefit to mankind.

Of late, the reports concerning the presence of tuberculosis in hogs have become alarmingly frequent. In nearly all of these reports the origin of the disease could be traced to the feeding of tuber-' culous products from infected cattle. The infection was most frequent when the hogs were fed with the centrifuge slime coming from creameries. The prevalence of tuberculosis among swine in certain parts of Germany and Denmark has been attributed to this system of feeding. To those still disbelieving in the possibility of tuberculous infection through ingestion of products coming from tuberculous cattle, this should be sufficient evidence.

Virchow, in his above-mentioned address (Nahrungsmittel[69]), thinks that in our combat against bovine tuberculosis we have lost sight of the fact of the frequent transmission of tuberculosis from tuberculous pork. Tuberculosis is much more readily diagnosed in the hog than in cattle, in the majority of cases being localized in the glands of the neck. Virchow admits that by removing these portions from the slaughtered hog the pork might be consumed without danger.

The same regulations which should govern the sale of beef should also hold good for the sale of pork. But farmers should be particularly urged not to feed their swine with refuse products from dairies without being assured that these come from non-tuberculous cattle; or, still better, to boil thoroughly all the food for swine which comes from cattle. They should also be advised to call in a veterinary surgeon when they notice a marked emaciation, especially among the young swine. Immediate isolation of such suspected animals is, of course, always advisable. .

Instances of tuberculosis in dogs, horses, goats, etc., can doubtless always be traced to an infection by tuberculous products from either man or cattle. Barrier[60] reported a case of intestinal tuberculosis in a dog contracted from his master. The most interesting point in this case was the presence of intestinal ulcers, swarming with bacilli, which had rendered the animal a dangerous centre of infection, inasmuch as innumerable germs were undoubtedly discharged with the fæces. Barrier therefore recommends that the same law be applied to dogs as is in force in France regarding bovine tuberculosis. Sheldon" has described an example of nodular tuberculous pericarditis in a dog of the large and powerful breed known as the "great Dane." There was tuberculosis of the peribronchial lymphatic glands, and undoubtedly this was a case of inhalation infection. Canine pets which cough and show symptoms of chronic disease, such as emaciation and weakness, should be killed before they have a chance to become a source of infection. Dogs should never be allowed in the rooms of consumptives or permitted to become their constant companions.

It is also well known that canaries and parrots frequently die of consumption, and the disease seems to be identical with tuberculosis in the human race. The utmost care and cleanliness should be exercised by persons caring for such birds, and they should be warned that in caressing and kissing them they are liable to become infected with tuberculosis. Consumptives should never have such animals in their rooms or be allowed to take care of them.

The managers of menageries and zoological gardens should also exercise great care in this respect. A tuberculous keeper might very easily infect the animals under his care, especially since their confinement makes them particularly susceptible to the invasion of the bacilli. The law which authorizes the sanitary authorities to kill tuberculous cattle should be extended to all other animals as well. There seems no reason why an apehouse, containing numerous consumptive animals, should not be as much a source of infection as a tenement house where ignorant or careless tuberculous individuals have expectorated indiscriminately. To visit the apehouse in the zoological garden and to remain there as long as possible is the delight of children. There is surely reason to be on guard against this possible source of infection of tuberculosis.

In stables where tuberculous cows are, or have been kept, in menageries where tuberculosis is the most frequent disease, the infection by inhaling the bacilli-laden dust of these places is perhaps far more frequent than is generally thought.

Laboratory researches, I think, have now definitely decided that the tuberculosis of chickens is not identical with that of man or the higher animals; but, of course, it is advisable that tuberculous fowl should not be used as food.

Predisposition and Preventive Treatment.

Direct hereditary bacillary transmission through the placenta is exceedingly rare, but it certainly cannot be denied. There are about forty cases on record in which direct bacillary transmission, while the child was still *in utero*, has been demonstrated beyond a shadow of doubt. Among those who reported such cases are Bang,[62] Birch-Hirschfeld,[63] De Renzi,[64] Galtier,[65] A. Jacobi,[66] Landouzi,[67] and Lannelongue.[68] These names are perhaps the best guaranty of the exactitude of the observations. The majority of cases of infantile tuberculosis are, however, due to postnatal infection occurring a short time after birth. Many of these cases are too often recorded as being due to direct hereditary transmission of the tubercle bacillus, while in reality the close contact of mother and child during the first few months of the latter's existence, and the ignorance on the part of the former are alone responsible for the infection. The remedy lies here again in education, the methods of which have been outlined in the section on special prophylaxis in childhood. Often a postnatal infection, though it may have taken place in early infancy, remains latent to manifest itself only in after years when aroused to activity by some disturbing factor in the economy of the individual. Some latent tuberculosis alone may constitute what we vaguely term a tuberculous predisposition. But, of course, I do not wish to deny the possibility of a transmission from one or both parents of a biological peculiarity which makes the offspring more prone to tuberculous disease. There is here a large field of research in biology and pathology yet before us, and it is to be hoped that future discoveries may teach us better to understand this vague term, tuberculous predisposition.

In spite of the discoveries in bacteriology and orrhotherapy our bacteriotherapeutists have thus far failed to give us any remedy which we might safely inject as an immunizing agent to prevent the development of tuberculosis. I should rejoice if such a boon were in store for mankind. However, we need not despair in the mean time. If the teachings of modern phthisiotherapeutists are followed, even the child of tuberculous parents may become a strong, healthy man or woman, and the accidental inhalation or ingestion of the tubercle bacilli will not suffice to make a consumptive of him or her. For it is the weak and enfeebled organism which becomes the easy prey of the bacillus tuberculosis. One in fair health, living a regular and hygienic life, has little to fear.

A predisposition to pulmonary tuberculosis may be inherited or acquired, but in either case the means to overcome this peculiar susceptibility are the same.   Let us examine, for a moment, an individual predisposed to consumption, and we shall be better able to understand the reasons for the therapeutic measures which I shall describe.   If a child, he is either undersized or presents an almost abnormal height for his age, with a narrow chest.   He is a bad eater, irritable, nervous, anæmic, with irregular digestive functions, at times constipated, at times suffering from diarrhœa, prone to all the diseases of childhood, and still mentally rarely behind his more robust companions.   He is averse to outdoor play, and, owing to his delicate constitution, he is often allowed to have his way, and his character is thereby spoiled.

The adult candidate for pulmonary tuberculosis differs from his younger brother but little: the physique is the same; the peculiar condition of mind is more pronounced; while sanguine at times, anxieties, disappointments, especially unfortunate love affairs and similar sorrows, often suffice to bring about a rapid development of the disease.   In sorrow one eats but little, the arterial pressure is low, the muscular weakness and depressed nervous state make the act of breathing incomplete.   The beneficial influence of natural and full breathing no longer exists; the heart is called on to do more work and a perpetual palpitation ensues.   The circulatory disturbances in the lungs impair the nutrition of this organ, and thus the field for the invasion of the bacillus of tuberculosis is prepared, or a latent tuberculosis comes to an outbreak.

The decreased power of resistance makes the anæmic individual especially prone to acute inflammations of either the mucous or serous membranes, and catarrhal conditions of the upper respiratory organs become alarmingly frequent and inclined to descend into the deeper air passages.   He takes cold easily because the vasomotor system is impaired, and the slightest change of temperature or insignificant exposure of some part of the body usually covered suffices to hinder the peripheral circulation to the extent of producing congestions and to impair the process of eliminating used-up substances, whose toxicity increases with the length of time they are retained.

It seems evident, then, that the insufficient air supply to the respiratory organs and the increased susceptibility to the slightest change of temperature are the principal factors in the production of consumptive individuals.   Therefore to prevent or improve the condition caused by an insufficient air supply we must resort to aërotherapeutics, and to arouse the vasomotor system to a more energetic action we have in hydrotherapeutics not the only, but, considering its salutary secondary effects, the most valuable therapeutic agent.

To prevent pulmonary tuberculosis, we must begin treating the child *in utero*, continue in the lying-in room, nursery, and school-room, and teach the young man or woman to keep the treatment up throughout life.

A woman who is to give birth to a child should abandon the corset and tight clothing in time to allow a continued, free abdominal and thoracic respiration. Better yet is it if she has never been addicted to the habit of tight lacing, for the experiments of Kellogg[69] and Mays have demonstrated that the so-called female or costal type of respiration which prevails among civilized women is the result of their restricting and unhygienic mode of dress, and is not due to the influence of gestation or to a natural difference in the anatomy and physiological growth of man and woman. For the mother to live as much as possible in pure, fresh air, to take frequent breathing exercises, to avoid crowded assemblies where the air is vitiated, to live, in short, as hygienic a life as circumstances will permit, will have a most salutary effect on the child's future health.

The newborn child is in need of pure, fresh air as much as the mother; and the lying-in room and the nursery should always be well ventilated. When in due time the child is taken for an airing, the thick, almost impermeable veil should be abandoned. These veils, often tightened around the little face, press against the nose and make it difficult for the child to breathe naturally, yet the mother wonders how the baby got into the habit of breathing through the mouth.

Frequently, also, mouth-breathing in children, and sometimes in adults, must be attributed to adenoid vegetation in the retropharynx, or to enlarged tonsils. These as well as all other causes of obstruction to a free, natural respiration, such as deviated septum, enlarged turbinated bones, hypertrophied mucous membrane, polypi, etc., must be removed if we desire to protect the child or adult from chronic nasal, pharyngeal, or laryngeal catarrhs, so often the forerunners of pulmonary disease. Only after the removal of all possible causes of obstruction in the upper air passages is a natural physiological respiratory function possible, and only under such conditions can we hope for real benefit from breathing-exercises.

I consider the air-bath and sun-bath for children at the earliest age most beneficial. Let the little ones toddle around naked every day for a short time; in cold weather in well-warmed rooms, and in summer in the room bathed by the rays of the sun, but always on a clean floor or clean Japanese matting. With their growing intelligence children should be taught by practice and example the value and the love of pure, fresh air. As soon as the age and intelligence of the child will permit, breathing exercises should be taught him. He should learn to like them, as the average child does general gymnastics. The following is a description of the exercises I recommend to all children and adults who breathe faultily, to the anæmic and those predisposed to consumption, and to the chronic tuberculous patient who is able to be about and for whom a modification is not indicated. These are also a part of the gymnastic exercises I should like to see incorporated in the curriculum of all schools, and not only in the se-

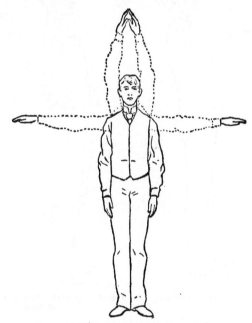

FIG. 27.—First and Second Respiratory Exercises.

lected few. I have prescribed them for years with very satisfactory results, and I can recommend them as practical, efficacious, and simple.

Presuming that the upper air passages are in a normal condition, the patient is taught to stand properly—that is to say, straight, chest out, and head erect—and to breathe always through the nose. He takes a deep inspiration slowly, beginning with the abdominal muscles, and then expanding the chest to its fullest capacity. During this inspiration he raises his arms from his sides to a horizontal position (Fig. 27). He holds the breath for a moment, and then lowers the arms during the act of expiration, which should be somewhat more rapid.

The second exercise is like the first, except that the upward movement of the arms is continued until the hands meet over the head.

In the third exercise (Fig. 28) the patient stretches his arms out as in the position of swimming, the dorsal surfaces of the hands touching each other. During the inspiration the arms are moved outwards and finally meet behind the back. They are brought for-

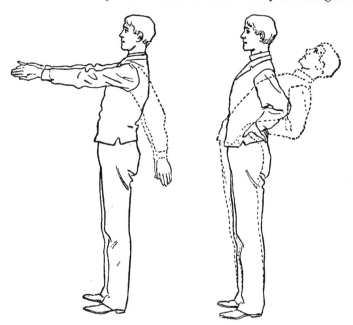

FIG. 28.—Third Respiratory Exercise.   FIG. 29.—Exercise for Patients in the Habit of Stooping.

wards again during the expiration. This exercise can be greatly facilitated and made more effective by the patient rising on his toes during the act of inspiration, and descending during the act of expiration. Each respiratory act should be followed immediately by a secondary forced expiratory effort. This is for the purpose of expelling as much of the supplemental air as possible, and may be effectually aided by supinating the arms and pressing the thorax with them.

Considering that the amount of tidal air—that is to say, the volume which is inspired and expired in quiet respiration—is only 500 c.c., the complemental air—the volume which can be inspired after an ordinary respiration—1,500 c.c., and the supplemental or reserve air—the amount which can be forcibly expelled after an ordinary respiration—amounts to 1,240 to 1,800 c.c., one can readily see the value of respiratory exercises, and also the utility of this second expiratory effort.

To consumptives, those predisposed to tuberculosis, and to children who have the habit of stooping, I teach an additional exercise, as follows (Fig. 29): The patient makes his best effort to stand straight; he places his hands on his hips with the thumbs towards the front and then bends slowly backwards as far as he can during the act of inspiration. He remains in this position a few seconds while holding the breath, and rises again, somewhat more rapidly, during the expiration.

When the patient is out walking it will, of course, not always be convenient nor possible to do these exercises with the movement of the arms. The patient should, under such conditions, content himself with raising his shoulders, and making a rotary movement backwards during the act of inspiration, holding the breath for a moment and then exhaling during a rotary movement forwards, assuming again the normal position. The secondary expiratory effort can follow this exercise also without attracting any attention.

For all classes of patients, candidates for consumption and bad breathers in general, the rules hold good never to take their breathing-exercises when tired, immediately after a heavy meal, or when uncomfortably or tightly dressed, never to continue them to the extent of becoming tired, never to take them in a bad atmosphere, and not to take them at their caprice, but according to the directions of the physician.

One exercise should be taught at a time, and only after it has been thoroughly mastered should the physician proceed to teach the next one. I have described them in the order of their difficulty. The first, a simple raising of the arms to the horizontal line during the act of inspiration, requires relatively little effort. The second one, in which the arms describe a circle by being raised outstretched until they meet above the head, requires a more prolonged inspiration and necessarily an increased muscular effort. The third, the swimming exercise, in which the hands should meet behind the back, is the most difficult. The necessary interval of time between learning the successive exercises will depend upon the aptitude, the expansive power, and the general condition of the patient. Some patients can be taught all these exercises within nine or ten days, while with others months often must intervene before the next exercise can be commenced.

The breathing exercises at school should be under the direction of the school physician or teacher of physical culture. In summer they should be taken out-of-doors, and on rainy, windy, or too cold

days in the well-ventilated school-room. To teach the children how
to breathe, sit, stand, and walk properly should be a part of the
every-day curriculum. Every school should have its large playground
or roof-garden, where, weather and season permitting, the classes
should alternately receive their instruction. In rural communities,
during the warmer season, instruction indoors should be the exception, not the rule. Singing and recitation especially should be encouraged out-of-doors. I have found that singing in pure air is an
admirable and most useful adjuvant in aërotherapeutics. Barth,[10] of
Koslin, who has made a careful study of the effects of singing on the
action of the lungs and heart, on diseases of the heart, on the pulmonary circulation, on the blood, the vocal apparatus, the upper air
passages, the ear, the general health, the development of the chest,
on metabolism, and on the activity of the digestive organs, has come
to the conclusion that singing is one of the exercises most conducive
to health. Considering the fact that it can be practised anywhere
(when the air is pure) or at any time, without apparatus, it should
be much more cultivated than it actually is. The German military
authorities, who have the reputation for instituting all exercises
which tend to invigorate the soldiers, have of late years encouraged
singing by the troops during marches.

Finally, it cannot be impressed too strongly on the minds of consumptives and of those predisposed to the disease that they should
always seek environments where the air is as pure as possible. Lord
Beaconsfield's celebrated words, "The atmosphere in which we live
has more to do with human happiness than all the accidents of for-
tune and all the acts of government," have, I think, a special meaning
for this class of sufferers.

Hydrotherapeutics, as a measure to prevent pulmonary tuberculosis, tends to develop to more vigorous action the vasomotor system; it also should be instituted at an early age. A child a few
months old can support with impunity a rapid sponging off with cold
water, followed by a relatively vigorous friction with a soft Turkish
towel after its warm bath. As the child grows older he should not
only be taught this use of cold water after his semi-weekly or weekly
warm bath, but he should wash at least the face, neck, and chest
every morning with cold water. Better yet, if he can accustom himself early to a daily cold douche. The utility of all-the-year-round
swimming baths, where old and young of all classes can, gratuitously
or for a moderate price, enjoy the salutary effects on body and mind
of a good swim, is too well known to need insisting upon.

For anæmic individuals who, as I stated above, are, in the majority of cases, candidates for consumption, a graduated course of hydro-

therapeutics seems to act almost as a specific. That there is never any danger from a judiciously applied affusion or douche has been demonstrated by years of practice. And why should there be? All that is necessary is to insure the proper reaction and an education of the skin and nervous system before the classical douche is employed. The surest sign of a proper reaction is the appearance of a red hue of the skin where the water has been applied. No exception should be made, whether the patient is simply predisposed, an anæmic, or a fully developed consumptive. It is always best to begin with massage for several days, and if the skin is particularly dry I prescribe, in addition, inunction with some fatty substance, preferably cod-liver oil. Next, for about the same period of time, comes friction with pure alcohol; then with half alcohol and water; finally friction with water alone. Then come the cold sponge bath, the affusion, and at last the douche. The friction with the hands directly in contact with the skin or over a large towel, after the douche, should always be kept up until the patient is thoroughly dry and warm.

Children and young people often develop tuberculosis for no other reason than that they are naturally bad eaters. Kind and persistent urging to eat a fairly hearty meal at least twice a day, combined with discipline in regard to regularity of meals and the proper kind of food; the exclusion of all delicacies and sweetmeats tending to impair the appetite or digestion, associated with a continued course in aérotherapy and hydrotherapy, will make, in a relatively short time, a well and strong individual out of a naturally bad eater. At times, of course, tonics, cod-liver oil, iron, phosphates, etc., may be needed to serve as adjuvants in this treatment.

What has been said of the value of air and sun baths—that is, the judicious exposure of the whole cutaneous surface of the body to the air and all except the head to the rays of the sun—for very small children is equally applicable to these bad eaters so long as they remain such. The tonic effects of sun baths are too often underestimated, even by medical men.

The excessively dry atmosphere in the majority of our American dwellings during the winter season is a not infrequent cause of chronic nasopharyngeal catarrh, so dangerous to predisposed individuals. As early as in 1836, Dr. Reid, of London, remarking upon the ventilation of the House of Lords, said that when water to the amount of seventy gallons was evaporated into the air at a single session, coughing among the members was much diminished.

Freudenthal, of New York, read an interesting paper on this subject before the American Medical Association in 1895." He holds that the excessive dryness of our houses, resulting from a bad heating system, is the cause of the frequent catarrhs of the upper air passages in winter. He says: "A heated room should not be warmer than 65° F. If we then feel cool, it is a sign that there is not enough moisture in the air; in other words, that the air absorbs not only from the upper respiratory tract, but from our lungs also humidity, and with that heat."

While simple evaporating devices, such as a vessel filled with water and a cloth suspended above it, touching the water so as to produce capillary attraction, will answer all practical purposes of rendering the atmosphere sufficiently humid, Dr. Barnes' humidifier

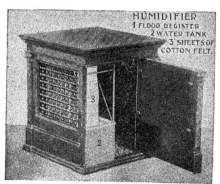

FIG. 30.—Barnes' Humidifier.

has certainly additional advantage. With the aid of this instrument (Fig. 30) the humidity of the atmosphere in an apartment can be regulated more precisely. It consists of an outer case covering a wall or floor register, with a tank for water, over which are suspended strips of cotton felt aggregating about twelve square feet of evaporating surface. I have ventured a little improvement of this instrument by placing a small pan filled with water in the upper portion of the humidifier, connecting the two tanks by the felt strips. Through capillary attraction these strips are thus kept constantly wet and impart to the hot air, flowing between them, from one to twelve quarts of water in twenty-four hours, depending on the percentage of moisture in the air entering the case. To further illustrate the usefulness of the humidifier, I will quote from Dr. Barnes' paper, read before the American Public Health Association," the following interesting passage:

"During sixteen days of February, 1897, I obtained in my office with this device a mean of 53 per cent. relative humidity, with ex-

tremes of 67 and 40 in a mean temperature of 65.3°, through the
evaporation of from two quarts to two gallons of water a day, the average being four and one-half quarts.   During this period the outside
mean temperature was 32° and relative humidity 73.5 per cent., with
extremes of 92 and 50.   I found 65° perfectly comfortable, whereas,
without the artificial supply of moisture, I required from 70° to 71°
temperature.

"I could have obtained a higher mean relative humidity by adding more strips to the humidifier, thus increasing the area of the
evaporating surface; but this would be attended with an excessive
deposit of moisture on the window panes, in the form of either vapor
or frost.   Where single window sashes are in use, the dew point—or
the saturation of the cold air near the windows, which causes the deposit of dew—takes place more abundantly than where double sashes
are employed, as a consequence of the cool air being unable to hold
in solution the volume of watery vapor that exists in the warmer air
of other parts of the room.   At zero temperature dew begins to be
deposited when the air contains but 0.564 grains of water in a cubic
foot; at 70° temperature it takes nearly sixteen times as much in a
cubic foot to cause a deposit.   This deposit of moisture on windows
serves as a valuable guide in determining the number of sheets, or
the area of evaporating surface, necessary to maintain a proper relative humidity in any particular room where artificial hydration is
employed.   When the required area of evaporating surface is once
known, the apparatus works automatically.   If the outside air supplying the furnace is comparatively warm and moist, but little water
is extracted from the sheets in its passage to the room; if cold and
dry, it takes water from the sheets with great rapidity."   Of course,
it must not be forgotten that the pans and felt should be cleaned as
often as the impurities in the water render it necessary.

We must mention also under prophylactic treatment the particular
care which should be taken with patients recovering from diseases
which might be called phthisiogenetic.   Nearly all eruptive diseases
of childhood and adult life, such as measles, scarlatina, variola, typhoid fever, and typhus fever, leave the patient only too frequently
predisposed to the invasion of the tubercle bacilli.   Severe grippe
should also be classed with the diseases predisposing to pulmonary
tuberculosis.   Such convalescents should be particularly warned not
to expose themselves to the possibility of infection.   They should
lead a most hygienic life, and be careful not to overexert themselves.

Of course, besides the phthisiogenetic diseases there are other
causes whereby one can acquire a predisposition to tuberculosis; for
example, a dissipated irregular life, excesses in Bacchus or Venus,

worry, overwork, unsanitary occupation, unsanitary dwellings, poverty, want, etc. Some of these can be avoided and thus treated by the efforts of the individual himself. Those appertaining to the social conditions are spoken of respectively under public prophylaxis and the social aspect of tuberculosis.

DIAGNOSIS.

In the present state of our knowledge of therapeutics and of phthisiotherapy in particular, one hardly needs to emphasize the importance of an early recognition of pulmonary tuberculosis in our combat.against this disease. Some authors claim fifty, some seventy, others ninety per cent. of absolute cures of early recognized and early treated cases. But the benefit which we derive from the fact that through early recognition and timely treatment a tuberculous disease may never come to the stage in which the invalid is a source of danger and infection to his fellow-men, surpasses in importance the curative results obtained, so far as the actual number of lives saved is concerned. Since of all tuberculous diseases pulmonary consumption is the most prevalent, we will deal first with the early recognition of tuberculosis in this form.

With the advent of Koch's immortal discovery of the bacillus tuberculosis it was thought by many that the problem of the early recognition of consumption had been solved. But the more careful physician soon realized that, while the presence of the tubercle bacilli in the sputum would confirm beyond a doubt his diagnosis of a tuberculous disease of the respiratory tract, not finding them at one, two, or even more bacteriological tests could not make him set aside conclusions arrived at by a careful physical examination.

Now, if we consider the matter carefully we must admit that in very early cases of pulmonary tuberculosis the expulsion of bacilli with the expectoration, which is at that time exceedingly scanty, can hardly be expected. There must be a disintegration of the tubercle before we can assume that the bronchial or pulmonary secretions will contain the specific organism of tuberculosis.

Koch's next most important discovery, the use of tuberculin as a test of the presence of a tuberculous condition, is certainly of the greatest diagnostic value in the bovine race, and thus indirectly of incalculable prophylactic benefit to mankind. But the utility and wisdom of the injection of tuberculin for the purpose of diagnosing the disease in the human race, I for one dare to doubt. I know that, in making this statement, I am at variance with many reputable and conscientious practitioners; but I also know that I do not stand alone.

in my convictions, and notwithstanding the criticisms which I have encountered, I do not hesitate to repeat what I have said before[12] in connection with this subject, that three, five, or even ten milligrams of tuberculin may in nine hundred and ninety-nine cases do nothing but reveal a latent tuberculosis; but in the thousandth case it may cause an unexpected generalization with a fatal result. When one has witnessed such a generalization, the desire to use tuberculin for diagnostic purposes in the human race is diminished.

It was no less an authority than Virchow who first warned against the use of tuberculin, for the very reason that he believed he had demonstrated the fact that this substance arouses the latent tubercle bacilli, causing a mobilization of an army of enemies which had slumbered peacefully. A drug or any other substance which, when introduced into the system, is capable of bringing about a rise of temperature sometimes as much as four degrees above the normal, and which through the circulation will reach the tuberculous deposits, if such are present, irritating these latent tubercles into an active process of inflammation, must be considered a dangerous thing. Ambler, of Asheville, N. C., in an article on this subject, asks whether any physician would be willing to risk the consequences of such a method of diagnosing a disease. And, addressing physicians directly, he says: "Do you believe you would carry out such a procedure in your own person under such possibilities? If you would not, you have no right to use it on your patients."[14]

And now let us ask, is the reaction obtained after the injection of tuberculin an absolute proof of the existence of a tuberculous disease? It is well known that a reaction can be obtained in cases of lepra. Joseph, Kaposi, Arning, Goldschmidt,[15] Babes and Kalendero,[16] and others have reported cases of that kind, but the analogy existing between lepra and tuberculosis probably accounts for this phenomenon. In a paper read before the Medical Society of the Hospitals of Paris, Netter[17] said that he had observed the characteristic reaction after injection of tuberculin in twenty-seven out of a hundred cases of individuals afflicted with other than tuberculous diseases of the lungs. Neumann, of Vienna, and Straus and Teissier, of Paris,[18] had occasion to see the tuberculin reaction in purely syphilitic subjects. Billroth and von Eiselsberg observed reaction in actinomycosis, and Trasbot in a case of cancer. Klebs, jr.,[19] claims to have had a reaction in every case of chlorosis. Would any one dare to say that every case of chlorosis must of necessity be of a tuberculous nature? Lastly, J. M. Anders,[20] of Philadelphia, an enthusiastic believer in tuberculin as a diagnostic means, nevertheless admits that he has seen cases in which there was no reaction to the tuberculin test, but in which the post-mortem examinations revealed tuberculous lesions. Cornet[81] in his recent book speaks also of cases in which tuberculosis existed beyond a doubt, and the injection of tuberculin caused not the slightest reaction.

The natural serums obtained from the dog or goat, or the artificial serum prepared according to Hayem's formula, which were used with the hope of being less dangerous and perhaps more certain than tuberculin, have proved in the hands of some[82] to be fully as dangerous, and in the hands of others[83] totally unreliable.

What other resources have we at our disposal to diagnose the beginning of *pulmonary tuberculosis?* These are still numerous, and we shall discuss them, not in the order of their importance, since really only the combination of several means can give us proof that our diagnosis is correct, but rather in the order of their adaptability to the use of the general practitioner who has not always easy access to bacteriological or electrical laboratories.

In the presence of an individual in whom we suspect the beginning of pulmonary tuberculosis we must first study the anamnesis and bear in mind all that past experience in phthisiology has taught us. Man is more disposed to consumption than woman, except a woman who has gone through many childbirths in rapid succession; the poor and underfed more frequently fall victims to consumption than the rich and well nourished; the single more often than the married. According to some authors, red-haired individuals are more exposed to pulmonary tuberculosis than those having brown, blonde, or black hair. While the notion that the red-haired individual is more exposed than one of the blonde or brunette type is erroneous, it is certainly true that persons with very white skin, no matter what the color of the hair of the head may be, if the chin, lips, pubis, and armpits are covered with reddish hair, very often have a predisposition to consumption. Hippocrates,[84] Galen,[85] Rhazes,[86] Daremberg the elder,[87] and of recent authors Behier and Hardy,[88] Beddoe, Landouzy,[89] Dewevre,[90] and Mahoudeau[91] have written on this subject; but the distinction between the red-headed and only partially red-haired individuals has not been made clear except in the works of Hippocrates and Rhazes. A recent article by Armand Delpeuch[92] decides this interesting question in favor of Hippocrates, and very strongly refutes the conclusions of Landouzy, who reports having found from seventy-five to one hundred per cent. of the red-haired individuals in his services at the Cochin and the Charité Hospitals to be tuberculous. Landouzy commits the same error as many others in calling these patients a Venetian type, red hair being not by any means characteristic of the Venetian population.* Delpeuch makes a clear distinction between the red-haired—erythrisme—and the red-bearded—erythrisme partiel—individuals. He found that many simply red-haired individuals were entirely free from a tuberculous taint, but among fifty-seven patients who had either blonde, brown, or black hair, and at the same time lips, chin, or pubis covered with reddish hair, he found fifty-two to be distinctly tuberculous. Long before Delpeuch, a Scotch author, John Beddoe,[93] had already demonstrated that red-headed individuals are not especially exposed to tuberculosis.

We may call to mind the professions and trades which are most exposed to consumption, and what has been said on this subject in the section on public prophylaxis, wherein we learned that the agriculturist is least and the printer most exposed to pulmonary tuberculosis.

We know that pulmonary consumption develops most frequently between the ages of seventeen and thirty-five.

In inquiring into the history of our patients we should deal delicately and carefully with the subject of a possible hereditary disposition, so as not to convey to the patient the idea that because some one in his family has died of consumption, he is doomed to succumb to it. I wish to remark here incidentally that in my experience nothing is often more difficult than to dissuade a tuberculous invalid from this preconceived idea, probably brought about by a popular notion and confirmed by questions asked him on that subject by every physician to whom he may have applied for counsel. Direct questioning as to the cause of the death of parents or near relatives should be avoided; one should rather endeavor to discern the hereditary tendency by exclusion. If we consider the rare occurrence of bacillary transmission on the one hand, and, on the other, how really few families there are wherein some one has not died from consumption or other tuberculous disease, I wonder if it is after all so very important to ply the patient with such questions, especially since an inherited tuberculous diathesis does not preclude the chances of recovery. Dr. H. P. Loomis, of this city, has expressed himself in this respect as follows: "My experience has led me to believe that tuberculous heredity has very little to do with the question of a person's recovery, all other things being equal. Of twenty persons known to me who have recovered from phthisis during the past year alone, nine have pronounced tuberculous histories. One had two brothers and one sister die of phthisis."[94]

The only direct question which I am in the habit of asking a new

* The denomination of Venetian type is probably to be traced to some paintings of famous Italian artists. A Baschet et Feuillet de Couches: "Les femmes blondes selon les peintres de l'école de Venice, par deux Venitiens." Paris, 1865, p. 7.

patient is: "Have you ever come in direct prolonged contact with a consumptive or a patient suffering from bronchial or pulmonary disease?" This question is important from two points of view. It may give a clew to show whether the disease has been acquired by infection, and at the same time it will be a topic to start on when directing the patient what to do to prevent transmitting the disease to others. On the other hand, I consider a careful inquiry into the mode of life of the patient, past and present, of great importance. The probably unhygienic environments, a dissipated life, a love for strong liquors, irregularity of meals, great disappointment in matters of love or business, or other depressing factors, all will often give a clew to the origin of an acquired, or to the awakening of a latent, pulmonary tuberculosis. It is well known that many a pulmonary consumption has been preceded by digestive disturbances or typical dyspepsia. Bad eaters are nearly always candidates for consumption. In an unmarried young woman a beginning of irregularity or a total cessation of menses is not infrequently a preliminary sign of approaching tuberculosis, just as much as the return of it in a patient under treatment should be considered as an evidence of the march towards recovery. But one should always be on guard when in the presence of a case with vicarious menstruation. Hemorrhage from the lungs in a young girl, even if it happens about the time for her menstrual period, often means the existence of tuberculous trouble.

Of the many phthisiogenetic diseases, that is, diseases which often prepare the field for the invasion of bacilli, first come all the severer types of bronchitis, pneumonia, and pertussis; next, all the eruptive diseases of childhood and adult life, such as measles, scarlatina, variola, typhoid fever, and typhus fever. Severe grippe, alcoholism, and syphilis rank no less high as phthisiogenetic diseases. Pleurisy, especially if followed by effusion, should always be regarded with suspicion; for I believe the majority, if not all, of such cases are of a tuberculous nature.

Bacterioscopical research in pleuritic effusion is often very unsatisfactory. Inoculation of a guinea-pig with the serous fluid drawn from the chest is a more satisfactory method when additional evidence of the existence of tuberculosis is desired.

One should also bear in mind that severe traumata can become predisposing factors in the development of pulmonary tuberculosis. Mendelsohn, Leyden, Ewald,[a] and others have reported cases of this kind. I have myself had a case under observation in which the first manifestations of disease showed themselves some time after a severe blow received in the back by some blunt instrument in the hands of a burglar.

What is said in the section on preventive treatment, of the psychical condition of an individual (whether adult or child) predisposed to any tuberculous disease, is, of course, also true of one in the incipient stage of phthisis. The patient will often himself confess to an increased irritability and an indifference or dislike for the performance of duties which he formerly loved; or, again, he himself or his friends may have noticed a decided neurasthenic condition or an inclination to melancholia. But one thing of which the patient hardly fails to speak is his increased tendency to nasopharyngeal or bronchial catarrhs. Cough, dyspnœa, superficial or deep-seated thoracic pains, and occasional night-sweats are other frequent early signs. Of the early cough in pulmonary tuberculosis, I may say that it is usually dry and irritating, observed at first only in the evening on reclining; later the patient has his regular morning coughing-spell.

In a very interesting article on "Personal Observations in Pulmonary Phthisis," [44] McLean explains the cough when reclining as follows: "The mere change of position from the erect to the recumbent has produced an immediate change in the circulation of the blood and air in the pulmonary structure, distributing the equilibrium which always exists in healthy chests, controlled by the natural tension through the vasomotors. A temporary passive congestion of hyperæmia is produced thereby, due to an insufficient expansion of the finer tubes and vesicles. The blood pressure being out of proportion to the air pressure, and the coats of the vessels being overdistended or varicosed from lack of support, the blood currents come under the influence of an extraneous force, gravity; this never occurs in vessels whose coats are normal, except by complete inversion of the body or in the hypostatic congestions of long illnesses. The change to the recumbent posture immediately causes an increase in the distending force within the blood-vessels and a decrease in the amount of air in the tubes and cells. As a result of this, a backwatering of blood into the bronchial vessels and a sensation of fulness or tickling are perceived in the region of the head of the sternum. The cough that occurs is Nature's own effort to remove this fulness, which it accomplishes at first with only a few long breaths and coughs. If this pathological condition is not relieved early, it goes on until it requires stronger and more prolonged effort in the act of coughing to remove it."

Coughing-spells are often brought about by a simple extra respiratory effort through laughing or excited speaking. After a little while the dry cough is superseded by one accompanied with more or less expectoration. From this moment careful bacteriological examinations for bacilli should be instituted. , Vomiting, or even the simple nausea concomitant with a coughing-spell, should be considered one of the early symptoms in pulmonary tuberculosis, and in taking the history of the case one should never fail to inquire whether such phenomena have ever taken place.

Of course, we ask the patient if he has observed that his sputum was ever tinged with red, or if he has at times actually expectorated blood. While I fully acknowledge the very important diagnostic value of pulmonary hemorrhage, large or small, when traumatisms or heart disease can be excluded, I do not think it wise to let the patient feel that we attach great importance to this occurrence. Rather let us embrace this opportunity to tell our patient that one, or even several pulmonary hemorrhages do not, of necessity, lessen the chances for his recovery.

While it should be an invariable rule to take the patient's temperature at the first examination, thermometry in early pulmonary tuberculosis is of value only when practised at regular intervals, for example, four times in twenty-four hours, and for several days in succession. It is of special value to note the rectal temperature before and immediately after a short rapid walk. Little, frequent, and persistent elevations of one degree or more must always be looked on as indications of a pathological process which may have its origin in a slight tuberculous infiltration.

A subnormal temperature, especially when observed in the evening hours, should also arouse our suspicion as being the probable result of the beginning of pathological changes of tuberculous nature. Murat's sign" of increased voice vibration may also help in the detection of an early phthisis. During loud and vigorous talking there is a vibration of the affected portion of the lung, recognized by the patient as a more or less disagreeable sensation. This symptom, which is entirely subjective, is explained by the physical law that a solid body is a better transmitter than air. At times, however, this condition may have escaped the attention of the patient, since its development is slow and not in the least painful. In order to discover it the physician should have the patient make prolonged expirations, accompanied by humming. If there is solidification, the patient will then perceive the vibration of his voice. If the left side is affected it will seem to him that there is a direct communication of the voice between the larynx and that side, while nothing whatsoever is perceived in the right, healthy side of his lungs, and vice versa. Dr. Murat has found this symptom in a number of cases of pulmonary tuberculosis before any subjective signs of infiltration could be elicited. I have since had occasion to confirm the presence of this sign a few times in early cases.

The *liséré gingival*, or reddish line along the edges of the gums, and the dilatation of the pupil on the diseased side—owing to the irritation of the sympathetic nerve at the root of the lungs—should, according to some writers,[98] be included among the important early signs of pulmonary tuberculosis. The fact, however, that one finds those conditions in a number of other affections leads me to regard these symptoms as of importance only when concomitant with others.

Before allowing our patient to undress for examination we should always make a careful inspection of the upper air passages. Not only may all the pathological conditions which stamp the patient as a candidate for consumption be located there, and by judicial treatment be removed, but a careful laryngoscopical examination will often, through the peculiar anæmic condition of the larynx and the general appearance of the mucous membrane, give, as Roe, of Rochester,[99] happily expressed it, "a very early hint as to the probable existence of tuberculosis of the lungs." The upper air passages should not only be examined very carefully by rhinoscope and laryngoscope, but the secretion, especially the nasal mucus, should also be submitted to microscopical examination. However, it must be borne in mind that the presence of tubercle bacilli in the nasal mucus in individuals habitually exposed to the inhalation of dust laden with micro-organisms may be of little significance unless additional evidence should corroborate the existence of pathological conditions. Straus, of Paris, whose experiments have already been referred to, found the nasal mucus of a number of nurses and employees of the Faculty's general hospitals and libraries laden with bacilli, and the most searching physical examination of these men and women did not reveal the slightest sign of tuberculous disease.[100] The observing physician will have discovered long before this, and without the aid of any instrument, a pronounced chloroanæmic condition, not infrequently seen in early tuberculosis, though this discovery will probably not prevent him from examining the blood later on for the number of red blood corpuscles and percentage of hæmoglobin.

We finally place the patient on the scales, take his height and ascertain whether there has been any loss of weight, and if so, since when this has been observed. Here we must bear in mind the splendid work done by Papillon, of Paris,[101] presented to the English-speaking medical world by H. P. Loomis, of New York.[102] I believe I cannot do better than quote, textually, Loomis' summary: "Weight, respiratory capacity, and chest measurement have no value in establishing the possibilities of the development of phthisis in themselves, but must be considered in relation to the height of the person, when they furnish three important aids to diagnosis.

"Corpulence is obtained by dividing the weight expressed in pounds by the height expressed in feet (in a normal man this should be twenty-six; in a woman, twenty-three). Thoracic perimeter is found by taking two measurements of the circumference of the chest —one at the moment of forced expiration, the other at the end of forced inspiration. The average of these two measurements should never be less than half the height.

"Vital capacity is the amount of air expressed in cubic inches, which can be exhaled after a full inspiration. Normally it should bear the relation to the height of three to one for a man and two to one for a woman"—i.e., for every inch of height there should be two or three cubic inches of vital capacity, respectively.

While some authors, such as Andvord, Loomis, and Wells, claim to have recognized a pulse characteristic of the incipient state, I confess that all I have been able to observe is that the pulse is chronically feeble, rapid, weak, and sometimes intermittent, which is characteristic of constitutional weakness of whatever cause. However, taking the arterial pressure with the aid of Potain's sphygmomanometer (Fig. 31) is a most valuable aid in diagnosing an early pulmonary tuberculosis. This instrument is composed of a rubber ball, a transmission tube, a reception tube, and the manometer proper. The rubber ball, distended by a pressure of 3 cm., becomes elliptic and has then a length of 3 or 4 cm., with a transverse diameter of 2.5 cm. The interior of the rubber ball is divided into four sections; three of these (A) are strong enough to resist a pressure of 30 cm., while the fourth (B) is much thinner, for the purpose of receiving the radial artery. The little receiving tube with the stopcock (R) serves to inflate the apparatus for the purpose of having a convenient tension. Professor Potain recommends a pressure of 5 cm. for that purpose. When it is not in use it is best it is to have the stopcock open. The manometer is constructed according to the principles of the metallic barometer inclosed in a case. The interior is in communication with the rubber bulb through the transmission tube. The manometer indicates the pressure to which the air in the ball is subjected.

Papillon's recent examinations in Potain's service at the Charité in Paris have shown that when the manometer showed less than 13 cm. arterial pressure, the subject was very frequently found to be in the incipient state of tuberculosis; but when there was a concomitant nephritis, it rose two or three inches above the normal, which is 16 or 17.

We now come to the *physical examination* proper. The patient is stripped to the waist, for neither percussion nor auscultation can be done with exactness when there are intervening layers of clothing.

We inspect the conformation of the chest, ascertain whether the heart-beat is displaced, and look for possible evidences of pleuritic retractions, especially for the supraclavicular depression or glandular enlargements.[103] In the early stages the inspection does not always reveal an emaciated form,[104] nor the typical *habitus phthisicus*—long, thin stature, stooping, hollow and narrow chest, pale countenance, and a tired look; but we may observe feeble respiratory movements, characteristic of nearly all candidates for consumption. The glistening eye, pasty skin, the bright color of the cheeks may be observed. Palpation may reveal an increased vocal fremitus. But there is another symptom revealed by palpation, which is not sufficiently emphasized in most of the text-books: By placing the palmar surface

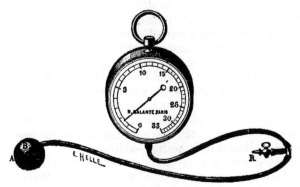

FIG. 31.—Potain's Sphygmomanometer.

of the two hands successively over the whole anterior region of the chest, the patient taking deep inspirations meanwhile, one can often feel the expanding portion of the lungs through the chest wall, and with a little practice differentiate the portions which are more or less involved. The motion or impulse given to the examining hand, by the inflation of the lungs during inspiration, is less in that part of the lung invaded by the tuberculous process or impaired by pleuritic retraction than in the still healthy lung substance. With a little practice one can educate his hands so as to render palpation a valuable additional means for localizing the beginning of a tuberculous process.

Katzenbach[105] suggests that, when making the physical examination of a person suspected to have a beginning pulmonary tuberculosis, the examiner should stand behind the patient and place his thumb on the scapula and the fingers under the clavicle, and, while making firm pressure, instruct the patient to take a deep inspiration.

If this respiratory movement causes pain on one side, it is quite probable that on that side the lung will be found diseased.

To learn all that can be learned from percussion and auscultation one should first examine the anterior portion of the chest, the patient's arms being in the ordinary position and his back resting solidly against the straight back of a chair or against the wall. Then one should examine him standing, with the arms above the head, so as to be able to percuss carefully and auscultate the lateral portion of the chest along the axillary line. In order to examine the posterior portion of the thorax, it will be advantageous to direct the patient to fold his arms across his chest, placing his hands on the opposite shoulders, and bend slightly forward.

Mediate percussion should be done with special care above and below the clavicle, and posteriorly in the supraspinous fossa and interscapular region, with a view of detecting possible dull areas in the apices. Immediate percussion, that is to say striking the clavicle directly with hammer or finger without a plessimeter, may help to reveal a beginning process of solidification in that region. Yet at a very early period of the disease the sound perceived through percussion may tell us little *per se;* but the experienced percusser, if he is accustomed to use his index finger as a plessimeter, may have noticed that the elasticity of the lung substance felt by the index finger is much less marked than in healthy subjects.

Auscultation may at a very early period give us a clew to the beginning of a tuberculous process. With Grancher, of Paris,[106] I consider the low inspiratory murmur, characterized by roughness when persistent and localized in one of the apices, one of the surest and earliest signs of pulmonary tuberculosis. Not infrequently the jerky or cogwheel inspiratory sounds, rhythmic with the heart, are also perceived. According to Professor Potain, of Paris, however, this wavy and jerky respiration is simply the respiratory murmur divided by the successive pulsations of the heart. In the opinion of this authority, it is by no means pathognomonic of pulmonary tuberculosis, but can be regarded only as a presumptive sign. - Potain has observed the cogwheel or jerky respiration in narrow-chested women where there has not been the least sign of pulmonary affection. When there is a pulmonary consolidation at one of the apices, even if but of slight magnitude, a marked transmission of the heart sound may not infrequently be observed in this region. Râles of a smaller magnitude may be heard, especially after the patient has coughed a few times. The prolonged expiratory sound is heard when the tuberculous process has been already in existence for some time, the prolongation of the sound being due to a contraction of the calibre of the finer bronchioles. If this prolonged expiratory sound is heard over both lungs it may be due simply to the fact that there is some obstruction in the nasal cavity.[107] To Da Costa we are indebted for having called attention to the fact that in a certain number of early cases of pulmonary tuberculosis a blowing sound in the subclavian or pulmonary artery may be heard, and that a murmur is sometimes present in the subclavian or pulmonary artery before any other physical sign is detected.

At times, during the early period of the disease, one may hear at the base of the lung, on the diseased side, more or less abundant mucous râles. These râles may be perceived with the inspiratory and the expiratory sound, or at the end of inspiration only. In the latter case the râles become crepitant. They are most probably due to a localized pulmonary congestion, since the patient hardly ever complains of pain or discomfort in that region. These congestive phenomena, which are not permanent, are explained by some authors[108] as being due to enlarged glands along the trachiobronchial tract.

I do not favor the giving of potassium iodide in order that the stethoscopic sounds may be revealed more rapidly and with more certainty. The fact that after the administration of the iodides râles of large magnitude can be perceived is evidence that a process of congestion and softening is produced, which must be considered harmful. Zeissl,[109] Vitvitsky, and others have reported cases of this kind. The case of Vitvitsky is particularly instructive and conclusive in this respect: The patient was a woman, twenty years old, who suffered from a cough, with a prickling sensation in the throat, and pain on deglutition; at the apices there were suspicious stethoscopic signs. However, the patient had no fever and her general health was excellent. A laryngoscopical examination revealed an intense congestion of the larynx and ulcerations of the vocal cords. As there was cause to suspect a syphilitic origin for this affection, ammonium iodide was prescribed in amounts of thirty grains a day. After eight days of this treatment the patient's condition was manifestly aggravated; the cough had increased, the temperature had become febrile in character, râles and a bronchial souffle were heard in the apices, Koch's bacilli were found in the sputum, which before had been free from them, and galloping phthisis set in, which terminated very soon in death.

Through Röntgen's discovery of the x-rays we have one more aid to the diagnosis of an early pulmonary tuberculosis. But while most highly appreciating the work done in this direction by such men as Bouchard,[110] Kelsch,[111] Espina y Capo,[112] Stubbert,[113] Williams,[114]

Crane,[118] and others, for the present I do not think that the fluoroscope will replace the ear, or that one can diagnose with it lesions that cannot be appreciated by physical examination. All that can be said of the x-rays up to this date, in relation to our subject, is that they may be considered an interesting means for corroborating a diagnosis made by ordinary physical examination. But the last word in radiography is not spoken, and research in this field of diagnosis should be highly encouraged.

Lastly, I wish to speak of agglutination as a means of discovering early pulmonary tuberculosis, and briefly give the result of some experiments which I made in the research laboratory of the New York City health department with the kind co-operation of Dr. William H. Park, the assistant director. The serum was very kindly furnished by Dr. Lambert, from his wards at Bellevue, and came from all kinds of patients.

The experiments with the pleuritic fluid drawn from a tuberculous guinea-pig were a decided success. The mixture of one part serum to nine of the bacilli emulsion showed the true adherent film after eighteen hours, and when agitated it broke up into thin large flakes characteristic of the positive reaction. The mixture of $1:20$ presented the same condition, but not quite so definite. In the hanging drop—under the microscope — the $1:10$ mixture, besides the small groups of bacilli which were originally present in the culture itself, showed numerous newly formed loose clumps of individual bacilli. These were absolutely motionless, having lost all Brownian movements. One part of horse serum plus nine of the watery emulsion of bacilli appeared identical with the simple watery emulsion. On lifting these tubes the sediment broke up into grains, and no true flakes appeared in the agitated fluid. According to Courmont, this is the absolutely certain sign of a negative reaction. In the hanging drop of both these mixtures, only tiny groups of bacilli, originally present in the culture, appeared; there remained many isolated single bacilli showing active Brownian movements.

The experiments with the serum from a number of patients suffering from various diseases were much less satisfactory. Of ten cases distinctly diagnosed as pulmonary tuberculosis, four reacted positively, two slightly, one gave a doubtful reaction, and three were absolutely negative. One case of miliary tuberculosis gave but a slight reaction. Of cases which, so far as we could tell, were free from tuberculosis, a positive reaction was obtained in one of postpartum hemorrhage—third day; a doubtful reaction was obtained in one of chronic hemiplegia, and also in one of alcoholic neuritis. Absolute negative reactions resulted from the examination of serum of a patient suffering from tertiary syphilis, and of two with acute articular rheumatism.

From our experience thus far we cannot subscribe to the claims of Arloing and Courmont,[116] that this method is of a very great diagnostic value in the early detection of pulmonary tuberculosis; but we realize that additional experiments may modify this conclusion and trust that further researches will continue in this interesting field.

In some rare instances the diazo reaction, which is of rather more importance in the prognosis of more advanced cases, may also be observed in the incipient stage and sometimes before the appearance of the bacilli in the sputum.[117]

Primary laryngeal tuberculosis is exceedingly rare, but we must acknowledge that at times the tuberculous lesions of the larynx predominate over the pulmonary affection, and the latter may not have been easily recognizable. The importance of an early recognition of laryngeal tuberculosis and a differentiation from syphilitic lupus or carcinomatous infections is thus evident. The early constitutional symptoms in laryngeal tuberculosis are virtually the same as in pulmonary tuberculosis. Huskiness or complete aphonia, constant pain intensified by swallowing, a spasmodic, whooping cough, dry or with expectoration, are early manifestations of the invasion of the larynx by the bacilli of tuberculosis. The laryngoscopical picture shows the characteristic pale mucous membrane, irregular reddish spots, and in addition a nodule or a monochorditis. At times an early ulceration in the interarytenoid space or at the base of the arytenoid cartilages[118] may be observed.

As regards the differential diagnosis we will give a few of the essential points. In carcinoma the pain is more constant than in tuberculosis, and in syphilis or lupus there is relatively no pain; but it is especially the laryngoscopical picture which usually clears up doubts. None but the tuberculous laryngitis has the pale mucous membrane. Syphilis has its clear-cut ulcer, lupus its nodular masses, carcinoma its indefinite growth in any portion of the laryngeal cavity. A syphilitic laryngitis will, of course, rapidly improve under the iodides, while this treatment will probably increase the tuberculous manifestation, but has no effect on either lupus or carcinoma.

Primary *tuberculous pharyngitis* is as rare as primary laryngitis, and its etiology can be explained only by the inhalation theory. Its earliest symptoms are those of an acute or subacute pharyngitis, and a positive diagnosis can be made only through bacteriological examination of the secretions, or after the formation of ulcers, through examination of the scrapings. According to Mayer,[119] the chief symptom is the pain usually extending to the ear, which becomes more and more distressing as the disease advances.

Tuberculous peritonitis, though perhaps never a primary disease, is very frequently the first manifestation of existing tuberculosis. The fact that recovery frequently follows simple laparotomy makes the early diagnosis most important in modern tuberculotherapeutics, though nothing is more difficult than the early recognition of tuberculosis of the peritoneum.

From Clavier's statistics[120] we learn that out of 135 cases there were 18 cases between the ages of 1 and 10 years, 29 between the ages of 10 and 20 years, 29 between the ages of 20 and 30 years, 28 between the ages of 30 and 40 years, 24 between the ages of 40 and 50 years, 7 between the ages of 50 and 60 years—total, 135 cases.

The development is always very insidious. Except a general failing and the occasional, by no means constant, abdominal pain and some meteorism, nothing of great import will perhaps be observed preceding the beginning of the effusion excepting a diarrhœa which occurs in some cases. Even the temperature may remain normal. But after all we can arrive at an early diagnosis of tuberculous peritonitis only by exclusion. If the constant failing of the health cannot be accounted for by a diseased condition of lungs, heart, liver, kidneys, or ovaries, and there are in addition chronic digestive disturbances with indefinitely localized abdominal pains, the thought of a tuberculous peritonitis must arise. Of course the bacteriological examination of the urine and of the pulmonary, cervical, or vaginal secretions is always essential in doubtful cases.

Joint tuberculosis and *tuberculous diseases of the bones*, which are most frequently seen in childhood, are more readily recognized in their earlier forms by an impairment of movement and localized acute pain on pressure in the epiphyseal regions and more or less marked local atrophy which may be accompanied by general malaise and often symptoms of a tuberculous diathesis. One can usually distinguish a tuberculosis of the bones and joints from an acute osteomyelitis or epiphysitis, as in the latter conditions the onset is more sudden, the pain more severe and permanent, and the destruction of bone and the appearance of suppuration are more rapid.

The early symptoms of *tuberculosis of the vertebræ*, when situated in the cervical regions, manifest themselves by a difficulty in deglutition and in breathing. The respiratory difficulties are sometimes accompanied by a dry cough. In the thoracic regions the diseased vertebræ are the indirect cause of encircling pains accompanied by digestive disturbances. If the tuberculosis is confined to the lower vertébræ, one will notice a marked irritability of the bladder and rectum, especially a desire for frequent urination. Tuberculosis of the sacral vertebræ is at times also the cause of radiating pains in the femoral regions. But in skilled hands the x-rays have been of incalculable value in the diagnosis of early joint tuberculosis. At a recent meeting of the New York German Medical Society, Dr. Otto G. T. Kiliani[121] demonstrated the importance of this means of diagnosis, and called attention to the fact that the negative alone, and not the print, would show the small glandular tuberculous foci. To use his own words, " one has to read the plates since prints are of no value." He succeeded in several cases in curing the disease by removing these early small granular foci, the location of which was indicated to him by the infallible dark spots revealed on the plate. Thus he also succeeded in photographing the rice bodies in a knee in a case in which a diagnosis of tuberculous infection was uncertain, and by the same process he discovered a tuberculous focus in the sixth cervical vertebra at a time when no other symptom existed except an indistinct pain in the neck.

The milder forms of tuberculosis in children are usually classed as scrofulous manifestations. One of the early symptoms is a more or less pronounced anæmia. The child usually manifests a phlegmatic condition, but we may also find some that are very nervous and irritable. Frequently one observes conjunctivitis and otitis media, which are apt to take a very chronic form. But the most characteristic symptom of all, and one that is rarely absent, is the swelling of the cervical glands. Much more rarely do we find swelling of the axillary or inguinal glands. The localization of tuberculosis in these glands should no longer be considered a manifestation of a tuberculous diathesis, but rather as the result of an infection from without, i.e., by inhalation or ingestion.

The early diagnosis of pulmonary tuberculosis during infancy and early childhood is extremely difficult. The history of the case is all-important. We must endeavor to find the source of infection. Phenomena which speak for tuberculosis are marked transformation of the child's temper, preservation of appetite and digestion with progressive loss of flesh and strength, and slight swelling of the supraclavicular glands. Paroxysms of cough are suspicious, but absence of cough does not preclude tuberculosis. The torpid course of simple, non-specific affections of the skin (boils, eczema), will strengthen the suspicion of tuberculosis in the presence of other evidences of the disease. The presence or absence of fever has no significance in the diagnosis of the disease under consideration; neither has the occurrence of enlarged spleen.[122]

When the disease runs an acute instead of a chronic course, another set of data supply information useful for diagnostic purposes. Some of the symptoms which point to acute tuberculosis are great unrest and agitation, convulsions, cyanosis, and accelerated breathing, sputum in large balls, transitory collapse in apparently healthy children, and râles differing in magnitude with extensive pulmonary infiltration.

Primary intestinal tuberculosis in childhood may be the result of the ingestion of tuberculous milk or other substances. Secondary intestinal tuberculosis, as in the adult, is the result of swallowing tuberculous sputum, especially since small children never expectorate. A tuberculous tabes mesenterica cannot be easily recognized so long as the glands are small. One has to rely on the constitutional symptoms and anamnesis to make a diagnosis. Intestinal tuberculosis in children is really difficult to diagnose with certainty at the earlier periods. The best characteristic symptom is perhaps a protracted diarrhœa, or frequent attacks of diarrhœa, which cannot be easily controlled by dieting or medication. A bacteriological examination of the fæces will often decide a doubtful case.

Lupus, which is the most prevalent form of skin tuberculosis, is treated of in the article on "Tuberculosis of the Skin" in the present volume, and for the details of its diagnosis and treatment we must refer our readers to that article.

TREATMENT.

Hygienic Treatment.

The method of treatment which we are about to describe is the one which has thus far proved the most efficacious, and which can be carried out in nearly all climates.

SANATORIUM TREATMENT.

In order to do the most good to the largest number of tuberculous individuals, I would place the sanatorium for consumptives within easy reach of a large centre of population, at no greater distance than from three to five hours by rail. It should be in a region known for its relative purity of atmosphere, where there is freedom from all miasmatic and malarial influences, and where the pathogenic microbes are found only in negligible quantities. If possible, it should be where the extremes of temperature are not too pronounced, and, if the region is a mountainous one, at an altitude of from one thousand to two thousand feet. The site should be a pleasant one, with a southern exposure and protected from cold winds by higher mountains or woodlands (pine woods should be given the preference). The ground, of course, should be dry and porous. But that all these conditions are not necessary has been proved in institutions which have the advantages neither of a favorable climate nor of a high altitude. There exists in Scotland an establishment devoted to the treatment of consumption, known as the "Victoria Hospital of Edinburgh" (at Craigleith). When I visited it, in September, 1894, it had only just been opened, and its latest reports show that it has had since hundreds of patients under treatment with most satisfactory results. What is possible in Scotland with its rigorous climate is possible anywhere else. In the United States I know of two institutions located but a few miles from two of the largest cities, and the results obtained are certainly most remarkable, for there are no special climatic advantages claimed for either of them. Both locations are exposed to the extreme heat as well as to the severe cold so frequently experienced in the Eastern cities of the United States. I refer to the Sharon Sanatorium, near Boston, and the Chestnut Hill Hospital for Consumptives, near Philadelphia.

The next question to be considered would be the choice of buildings and their mode of construction. Which plan would it be best to adopt—the European system, in which they house as many as seventy-five to one hundred patients under one roof, or the American cottage system, with no more than from four to eight in each cottage? To make so large an aggregation as one finds in some of the European institutions seems certainly not a good plan, since the hygienic measures are almost sure to suffer in such a house. On the other hand, the cottage system, while it may be the ideal for some diseases, is, on the whole, not the most desirable for a sanatorium for consumptives. The constant medical supervision—one of the most important features in the sanatorium treatment—can hardly be carried out in a village of twenty or thirty small cottages several hundred feet apart, not to mention the increased expense such a system involves.

To give an idea of what is meant by the European system of one house and by the cottage system, I reproduce here for illustration the Hohenhonnef Sanatorium with plan (Figs. 32 and 33) and also the Adirondack Cottage Sanitarium with groups of cottages and the ground plan of one of the cottages (Figs. 34-37).

In visiting the numerous institutions I endeavored, by taking comparative notes, to form a plan of what would seem an ideal sanatorium for the treatment of tuberculous patients in all stages, and under varied climatic conditions, and adaptable to nearly all localities. I conveyed my ideas to my friend, Mr. John Van Pelt, an

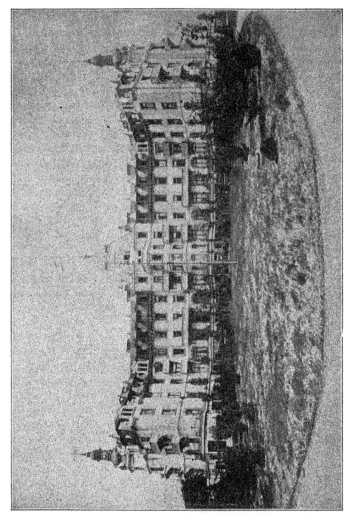

Fig. 32.—General View of Hohenhonnef Sanatorium.

architect, with instructions to draw the plans necessary to illustrate my conception of a model sanatorium* for the treatment of patients

* Contrary to the custom of many English-speaking people, especially in the United States, I call these establishments *Sanatoria*, and not *Sanitaria*. The

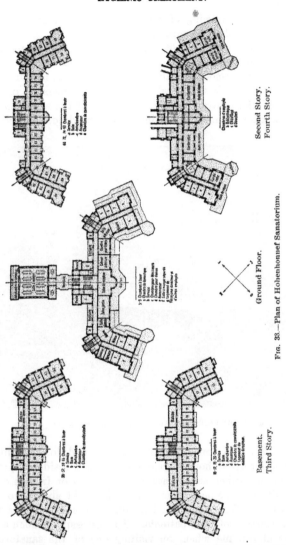

Fig. 33.—Plan of Hohenhonnef Sanatorium.

Ground Floor.

Second Story.
Fourth Story.

Basement.
Third Story.

suffering from pulmonary tuberculosis. I show here the general view, the general plan, the detailed plan of the first story of one of

former (sanatorium), from *sanare*, to heal, gives a better equivalent to the German "Heilanstalt," the word used by the originator of this system (Brehmer). Secondly, the word "sanitarium," from *sanitas*, health, is usually employed to designate a place considered simply as especially healthy, a favorite resort for convalescent patients.

the pavilions, and a drawing of the corner of the veranda, with an adjustable chair for the rest cure (Figs. 38-41).

As will be seen, I have adopted a plan between the European and the American; in other words, the large pavilion system. Three pavilions, each accommodating about twenty patients, are united by galleries one hundred feet long, which serve for promenades on rainy days. Behind the central building are situated the winter garden, dining-room, kitchen, and the administration building, connected by

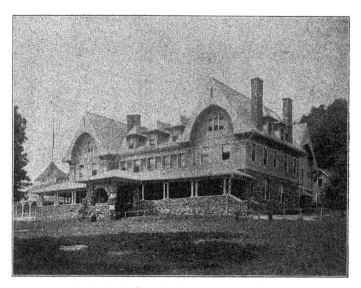

Fig. 34.—Main Building of Adirondack Cottage Sanitarium.

covered passages. At some little distance we find, to the right and left, two medium-sized houses, one serving as a residence for the medical staff, the other as a place where visitors or friends of the patients, desiring to be near them, may reside. At about two hundred and fifty feet from the main building, to the left, is a pavilion for the purpose of isolating patients. The necessity of such a precaution was shown me when, on visiting one of the sanatoria in Switzerland, I learned that a short time before a case of scarlatina had been discovered among the inmates of the one existing building, and as a consequence everybody who could had fled. Besides, even among the ordinary pulmonary invalids, the occasion for the need of isolation may arise. (In cases of gangrene, temporary insanity, etc., a separate smaller pavilion will be indispensable.) On the opposite side of the other buildings, at a considerable distance, is situated the recreation pavilion, constructed so that two sides are always entirely

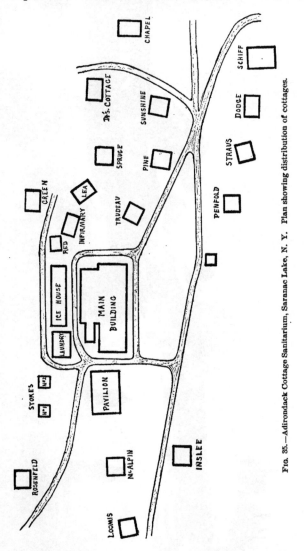

FIG. 35.—Adirondack Cottage Sanitarium, Saranac Lake, N. Y. Plan showing distribution of cottages.

open. The closed sides can be changed according to the direction of the wind. The other buildings are houses for the gardener, stables for the horses, etc.

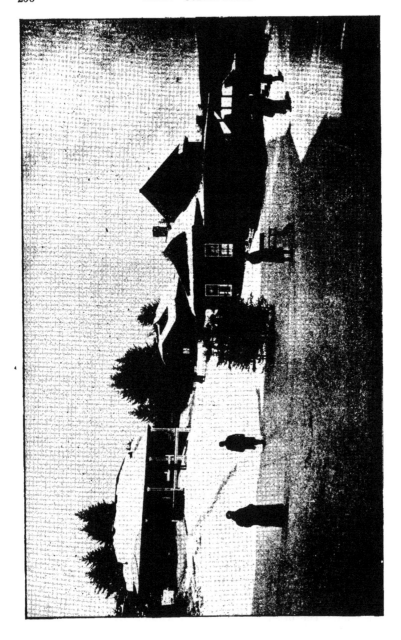

In front of the pavilions, on the south side, is the park, with its turning kiosks, sun boxes, graded paths, benches, etc. On the first floor of each pavilion are fourteen comfortable, well-lighted, well-ventilated sleeping-rooms for the patients, with two more rooms for the nurses; also the toilet-rooms, etc. On the ground floor are the sitting-rooms, library, parlor, consultation-rooms, and the room necessary for the hydrotherapeutic applications, and also several bed-

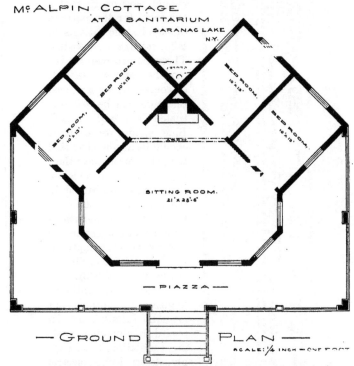

Fig. 37.—Ground Plan of one of the Cottages of the Adirondack Cottage Sanitarium.

rooms for patients. The verandas, each one hundred and thirty-five feet long and fifteen feet wide, extend along the length of the pavilions; they are protected by a roof made partly of glass, provided with curtains, and arranged to make the prolonged stay of the pulmonary invalid as pleasant as possible; for it is here that he will have to pass the greater part of his time. For weaker patients, not yet able to go down-stairs or take their rest cure on the veranda, there is ample room to place a lounge, or even a bed, on the balcony opening directly from the rooms.

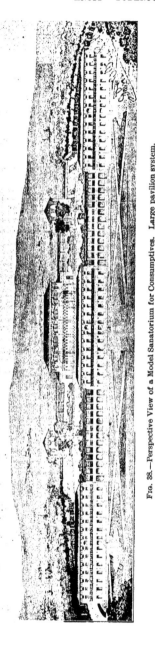

Fig. 38.—Perspective View of a Model Sanatorium for Consumptives. Large pavilion system.

The reclining chairs on the rest-cure veranda should not be placed too close to each other; a space of at least five feet should intervene.

Each large pavilion should have on its roof a sun-room for the purpose of enabling the patients to take their sun-baths. These sun-rooms, in the model sanatorium, should, of course, be so arranged that they can be well ventilated and well heated. Blue shades or curtains should be arranged so that the patients can have their heads in the shade while their bodies are bathed in the rays of the sun. Of the value of the sun-bath as a therapeutic agent in the treatment of consumptives, we shall speak more in detail below (page 278).

Besides the ordinary hygienic precautions and modern installations in regard to plumbing, heating, ventilation, water supply, electric lights, electric fans in dining-rooms, sitting-rooms, etc., all angles throughout the house are rounded to prevent the accumulation of dust. The walls are painted so that they may be easily disinfected; the floors are of hardwood and may be easily mopped, as sweeping or raising dust should be absolutely forbidden, not only in a well-conducted sanatorium or special hospital, but in the home of a tuberculous patient as well. Unnecessary commotion whereby dust

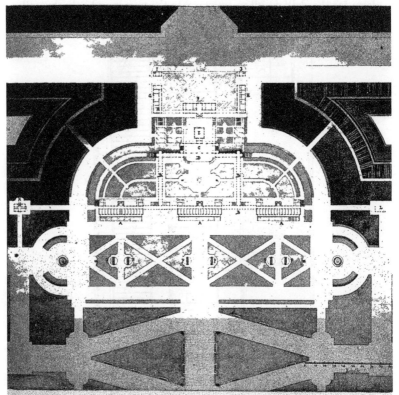

Fig. 39.—Plan of the Model Sanatorium. *A*, Pavilion for patients; *B*, galleries uniting the pavilions; *C*, dining-hall; *D*, winter-garden; *E*, kitchen; *F*, administration building; *G*, physician's house; *H*, house for visitors; *I, J*, janitor and gardener; *K*, house for isolation; *L*, recreation pavilion; *M*, disinfecting-room; *N*, stables; *P*, revolving pavilions.

may be raised should be avoided wherever there are sick persons, but especially pulmonary invalids.

In large buildings where many invalids congregate, of whom some may even be helpless at times, great precaution should be taken to prevent possible accidents by fire. There should be large staircases and hallways, lighted all night, a sufficient number of exits and well-kept fire-escapes, and, besides the ordinary fire hose on each floor, portable fire extinguishers should be distributed throughout the building. But equally important is the training of the nurses and

other help for such emergencies.   During my service at the Falkenstein Sanatorium I witnessed a few drills of the sanatorium fire bri-
gade, composed exclusively of the *personnel* of the institution.   The
alarm for the drill is given unknown to the nurses and help, but all

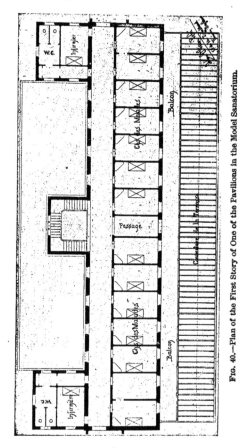

Fig. 40.—Plan of the First Story of One of the Pavilions in the Model Sanatorium.

patients were previously notified that at a certain time the fire-alarm
bell would be sounded.   These drills serve not only as a pleasant
diversion to the patients, who could calmly look on upon the interesting feats performed by the firemen, but they also serve to give them
a feeling of security.

Since it is the duty of the modern phthisiotherapeutist and sanitarian to avoid by all possible precaution the tuberculous infection
of man through beast, he must also necessarily institute measures to

protect the beast from tuberculous infection through man. The necessity of such precaution was strongly impressed upon me when visiting an institution in a State where much is done in the direction of prophylaxis. The institution receives nearly two hundred patients annually, the majority being consumptives.

The following is one of the rules conspicuously posted throughout the house: "Patients must at all times, when in the institution or on

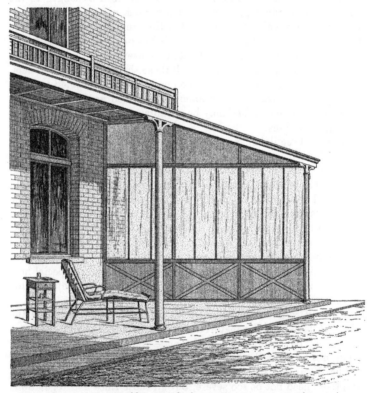

Fig. 41.—Corner of Veranda with Adjustable Chair for Rest Cure in the Model Sanatorium.

the verandas, expectorate in the sputa-cups provided. They must never expectorate in the sinks, wash-basins, closets, or on the floor, or in their handkerchiefs." Outside the institution the patients are not restricted; they may expectorate wherever they please, and I have no doubt they do. I was told that a neighboring farmer, who had some time ago bought five healthy cows, had them recently tested, with the result that three were found tuberculous. It seems thus to me unwise to have the dairy on or too near the premises of a sanatorium for consumptives. There will be occasionally a careless, unconscientious patient in all institutions of this kind who may expectorate on the surrounding grounds, where animals are likely to come in contact with the sputum on the grass.

In an institution for the treatment of consumptives there will be, of course, the strictest precautions concerning the tuberculous expectorations and other secretions. We have described at length in the chapter on individual prophylaxis the various spittoons now in use and need not speak of their construction in detail again. There should be the elevated spittoons in dishes or on stands; the small, mug-like spittoon, which the patients may use during their rest cure, and, finally, the pocket flask. Of all these there should be two sets, so that they are never wanting when one set is being cleaned and disinfected. If for reasons of economy clean linen napkins cannot be given with each meal, they may be advantageously replaced by Japanese paper napkins.

Each well-regulated sanatorium should have special facilities for disinfecting spoons, knives, and forks, which should be done after each meal. At the Falkenstein Sanatorium an especially constructed sterilizing apparatus is used for this purpose. All table-linen should be steeped in boiling water before being given to the laundry, and the same precaution should be exercised with the bed and private linen of the patients. The rooms in an ideal sanatorium for consumptives should be submitted to a thorough disinfection by formaldehyde gas at regular intervals, and not only after the death or removal of a patient. As an additional precaution in a sanatorium or special hospital I would suggest the disinfection of the patient's clothing on his arrival, and at periodic intervals.

While it will not be possible to enforce a rule concerning the toilets of ladies in a sanatorium, the wearing of trailing dresses should not be permitted, and the male inmates of the institution should not be allowed to smoke inside the buildings.

The discipline in a model sanatorium for the treatment of consumptives need not be too severe, but all those rules and regulations enacted in the interest of the patient and his surroundings should be religiously obeyed. A patient should not absent himself from the sanatorium without permission from the doctor.

It may not be amiss, in speaking of an ideal sanatorium, also to say a few words regarding the ideal management. Some of the European institutions are managed in two departments, presided over by a medical director and a general superintendent, respectively. In some the former, in others the latter would be considered the superior in cases of conflict. While visiting the European sanatoria it has been my lot to witness such a conflict between the two heads of a sanatorium, and the lesson I learned therefrom was most valuable. In a sanatorium for the treatment of consumptives the medical director should always be the final court of appeal, as well in the general as in the medical affairs of the institution.

SPECIAL HOSPITALS.

So much for the general and special hygiene in a sanatorium. What would be the requirement for a special hospital which should be particularly established with a view of taking care of the more advanced cases of pulmonary tuberculosis, or of receiving temporarily those from which the invalids for the mountain sanatorium are to be selected?

Since the special hospital is situated in or near a city, in it much that can be had with ease in the country sanatorium can be obtained only with difficulty.

The first requisite for the special hospital is a location as quiet as possible. The building should be erected on high, porous ground, and, of course, in accordance with the modern conceptions of hygiene and sanitation. While many of the patients will perhaps be in bed most of the time, there should, nevertheless, be plenty of verandas and balconies, wide enough to hold beds or couches, which can be placed there on warm days with their inmates. In a city. hospital for consumptives it will be wellnigh impossible to have a separate room for each patient, but too large wards also have their disadvantage. Rooms to accommodate from four to six patients, with a number of single ones for special cases, seem the best arrangement for such an institution. The temperature throughout the hospital should rarely be higher than 60° to 65° F., and as nearly as possible uniform throughout the establishment. In winter as well as in summer the atmosphere of the rooms must be frequently renewed by opening the windows, or by ventilators.

What was instituted by Unterberger[123] in the Military Hospital of Tsarskoye Syelo near St. Petersburg, would be an excellent addition to the equipment of a special hospital. Pine trees, planted in tubs of wet sand, are placed throughout the hospital, more numerously in the bedrooms and sitting-rooms. Towards evening, when the odor of the pine grows weak, the trees are sprayed with the following solution:

℞ Ol. pini sllv. (Scotch fir), ... 10 parts
Ol. terebinth. pur., ... 30 "
Aq. font., ... 300 "

Through this combination the air becomes more impregnated with ozone, and for a consumptive to live and take frequent respiratory exercises in such an atmosphere is certainly beneficial.

Frankel's mask, as a protection against the expulsion of bacilli, should be worn by the patients whenever practicable in the wards, and a respirator by the nurses while cleaning. It should be the duty of the nurse in charge to make the rounds at stated intervals among the patients assigned to her or his care, not only for the purpose of looking after their wants, but to see that they have not, owing to their feebleness or carelessness, expectorated where the sputum may constitute a danger. An ample supply of moist rags should be at the bedside of patients too far advanced to make use of a spittoon.

HOME TREATMENT.

Just as in a sanatorium or special hospital, so also in the home treatment of consumptives the largest, pleasantest, sunniest, best-ventilated rooms should be given up to the patients. In the room mainly occupied by the invalid, whether in the sanatorium or at home, velvet or plush covered furniture should be replaced by such as will not accumulate dust. There should be no carpets, heavy curtains, or superfluous furniture, and the indispensable furniture should be so constructed that it can be wiped off with a moist cloth every morning. Very tall pieces of furniture are always dust collectors. But even with this sanitary arrangement, the room need not be cheerless. Easy chairs, small rugs, and curtains that can be washed may be allowed.

A tuberculous patient should always sleep alone and in a bed which should be freely aired during the daytime. A very weak patient who is unable to sit up should, whenever it is possible, have a second bed placed in his room so as to be able to change. A brass or iron bed with wire springs is preferable. Feather beds should not be used, and the bed should be placed, whenever possible, with the head against an inside wall. Draughts should be avoided as far as possible, but this precaution must not be carried to extremes so as to make the patient afraid of a breath of fresh air. If the bedroom is too small to make it possible to place the bed so as to avoid the direct draught from the open window, a substantial screen should be used as a protection. In short, the special and general hygiene at home should be the same as in an ideal sanatorium.

During the day the lounge or reclining-chair should be moved near the open window if there is no porch or balcony. In summer, or on not too cold or windy days in winter, the patient may be placed, warmly wrapped, on his chair on the flat roof, protecting his

head from the sun by an umbrella or a small, improvised tent. If
there is a yard or garden, a small platform of boards may be arranged for the chair in a spot sheltered from the wind. A plain
steamer-chair, padded with a quilt or blanket, will answer the purpose just as well as a costly reclining-chair. Another good and simple method of carrying out the "Liegekur," or rest cure, in the open
air is the one suggested by Daremberg.[124] A large beach-chair of
wicker work, such as is seen in our fashionable seaside resorts, is

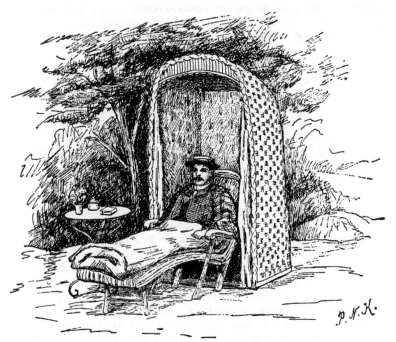

Fig. 42.—Portable Rest-Cure Arrangement for Private Patients.

procured. After the seat has been removed the inner walls are lined
with padding. A reclining-chair is placed with its back in the interior, and the whole arranged so that the patient is protected from the
wind and sun. There the patient installs himself for the day, with
his books or writing materials at his side, placed on a little table, on
which his meals may also be served. The accompanying illustration
(Fig. 42) will show how easily such an arrangement can be effected.
Being light, the whole can be shifted whenever the wind changes and
according to the position of the sun, so that the invalid's body may be
bathed by the rays of the sun, while the head remains in the shade.

Aerotherapy and the Pneumatic Cabinet.

In this section we shall describe the rest cure, the breathing and walking exercises, and the pneumatic cabinet treatment, as best adapted for the average tuberculous invalid. That these must vary according to the environments and the condition of the patient is self-understood. There can be no one scheme of therapeutics for all consumptives. We must adapt our curative means to the patient, not to the disease, and more than in any other ailment the treatment must be individual. Thus I venture to give the following method as carried out in a sanatorium only as a general guide:

The main object of aërotherapeutics is to oblige the patient to live as much as possible in the open air. A patient arriving at a sanatorium and having a high temperature—for example, above 102° F.—should be left in bed and moved, during the day, towards the open window or on to the balcony. When his temperature goes down he is allowed to begin his rest cure (Liegekur of Dettweiler) on the veranda, on a lounge, steamer-chair, or, better yet, on a reclining-chair especially constructed for the purpose, such as illustrated in Fig. 41. The back of this chair can be given any desired inclination.

It is needless to say that a patient, especially one coming from a sick-room in a large city, must be submitted only gradually to the exhilarating influence of a constant sojourn in the open air; but the endurance which may be arrived at in this respect is wonderful. In Falkenstein the patients remain out-of-doors in their chairs from seven to ten hours a day all the year round, in spite of fog, rain, wind, snow, and even with the thermometer at 12° C. below zero (10° F. above zero), and often no sunshine. Dr. Andvord, of Tonsaasen, Norway, wrote me that he leaves his patients on their chairs, wrapped up in furs, from five to nine hours a day at a temperature of −25° C. (−13° F.).

It is to this prolonged stay in the open air (Dauerluftkur of the Germans) that the marvellous results obtained in sanatoria may be attributed. Besides the rest cure in the fresh air, there is moderate exercise on gradated walks in the garden—that is to say, on paths varying in inclination from one foot in three-hundred to one in sixty. At night the patient sleeps with his window open, rain or shine, warm or cold; wide open in summer, less so in winter. The only excuse for closing the window might be a very strong wind or a thick fog.

For the benefit of patients who cannot go to a sanatorium, it may be said that night air in towns and cities is, if anything, even purer than day air, and they should not fear it. If circumstances compel them, for example, to remain in their city homes during the sweltering heat of our Eastern summers, I would encourage them to instal themselves for the night on the roof, with an improvised shelter of canvas or boards over them. In towns and villages where patients often own their own homes an addition to the building to serve as a house sanatorium might be advantageously erected. I take pleasure in reproducing here such a home which has been illustrated in an article by Millet

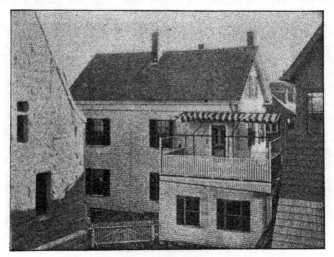

Fig. 43.—Permanent Arrangement for Open-Air Treatment at Home.

on "The Night Air of New England in the Treatment of Consumption."[125] A consumptive, if he wishes to get well, should live every moment of his existence in the purest and freshest air possible. If feasible he should even take his meals outdoors. During the rest cure on the reclining-chair the patient is allowed to read or write, and is made as comfortable as possible. The main point to be attained is an almost complete muscular relaxation, in order to economize and store up strength and reduce the fever. When on their chairs on the veranda (Fig. 44) patients should always be covered with blankets or lap-robes, in accordance with the season; furs in winter are indispensable.

In sanatoria there is always an attendant attached to the service to see that the patients do not become uncovered while asleep. Short naps after meals are allowed, but they should not exceed ten minutes or so. Consumptives are so apt to perspire when asleep any length of time, and especially when warmly dressed, that this might be the cause of their taking a severe cold. Patients are warned, when taking their rest cure, never to let the sun shine directly on their heads. Congestion, headache, and other troubles often follow if this precaution is neglected. But the rest cure should not be carried out exclusively on the veranda. Whenever it is practicable chairs should be placed in the grounds, in the parks or gardens surrounding the institution or home, and thus make the rest cure a veritable open-air treatment. The accompanying illustration (Fig. 45) gives a good

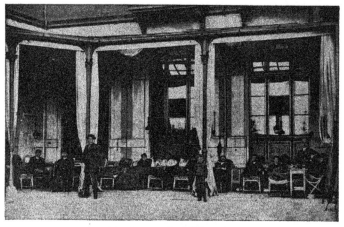

FIG. 44.—Veranda at Falkenstein.

idea how such an arrangement may be carried out. In some sanatoria there are also revolving kiosks, large enough to hold four or five reclining-chairs. These kiosks turn easily on a pivot in any direction desired.

The good results which are obtained at times by the rest cure in the open air are indeed wonderful; and still it is not without danger, as it is practised in some European sanatoria. To have a patient recline on his back for three or four hours at a time without rising, and repeating this two or three times during the day, seems to me dangerous, for it facilitates hypostatic congestion of the lungs. I know of several cases in which this condition has been brought about by thus remaining too long in the recumbent position. There is another reason why I do not favor one remaining undisturbed for hours on the reclining-chair. The local temperature of the back, being in constant contact with the warm cushions, will cause this part to become more sensitive to temperature changes than it had been, perhaps, ever before; and it seems to me easy to explain thereby why patients

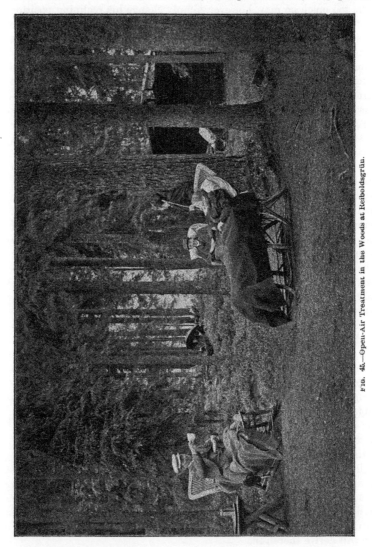

Fig. 45.—Open-Air Treatment in the Woods at Reiboldsgrün.

in institutions where the cure is practised as just described always complain of cold backs.

It is for this reason that I think respiratory exercises should be made to alternate with the rest cure outdoors. The patient should' rise every hour, or half-hour, to take these exercises. If this tires him too much he may, however, simply change his reclining position for the straight sitting position, raise his arms and go through the first and second respiratory exercises a few times. Should even the raising of the arms tire him, he may go through the exercise by simply moving his shoulders upwards and backwards, which is the exercise prescribed for pulmonary invalids when the raising of the arms is not practicable. Experience has taught me that these exercises are of value in nearly all cases except in acute inflammatory processes, in frequent active pulmonary hemorrhages, and whenever there is a constant temperature of 100° or more; or, again, when the disease is in active evolution, and absolute rest is to be preferred.

I have described in full, and endeavored to illustrate, my system of breathing-exercises in the pages on preventive treatment. As I stated there, they are alike beneficial for the predisposed and for the patient with developed pulmonary tuberculosis. For the latter a more strict medical supervision and a more careful gradation is, of course, necessary. It is true that whenever there are old pleuritic adhesions these extra-respiratory efforts may cause moments of pain; the patient must, however, bear in mind that these pains are not lasting and are in reality salutary, being caused by the loosening of the fibrinous bands. By these breathing-exercises the respiratory muscles are developed, the process of hæmatosis becomes more complete, and the increased respiratory function helps to dissolve the mucus and makes cough and expectoration more easy. More advanced and very weak patients must content themselves with deep but quiet respirations without movements of the arms. Placing a pillow under the back of such a patient so as to realize somewhat Sylvester's position, employed when artificial respiration is necessary, will be found a valuable adjuvant. But there is another matter in relation to the rest cure on the reclining-chair which, I regret to say, I saw sadly neglected in the majority of the sanatoria I visited. Women lie on their chairs with their tightly laced corsets on, men with stiff shirts and high collars, and they were expected to take deep breaths in order to expand their lungs. The fallacy of such methods is evident. There must not be any restriction to free full abdominal and thoracic respiration while taking the "Liegekur." The more comfortably the patient is dressed, the more he will enjoy his cure, and the more benefit he will derive therefrom.

Much has been written on the question of exercise in the open air for pulmonary invalids. Brehmer was much in favor of it and as much as possible of it in order to strengthen the heart, and some of our American phthisiotherapeutists are of the same opinion. Dett-weiler and his pupils, on the contrary, are opposed to it, except under restriction and the most careful supervision. The rest cure on the reclining-chairs, as above described, is now admitted in the sanatorium created by Brehmer. It seems to me that the wisest course to pursue would be to consider each individual case, and pre-scribe or forbid exercises according to the condition and the strength of the patient.

We have already spoken of gradated walks of various inclination to test the patient's strength in regard to his climbing-powers. The duration of a promenade should be graduated with equal care. One should commence with a walk of a few minutes until a walk of an hour or an hour and a half can be taken without producing fatigue. Wherever it is practicable these excursions should begin up-hill, so that the return is easy. After his promenade the patient's tempera-ture should be taken. If it exceeds the normal it is an indication that the patient has overtaxed his powers. Whether complete rest or simply shorter walks are then indicated will be decided by the variation of the temperature before and after exercise. When the temperature of the patient rises only slightly in the evening (99°–99.5° F.), short walks in the morning, while in the apyretic state, may be permitted. A lasting temperature of 100° F. or over is an absolute. contraindication to exercise. Tachycardia should also be considered as such. If there is, however, a chronic tachycardiac condition, absolute rest might not be the best policy. But these patients, more than any others, should be warned against the slight-est overexertion. Breathing-exercises and walks may be combined, the patient taking three to five of the exercises above described, with or without moving the arms, in every one hundred and fifty to two hundred steps.

The Pneumatic Cabinet.—In the modern therapeutics of pulmo-nary diseases the pneumatic cabinet takes its place in importance immediately after general aërotherapeutics. To the physicians who have used it persistently and studied its effects, it certainly has rendered valuable services. Still I am aware that it is relatively little known, and thus it may, perhaps, not be amiss to describe its construction somewhat in detail.

The pneumatic cabinet has the form of a tall safe, somewhat larger at the bottom than at the top. Its doors and apertures close hermeti-cally. It is large enough for a patient to sit comfortably inside. The front is composed, in part, of a large plate of glass through which the operator, manipulating the lever, watches the patient. By a system of valves, bellows, and lever, compressed or rarefied air can be produced. An opening through the frontal glass-plate serves for communication with the outside air, which the patient inhales through a rubber tube. The amount of incoming air can be regulated by the stopcock of a faucet. The degree of rarefaction or compression is indicated by a manometer in communication with the inside atmosphere of the cabinet. I append a drawing of the pneumatic cabinet

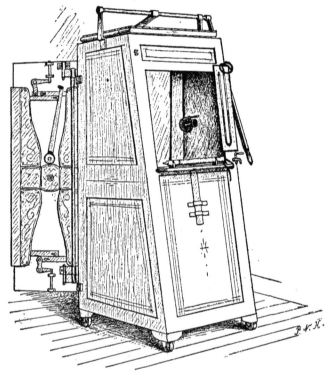

FIG. 46.—Pneumatic Cabinet.

in my possession, which is the model now used by nearly all phthisio-therapeutists who employ this instrument.

The principle of the cabinet in the treatment of pulmonary tuberculosis is to diminish the weight of the atmospheric pressure, which at the sea-level, under normal conditions, is about fifteen pounds to the square inch. With the aid of the cabinet it can be reduced nearly to fourteen pounds to the square inch.

The action of the pneumatic cabinet has been described by many authors, such as Bowditch,[126] Fox,[127] Houghton,[128] Hudson,[129] Jensen,[130] Ketchum,[131] Westbrook,[132] Williams,[133] and others.   In perusing the extensive literature on the subject I found Platt's[134] exposition one of the clearest.   His experience agrees with mine in almost every detail.   He describes the action of the pneumatic cabinet as follows: "Such portion of the thoracic cavity as is not occupied by tissue—muscular, glandular, the parenchyma of the lung, etc.—consists of air space and blood space, and it is obvious that the increase of one of these will tend to the diminution of the other. The respiration of air at the normal tension while the body is immersed in a rarefied atmosphere is, in effect, the same as the introduction of a compressed atmosphere into the air space of the lungs; it will increase the air space and tend to diminish the blood space, driving a certain portion of the blood from the lungs into the general circulation, which is subjected to a diminished pressure.   The pulmonary congestion is diminished in exactly the same way as the congestion of an inflamed joint or of an ulcer by bandaging.   Or, to put it in another way, the blood is sucked or drawn out from the lungs into the general circulation, as it is sucked into the space beneath a cupping-glass.

"Thus I believe the main action of the cabinet to be the reduction of pulmonary congestion, and the theory is practically verified by our experience with regard to blood-spitting and bronchial hemorrhage. Time and again, patients have come into the office complaining of the sputa being blood-streaked, and, almost without a single exception, the use of the cabinet has relieved the symptom in the course of a few minutes.

"In addition to the effect it has upon the pulmonary congestion it undoubtedly acts beneficially in other ways.   The thoracic gymnastics afforded by expiration against increased resistance will probably be of benefit to the weak-chested.   The increased oxygenation of the blood will, doubtless, improve the nutritive processes.   Then the spray, if proper medicaments are used, may be expected to act beneficially upon the accompanying bronchitis."

Quimby,[135] who is, perhaps, the best authority on the subject of cabinet treatment in pulmonary tuberculosis—for he has used the cabinet longer and more persistently than any other phthisiotherapeutist I know of—gives as the conclusion of a most remarkable paper on this subject, read before the American Climatological Association in Richfield Springs, N. Y., June 24th, 1892, the following interesting table:

RELATIONS OF THE PNEUMATIC CABINET TO THE DESTRUCTIVE FORCES OF PULMONARY PHTHISIS.

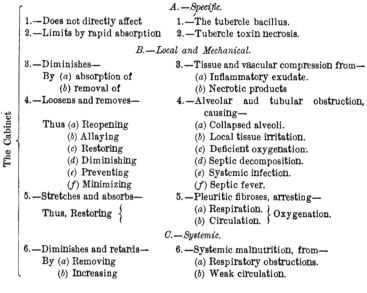

The Cabinet

A.—Specific.

1.—Does not directly affect
2.—Limits by rapid absorption

1.—The tubercle bacillus.
2.—Tubercle toxin necrosis.

B.—Local and Mechanical.

3.—Diminishes—
  By (a) absorption of
    (b) removal of
4.—Loosens and removes—

  Thus (a) Reopening
    (b) Allaying
    (c) Restoring
    (d) Diminishing
    (e) Preventing
    (f) Minimizing
5.—Stretches and absorbs—

  Thus, Restoring

3.—Tissue and vascular compression from—
  (a) Inflammatory exudate.
  (b) Necrotic products
4.—Alveolar and tubular obstruction, causing—
  (a) Collapsed alveoli.
  (b) Local tissue irritation.
  (c) Deficient oxygenation.
  (d) Septic decomposition.
  (e) Systemic infection.
  (f) Septic fever.
5.—Pleuritic fibroses, arresting—
  (a) Respiration. }
  (b) Circulation. } Oxygenation.

C.—Systemic.

6.—Diminishes and retards—
  By (a) Removing
    (b) Increasing

6.—Systemic malnutrition, from—
  (a) Respiratory obstructions.
  (b) Weak circulation.

RELATIONS OF THE PNEUMATIC CABINET TO THE CONSTRUCTIVE FORCES OF PULMONARY PHTHISIS.

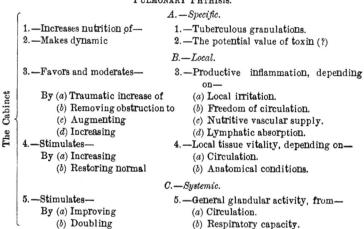

The Cabinet

A.—Specific.

1.—Increases nutrition of—
2.—Makes dynamic

1.—Tuberculous granulations.
2.—The potential value of toxin (?)

B.—Local.

3.—Favors and moderates—

  By (a) Traumatic increase of
    (b) Removing obstruction to
    (c) Augmenting
    (d) Increasing
4.—Stimulates—
  By (a) Increasing
    (b) Restoring normal

3.—Productive inflammation, depending on—
  (a) Local irritation.
  (b) Freedom of circulation.
  (c) Nutritive vascular supply.
  (d) Lymphatic absorption.
4.—Local tissue vitality, depending on—
  (a) Circulation.
  (b) Anatomical conditions.

C.—Systemic.

5.—Stimulates—
  By (a) Improving
    (b) Doubling

5.—General glandular activity, from—
  (a) Circulation.
  (b) Respiratory capacity.

When I first began to investigate the pneumatic cabinet treatment, I saw it used as I believe it is now still used by the majority of physi-

cians. The patient enters the cabinet completely dressed, he inserts
the tube into his mouth, and the operator manipulates the lever from
five to ten minutes, retaining the manometer at the height of about
an inch. The good effect of this treatment, it seemed to me, could
be heightened by some modifications which suggested themselves to
me in the course of my own experience with the cabinet.

With the exception of the very weakest and highly febrile cases,
nearly all tuberculous patients can take the pneumatic cabinet treatment. However, before admitting my patients into the cabinet I
teach them how to breathe. They must first take a course of respiratory exercises, such as described under Preventive Treatment, and
only after they have learned to use their respiratory muscles to the
best advantage do I begin the treatment, with short *séances* at first.
Any mechanical obstruction to proper breathing has, of course, been
looked after previous to the commencement of the respiratory exer-

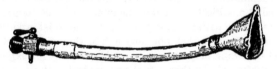

Fig. 47.—Tube with Nose-mask.

cises. Any intercurrent acute coryza must be attended to before putting the patient in the cabinet. Besides the general treatment these
coryzas should be treated locally either by the application to the
nares of a one- or two-per-cent. solution of cocaine, or by cleansing
with and spraying of liquid albolene, benzoinol, alphasol, or other
mild antiseptic solution. I insist upon proper breathing through
the nose, and the conditions necessary thereto, for the reason that
I have abandoned the custom of having the patient put the rubber
breathing-tube in his mouth. To this end I had nose-masks constructed, which, owing to the malleability of their posterior portion,
can be moulded to fit the form of any nose. The patient either holds
the mask, pressing it to the face, or it is fastened by a strong elastic
band encircling the head. A little cotton or a thin cloth placed between the nasal bones and the malleable portion of the mask will prevent the possibility of the outside air entering the cabinet. The anterior portion of the mask is attached to the ordinary rubber tube,
which, in turn, is fastened to the cabinet end of the faucet. The
accompanying drawing illustrates both (Fig. 47).

I have found this system of natural breathing superior to mouth-
breathing, and many of my hospital patients who had been also
treated by my predecessors, but with the mouth tube, have again

and again assured me that they not only liked the nose-breathing better, but that they felt better after it than when they breathed through the mouth. They felt that they got just as much air into their lungs as with the old system. I mention this to answer the objections which were made by some of my colleagues at the hospital, who claimed that the patient does not receive enough air through the nose-mask. After having placed my patient in the cabinet, I open widely the window of the room in which the cabinet stands. I do this in office as well as in hospital practice, be it summer or winter, rain or shine, to assure my patient the purest and freshest air obtainable. Since the patient breathes through the nose, the possibility of catching cold is removed, though the outside temperature may even be severely cold. In very anæmic individuals I occasionally combine oxygen or ozone inhalations with the cabinet treatment. If it is desirable a nebulizer can also be placed in front of the faucet, and medicated inhalation be combined with the cabinet treatment.

My second modification in the pneumatic cabinet treatment consists in having the patient enter stripped to the waist, and the trousers or skirts loosened, that not only a free thoracic but also a free abdominal breathing may be possible. My reasons for exposing the cutaneous surface of the thorax to direct contact with the rarefied air are threefold:

1. There is no outside restriction whatsoever to fullest expansion of the lungs—a thing which is not possible for a woman wearing a tightly laced corset and numerous skirts tight around the waist. Even a man will breathe easier with trousers loosened and suspenders removed.

2. The cupping effect, if I may call thus the action of the cabinet which relieves nearly one pound of atmospheric pressure per square inch, is heightened by removing several intervening layers of clothing.

3. It does the cutaneous surface good to get a chance to breathe directly, as it acts also as a respiratory organ; in other words, the skin of the chest, made especially sensitive in nearly all consumptives through exaggerated warm dressing, will become less sensitive by systematic exposure to the air.

To prevent the patient from taking cold the window is closed before he is allowed to leave the cabinet; and if he should feel very warm, or if he should perspire, as patients sometimes do, a large Turkish towel is thrown around his shoulders, wherewith he produces vigorous friction over chest and back before dressing.

To make the use of the cabinet as comfortable for the patient and at the same time as effectual as possible, I have added two minor modifications in its use. I had a stand constructed with a semi-circular board top, which, placed in the cabinet in front of the chair, enables the patient to rest his arm when holding the nose-mask. This stand can be fixed at any desirable height. The other minor modification consists of a little cap made of two layers of metallic gauze, placed over the external opening of the stopcock communicating with the tube. Between the two layers absorbent cotton can be placed in order to filter the air which enters the tube when the patient inhales. The cotton can also be impregnated with whatever medicinal substance the physician thinks most appropriate. I give the essence of peppermint the preference for such purposes, as it has a soothing, cooling influence on the irritated membranes.

Like all respiratory exercises, the pneumatic cabinet treatment should be begun carefully and gradually. I usually commence with a *séance* of two minutes, increasing the duration from day to day up to six or eight minutes. At first the *séances* should be given once every day. As the patient's respiratory function becomes more perfect and the disease tends toward recovery, the sittings need not be quite so frequent. Longer *séances* than eight minutes are seldom indicated. About one inch of elevation, shown by the manometer, suffices to reduce the atmospheric pressure from 15 to about 14 pounds to the square inch. This reduction is all that is needed to procure the desired effect.

My patients, with rare exceptions, look forward to their *séance* with pleasurable anticipation, especially when there is a tendency to dyspnœa. I have entered the cabinet myself, my assistant working the lever, in order to experience the sensation so vividly described by some of my patients. I cannot say that at first the feeling of being inclosed in such a small space, with only a tube to breathe through, is a pleasant one. The first movements of the pump produce an almost painful sensation ·in the ears, but, by and by, with the exhaustion of the air, and by swallowing a few times, this ceases and there comes a feeling of freedom. The respiratory muscles seem to expand to a much greater degree; the fresh, cool air, entering through the nose, arrives in the lungs sufficiently warmed not to be harmful, penetrating habitually unused portions of lung substances. There comes, and remains for hours afterward, a feeling of exhilaration analogous to that experienced on mountain tops. Regarding the action of the cabinet on the various pathological conditions in pulmonary tuberculosis, I have cited the experiences of Platt and Quimby; as stated above, I may repeat that they coincide in nearly every respect with mine, and I can recommend the judicious use of this method of aërotherapy most earnestly. I think that the few

modifications which I have instituted in connection with the employment of the cabinet will tend to increase its usefulness.

Solar Therapy.

We will now speak of solar therapy or sun baths, as they may
be advantageously applied in phthisiotherapy. In describing our
model sanatorium, we spoke of the construction and arrangement of
the sun-room as it should exist over the pavilions designed for the
respective sexes. In private practice, the sunniest room should be
selected for that purpose. Fixed carpets should, of course, not be
placed in such a room, and the floor must be kept scrupulously clean.

In a private home where neighboring windows are often near, the
arrangement will be more difficult and low screens may have to be
used. In winter the room should be heated to from 70° to 75° F.
By and by the patient's skin will be less sensitive to the air, and the
temperature of the room can be decreased. The room must always
be well ventilated. · In summer the upper part of the windows can be
left open.

As to the *modus operandi* of the baths, I recommend the following:
The patient undresses entirely, but if he complains of cold feet he
can keep his stockings or even his shoes on until he has become
warm enough, and desires to take them off. He places first a
warmed sheet around his body and then a large blanket; he then lies
down on the floor in the sun, his head in the shade and slightly elevated by a cushion. As he begins to feel the warmth of the rays of
the sun, he uncovers himself gradually until the whole of his body is
exposed to the rays of the sun; he exposes his back by turning on
his chest. He remains in the sun-room for from half an hour to two
hours, according to the direction given him by his physician. He
may change the recumbent to the sitting position or walk about.
Like all the curative agents in the treatment of phthisis, the carrying
out of this solar therapy should never be left to the caprice of the
patient. Too much exposure to the hot rays may cause an erythema,
an urticaria, or other cutaneous troubles. To prevent these latter, I
tell my patients to cover themselves with one or even two layers of
their sheet when the sun's rays produce a slightly burning sensation.
Should these cutaneous complications occur nevertheless, the sun
baths must be omitted for a time and the skin bathed in warm water,
and friction with lemon juice applied. Headache, or a feeling of
discomfort, is the signal to stop, no matter how short a time the bath
has lasted. A high temperature is, of course, a contraindication to
sun baths. Such patients must remain in bed. Slightly feverish

patients may be allowed to try solar therapy, but when experience shows that these are followed by an elevation of temperature, the baths must be discontinued.

While taking his sun bath, the patient should perform frequent abdominal and thoracic breathing exercises.

Of the value of carefully conducted solar therapy, I cannot speak too highly. The exposure of the whole body in its nude state to the air and the rays of the sun at the same time, has a remarkably favorable influence on metabolism, oxygenation, and the general condition of the phthisical patient, aside from the fact that thereby his cutaneous system will be educated to a greatly diminished susceptibility, and intercurrent colds will be much rarer.

Dress and Personal Hygiene.

Consumptives should dress sensibly, comfortably, and according to the season. They should avoid heaping successive layers of clothing upon themselves, especially in the line of so-called chest protectors. These latter, or the numerous woollen undershirts, often worn by the pulmonary invalid, are in many cases the very cause of contracting repeated colds by rendering the individual too sensitive. As to what is the most suitable and rational underwear in general, and especially for a consumptive, there is as much difference of opinion among physicians and sanitarians as there is concerning the most disputed points in medicine. To suit the individual case seems to me as essential here as in other branches of phthisiotherapy. The climate in which the patient lives must be, of course, also taken into consideration. Moderately thick and loosely woven wool of different grades, according to season, has been perhaps most frequently recommended for the inhabitants of countries suited in the temperate zone; yet, in many portions of Germany, Austria, and Russia, sick and well people wear nothing but coarse linen next to their skin. Many people, sick and well, in this country wear cotton and would not wish to wear anything else, others wear nothing but half cotton and wool, others nothing but silk.

The advocate of any of these systems will be able to say something in favor of his particular one. There seems to be a great deal of truth in what Professor Rubner stated in his article on "Bekleidungsreform und Wollsystem," [135a] that one can clothe one's self sensibly with other material than wool, if one keeps in view the principles of rational clothing; no overwarm garments and good ventilation of them, homogeneous evenly woven tissues, the layer next to the skin not too thin, and as little difference as possible in conductibility in the tissue in its dry and moist condition. Thus, I believe, so long as our patients do not wear absolutely too warm or too much underwear, we can well afford to let those who are accustomed to wear this or that brand of woollen or half woollen undergarments abide by them, especially when these patients are in the more advanced stages of the disease. When through a proper course of hydro-, aéro-, and heliotherapy, the patient has become less susceptible to temperature changes, lighter or different underwear may be thought of. Yet we should be careful in selecting the proper season for such a change, and the most opportune time for a change from heavier to lighter underwear is, of course, when the weather is becoming warmer.

A substance which is not overwarm, as Professor Rubner puts it, and which assures good isolation, would certainly be linen if it could be woven thick and porous enough to meet the other requirements concerning the conductibility in its dry and moist condition, and porosity. Such thickly woven and wide-meshed linen underwear has been manufactured in Germany under the direction of that strange genius Father Kneipp, who, in spite of being an empiric, had certainly some very sound ideas on hygiene. I experimented with Kneipp's underwear on myself some years ago, and found that, when one gets accustomed to it, it is, as a rule, warm enough for any season. These garments should be warm enough here, where our houses are nearly always overheated, especially as there are heavier grades made for the winter. When going outdoors, one can protect one's self against the rigorous cold by proper outdoor garments.

This linen underwear produces a pleasant constant friction on the cutaneous surface, which counteracts rapidly the first sensation of chilliness which one experiences when the linen touches the skin. As a means of hardening a tuberculous invalid, or as a prophylactic factor in a predisposed individual, I recommend a trial of this kind of linen underwear; but, of course, as I said above, not without having prepared him for the change by cold douches, open-air treatment, etc. Babcock of Chicago, Tilden of Denver, and Ambler of Asheville, have of late become quite enthusiastic advocates of the linen-mesh underwear, which is now manufactured in this country by Dr. Deimel. In a recent paper on the subject, Ambler[136b] expresses himself as much pleased with the experience he has had with the linen-mesh underwear with a number of his tuberculous patients.

Consumptives should have warm outer garments for winter, but not so heavy as to hamper their movements.

Whenever and wherever conventionalism does not reign supreme, the starched linen should be replaced by the light, woollen, negligée shirt. It permits better ventilation and freer respiratory movements. Men with a good head of hair need not fear to go uncovered at times, but all, even those with thin hair or bald heads, should not wear too heavy hats or caps, and should always have them well ventilated.

In speaking of infection by ingestion, we said that to wear no beard and no mustache would be the most hygienic practice on the part of the consumptive; but since it is very hard to enforce rules, the carrying out of which would change the appearance of a person often to a considerable degree, it is best to simply advise the tuberculous invalid to keep his beard and mustache as short as possible, and to wash the same with warm water regularly a few times each day.

Whether a consumptive uses a pocket-flask, squares of muslin, or a paper spittoon for the purpose of expectorating therein, it is well to repeat here that he should be enjoined to wash his hands always most thoroughly before touching food.

As a matter of personal hygiene for pulmonary invalids, I should again suggest not to make use of tobacco in any form whatever. There is no doubt in my mind that the congested condition of the mucous membrane of the upper air passages (nose and throat) so frequently found in smokers, is exclusively due to the excessive use of tobacco. Smoking of cigarettes should be considered particularly dangerous for the pulmonary invalid. Patients who were addicted to the use of cigarettes have confessed to me that when smoking they no longer had any desire to breathe deeply. It seems as if the smoke thus inhaled partially paralyzed the respiratory centres.

For women I would recommend the Lady Habberton or Jenness Miller system of dress reform.[136] It may not be amiss to give a short description of the system here, for, while it may enjoy a certain popularity among sanitarians, I cannot say that the majority of ladies seem to be very familiar with this reform. "Dame Fashion" has, no doubt, a great deal to do with the seemingly total ignorance of this most healthful mode of dress among otherwise well-informed ladies.

According to the fundamental rules for dress reform as advocated by Lady Habberton, Mrs. Miller, and others, the garments are arranged so that they follow the symmetrical lines of the female form, and in all possible cases are made of one piece. Each limb is properly clothed in its turn. Legs, arms, and neck are comfortably and closely protected, while the body is wrapped a little tighter. The under-garment is made all in one piece, and with no bands around the waist. If a corset must be worn it should be corded or stiffened with a few whalebones and never tightly laced, for that, with the weight of the heavy skirts fastened tightly around the waist in the usual manner, renders all abdominal breathing impossible. As has been already stated in our chapter on prophylactic treatment, abdominal breathing is as natural to women as it is to men and animals.

Next to this undergarment, or union suit, a so-called "chemisette" is worn, made on the same principle as the undergarment, but of looser and lighter material. The third in order is the so-called "leglette," a divided skirt and waist attached, which gives the wearer great comfort and freedom of motion. It can be made of almost any material. And now as to the outside dresses; they are made as nearly as possible in the styles in vogue, but never with trains, and in them all are preserved the physiological features of the female form. In the complete toilet all garments are so arranged that their whole weight is supported by the shoulders, and no pressure whatever is brought to bear upon any of the vital organs in either thoracic or abdominal cavity.

I have frequently seen ladies dressed according to this sensible mode, and they looked to me and to others more becomingly dressed and more graceful than those arrayed in the very latest fashion, whose waists have been reduced by tight lacing, changing their appearance, perhaps, from the figure of a Venus to something resembling two cones placed with their summits in apposition.

Men and women alike should never wear anything tight around the neck. This constricting mode of dress is not only often productive of headaches but is a hindrance to free and deep breathing.

Phthisical patients should keep their feet warm and dry, and should never wear tight shoes. Rubber shoes when it is wet, fur-lined ones when it is cold, and hot-water bags or bottles at their feet when lying on their chairs in winter, should be recommended to attain this end. On rainy days patients should not fear to go out for a constitutional walk, but they should wear a light rubber cloak.

The care of the skin is an essential part in phthisiotherapy. As a rule a tuberculous patient should take his hygienic bath regularly once or twice a week. It should be of short duration, pretty warm, and followed by a rapid sponging off with cold water. The best time to take the hygienic bath is in the evening, before retiring. A pulmonary invalid should never take his bath without there being some one within call, in case he requires any assistance. When the skin is especially dry, nothing will be better than an occasional massage with vaseline or some other oily, non-irritating substance.

Hydrotherapy.

Of the tonic effects of cold water and its stimulation of the general system, we have already spoken under prophylactic treatment. The general education of the cutaneous and nervous systems of a patient whose body has not been accustomed to the extensive application of cold water is especially imperative in the case of a consumptive. How this should be done has been described before. Presuming, then, that the patient has gone through the usual preparatory course of dry friction, friction with alcohol, with water, etc., we come to the douche. So as not to produce too great a shock, I begin by directing a gentle stream towards the feet, then rapidly upwards as far as the hips; then I apply the spray uniformly all over the body, and direct also a small jet with little more force over the apices. Apparatus for this kind of douche can easily be constructed in a sanatorium, or even in a private dwelling.

There is one thing, however, which I would insist upon in the arrangement of a douche-room. A patient should be taught to exercise as many muscles as possible during the application of cold water. To this end he should take hold of a bar fastened across the room at about the height of his shoulders. This prevents his slipping on the wet floor while he moves his thorax from side to side, raises his feet alternately, moves his arms, and, in short, agitates his whole body as much as possible. The shock produced by the cold water is thus much lessened and a more speedy reaction assured. Of course, the large towel to envelop the patient from head to foot is necessary, over which the bath attendant uses vigorous friction to favor a proper reaction and return to warmth. The head should always be dried first. If the patient dislikes the spray douche on his head or suffers from headache or other discomfort afterwards, it is better to direct the spray douche from the front or back and only have the jet on the apices directed from above. In some cases of tardy reaction warming the towels is indicated.

Baruch's ingenious douche apparatus, of which I give a reproduction, could, with a few additions, become an ideal installation for a large sanatorium for consumptives. These additions should be the cross-bar, just mentioned, in front of the circular douche apparatus, and an arrangement permitting direct jets to be given from above over the apices. For this purpose two apertures could be conveniently placed one on each side of the rain douche (R). A detailed description of this apparatus will be found in Baruch's excellent book on "The Principles and Practice of Hydrotherapy."[37] The legends

under the two pictures will give, however, a fair idea how this apparatus can be arranged.

When the visit to the douche- or bathroom is either inconvenient
or not safe, I resort to the following simple method: A wooden chair
is placed in a large, circular, English bath-tub, and the patient sits
astride the chair, holding the back with his hands and bending his
head slightly forward. Then two, four, or more pitchers of cold or
tempered water are rapidly poured over the shoulders. In cases

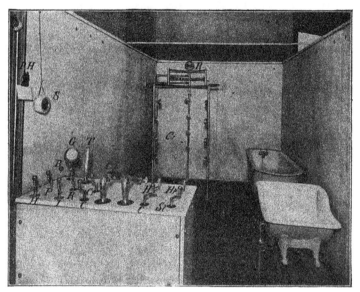

Fig. 48.—Baruch's Douche Apparatus. *PH*, Prescription-holder; *S*, "second" clock; *H*, hot
water; *I*, ice water; *C*, cold water; *P*, pressure regulator; *B*, bell; *G*, gauge; *T*, thermometer;
R, rain douche; *Cr*, circular douche; *CJ*, cold-jet douche; *HJ*, hot-jet douche; *H*, hot water for
Scotch douche; *C*, cold water for Scotch douche; *Hp*, hip-bath; *St*, steam douche.

in which the reaction is feeble the patient is quickly put back into
his warm bed, even if not thoroughly dry.

The best time to take the hydrotherapeutic application is in the
morning, half an hour or so after a very light breakfast. Patients
accustomed to heavy breakfasts should take such after their douche
and morning walk, but should take a glass of milk with a slice of
buttered toast before leaving their room. A morning walk should,
if possible, always precede the douche. This is for the purpose of
creating what French hydrotherapeutists call a preaction.

Every douche or affusion should also be followed by a short walk
or a return to bed, according to the indication of the case. The cold

douche should never last longer than twenty to twenty-five seconds, and should always be begun gradually, not lasting more than five sec-

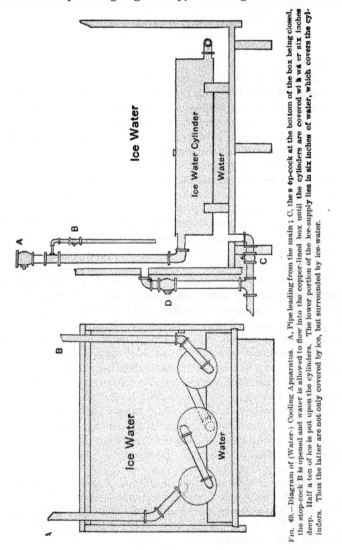

Fig. 49.—Diagram of (Water-) Cooling Apparatus. A, Pipe leading from the main; C, the stop-cock at the bottom of the box being closed, the stop-cock B is opened and water is allowed to flow into the copper-lined box until the cylinders are covered with water six inches deep. Half a ton of ice is put upon the cylinders. The lower portion of the ice-supply lies in six inches of water, which covers the cylinders. Thus the latter are not only covered by ice, but surrounded by ice-water.

onds at first. The temperature may vary from 60° to 40° F. Only in exceptional cases would one need a more precise graduation of the temperature.

The complicated procedure of the dripping sheet seems to entail too great a strain on the patient, and I do not favor it in phthisiotherapeutics. Wet packs, on the contrary, over the thorax, seem to exert a soothing influence whenever there are pleuritic or intercostal pains, or that vague and undetermined feeling of discomfort in the chest. Lateral douches, not too strong, directed toward the seat of old pleuritic adhesions, often aid considerably in the resorption of the fibrinous bands and a consequent free chest expansion.

In patients above fifty, it must be remembered that the usual reaction after a cold douche is slow to come, and in such cases it is best not to use the water too cold. A chilly sensation, continuing even after thorough drying and friction, should in all cases be a warning and a guide regarding temperature and duration of the douche. There are idiosyncrasies which must also be considered with some patients in regard to the application of the cold douche.

Of the other uses of cold water in pulmonary tuberculosis we will speak under symptomatic treatment.

An apparatus for taking steam baths becomes also part of an hydrotherapeutic establishment. Such are now made portable and constructed cheap enough to become an adjuvant even to the home treatment. I certainly think that a steam bath, or hot-water bath, of not too long duration, taken once or twice a week and followed by a sponging off with cold water and vigorous friction of the body with a rough towel, is to be recommended. Of course, cases for this treatment must be selected and extremely feeble invalids must be excluded. The therapeutic effects of the short steam or hot-water baths in pulmonary tuberculosis are their tonic action on the skin and the general system, and secondly, the elimination of toxic products, probably constantly generated by the tubercle bacillus or its associates, the streptococci, staphylococci, etc. It is essential that the hot-water bath should be as hot as the patient can stand it. Tepid baths are weakening, hot baths stimulating. The duration of such a bath should never be longer than about fifteen minutes, and always be regulated according to the strength of the patient. It is an absolute rule that the patient must be put to bed immediately after his steam or hot-water bath, and thus, of course, the most convenient time for such a bath would be in the evening. If the steam bath is taken the sudorific action will be facilitated by taking beforehand a hot foot bath. Headaches, which often follow the steam baths, are thus also avoided.

Dietetic Treatment.

Dettweiler is in the habit of saying "la cuisine est ma pharmacie." [134] To nourish the patient, to feed him well with good food, or rather overfeed him so that he assimilates more than he expends, forms indeed a most important part in the treatment of phthisis. The patient should have an abundance of proteids, carbohydrates, and fats, but in proper proportion; thus the menu for a tuberculous invalid should be much varied. He should never have a diet exclusively of meat or of vegetables; a mixed diet, with some eclecticism as to the more digestible substances, should be the rule. Meat, milk, fats, eggs, vegetables, bread (cereals), fruits, especially grapes, should all contribute to the diet of the patient.

Consumptives, as a rule, have small appetites, and it requires sometimes no little art to make them eat. The one important truth that they should be made to understand is that their digestive powers are far greater than their appetite indicates. Leaving exceptional cases aside, such as absolute anorexia, hyperacidity, or lack of gastric secretion, of which we will speak later, one usually succeeds in making the patients eat by persistent persuasion, and by offering them a variety of food arranged as appetizingly as possible.

The meals given the patients in the leading European sanatoria are about as follows: In the morning—half-past seven to half-past eight o'clock—they have bread and butter and honey, with cacao, coffee, or chocolate, and two or three glasses of milk taken slowly in small swallows. At ten o'clock they have bread and butter, cold meats, fruit, etc. At one o'clock the dinner—soup, fish, three kinds of meat, vegetables, salad, preserves, dessert, and fresh fruit, with one or two glasses of wine. At four o'clock they have a glass of milk, with bread and butter. At half-past seven there are thick soup, meat or potatoes or rice, cold meat, bread and butter, salad, and cooked fruit, with again one or two glasses of wine. At nine o'clock they take a glass of milk with two or three teaspoonfuls of cognac.

To eat a great deal of butter and cream is especially to be recommended to pulmonary invalids, and milk should be allowed at any time without restriction. However, some patients, in their eagerness to get fat, overdo in this respect. When drinking numerous glasses of milk between meals interferes with the proper appetite at mealtimes, the number of glasses should be reduced accordingly. Again, neither milk nor cream agrees well with some consumptives. To make the former more digestible, one may add to each wineglassful one-half of a teaspoonful of cognac, kirsh, or rum, with or without hot

water. Milk may also be rendered more digestible by adding to each
tumblerful about six grains of bicarbonate of soda and five grains of
common salt dissolved in two tablespoonfuls of hot water.   There is
little fear that the patient will ever overdo in regard to the eating of
butter. He should be urged to take it with all his meals, fresh or
salted, whichever he likes best.

The pulmonary invalid must be treated and fed in accordance
with what he was accustomed to before being taken sick, for meal-
times and number of meals differ among different nations.

For average cases I would suggest the following regimen, to be
adhered to as nearly as possible during the course of the disease: As
soon as the patient awakes in the morning, while yet in bed, a glass
of hot milk, half tea and milk, or half coffee and milk, with a slice
of milk toast, or dry toast, should be given him.   After a little while
he will rise to prepare for his douche, friction, or massage, whatever
the physician's prescription may call for.   After this it will probably be nine o'clock, and the patient may take his ordinary breakfast. He should have eggs, and may have his choice as to the way
they may be prepared or served — soft-boiled, poached, raw, in
form of eggnog with a tablespoonful of sherry or a teaspoonful of
whiskey, or stirred into his coffee. If he is accustomed to a meat
breakfast, he should have broiled steak, chops, poultry, sweetbread,
etc., or raw chopped beef. Bread a day old—preferably whole-wheat
bread or French rolls, but not hot—with plenty of butter or honey,
either milk, cacao, coffee with milk, but not too strong, or a cup of
bouillon, may also form part of the meal. The whole-wheat and the
rye bread are certainly more nourishing than the ordinary wheat
bread. Whether the patient likes to have his mush (cereals) for
breakfast or supper, may be left to his choice; some fruit should always precede his eggs or meat in the morning. If fish is served in
the morning it should be either broiled, boiled, or baked. As a beverage besides milk, pure water is certainly the best. If one is not
certain as to its purity, it should be filtered. It should be rendered
cool by being placed on ice, but the ice should never be put in the
water.

The patient should take the heartiest meal between the hours of
twelve and two o'clock (four hours after his breakfast). Broth or
soup should constitute the first course. Any kind of fresh fish may
be served again at dinner, and in any form except fried; and there will
be, of course, roast meat of some kind, rare roast beef, mutton, poultry, etc. Of vegetables, spinach is particularly to be recommended
on account of the large proportion of digestible and assimilable iron.
Next to this in nutritive power come lentils, peas, beans, cauliflower,

and potatoes. Fresh vegetables should be given whenever it is possible to have them. Lettuce and other salads, preferably prepared with lemon juice instead of with vinegar, and plenty of good olive oil, are permitted. Light puddings, fruits, and nuts may constitute the dessert. Whenever possible the dessert should be seasoned with cinnamon, for this spice seems to have peculiarly stimulating properties without being harmful; perhaps also the cinnamic acid contained therein exerts a favorable influence on the general condition of the patient through its direct action on the bacilli or their toxins.

At about four or five o'clock some milk with toast may be taken, or, if the patient cares for it, he may have a cheese or meat sandwich. At this time the milk may be replaced by bouillon or chocolate.

The supper should not be quite so voluminous as the dinner. Cold or warm meats, rice with milk or gruel, and jellies, fruits, etc. At bedtime again a glass of milk or some milk toast. If there is no tendency to diarrhœa, the patients should accustom themselves to drink a few glasses of pure fresh water during the day.

It is, of course, impossible to lay down an absolute rule of what to allow and what not to allow. One must consider the patient's likes and dislikes; there are idiosyncrasies for certain dishes as well as for certain medicines. I have learned to allow my patients occasionally such things as ham, smoked tongue, and even pickled or salt herring, sardines, and sardelles, and I have not yet found any occasion to regret this practice, for they seem at times to stimulate the appetite.

In a sanatorium the menu should be submitted to the medical director previous to its preparation. I will give a few receipts for particularly useful dishes which I have seen served or eaten myself in sanatoria, during my *voyages d'étude*, and have tried since with my private patients with most satisfactory results.

First, I will describe a good method of preparing the raw beef, or the so-called *Hamburg steak:* With a knife, not too sharp, scrape the surface of the meat (rump steak). Put the fine scrapings thus obtained in a stone or glass mortar and grind them. Then spread the mass on a sieve and press it gently with a spoon. What passes through is a meat pulp without fibres or gristle, perfectly digestible and very nutritive. I have found, however, that for all ordinary cases the scraped meat suffices without being ground.

The supply of meat pulp for the day may be made in the morning, but it must be kept in a cold place, as it taints easily. It is better, however, when possible, to make it fresh just before it is to be eaten. The patient may take the pulp in any way he pleases. It can be eaten plain with pepper and salt, mixed with milk, with warm bouillon, with mashed vegetables, or with sweets. The latter method will make it tempting for children. It can be rolled into balls easy to swallow, or made into sandwiches with a few anchovies, or a little anchovy paste, pickled herring, or some other relish, according to the patient's taste. The yolk of a raw egg added increases the nutritive quality of the meat pulp. Thus it will be seen that the ways in which the raw meat may be taken are so numerous that it can be made palatable to almost any patient.

To make a good *mucilaginous soup*, take five pounds of veal bones and ten quarts of water or weak bouillon. Bring it to a boil and then skim. Add two pounds of barley and a little salt, cook slowly for five or six hours, and then strain off the liquid. A cupful should be taken mixed with the yolk of an egg. If the soup is too thick, dilute it with a little bouillon.

To prepare a good *milk jelly*, boil two quarts of milk with a half pound of sugar for five or ten minutes. When the milk is cold add one ounce of gelatin dissolved in a cup of water, the juice of three or four lemons, and three glasses of good Bordeaux wine.

It is often very convenient to have a bottle of *beef essence* on hand. The following is an easy way to prepare it: Put two pounds of round steak, cut in small pieces, into a jar without water. Place the jar, covered closely, on a trivet in a kettle of cold water. Heat gradually, and keep it not quite at the boiling-point for two hours, or till the meat is white. Strain, pressing the meat to obtain all the juice, season with salt. Or place the jar in a moderate oven for three hours. The liquid thus obtained contains all the nutritive parts of the meat. It may be kept in the refrigerator, and a small portion heated (not boiled) as wanted. Or it may be made into beef tea by diluting with boiling water. The essence can also be given ice cold to febrile patients.

Bouillons and soups taken regularly at the principal meal increase the appetite and aid the digestion by stimulating the gastric secretions.

A patient who has fever should eat when his temperature is lowest, and only the most easily digestible substances. All pulmonary invalids should be taught to take their meals at regular intervals, to eat slowly, and to chew their food well. The patient should be weighed and carefully examined every month or two weeks, according to his condition, and thus the progress of the cure can be ascertained.

The good condition of the teeth is, of course, essential, and a well-conducted sanatorium should not be without its dental chair, and should receive the regular visits of an experienced dentist. The physician should teach his consumptives that it will increase their appetites to brush their teeth and rinse their mouths after each meal with some refreshing, mildly antiseptic mouth wash.

Opinions in regard to giving alcohol to consumptives differ very largely, and it is extremely difficult to lay down any rule on this subject. My own experience has taught me that alcohol is indispensable in some cases, but it should be given preferably in the diluted form of wine or beer, or good cognac in small quantities mixed with milk. It should rarely be given as an antipyretic remedy. When prescribed in the form of cognac or whiskey, it should be dealt out carefully like a powerful drug.

This is another advantage of treating the patients in a sanatorium where they are seen several times a day. The effect of the alcohol or any other medicine can be watched. The physician of a sanatorium, seeing his patient almost constantly, will soon be able to judge whether the improvement the patient may confess to feel after taking the alcohol is physiological or pathological (intoxication). Especially in treating the laboring class either in institutions or at their homes, it seems to me better to discourage the use of alcohol as a therapeutic means in phthisis than to encourage it.[139]

Of the many food substances which have been recommended recently as especially valuable in the dietetic treatment of tuberculosis, I have used most extensively and with most satisfactory results the new product, tropon. It is a tasteless and odorless albuminous preparation in the form of a yellowish-brown powder, obtained by a complicated chemical process from animal and vegetable substances.[140]

Considering that tropon is really an able substitute for the albumen in other foods, that it rarely causes digestive disturbances, that it can be taken for a long period of time without aversion, and that it is excessively cheap, we may look upon this new product as a most valuable adjuvant in the dietetic treatment of phthisical patients.[141]

Medicinal and Symptomatic Treatment.

There is hardly any substance in the materia medica, which at some time or other has not been recommended as an antituberculous remedy. While I do not believe in going to extremes, saying that we can treat pulmonary tuberculosis without any medicinal substances, I think, nevertheless, that we may reduce their number to relatively few. To build up the system cod-liver oil may be given whenever the stomach can support it. A good method for its administration is that of Bricemoret, which is to mix it as follows:

℞ Cod-liver oil, ...	fl ℥ xij.
Syrup of tolu, ...	fl ℥ vi.
Tincture of tolu, ...	gtt. xij.
Oil of cloves, ...	gtt. ij.

At the moment of administration the mixture is to be well shaken, and a tablespoonful taken two or three times daily. Taken thus, the taste of the aromatic syrup only remains after the ingestion of the oil. In younger subjects and children, cod-liver oil seems to have a particularly gratifying action. Some of the cod-liver oil emulsions, such as Russell's, may also be advantageously administered when there is too great a dislike for the pure oil.

The various malt preparations, as maltzyme, malt extract, and maltine, may be given with benefit in either the pure state or combined with cod-liver oil or hypophosphites. For the summer months the combination with the hypophosphites is to be preferred, especially for young people and children. The hypophosphite combination should, however, always be given when the cod-liver oil in its pure or the combined state is not well borne. To mix the maltine and hypophosphites with a little lemon juice and water will make them still more palatable. Next in efficacy come the arsenical preparations, strychnine, iron (ferratine is especially well borne by phthisical invalids), and the phosphates.

Iodoform has given much satisfaction in the hands of many phthisiotherapeutists such as Flick,[142] Daremberg,[143] Ransom,[144] de Renzi.[145] It has been recommended for nearly all degrees of phthisis, given as an inhalation in the form of one part of iodoform to ten parts of ether (twenty minims of the mixture for each inhalation with respirator inhaler). It is given in pills according to the following formula:

℞ Iodoform, . ·	gr. iss.
Codeinæ, ...	gr. ⅓.
Ext. cascaræ, ...	gr. ¼.
M. et ft. pil. i.	

Flick gives iodoform as an inunction. De Rènzi's method of its administration is especially recommendable. If the patient is suffering from diarrhœa he gives the following prescription:

℞ Iodoform, ...	gr. xxx.
Tannin, ...	gr. lx.
M. Divide into forty powders, from two to four to be given daily.	

If there is a tendency towards constipation, de Renzi replaces the tannin by naphthalin.

The various modern preparations of creosote and guaiacol seem in most cases, when given in small doses, to exert a favorable influence on the general condition of the patient, especially when there is a mixed infection. I prefer to give the creosote in milk, beginning with two or three drops thrice daily, gradually increasing to about twenty-five drops per day. The moment there is the slightest digestive disturbance I stop the creosote; and if I find then that the patient does as well without as with it, I do not recommence its administration. In order to protect the consumptive invalid as far as possible from his greatest foe, dyspepsia, I follow this rule with all medicinal remedies.

Creosotal (creosote carbonate) is seemingly more easily borne than creosote. It has been strongly recommended by von Leyden,[146] de Planzoles, Cornet,[147] and others. Creosotal contains ninety per cent. of its weight of pure creosote. It can be taken pure or as an emulsion with the yolk of an egg, with milk, or with cod-liver oil. For an adult fifty to sixty minims may be given two or three times daily; this should, however, be considered a maximum dose. It is best in all cases to begin with small doses, as, for example, five to ten drops per diem; then gradually increase and return again to smaller doses.

According to Stubbert,[148] ichthyol prepared as enteric pills, two grains each (three to fifteen per day), has been used with considerable success at the Liberty Sanitarium. One may also combine the ichthyol in the following way:

℞ Creosote-carbonate,
Ichthyol, ... āā 15 parts.
Glycerin, ... 30 "
Peppermint water, ... 10 "
M. S. Ten drops, to be gradually increased to thirty. To be given in a wineglassful of water or lemonade.

The extract of kalagua has, in the hands of Stubbert and others, also given satisfactory results. It is administered in pill form of one and one-half grains each, two pills three times daily, and increasing gradually to four pills four times daily.

Guaiacol has also found favor with some phthisiotherapeutists as a valuable remedy in tuberculosis. It has the advantage over creosote that it is less irritating and that it deranges the digestion more rarely than the former. It is best given diluted with milk, beginning with five drops three times daily, gradually increasing this dose to fifteen. The patients who have too great a dislike for its peculiar and unpleasant odor can sometimes be induced to take guaiacol in capsules. Goldmann, in the *Riforma Medica* of December 22d, 1898, recommends guaiacol and ichthyol in the following combination:

℞ Carbonate of guaiacol,
  Sulphichthyolate of ammonium, ... āā gr. ccv.
  Pure glycerin, ... ℳ dc.
  Peppermint water, ... ℳ cl.
  M. Twenty to thirty drops to be taken daily.

If guaiacol is not well tolerated by the stomach, Bouteron's[149] guaiacol enema or suppositories may be advantageously employed:

℞ Guaiacol (in crystals melted at a low temperature), gr. v.–xv.
  Olive oil, ... 3 iss.–ℨ ij.
  Inject at a temperature of about 90° F.

℞ Guaiacol, ... gr. iij.–viij.
  Cacao butter, ... 3 i.
  For two suppositories, to be applied within twenty-four hours.

As an external medication to improve the general condition, Flick[150] recommends europhen by inunction, using the following formula:

℞ Europhen, ... 3 i.
  Oil of rose, ... gtt. i. „
  Oil of anise, ... 3 i.
  Olive oil, ... ℨ iiss.
  M. S. Rub about a tablespoonful into the inside of the thighs and into the arm-pits before retiring at night.

Oil of camphor (oleum camphoratum, Ph. G.) has in the hands of Alexander[151] and Kobert[152] done considerable good, especially in the more advanced cases with cavity formations. Alexander administers it in the form of subcutaneous injection and as much as fifteen minims at a time. One injection every day for four days, followed by a suspension of the treatment for ten days.

Gomenol, the product of the distillation of the leaves of the Melaleuca Viridiflora (New Caledonia) hypodermically injected, has according to the reports of some French phthisiotherapeutists[153] given excellent results. The dose is from 1 to 20 c.c., gradually increased, and diluted with five times its bulk of sterilized olive oil.

Cinnamic acid has been recommended by Landerer[154] and others as a specific in pulmonary tuberculosis. He recommends it to be administered in the form of sodium cinnamate by intravenous injection. Mann, of Denver,[155] who tried it on himself, attaches to it great therapeutic value. However, this form of administering any remedy is not without danger and is always difficult and complicated. As already mentioned under dietetic treatment, I give as much of the cinnamon as I can with the food, and if the progress toward recovery seems to be too slow by the ordinary hygienic and dietetic methods, or if there are some fears of the disease taking a hectic type, I give for as long a period of time as possible the following mixture:

R Quininæ sulphat., ... gr. vi.
Tr. cinchon. comp.,
Syr. aurantii, ... āā ℥ iss.
Aquæ cinnamomi, ... q.s. ad ℥ viij.
M. S. One tablespoonful three or four times daily.

Another method of administering the cinnamon is that of Mendel (quoted by Flick [156]), of dropping 45 minims of the following mixture directly into the trachea:

R Ess. of thyme,
Ess. of eucalyptus,
Ess. of cinnamon, ... āā ℳ lxxx.
Sterilized olive oil, ... fl ℥ liiss.
Iodoform, ... gr. lxxv.
Bromoform, ... ℳ xxx.

Mendel, however, ascribes the good results derived from this mode of treatment rather to the oil of thyme than to the cinnamon. He regards the other ingredients of this mixture as of secondary importance.

Ordinary salt has often been found of value by me as an alterant in the treatment of pulmonary tuberculosis. While it may be given in solution as an inhalation, it is most easily and effectually administered in large doses with the consumptive's daily meals. Drozda[157] ascribes to chloride of sodium a remarkably stimulating and eliminating effect on the pulmonary secretions. Besides this, I have no doubt that the ingestion of large quantities of salt aids to quite a considerable degree in the calcareous transformation of tuberculous lesions.

The old idea of ingestion of the fresh blood of bullocks as an antiphthisical remedy has been recently revived by Whittaker.[158] He, however, recommends it administered in the form of enemata. To each quart of blood he adds half an ounce of bicarbonate of sodium and sugar of milk and one grain of common salt. Two pints of a mixture consisting of equal parts of water and blood are thrown high up in the rectum. Whittaker has found marked increase in weight and gain in nutrition to follow the repeated use of such blood enemata in tuberculosis.

Organotherapy, such as the administration of Brunet's suc pulmonaire[159] (lung juice) or Hofmann's extract of bronchial glands in pulmonary tuberculosis is still too much in an experimental stage,[160] and I prefer to refrain from expressing any opinion as to its future in phthisiotherapy.

Lastly, I would mention the treatment by inhalation of "formalina," recently instituted by Professor Cervello, of Palermo. Formalina is said to be a powerful antiseptic gas. The experience with it has thus far not given results which would substantiate the claims of its inventor.

These are probably the most important medicinal substances which at the present time are used in tuberculous diseases with a view of building up the system, of changing the tuberculous diathesis, or perhaps of acting more or less directly on the bacilli or their secretions.

SYMPTOMATIC TREATMENT.

Anorexia.—Coming now to the symptomatic treatment, we have, of course, first as the most serious symptom the anorexia, or lack of appetite and other dyspeptic conditions. If the dietetic and hygienic measures already described have not been sufficient to combat the anorexia, it will be necessary to resort to the judicious administration of pepsin or pancreatin preparations.

As a general tonic the following composition has given me much satisfaction:

```
℞ Tinct. nucis vomicæ, .    .    .    .    .    .    ℨ ij.
   Tinct. cinchonæ,
   Tinct. calumbæ,    .    .    .    .    .    . āā ℥ i.
   Tinct. gentianæ,    .    .    .    .    . q.s. ad ℥ iv.
M.  S. One teaspoonful in a little water before each meal.
```

A milk diet often helps to bridge over a period of anorexia; but some people cannot or will not take milk. Raw eggs stirred into substantial soups may be made to take its place. Kumyss (fermented mares' or cows' milk) is also a most valuable substitute whenever there is an aversion to milk in its natural state. In absolute anorexia one must endeavor to find out the cause by an analysis of the gastric juice, and direct the medication accordingly. A good preparation for excessive acidity of the stomach is five grains each of bismuth, bicarbonate of sodium, and salol or benzonaphthol, to be taken before meals. Not infrequently, however, this hyperacidity seems to be of a purely nervous origin, and persuasion and suggestion or electricity will prove the best remedies.

In undetermined troubles to wash out the stomach a few times often gives relief. I have also learned that there are certain dyspeptic conditions which will disappear upon replacing wine or beer by pure, fresh water, even in persons who only drink moderately and with their meals.

At times it may become necessary, in order to convince the patient of his digestive power and not to let him starve, to resort to Debove's method of tube-feeding.[1] His *poudre alimentaire*, or meat powder, is prepared in the following manner: Beef is taken and all the fat possible removed, and also the tendons. It is hashed rather coarsely and spread on plates, to be dried in an oven at a temperature of 194° F. When the meat has dried hard, it is ground in a mortar and then strained through a fine silk sieve. The powder thus obtained is impalpable and will keep indefinitely if preserved from dampness. It represents four times the weight of fresh meat. The best vehicle for the introduction of meat powder is bouillon, to which may be added the whites and the yolks of two eggs, previously beaten. If there is an aversion to the powder, fresh meat juice will prove of great value in absolute anorexia. But the juice should always be freshly pressed out and used at once.

Dilatation of the stomach depending merely upon functional causes often yields rapidly to the dry diet so highly recommended by Bouchard, of Paris.

Diarrhœa.—Acute attacks of diarrhœa, if not due to tuberculous intestinal lesions, are best treated by first cleansing the intestinal canal and then giving the patient appropriate food, such as cacao, toast, eggs, rice with cinnamon and but little sugar, mucilaginous soup, and Bordeaux wine with arrow root. If the diarrhœa is due to tuberculous intestinal lesions, the case is more difficult. Mere diet does not suffice to stop it, and even large doses of opium and bismuth have no lasting effect. Hot claret with cinnamon, or tannic or gallic acid in large doses, sometimes gives more lasting relief. As a medicinal remedy for chronic diarrhœa in tuberculosis, de Renzi's combination of tannin and iodoform, mentioned above when speaking of iodoform, should be recalled.

Washing out or rather irrigating the lower bowel from time to time with warm soap suds, made of good Castile soap, has given me good results in a number of cases in procuring at least a temporary relief. I use for this purpose a large fountain syringe, elevating it as much as possible, so as to reach the higher portion of the lower bowel.

The accumulated irritating microorganisms and their toxins are thus removed from at least a portion of the intestinal tract.

Phthisical patients suffering from frequent diarrhœa should keep the abdomen warmly covered. They should avoid such articles of food as cabbage, salads, sweetmeats, or substances which their experience has taught them tend to increase the frequency of stools. They should adhere strictly to the antidiarrhœic diet just described for acute attacks. In the severer forms of diarrhœa, absolute rest in bed must be insisted upon.

Of course, there are also diarrhœas in phthisical patients which are due neither to a mistake in diet nor to tuberculous lesions, but simply to the ingestion of medicinal substances, such as cod-liver oil, creosote, sodium salts, arsenic, etc. The temporary or permanent omission of these substances will often cure such intestinal disturbances.

Constipation.—It should be impressed upon the patient that his bowels must move freely once every day. Any tendency to constipation he should at once report to the physician. Great effort during the act of defecation may bring about a severe hæmoptysis or cause the development of hemorrhoids. Carlsbad salt and the California cascara sagrada are favorite remedies in the European sanatoria when prunes and other fruits are of no avail. For the more obstinate forms of constipation in fairly strong patients the judicious administration of hydrargyrum chloridum mite—as, for example, ten grains in fractional doses of one grain every hour, with sugar of milk as a vehicle — often renders valuable service. Not to weaken the patient unnecessarily I have him stop the calomel powders the moment he has had a free evacuation, which in many cases is effected by the fifth or sixth dose. I do not favor too frequent enemata; they tend to lessen the contractile power of the large intestine. At times a glycerin suppository will do the work of an evacuating enema. If the constipation assumes a chronic character, abdominal massage is usually resorted to with good results. The application of the wet pack over the abdomen for a few hours, followed by a gentle friction with alcohol, also rarely fails to help.

Cough.—Painful coughs seem best relieved by small, repeated doses of codeine in solution, but the dry cough, which is often the result of habit, and with which there is really nothing to expectorate, should be suppressed by discipline. Sips of cold water, orange juice, or milk, small pieces of ice or tablets of Iceland moss (cetraria), will help to overcome tickling sensations in the throat until the patient has fully become master of the cough. Holding the breath for a few seconds will often help also. It is really wonderful how much it is possible to accomplish in this respect by discipline. In Falkenstein I have dined for months with a hundred and more consumptives in one large dining-hall, and it was a rare occurrence to hear a single cough during the dinner-hour.

To relieve the not infrequent morning attacks of coughing, a glass of hot water with some lemon juice, with but little or no sugar, or with five to ten drops of the ammoniated spirit of anise (liquor ammonii anisatus), often suffices. Occasionally it becomes absolutely necessary to give expectorants regularly to relieve a distressing cough and the tenacious expectoration. The following prescription has rendered me good service in most such cases:

R Codeinæ, ... gr. vi.–viij.
    Acidi sulphurici diluti, ... ℥ iss.
    Glycerini,
    Aquæ laurocerasi, ... āā fl ℥ i.
    Syr. pruni virginianæ, ... fl ℥ ij.
    Syr. tolutani, ... q.s. ad fl ℥ vi.
    M. S. A teaspoonful whenever the cough becomes distressing; more than six teaspoonfuls should, as a rule, not be taken in twenty-four hours.

At times I change this prescription for Murrell's cough mixture, which is also very good. It is as follows:

R Codeinæ, ... gr. iv.
    Acid. hydrochlor. dil., ... ℳ xxx.
    Spirit. chloroformi, ... ℥ iss.
    Syrup. limonis, ... ℥ i.
    Aquæ, ... q.s. ad ℥ iv.
    M. S. One teaspoonful as occasion demands.

In a number of cases I have tried the new remedy, heroine, recommended by Dreser and Floret and by Manges.[162] It has given satisfaction with quite a number of patients, relieving dyspnœic sensation and seemingly allaying the irritating cough. I have given it in tablet form as well as in solution, but in smaller doses, as recommended by Manges. From $\frac{1}{6}$ to $\frac{1}{10}$ grain, taken several times during the day, seems to render the patient drowsy. I give gr. $\frac{1}{15}$ to $\frac{1}{20}$ preferably, in solution, and I have found diluted sulphuric acid just as good a solvent as acetic acid, recommended by Manges. Replacing the codeine by three grains of heroine in the six ounces of cough mixture given above will render good service. When the cough does not yield to these medications, or when there is a marked bronchorrhœa, daily intratracheal injections of ℳxx. of the following liquid often give relief:

R Guaiacol,
    Menthol, ... āā ℳ x.
    Olive oil, ... ℥ i.

If violent coughing-spells cannot be repressed, tying a wide flannel band around the chest will lessen the painful concussions.

Vomiting in consumptives may be due to a purely nervous condition or to actual digestive disturbances from injudicious dieting or the administration of medicinal substances. Most frequent of all is the vomiting due to the reflex action brought about by coughing-spells. The latter can best be controlled by an enforced absolute quiet after eating, and sojourn in the open air, aided by will-power. Quiet, deep inspiration with head tipped backward, small swallows of very cold or very hot water may also help to overcome this troublesome symptom. But of paramount importance should be the instruction to the patient not to be discouraged if he has vomited, even the whole meal, but to take soon afterwards another light repast. If the cause of vomiting is injudicious overfeeding, the remedy is self-evident. Of the medicinal substances which are at times the cause of vomiting we must mention creosote and other coal-tar preparations, quinine, and heroine. The suppression of these or the substitution of other remedies becomes necessary in such cases.

Intercostal Neuralgia.—Besides the pain in the side, of which we will speak in connection with pleurisy, tuberculous patients suffer intensely at times from intercostal neuralgia or deeply seated pain in the lungs. Hot-water compresses, frequently repeated, or the Priessnitz compress, will render good service. When the suffering becomes unbearable in spite of local applications, a subcutaneous injection of gr. ¼ of morphine at the seat of pain should be given. But before I resort to opiates I invariably try a counter-irritant. It often gives instant relief, and is of value in nearly all the stages of the disease. The counter-irritants seem to draw from the delicate respiratory and circulatory organs countless dangerous micro-organisms into the less delicate cellular tissue, where by the action of these irritants the number of the phagocytic white corpuscles is increased; thus an actual destruction of pathogenic microbes is brought about by the simple mustard plaster, the old-fashioned dry cups, or the "points de feu" (ignipuncture).

The counter-irritants as a means of producing revulsion in chronic pulmonary tuberculosis have of late gone somewhat out of use, especially in this country. I fear their therapeutic value has been underestimated in the eager search for something specific. In France, counter-irritants are yet quite extensively resorted to, especially in hospital practice. In the *Archives Cliniques de Bordeaux* Arnozan has taken up the study of the influence on the kidneys of the application of cantharidized blisters to the thorax. The patients selected were only those with normal urine. The latter was tested before and after the application of the blister, and it remained normal; no other inconveniences were observed in any case. As a result of these observations, Arnozan agrees with Grancher,[169] of Paris, that small blisters applied repeatedly furnish one of the best means of arresting the progress of chronic pulmonary tuberculosis, although if the urine proves abnormal in preliminary examination, some other revulsive than cantharides should be employed. Whenever a stronger revulsion than dry cupping or the external application of the tincture of iodine is indicated, and the patient's fear of the hot iron can be overcome, I give ignipuncture the preference, it being the cleanest and safest revulsive. After its application I sprinkle over the parts some inert powder as a protective.

Pulmonary hemorrhage is one of the most important symptoms to be considered in the treatment of consumption. We cannot here enter into the pathological significance of the various types and degrees of hæmoptysis, from almost imperceptible bloody expectoration to a profuse flow of bright red or dark colored blood, at times from mouth and nose at once. When called to see a patient with a considerable hemorrhage, it is not always easy to say whether it is due to a congestive or an ulcerative process, and I really do not think that the treatment can differ very much. In profuse bleeding, absolute rest is the all-important indication. The patient must not be allowed to talk and should be placed in a semi-recumbent position. He should be enjoined to refrain from an attempt to hold back the flow of blood. Suffocation or ensuing pneumonia is to be feared when such attempts are made. All persons not needed in the room should leave and everything should be kept as quiet as possible. The physician will have at his disposal four important remedies—morphine, ergotin, atropine, and hydrastis canadensis—all of which he may need before being able to obtain a stoppage of the flow of blood. Starke[164] and Solly recommend the hypodermic injection of large doses of atropine (gr. $\frac{1}{70}$) in all serious cases, particularly in those in which ergot has proved a failure. Nitroglycerin in one-half-drop doses of one-per-cent. alcoholic solution every half-hour has, in the hands of Dr. Flick, of Philadelphia, rendered excellent service as a bæmostatic in hæmoptysis.[165] In the mean time the patient is given small pieces of ice or small sips of ice water. Brannan[166] recommends aconite as a direct cardiac sedative. According to the experiments of Andrew,[167] this produces a fall in the pressure in the pulmonary artery.

The assurance that a pulmonary hemorrhage is in itself not by any means a symptom necessarily dangerous to life, and still less excluding the possibility of a good recovery, will have the best effect on the usually much-alarmed patient. Right here I wish to say that I think Wolff's[168] policy, to tell all patients of the possibility of the occurrence of a hemorrhage, even if they have never had one, will have, so far as mental agitation and excitement are concerned, a most beneficial effect. Especially will this be so when the warning is accompanied by the assurance that pulmonary hemorrhage is one of the phases rarely absent in the development of the disease, and is a symptom which, while needing careful attention, is not more dangerous than many others. After the injection of either morphine, ergotin, or atropine, or the administration of hydrastis canadensis, bags of cracked ice may be placed over the pectoral region or the apices. But since ice may not always be had when it is most urgently needed, and the weight of the bag becomes sometimes oppressive to the patient, the following method of applying cold water when in presence of hemorrhage from the lung is, I think, well worth remembering. It was, I believe, first instituted by Winternitz. One procures the water as cold as possible and soaks in it a part of a sheet or a piece of rather coarse linen. When wrung out so that it does not drip, the cloth is folded in the shape of a triangle, placed closely over the patient's chest, and is pressed into the supraclavicular spaces. The apex of the triangle reaches over the pit of the stomach, and the base touches the neck. Whenever the compress becomes warm it can be rapidly changed without disturbing the patient's position. The cooler and more frequent the application, the more rapid is the action of the vasoconstrictors.

When the shock from the hemorrhage has been very severe a hypodermic injection of ether, digitalin, or caffeine is well indicated. I should also suggest in cases of severe shock, as a result of a profuse hæmoptysis, Kemp's method [169] of rectal irrigation with hot salt solution (one teaspoonful of chloride of sodium to a quart of water at a temperature of 100° to 120° F.) by means of his double catheter. The warmth thus conveyed to the body, and in addition the absorption of the saline solution, will help to bring about a favorable reaction. The irrigation can be kept up for an hour or more without the patient being inconvenienced.

Of the physical means to control pulmonary hemorrhages, I desire yet to mention the sometimes very useful ligation of the lower and upper limbs to prevent, in a measure, the blood from returning to the lungs. During my visits to the European sanatoria I saw some very elaborate and expensive instruments devised for that purpose (Assalinische Schnallen), but any flannel band, muffler, or large handkerchief will answer the purpose just as well. These ligations of arms or legs are made as near the trunk as possible, and just tight enough to hinder the return of the venous flow, but not to compress the arterial pulse. Every half-hour or so the bands should be loosened, provided a too painful compression of some nerves or a threatening anæmia of the brain does not demand an earlier removal of the ligatures. Under ordinary circumstances these constricting bands can be renewed after short intervals, and as often as the condition of the patient may indicate. A hot-water bag should, at the same time, be placed at the feet.

After the stoppage of an acute hemorrhage, the administration of astringents, such as the fluid extract of ergot, or, better yet, gallic acid in ten-grain doses, and of iced drinks must be continued for some time. Cold food, liquid or semi-liquid, should also be insisted on for a while after acute attacks. The meals should be small but frequent, to attract the blood to the alimentary canal. The drinking of quantities of pure cold water should be encouraged. The patient should also be instructed to refrain from coughing violently, to avoid a renewal of the hemorrhage.

Lastly, I wish to speak of the value of deep, quiet respiration, of course, without any extra effort or movement of the arms. When instituted an hour or so after the acute attack has subsided, two or three deep respirations every thirty or sixty seconds will hasten the complete cessation of the bloody expectorations which have so frequently a tendency to become chronic. It is often the custom to continue the absolute rest necessary during the acute attack too long. I see in this habit a certain danger of hypostasis; in fact, I think, we should permit a patient to leave the bed or couch a few days after the cessation of the hemorrhage to take short walks, according to his strength, around the room or on the veranda.

It goes without saying that those patients whose bloody expectoration is of a distinctly chronic character, when the congestive origin is evident and the general condition is relatively good, should rather be as much as possible out-of-doors; and for them respiratory exercises are of special value. No less an authority than Traube instituted this mode of treatment for chronic hæmoptysis due to congestion of the respiratory organs. For the same class of patients the pneumatic cabinet treatment, persistently carried out, is most valuable in arresting chronic pulmonary hemorrhages. The repeated but careful administration of saline cathartics also renders good service in relieving the thoracic organs of their congestion.

Pyrexia.—To combat fever in pulmonary tuberculosis requires close study and observation. There is the chronic type and the acute type. We will speak first of the most frequent—the chronic form.

Some phthisiotherapeutists recommend that the temperature of their ambulant or non-ambulant patients be taken by the invalids ·themselves every two hours. I do not approve of this method, for, to my mind, it has a tendency with many patients to increase uselessly their anxiety, and, *ipso facto*, their temperature.

Non-ambulant febrile patients should never be allowed to take their own temperature; in fact, the nurse who attends to this should use all possible tact not to reveal to the patient any marked elevation. Mercier's or other so-called automatic thermometers will be of use with this class of patients. It seems to me that, even with a patient seriously ill, to take the temperature at about eight o'clock in the morning, about one and five o'clock in the afternoon, and at nine o'clock in the evening, would suffice as guidance to the physician in his antipyretic treatment. In milder cases, taking the temperature at about nine in the morning and five in the afternoon will be usually all that is needed. In all severer cases the nurse should take the rectal temperature; this method is less trying to the patient and more exact.

As to the therapeutic means at our disposal, we will divide them into five classes: prophylactic, physical, dietetic, general medicinal, and bacterio-medicinal.

Prophylactic.—A febrile patient arriving at a sanatorium, hospital, or health resort, should be put to bed, or at least enjoined to take absolute rest on a reclining-chair in the open air or in a well-ventilated room, according to the degree of the fever. In private practice, when the patient cannot be constantly observed, he should be warned, even if only in the incipient state or on the way to recovery, to avoid climbing many stairs or other temperature-increasing physical exercise, late dinners, theatres and all exciting amusements. Even the reading of exciting novels can produce an elevation of temperature in a tuberculous invalid.

The physical means at our disposal to combat the pyretic condition in pulmonary tuberculosis are numerous. Here, again, rest stands first, and, above all, rest in bed in well-ventilated rooms. Turban showed to the Congress for Internal Medicine, held at Munich in 1895, a number of fever charts of his phthisical patients, in whom he succeeded in reducing the temperature to normal by prolonged uninterrupted rest in bed. Next in importance comes the rest cure in the reclining-chair in the open air; the details of this procedure we have already described in the chapter on aërotherapeutics.

As the next most important physical means to reduce temperature, comes water, administered internally, pure or in the form of lemonade, and externally, tepid, cold, or in the form of ice. The most pleasing of all antipyretic drinks are lemonade and orangeade. The best method of preparing them is as follows: Take three tablespoonfuls of lemon or orange juice and half of the peelings of one lemon or orange; pour over this ten ounces of hot water; before putting the beverage away to cool, remove the peels; add a few spoonfuls of sugar to suit the taste.

The external application of water as an antipyretic remedy is most important. As a rule, we may say that the weaker the patient and the higher the temperature, the more decidedly tepid should the water be (68° to 78° F.). For the average patient sponging—first partial, then entire—with water varying from 55° to 65° F. is indicated. With timid patients the sponging should always be gradual and partial at the beginning, and in the following order: Hands, forearms, face, throat, neck, armpits, arms, back, stomach, gluteal region, finally the lower extremities from the hips downward. This order of procedure has been given by no less an authority than Winternitz. [70] This sponging should be done under cover, and with as little exposure to the air as possible. Each portion, after being sponged off, should be rapidly covered without being dried, so that the water, through its evaporation, may add to the cooling effect. The effect of the first application will be a guidance to the physician for further procedures. This method of applying the cold water can be repeated three, four, or more times daily, until a perceptible reduction in the temperature is obtained. In the use of wet-packs the same gradual procedure and the same care as to the temperature should be exercised.

I do not favor the entire enveloping of a phthisical patient in a cold sheet, but prefer the partial application of compresses to either lower or upper extremities, or over the chest. I resort to this especially when the sponging seems to disturb the patient too much. I apply, for example, the wet-pack first for a while to the lower extremities, next to the upper, and so on alternately every half-hour. The wet-pack can be rapidly improvised with a couple of ordinary towels as pack, and a few larger Turkish towels as cover. When the temperature is very high an ice-bag over the heart will render excellent service; but still better would be the application of a coil of rubber tubing over the head or over the heart. The water can be made as cold as desired, and the rubber coil is not nearly so heavy as the ice-bag and is more easily applied.

The dietetic treatment in fever is, of course, important. We have touched already on the subject in speaking of diet in general, and there mentioned that the febrile patient should eat when his temperature is lowest. When the fever is not excessively high, these patients eat often with more appetite on the reclining-chair on the veranda, where it is quiet, than in the dining-room, where they perhaps cannot eat with the same ease and comfort. Cold dishes are, of course, also more suitable than hot ones for any fever patient. Cold milk will constitute an important factor in the nutrition of febrile consumptives, especially when they are confined to bed. Other drinks of the nourishing kind which should be permitted are light beers and moderately alcoholic wines largely diluted with water. More nourishing are iced barley-water and milk-lemonade. The latter may be prepared as follows: Have in readiness two ounces of sugar, five ounces of boiled milk, half a lemon or two ounces of white wine, five ounces of boiling water, and the fine peelings of half a lemon. Pour the boiling water over the peeling and the sugar, let this cool off, and then add the milk and the lemon-juice or the wine, and strain the mixture after ten minutes.

General Medicinal Treatment of Fever.—The antipyretic medicinal substances at our disposal are here named in the order of their seeming efficacy to reduce the temperature, at the same time doing the least harm to the patient:

Lactophenin,	.	.	.	5 to 10 grains,	1 to 3 times daily.			
Phenacetin,	.	.	.	3 " 5 "	1 " 3 "	"		
Antifebrin,	.	.	.	3 " 5 "	1 " 3 "	"		
Antipyrin,	.	.	.	10 " 15 "	1 " 3 "	"		

In the administration of any of these four substances just mentioned, it must be remembered that they should not be given as a means to lower the temperature, but rather to prevent it from rising. I have found Daremberg's method [1] in this matter a good one to follow. If the fever commences at two o'clock and declines toward seven in the evening, and by five o'clock it has not risen over 100° F., Daremberg gives about ten grains of antipyrin at half-past three o'clock in the afternoon of the following day. If the temperature at three o'clock has already attained 100° F., he gives the following day ten grains of antipyrin at noon and the same dose at three o'clock. If the temperature at three o'clock is 102°, he increases the two doses to fifteen grains each. As above mentioned, I prefer to give the lactophenin or phenacetin in appropriate doses in place of the antipyrin. If any of these remedies cause too much digestive disturbance, they should be administered per rectum. Quinine in large doses is of little avail in the chronic fever of tuberculosis. But in some cases the small doses—for example, two grains, several times repeated during the day—act quite favorably. Quinine in larger doses seems to be of more value in the acute exacerbations, characterized by high temperature and suddenness of onset.

Bacterio-medicinal Treatment of Fever.—One of the most surprising things which I noticed in my studies of the sanatorium treatment, especially in institutions situated in higher altitudes, was the almost total cessation of the fever of many of the newly arrived consumptives after a few days, without the administration of any antipyretic whatsoever. The only explanation was the almost total absence of pathogenic microbes, especially the streptococci, in these higher altitudes, and consequently a cessation of the association of microbes. This conclusion led me to experiments with Marmorek's antistreptococcic serum.[112] Through the courtesy of Professor Biggs, I have been allowed to test the antistreptococcic action in the New York City Laboratory by a series of experiments on animals.

I will briefly summarize the results obtained at that time and in subsequent clinical experience with this serum. With patients whose temperature rose above 102.5° F. for several days I did not obtain any results. When, however, there was a temperature of only 101.5° F., or a trifle over, with streptococci in the sputum, a first injection of 10 c.c. reduced the temperature from one to one and one-half degrees. A second of 10 c.c. brought it down to nearly normal. A third, fourth, fifth, and sixth of 5 c.c. each, given first every twenty-four hours, then at longer intervals, helped to maintain the normal or nearly normal temperature, and a general better feeling was experienced by the patient.

Others who have used the same serum, such as Bermingham, Weaver,[113] and Stubbert,[114] have had relatively better success than I. So, for example, Weaver succeeded in reducing a temperature of 105° to nearly normal with a single dose, and maintained it there by repeating the injection every second day for some time.

If these experiments have taught us anything, it is that the action of the serum is not always uniform, and that there are evidently other associations with the bacilli besides the streptococci which cause the hectic condition of a patient. More experimentation will be necessary before we can fix the real value of the serum.

Whenever there is a distinct mixed infection a few inunctions of unguentum Credé (ointment of soluble metallic silver) may also be advantageously used, especially when serum treatment is not indicated or has proved of no avail. Some authors still recommend intrapulmonary injections of carbolized iodine in the treatment of septic conditions arising from the presence of pyogenic organisms in existing cavities. John Blake White in a paper[115] on this subject recommends for well-selected cases the following formula, with which he has obtained the most satisfactory results:

℞ Atropine, ...	gr. ¼
Morph. sulph., ...	gr. ij.
Tinct. iodine, ...	ʒ iij.
Carbolic acid (pure), ...	gtt. xx.
Glycerin, ...	ʒ iss.
Diluted alcohol, 20 to 30 per cent., . . .	ʒ iss.

M. S. Fifteen to thirty minims by injection.

It seems to me that one must use great care in the selection of cases for this surgical intervention, and it should be resorted to only when all other means have failed.

Hyperidrosis.—The control of nightsweats will largely depend upon the success of the antipyretic treatment. Frequently, however, they need special attention, and an antisudorific treatment must be instituted. The prophylactic treatment of hyperidrosis is, of course, the rest cure in the open air during the day, and sleeping in a cool room at night where the fresh air enters constantly through the open window, the patient being protected from the draught by a screen. The bed-clothes should not be too heavy; all underwear should be left off; a muslin nightshirt should be worn instead of a woollen one. If the patient can train himself to leave his arms outside the covers, he will find this a help, even if he has to have them protected by extra sleeves. Besides these hygienic precautions the patient should take as a dietetic treatment for nightsweats one or two glasses of cold milk with a teaspoonful of cognac before retiring. He should never retire hungry, and should always have some light lunch on a table near his bed, so that he may eat something if he wakes in the night feeling faint. Again, if the patient is in the habit of waking up at a certain hour in the morning bathed in perspiration, he should be waked two hours earlier and given egg-nog or other light lunch. Sometimes it will be necessary to give him a sponging with pure alcohol or water and alcohol, or water and vinegar, or water and lemon-juice. But often, when these remedies fail to control the nightsweats, the following hydrotherapeutic procedure works well even in cases of severe hyperidrosis. Several thicknesses of rather coarse linen, folded in the form of a shawl, or, better yet, three different cloths,—one narrow one for each apex like a broad shoulder-strap, and another wider one to wrap around the chest,—are soaked in water at a temperature of about 55° F., wrung out and then closely applied over the apices and around the thorax. A thick flannel band, somewhat wider than the compress, is wrapped over this, and the whole is fastened in place where it remains all night. The patient usually feels no discomfort, sleeps well, and sweats but slightly, if at all. In the morning the compress is removed, and the chest and shoulders are rubbed thoroughly dry. If the consumptive is relatively strong and experience has demonstrated to the attending physician that an occasional sweat-bath does not exhaust the patient too much, but, on the contrary, lowers his temperature and improves his general condition, this method of combating a hyperidrosis is perfectly justified. Through the sweat-bath the excretory action of the skin is considerably increased, and a larger quantity of toxin is thus more rapidly eliminated. Of the details of the procedure we have already spoken in the paragraph on hydrotherapy. Aside from the aërotherapeutic, hydrotherapeutic, and dietetic means there exist two medicinal substances to which we must resort sometimes. These are, first, agaricin in doses of gr. $\frac{1}{30}$ to $\frac{1}{15}$, and atropine in doses of gr. $\frac{1}{100}$ to $\frac{1}{60}$.

Chills, not of a malarial type, which appear in some patients at regular intervals, should be anticipated by the patient remaining in bed and taking a hot lemonade, etc. The room should be kept warmer than usual, and everything which is apt to cause a chilly sensation, as washing in cold water, changing of linen, touching of cold metallic objects, should be avoided. Windows should never be opened before half an hour after the complete cessation of the chill. In the endeavor to combat chills the physician should strive to postpone the usual hour of its appearance from day to day. In summer, the patient should be placed out-doors during his attacks, in a sunny, windless spot.[176] If the nature of the chills suggests the administration of quinine it should be given per rectum, so as not to disturb the digestive function.

Extreme states of *weakness* must be treated by careful stimulation with champagne, wine, whiskey, milk-punches, or kumyss; and, if this condition becomes chronic, the hypodermic injection of camphorated oil or caffeine is indicated. General massage has at times also rendered excellent services in such cases, rest in bed and judicious feeding being combined with it, thus imitating, in a measure, the rest cure of Weir Mitchell. Of course, all patients suffering from such attacks should be enjoined to avoid all mental and physical exertions of whatever nature. If there is an acute tachycardia, local applications of ice over the pectoral region may become necessary.

For acute attacks of intense *dyspnœa*, besides a hypodermic injection of morphine, the inhalation of oxygen or of Walton's oxygen compound (oxygen, two parts; nitrous monoxide, one part; ozone, one per cent.) seems still the best remedy, and every well-equipped sanatorium or special hospital for consumptives should have a supply of oxygen cylinders on hand.

Insomnia in tuberculous patients is an important symptom, and when confronted with it one should not rashly resort to the hypnotics of the pharmacopœia. In phthisical patients insomnia may be due to irritating cough, to pyrexia, or to digestive trouble, or it may be a purely nervous manifestation. The therapeutics of fever and cough have been sufficiently dealt with in the preceding pages, and, as a dietetic means of preventing insomnia, I would only suggest that the patient's last meal before retiring should be light and very digestible. Tea and coffee should be strictly forbidden at the evening meal. As a sleep-inducing dish before retiring, buttermilk is most highly to be recommended; kephir and kumyss may take its place. The nervous insomnia of phthisical patients is less frequent in sanatoria than anywhere else, for there the open-air treatment is more systematically carried out. Nothing is more conducive to sleep than remaining out-of-doors. If the patient is able to add a moderate amount of physical exercise to his rest cure, he will be almost certain of a good night's rest. Of course, regularity in his hours of retiring and rising will be essential. Absolute quiet should, as much as possible, be assured within and in the vicinity of the consumptive's bed-room. The bed should be comfortable, not too soft, not too warm, and, of course, the room must be well ventilated. For the average patient the temperature of the bedroom in winter should be about 60° F. Whether to sleep on the right or left side, or on the back, is a matter of choice and habit. The only thing which I recommend my patients in this respect is to accustom themselves to sleep with as low a head-rest as possible. Feather-beds as covers should be banished from the bedroom as unsanitary.

As hydrotherapeutic means to induce sleep we must again mention the wet-pack over chest or abdomen. Bathing the face with cool water or lightly sponging off the whole body is sleep-inducing. Also vigorous friction of the feet with a rough towel soaked in cold water, or "effleurage"—that is to say, gentle strokes with the palm of the hand from the neck downward and over the spinal column—may produce the desired effect. General massage should be applied only early in the morning or during the day; the same rule should hold good with the light gymnastics, which may at times be permitted in early cases. All these more or less energetic exercises are just as much conducive to sleep, and in fact more so, when done in the morning or in the afternoon as when done in the evening; thus, the exciting effect of the exercises will have passed away by bedtime, and only the desired feeling of fatigue needed for sleep remains.

Rose[177] recommends, as a physical means of producing sleep, energetic and frequently repeated opening and closing of the eyelids; but this seems to be effective only in the very mildest cases of insomnia. In the following number of the same journal, Buxbaum[178] recommends auto-suggestion in insomnia with all patients inclined to neurasthenia —in other words, he tells the patient not to fear insomnia, but to go to bed with the firm determination to sleep.

The medicinal hypnotics, which must be resorted to in extreme cases, are trional, morphine, and chloral. Trional seems to be a peculiarly suitable hypnotic in cases of phthisis. It should be administered in doses of from 5 to 15 grains in a warm fluid half an hour before retiring.[179] If there is physical pain gr. $\frac{1}{12}$ to $\frac{1}{20}$ of heroine may be added. Morphine injected hypodermically, and chloral by the rectum, in the smallest possible doses, will prevent digestive disturbances apt to arise from the administration of these drugs by the mouth. While I desire to repeat that sleep-producing drugs should be administered in pulmonary tuberculosis only after all physical means, single or combined, have failed, I would apply this rule only to cases in which a cure or decided improvement may be looked for with reasonable certainty. Phthisical patients in the last stages of the disease, suffering from insomnia or pain, should be made comfortable even at the price of making them depend, toward the end of their lives, upon the administration of larger doses of morphine than would be advisable under ordinary circumstances. In some phthisical patients an extreme nervousness enters as an important factor into the symptomatology. Judiciously prolonged rest, open-air treatment, suitable diet, and gentle sponging off with cold water are the best means for combating such conditions. The bromides should be resorted to only when all other means have failed. A change of environments is often all that is necessary. A patient may be restless in one place and quiet in another. But fatiguing travel should, of course, not be encouraged.

Anæmia.—Not infrequently the anæmic condition of the tuberculous invalid causes him to suffer from dizziness, headaches, etc. When the dietetic treatment, combined with hydro-, aéro-, and heliotherapy, does not suffice to overcome this condition or when improvement is slow, iron and strychnine should be given in addition. Landon Carter Gray[180] combines the two substances in the following convenient way:

R Ferratin, ... gr. iij.
Strych. sulph., ... gr. $\frac{1}{30}$
Ft. in capsul. No. 1. Mitte xv. S. One three times a day just after meals.

Treatment of Complications and of Special Forms of Tuberculosis.

One of the gravest of all complications in phthisis, and, alas! also the most frequent, is *laryngeal tuberculosis*. Heintze reports that in 1,226 cases of pulmonary phthisis he found an involvement of the larynx 376 times. Kruse saw laryngeal affections 123 times in 742 cases of pulmonary tuberculosis, and Chiary gives the frequency in the Vienna hospitals as varying from 6 to 12 per cent.

Laryngeal tuberculosis must be treated locally and generally. The vocal organs should be given absolute rest, and the patient should avoid all exciting occupations which will make him talk in spite of his best resolutions, and, of course, he should avoid strong winds, heavy fogs, sudden temperature changes, and all places where dust is raised or irritating odors fill the air and cause coughing-spells. For such patients the selection of a warm, moist climate is recommendable (warm sea-coasts), for they really suffer in cold and dry regions. As a rule high altitudes are less suitable for them. The throat should be protected so as to keep that portion moderately warm. Schmidt [181] insists, however, that the covering around the neck should always be loose.

The diet for patients suffering from laryngeal tuberculosis need not differ materially from that described for the pulmonary invalid. Of course, hard substances, such as bread-crusts and dry toast, should be avoided, and also much seasoning, as through their ingestion irritation and pain may ensue. For painful deglutition, weak solutions of codeine, or better yet cocaine, should be applied before meals. A tablet of gr. $\frac{1}{24}$ of hydrochlorate of cocaine placed on the back of the tongue is a good way of administering the cocaine, since the patient can do this himself without any danger. When the dysphagia during deglutition becomes too intense, nutritive enemata should be given. At times hot inhalations with a steam atomizer give decided relief. These steam sprays can be medicated according to the indication with astringent, balsamic, disinfectant, or analgesic substances. A simple cold spray or the external application of cold in the form of ice-cravats or cold-water compresses seems to be beneficial in many cases. Intratracheal injections of guaiacol, menthol, and olive oil, as described above for persistent cough in pulmonary tuberculosis, are well adapted to the treatment of this distressing symptom in laryngeal tuberculosis, when simpler remedies, such as codeine or heroine, do not suffice.

These injections must in some patients be preceded by the application of a cocaine solution. The new product, orthoform, has in the hands of some laryngologists yielded better results as an analgesic in the dysphagia of tuberculous laryngitis than cocaine. Orthoform, a benzoic-acid derivative, is a clear white powder of powerful analgesic action on the denuded mucous membrane, and is free from toxic effects. Freudenthal, [182] who has used it extensively, observed after an insufflation of five to ten grains not only the disappearance of the dysphagia, lasting for hours afterward, but also a diminution of purulent exudation and a gradual healing of the ulceration without the application of other local remedies. The same author also recommends orthoform (12.5 gm.) combined with menthol (10 gm.), sweet almond oil (30 gm.), distilled water (100 gm.), and the yolks of two eggs as an emulsion, to be used for injection with the aid of the ordinary laryngeal syringe.

In my experience I have found the inhalation, by means of a steam spray, of cinnamon water, diluted according to the susceptibility of the patient, particularly soothing and alleviating in moderately advanced laryngeal tuberculosis. When the hot spray is not well borne, the cinnamon water may be applied cold with the aid of the nebulizer.

Aërotherapy, of course, must not be neglected in these cases. Breathing-exercises should be instituted in this disease as well as in pulmonary tuberculosis. They should be taken judiciously, according to the strength of the patient. The milder the air these patients breathe, the better they will feel. The addition of the nose mask in the pneumatic cabinet treatment will permit the sufferer from laryngeal tuberculosis to enjoy the benefit of this valuable adjuvant in aërotherapeutics just as well as the sufferer from pulmonary consumption. In breathing through the nose with the aid of the adjustable mask, instead of through the mouth tube, the air is warmed sufficiently to cause no irritation whatsoever, and the increased air supply thus entering the respiratory organs has its beneficial effect.

As a curative measure the lactic-acid application, varying in strength from ten to seventy-five per cent., has thus far been most universally used. The most frequent way of applying this acid is directly upon the tubercles or ulcerated surfaces. It may, however, be also injected under the mucous membrane. At the recent Spanish laryngological congress, iodoform in the treatment of laryngeal phthisis was again advocated. Dr. de Aresse[192a] claimed that Newman's method of applying the saturated solution of iodoform directly to the tuberculous laryngeal lesions had given him excellent results in eighteen cases. He uses for his solution pure alcohol and sulphuric ether in equal proportions.

At times, surgical interference is inevitable, and no large institution devoted to the treatment of tuberculous patients should be without its competent laryngologist.

The removal of tuberculous growths in the larynx by means of curettage seems to be indicated in a certain number of cases. Gleitsmann,[193] in his excellent report to the Section on Laryngology and Rhinology of the Twelfth International Medical Congress at Moscow, has promulgated the following indications and contraindications of the curette in laryngeal tuberculosis:

Indications: (1) In cases of primary tuberculous affections without pulmonary complications; (2) in cases with circumscribed ulcerations and infiltrations of the larynx; (3) in cases with dense, hard infiltrations of the arytenoid region of the posterior wall, also of the ventricular bands and tuberculous tumors of the epiglottis; (4) in the incipient stage of pulmonary disease with but little fever and no hectic symptoms; (5) in advanced pulmonary disease with distressing dysphagia resulting from infiltration of the arytenoids, as the quickest means of giving relief.

Contraindications: (1) Advanced pulmonary disease and hectic; (2) disseminated tuberculosis of the larynx; (3) extensive infiltrations producing severe stenosis when tracheotomy is indicated or laryngotomy can be taken into consideration.

Gleitsmann, as well as Heryng, does not advise the operation in timid, distrustful patients lacking the necessary nerve-power, and both prefer to operate on the patient in a hospital, where he is under absolute control, and the after-treatment can be carried out more satisfactorily.

For the operation of curettage various instruments have been devised, such as Krause's curettes, Gougenheim's "emporte pièce," and Heryng's rotary double curette. The last one mentioned is given the preference by Gleitsmann, beause it enables the operator to remove a greater amount of tissue.

At times tracheotomy may become necessary to prolong life.

Concerning the curative effect of solar or electric light on tuberculous ulcerations of the larynx and elsewhere, interesting observations have been published by Abrams,[184] Gebhard,[185] Bellow, Kellogg, and Freudenthal, but we have still too little evidence to express a definite opinion on the subject.

Obesity.—Occasionally we meet a consumptive with more adipose tissue than is good for him, and in such cases a fatty degeneration of the heart is to be feared. Extreme dyspnœa and feeble heart-action are frequently the alarming symptoms. To attempt to reduce the fat by such diet as prescribed by Ebstein, Harvey, or Schweninger would be dangerous. The dieting must be done much more gradually, and, while it is essential to relieve the heart from its too fatty environment, such patients should not lose more than about two pounds in the course of one month. Moderate exercise and massage will aid in replacing the adipose tissue by muscular tissue.

Bronchitis must be treated first prophylactically by the aëro- and hydrotherapeutic measures described in the chapter on prophylactic treatment. The inhalation of impure, dusty, or irritating atmosphere is productive of bronchitis, especially in consumptives whose

point of least resistance lies in the respiratory tract.   An unob-
structed nasal breathing is one of the essential conditions to avoid
bronchial catarrhs.

The use of opium is certainly a valuable means of aborting an attack
of bronchitis.   Charbonneau says a full dose of Dover's powder will
frequently abort an attack.   Osler is of the same opinion, saying that
no remedy can take its place.   English[188] explains the therapeutic
action of opium in such cases when given in full doses as follows:
"Reaction of irritability, congestion, or inflammatory activity.
Alteration in the character and limitation of the amount of secretion.
Increase in the general comfort by relief of pain and soreness, and
removal of cough and incidental insomnia."

Counter-irritants, as mustard plasters or dry cupping, are good
local remedies.   The inhalation of thymol (one grain to one ounce of
liquid albolene) or other antiseptic or balsamic preparations is also
useful.   As an antipyretic in acute bronchitis I give quinine the
preference.

If the cold-pack—that is, cold-water compresses—is applied, it
should be as described for excessive hyperidrosis.   Care should be
taken, in removing the compresses, not to chill the patient.   It is
prudent to remove the wet-pack under the bed-cover, and rub the
chest dry with a somewhat rough towel, and follow this by vigorous
friction with alcohol.   To control the cough I give the codeine or
heroine in the manner already described when speaking of the cough
in pulmonary phthisis.

Pleurisy may manifest itself in a consumptive as a concomitant
or an intercurrent disease.   The acute forms, arising as a new complication, must, of course, be treated by rest in bed and milk diet.
If there is a large exudate, absolute quiet before as well as after
thoracentesis must be insisted upon.   If there is but a small amount
of liquid in the chest, dry cupping and mustard applications often
suffice to cause absorption.   Judiciously directed respiratory exercises are of value chiefly in the subacute and chronic forms, if there is
no intense pain.   To relieve the sometimes acute suffering from intercostal or pleuritic pains, cold applications are indicated; if they
are not well borne warm poultices may be substituted.   Of medicinal
substances opiates are at times indispensable.   Diuretics, such as
potassium acetate, digitalis, squills, etc., may be indicated.   The
patient's strength must be kept up by tonics.   If the pleuritic exudate becomes purulent (empyema), the case belongs to the domain of
surgery.   In the speedy and thorough evacuation of the pus lies the
only hope for the recovery of the patient.   Of the value of lateral
douches and respiratory exercises to aid the absorption of chronic

fibrinous adhesions, the residual of an old pleuritic inflammation, we have already spoken.

Emphysema.—For chronic forms of emphysema and other moderate but frequent *dyspnœic conditions*, I have found the pneumatic cabinet most valuable by letting the patient exhale in the rarefied atmosphere. To this end the patient should be made to inhale the outside air, but exhale into the rarefied atmosphere of the cabinet. With a little practice the patient will soon learn to alternate the respiratory movements, and will derive real comfort from his sojourn in the cabinet. The modus operandi of this inhaling from without and exhaling into the cabinet is as follows: The patient holds the nose mask in place with his hand; he takes his first inspiration while the physician begins to manipulate the lever. During the first expiration the patient removes the nose mask. The operator, while continuing with one hand to manipulate the lever, places the palm of his other hand tightly over the funnel of the faucet during the patient's expiratory movements, and thus there is an almost perfect occlusion, and little if any outside air can enter the cabinet. With a little practice these manipulations enable the patient to breathe with ease and comfort, and gradually he loses his distressing symptom to a considerable degree. At first, expiration through the mouth may be permitted, so as to give the patient rapid relief with the least possible exertion.

Respiratory exercises are also of great value in emphysema of the lungs. They must, however, be differently executed from those I have recommended as prophylactic and curative measures in simple pulmonary tuberculosis. There should be more abdominal breathing; instead of the inspiratory the expiratory act should be prolonged, and particular attention should be paid to the second expiratory effort. During the inspiration a considerable pressure with the palms of the hands should be exerted over the lateral portion of the chest, and holding the breath after the inspiration should be omitted.

If the patient suffers intensely, and is obliged to remain in bed, Gerhardt's method [187] to help expiration is to be highly recommended. I will briefly describe this method: The patient lies down on his stomach, crossing the arms behind the back and planting the soles of his feet firmly against the foot of the bed. Then a small pillow is placed under the upper portion of the thorax, a second one under the forehead. Now the patient begins to breathe deeply, and at every expiration he makes a vigorous movement of extending his lower extremities. Through this movement the chest is pressed against the pillow, and in a few minutes considerable relief is obtained.

Of course, all such patients must also be especially careful regarding overexertion. Walks taken with judgment and care on graduated paths of various inclinations are, however, to be recommended. Too long and animated conversation should be avoided. The diet of these patients should be superintended with particular care, and all such food as beans, peas, cabbage, etc., which tend to distend the intestines and push up the diaphragm, should be strictly forbidden. With emphysematous patients the so-called "suralimentation," or over-feeding, should be carried on only gradually, since, as a rule, they feel uncomfortable when they gain flesh and adipose tissue too rapidly. Too voluminous meals are especially contraindicated. They often cause veritable distress to the patient. The proper way of feeding this class of pulmonary invalids is in small but more frequent meals, avoiding too much liquid.

The very serious complication of *œdema of the lungs* must be treated by hypodermic injections of morphine (gr. ¼), cardiac stimulants, and counter-irritation over the chest and back.

Pneumonia, which in consumptives is usually of the lobular kind, must, when arising in the course of pulmonary phthisis, be treated as in any other patient. Rest in bed, careful antipyretic medication (quinine or lukewarm-water baths), and, above all, remedies to keep up the proper heart-action—digitalis, alcohol, etc.—are essential. A. Jacobi counsels giving, from the very onset, two drops every four hours of the fluid extract of digitalis (Squibb's), thus strengthening the heart, and by the cumulative effect of the drug putting the heart in a condition of defence at the most critical stage of the disease. Counter-irritation over the whole of the chest renders also great service. The administration of ammonium carbonate and ammonium iodide will aid materially in the removal of the inflammatory products during the stage of resolution. E. G. Janeway's method of putting the pneumonia patient on a milk diet has rendered me excellent service on various occasions. In all cases the diet should be in liquid form, not too concentrated, and water should be given freely. For severe pains, carefully administered doses of morphine (hypodermically over the seat of pain) are the best analgesic.

Pneumothorax, during the course of pulmonary tuberculosis, is most frequently the result of some sudden physical overexertion or traumatism, such as jumping, running, rapid mounting, loud singing, or a sudden blow against the chest. Again, a violent coughing-spell may be the cause. It is most important to prevent such accidents. However, patients cannot always control their coughs, and a pneumothorax may occasionally develop in a consumptive without any apparent traumatic origin. As in pneumonia, rest in bed is essential. Liquid diet and stimulants of all kinds are strongly indicated. Leyden,[188] of Berlin, favors "gavage," or feeding by the tube, in such cases. Locally, cold-water compresses or ice-bags often give relief. Of course, frequently surgical interference must be resorted to. Immediate relief may often be obtained by aspirating carefully the accumulated air.

Pulmonary gangrene, which is one of the distressing intercurrent troubles that may appear during the course of pulmonary tuberculosis, should be treated vigorously by tonics, digitalis, caffeine, alcohol, etc. Jaccoud recommends to give the patient from eight to ten grains of salicylic acid a day. For antiseptic inhalation a few teaspoonfuls of the essence of turpentine poured into hot water is to be recommended (Trousseau). The vapor of a five-per-cent. solution of carbolic acid can also be used for the same purpose. If there are several foci, medicinal treatment is all that is possible; but if the gangrene is circumscribed and this treatment is ineffectual, pneumotomy and drainage are indicated. The part of the lung involved has been resected in some cases with satisfactory results.

A *fistula in ano* is not an infrequent occurrence in the later stage of consumption. There is still a variety of opinion as to the advisability of operating. It seems to me that if conservative treatment, such as iodoform injections and suppositories, does not suffice to cure the fistula, operative treatment should be resorted to. Especially is an operation indicated if a patient is fairly strong, but cannot walk with comfort on account of the fistula, and suffers from pain and discomfort during defecation.

When *diabetes* complicates phthisis, the hygienic and dietetic measures combined with aéro- and hydrotherapy should be continued with such modification as the diabetic condition demands. Alcohol should be given somewhat more freely, but preferably in the diluted form of light white wines at meal-times. The main point, in such cases, is to strive to maintain the strength of the patient by a judicious over-feeding with the exclusion of sugar, sweetmeats, pastry, preserves, sweet jellies, macaroni, peas, beans, etc. A small amount of bread and potatoes should be occasionally allowed.

While *pityriasis versicolor* (tinea versicolor, pityriasis of Eichstedt) can hardly, in the light of modern research, be considered symptomatic of pulmonary phthisis, it is, nevertheless, met with frequently enough in phthisical patients to merit some consideration here. It is most usually found in patients whose skin has not received proper hygiene. The disease is due to a vegetable parasite (microsporon furfur); the eruption is superficial, of yellowish or reddish color, and the itching sensation is most intense when the patient gets overheated. It is usually located over the sternum; sometimes, however, it is scattered over the front of the chest and the back. The edges of the patches are rounded and somewhat elevated.

The treatment consists in first removing these patches by warm baths with soap, preferably sapo viridis, and then applying the antiparasitic remedy. As an antiparasitic pure ichthyol has given me much satisfaction in such cases. After having bathed the affected parts as above described, I apply a good coat of the ichthyol over night, removing it in the morning by the aid of a weak solution of bichloride (1:5,000 to 1:10,000). Other applications, such as salicylic acid, carbol, or resorcin salves, will also rarely fail to destroy the parasite. One precaution must be insisted upon, otherwise the trouble is sure to recur: that is, the thorough boiling and disinfecting of the patient's underwear.

Acute miliary tuberculosis can, in the present state of our knowledge, be treated only symptomatically. A remedy which I have seen do excellent service, and under which I have observed a few apparent recoveries, is tannic acid, administered in large doses of from ten to fifteen grains three or four times daily.

The treatment of *tuberculous peritonitis* will have to be surgical in the majority of cases. Still, circumstances may arise when, at least for a time, a medical management must be resorted to. Aside from the judicious hygienic changes in the environments, and a careful installation of aërotherapy, I think Byford's non-operative method of treating tuberculous peritonitis may be safely recommended for such cases, especially when the attack seems a sudden one.

During the first few days of an acute attack Byford[189] recommends that the patient should receive the treatment that is suitable for an acute peritonitis. After the first few days no opium should be allowed, but hot fomentations should be applied to relieve pain. Enough calomel should be given to turn the stools to a dark green, and afterward divided doses of salines sufficient to produce two or three soft stools should be administered each day. The diet should be fluid, in small quantities, so as to avoid the production of intestinal gases. Later such solids may be given as will neither produce gas in the stomach or bowels nor leave a solid residuum. The patient should be kept in bed until all abdominal tenderness is gone and the evening temperature is almost normal. Later, when there is any rise in temperature or indication of abdominal tenderness, he should again remain quiet. Salol, guaiacol, and creosote are helpful in keeping down intestinal fermentation. For several months the diet should be carefully regulated. It is Byford's belief that the rest in bed and scanty diet are responsible for the cures of tuber-

culous peritonitis which sometimes follow operations performed upon
patients suffering with this disease.

It goes without saying that if the patient is to be guarded against
a relapse even after a successful laparotomy, the hygienic and dietetic
treatment indicated for pulmonary tuberculosis must be insisted upon
for at least several months. To judge from a number of cases I have
had occasion to observe, even a moderately advanced pulmonary
tuberculosis or a tuberculous pleurisy offers no contraindication to
laparotomy for a concomitant peritonitis.

Local Tuberculosis.—At times, in a patient suffering from pulmonary tuberculosis, even in the earlier stages, there will be found manifestations of local tuberculosis in the joints, testicles, etc. I do not in-
tend here to treat the subject from a surgical point of view, but only to
indicate the newer methods of treatment applicable to the earlier stages
of joint tuberculosis. First in this respect stands Bier's method of
producing local venous hyperæmia. Shortly after the publication of
Bier's monograph [100] on this subject, I had occasion to watch, together
with Dr. Franz J. A. Torek, of New York, the result of this treatment
in several cases of early joint tuberculosis, and the decided relief from
pain and the general amelioration were certainly encouraging. This
method consists in ligating the member above the affected joint by an
elastic band of medium width. This is done several times a day for
a period varying from ten minutes to one hour at the beginning, and
increasing the duration of time, according to the patient's susceptibility and power to endure the pain and tickling sensation produced
by the constricting band, up to four or six hours, or even a whole
night. The band is applied only tight enough to impede the venous
circulation, and if the pain becomes too intense, the band must be
removed. It is essential to see that the constricting band does not
produce anæmia, but hyperæmia and swelling. To protect the skin
it is advisable to envelop the part first by a band of linen or other
soft material, and also to change the place for ligation at successive
applications. The curative principle of this method seems to lie in
the fact that the locally increased carbonic-acid gas, and, perhaps,
also an increased phagocytosis, both attack the micro-organisms.
Dr. Torek also had a case of advanced tuberculous disease of the
testicle treated by the same method, with gratifying results. Of
course, any tuberculous joint must, in addition to this treatment,
be given as much rest as possible. During the last few years I have
had occasion to treat several cases of early tuberculous joint diseases
in this way; but I have alternated the séances of ligation with local
hot-air application, by the aid of Betz's hot-air apparatus. The
relief which is given to a painful tuberculous joint by Bier's applica-

tion of the elastic band is almost instantaneous; in all other joint affections the cessation of pain after this treatment is much slower, if it is at all effective. This has led some observers to make the statement that the rapid cessation of pain in a joint is a pathognomonic sign of tuberculosis.

The idea of treating tuberculosis of the joints by hot air originated with Verneuil, of Paris, in 1890. The hot air is to be applied to the affected member with the usual precautions. Two layers of Turkish towelling should always be wrapped somewhat loosely around the arm or leg to be treated, and the temperature should not be higher than about 275° F. The hot-air treatment can be taken twice daily, alternating with the Bier application, but the former should not last longer than an hour. Local venous hyperæmia, followed by the hot-air treatment, seems to be for the present our best therapeutic means of dealing with early tuberculous affection of the upper or lower extremities.

We have spoken of the value of solar therapy in the general treatment of tuberculosis, but the sun bath can be advantageously utilized even for local tuberculous lesions. Finsen uses the ultra violet rays of the spectrum in the treatment of lupus, and De Millioz, a pupil of Poncet, recently presented an excellent thesis before the faculty of Lyons on the subject of "Continued Sun Baths in the Treatment of Tuberculous Joint Diseases." [190a] Unlike Finsen, De Millioz employs all the ray of the sun to act upon the diseased joint. He justly disapproves of the systematic fixation of the limb in which the tuberculous lesion is located. He exposes the afflicted member in the following manner:

The patient is placed on a suitable couch in the sunniest part of a garden or other open place, with the affected joint fully exposed to the rays of the sun. To protect the head of the patient, some sort of sun shade should be improvised. If the upper limb is the seat of the disease, the patient may preferably be allowed to walk about in the garden. The duration of the sun bath should be several hours a day. During the intervals, the joint is covered with wool and rather firmly bandaged. Sometimes, after the first or second bath, the joint becomes more painful. This soon passes away in most cases; but if it should not, it may be necessary to discontinue the treatment for several days. Rapid pigmentation of the skin by the sun's rays has been noticed to coincide with comparatively quick recovery. It would seem to me a good precaution, at least for the first few séances, to protect the usually very tender skin of the affected joint with a layer of wool or cotton held in place by a gauze bandage.

De Millioz observed that under this local solar treatment swollen tuberculous joints become smaller, the skin healthier looking, and the discharges, if such were present, less purulent; and the fistulæ gradually close. To obtain such results it requires, however, months of continuous treatment; and I would hesitate to allow an accumulation of pus to discharge so slowly. Rather apply the sun baths after the surgeon has attended to a thorough evacuation of the pus, and has left the joint in a fairly aseptic condition. Except in the early stages of tuberculous joint diseases, local solar therapy should rather be considered an adjuvant to the most approved orthopædic or surgical treatment.

We will finally mention Hoffa's soap treatment of local tuberculons processes. Hoffa[191] uses the sapo kalin. venalis transparens of linseed-oil and crude caustic potash solution without alcohol; twenty-five to forty grams are rubbed into the skin of the back from the neck to the knees, with a sponge or the palm of the hand, two or three times a week, usually at night. The soap is washed off with a sponge and warm water after half an hour. He has treated over two hundred patients in this way in the last years, with the most satisfactory results. With this general treatment Hoffa combines the local treatment required. He reports most remarkable cures in cases of multiple bone and joint tuberculous processes.

That all the other organs of the body, such as skin, ear, eye, the genito-urinary system, etc., can be invaded by the tubercle bacillus is well known, but the treatment of these infections, mostly secondary, belongs to the domain of surgery. Scrofulous and all other tuberculous manifestations in childhood, if they do or do not demand surgical interference, must be treated by hygiene, aëro- and hydrotherapy, judicious dieting, and medicinal treatment. All these therapeutic methods are virtually the same for children as those outlined for adults. Seaside sanatoria are particularly well adapted to cope with tuberculosis in childhood. Brine baths, cold or hot, which are such a valuable adjuvant in the treatment of scrofulous and tuberculous diseases in children, should be more universally used in children's hospitals, and in the homes where there are children suffering from such diseases.

Education, Discipline, and Marriage Relations.

The first point in the education of a patient is, of course, the instruction concerning the care of the expectoration, of which we have spoken in detail in the preceding pages. Next in importance comes teaching him how to avoid taking cold. Consumptives should be particularly careful not to face the wind when taking breathing or walking exercises, and should always keep their mouths closed. When taking the rest cure on reclining-chairs out on the veranda, they should avoid much conversing on cold and windy days. In a sanatorium gradated walks and the distribution of numbered benches will make the method of carefully testing one's strength from day to day especially interesting. The consumptive should never start out with a determination that he must reach a certain spot. Over-exertion is to be feared. The pulmonary invalid must, more than any other, be careful not to get in a perspiration through exercise; he should stop before he is tired, and learn from day to day what he can do and what he cannot do. Should he, in spite of these precautions, begin to perspire freely during one of his daily walks, he should not sit down and rest to cool off, but return home at once, without any increased speed, however, ask to be rubbed off, and go to bed. A hot lemonade or grog is administered, and the doctor notified. If the patient has perspired but slightly, he should at least enter the house after his excursion and change his under-garments. In all well-equipped sanatoria special accommodations for this purpose are established. Carrying out rigorously all the instructions concerning the prevention of taking cold will save many an intercurrent bronchitis, or pleuritis, or even pneumonia. Patients often take cold and the cause escapes the most careful attention until it is discovered that they are in the habit of rising at night in the cool room, bathed in perspiration, in order to urinate. I always insist that such invalids have a urinal placed near their bed, of which they can make use without uncovering themselves. Or, again, the patient takes cold by uncovering himself during the act of expectorating. As a rule, he raises himself for that purpose to a sitting posture, leaning over, and thus the cold air of the room strikes the whole thorax. To avoid this I tell my patients to place their pocket-flask under their pillow at night. If the necessity of its use arises, the act of expectorating in the pocket-spittoon can then be done with little inconvenience, and without there being a necessity of uncovering themselves.

Some patients have, before entering the institution or submitting themselves to treatment, acquired bad habits which are often the cause of taking colds. One of them, not common to the fairer sex alone, is that of spending half an hour or more every morning in a cool bedroom, half dressed, to complete their toilet. Ladies will sometimes sit for hours scantily dressed in their cool bedrooms, just to do a little mending. All such habits must be stopped; also reading in bed at night. Patients should not leave the house before sunrise, and they should always remain within doors during the hour of sunset, especially in localities where that phenomenon is accompanied by a rapid saturation of the atmosphere (Riviera, Southern California, etc.). Tuberculous patients should have at least nine hours' sleep in the twenty-four. Ambulant patients, who are often either unable or unwilling to give up their usual vocation, and thus do not get their full nine hours' sleep, should remain in bed all Sunday morning in order to get thoroughly rested.

Light occupations or distractions, quiet drives not lasting too long, reading, writing, unexciting games, and music should be allowed the patient. Little writing-desks, which can be attached to the reclining-chair, make reading and writing especially convenient during the rest cure in the open air, and prevent the patient from bending over. Ladies should not be allowed to do fancy work which necessitates leaning over. I make it a rule to control, in a measure, whenever it is possible, what books the patients read. Feverish patients should not read exciting literature. Quiet entertainments, musicales, and, if possible, an open-air performance, instructive lectures on hygiene in general, and especially on the hygiene of the tuberculous patients, and the mode of life of the cured consumptive, etc., should form the pleasant features of sanatorium life.

The patient's tastes and inclinations, so long as they do not conflict with his own welfare or that of the other inmates of the institution, should be indulged. Large establishments should facilitate holding religious services of the various denominations, so that religiously inclined people should not miss what may be dear and needful to them. All that tends to make the patient happy and cheerful should be permitted; all that is cheerless and depressing should be banished from his surroundings. Some pulmonary invalids cannot bear the idea of entering a sanatorium; they fear the association, and others fear the discipline. From my experience as assistant physician at Falkenstein, and from many conversations which I have had with the inmates of sanatoria, who had come from all classes of society and from many different countries, I learned that each soon became so interested in his own case that he forgot all trifles, and the attention bestowed upon him by the physician and his assistants made him feel that everything in the sanatorium was done to make him comfortable, and to hasten his restoration to health. This feeling predominates over all others, and the new arrival usually soon accommodates himself to his environments.

Now as to that much-feared word, discipline, in sanatoria for consumptives. The whole thing consists in the good will and the earnest determination on the part of the patient to follow the rules of the house, which have been created in his interest, and to obey the counsel and carry out the prescriptions of his physician; and, on the part of the physician, a never-failing kindness, combined with an unmoved firmness when occasion demands.

The doctor's advice will and should be sought in many of the most secret family matters—in all the subjects of sexual relation, marriage, childbirth, nursing the infant, etc.—and it is the duty of the true modern phthisiotherapeutist to enlighten his patient on these vital issues, whether consulted about them especially or **not.**

At times a rise of temperature will be observed in spite of the patient's assurance that the physical and mental rest has been observed. The increased pyretic state may then find its explanation in an over-indulgence in sexual pleasures, which a tuberculous invalid should exercise only at the rarest intervals.

Some tuberculous women suffer, at the time of their monthly period, from pulmonary congestion and hæmoptysis. To these, absolute rest, beginning three or four days before and lasting throughout the period, should be the rule. Daremberg recommends, in addition, a mustard plaster over the lower abdomen, and gives some bromide with digitalis to quiet the pulmonary condition.

As a rule, the tuberculous patient should not marry; but I have no hesitation in giving my consent to marriage when the patient has been cured, or, since some authorities do not accept this word in the *ad integrum* sense, if he has remained in good health for two successive years. He should, however, be impressed with the importance of living a quiet, regular life, free from excesses of any kind. There are times, however, when we must deviate from the iron rule not to allow a tuberculous patient to marry. If we are in the presence of a young, highly impressionable woman in the first stages of pulmonary tuberculosis, who is engaged to be married, it would be cruel and unwise to put a stop to the union; the consequent sorrow brought upon this young woman would simply mean hastening a fatal termination of her disease, while, as a happily married woman, she has a fair chance of getting well. This is one of the few instances in the practice of medicine in which it becomes the duty of the physician to tell the husband that, if his wife becomes pregnant before her complete recovery, it means danger to her and to the child, and the husband should be instructed to that effect.

When, nevertheless, a tuberculous woman has become pregnant, should we interfere with a view of saving the woman's life? To judge from what I have seen in the large maternity hospitals of the Old and the New World, and from my own personal experience, such procedures are, in the light of our present knowledge, no longer justified.

Tarnier,[192] Hergot, Gaulard,[193] and others have, in accidental or induced abortions, seen the mother's tuberculous disease take, nevertheless, the rapid course so frequently observed after an apparent improvement in cases which go to full term. During my visit to the various sanatoria,[194] I inquired into the results obtained by the hygienic and dietetic treatment in these institutions with pregnant tuberculous women. Dettweiler, Meissen, Wolff, Roempler, Turban, and Trudeau had observed cases in which the patients did remarkably well for years after, as also did their children. Sabourin, Achtermann, and Weicker, on the other hand, had only observed an apparently much improved state before the birth of the child, followed by a rapid decline after confinement. To summarize this important question we would say: Prevent conception in a tuberculous woman; if conception has taken place, institute hygienic and dietetic treatment, preferably in a sanatorium near the home of the patient. But, as Trudeau says, it is essential that the treatment be continued for a long time afterward; and I should like to add that a repetition of pregnancy must be prevented. Never bring about abortion, for it does not save the life of a tuberculous mother.

It goes without saying that a tuberculous mother should not nurse her child. A child whose father or mother is, or has been, phthisical should be, from its very earliest age, surrounded by the best hygiene. Especial care should be given to its nutrition. A healthy wet-nurse would, of course, be the best guaranty for the child's normal development. If the procuring of a healthy fostermother is impossible, sterilized cow's-milk, carefully diluted with boiled water, etc., must constitute the child's food.

The treatment of tuberculosis in the private home by the family physician should be educational and prophylactic in the broadest sense of the word. It is the family physician who will see the incipient cases first; it is he who will discover a predisposition to phthisis when a wise and judicious treatment will save the patient and instructions to the other members of the family prevent them from acquiring the disease. The intimate relation which exists between the family physician and all the members of the family give him superiority even over the sanatorium physician. The latter can help only the patient placed under his care, while the family physician can at the same time prevent the breaking out of tuberculosis among the other members of the family.

All offspring of tuberculous parents should choose out-door occupations by which to earn their livelihood, and live and work in places where they are as little as possible exposed to the inhalation of dust and other irritating substances. The cured or ameliorated patient, upon his return home, should lead a very regular life. He should avoid crowded assemblies and violent physical exercises; in short, use his experience and training while sick as a guide to keep well.

Hypurgy.

Hypurgy is a word derived from the Greek ὑπουργεῖν, which means to make use of adjuvants. It was used in the early works of Hippocrates,[195] and has recently been adopted by Mendelsohn,[196] to show the difference between the services rendered by the nurse to the patient (Krankenwartung) and the services rendered by the physician —not by the administration of medicinal substances, but by the scientific application of the various therapeutic agents, such as hygiene, diet, comfort, rest, exercise, etc., which may help the patient on to recovery (Krankenpflege).

There is no occasion in which hypurgy must be more thoroughly studied than in connection with phthisiotherapy. First of all, the physician must know how to occupy his patient all day with something which has the cure of the disease for its definite object—at this hour his meals, at that his rest cure, at this his respiratory exercises, at this his sunbath, at that his walk, at another his douche, etc., etc. In private practice a leaflet of instruction should be left each day with the nurse or the patient himself.

The peculiarities of each patient should be studied. In no other disease does the temperament differ so much as among phthisical patients. I have found many overcareful, others criminally careless, some sanguine, some morose, some hopeful one day and deeply depressed the next, some always indifferent, and so on. To those who are very depressed and doubt the possibility of a cure, the physician should hold out living examples of cured tuberculous patients.

Modern phthisiotherapeutics must be practically studied, and the place to study it best is undoubtedly the sanatorium or special hospital. The custom, recently instituted by Curschmann, of Leipzig, and Penzoldt, of Erlangen,[197] of making excursions with their students to neighboring sanatoria as a practical demonstration of their lectures on phthisiotherapeutics, seems to me well worth imitating. There is much to be seen in such institutions which will be of value to the young practitioner.

Nurses who undertake to help the physician in his care of the consumptive invalid should be physically strong and of a cheerful disposition, and also especially prepared for this kind of work. Nurses' training-schools might advantageously be attached to some of the larger sanatoria.

Chronic pulmonary consumption is not an easy disease to treat. It requires not only a thorough knowledge of the etiology, pathology, and therapy, and a familiarity with all the symptoms of the disease, but also a great deal of devotion and patience, combined with great strength of character. The peculiar psychological state of nearly all phthisical patients, we repeat once more, makes it necessary for the true phthisiotherapeutist, not only to be to his patient a devoted physician, but also his best and most confidential friend.

Treatment by Culture Products.

In the chapter on early diagnosis I have stated my views in regard to the use of tuberculin as a means of discovering pulmonary tuberculosis. Regarding its employment as a curative means I am also of the opinion that it is a dangerous drug and capable of doing more harm than good. I know that in some sanatoria and special hospitals small doses of tuberculin, much smaller than formerly recommended by Koch, are continually used as a curative agent, and good success reported, especially in the early cases. But may we not ascribe these good results just as much to the hygienic, dietetic, and symptomatic treatment so rigorously adhered to in these institutions, where such good results were obtained before tuberculin was ever used? At any rate, the results published by institutions using culture products as curative means are not better than those which refrain from the use of tuberculin as a therapeutic agent. There are numerous general practitioners, and among them such men as Whittaker,[198] of Cincinnati, Spengler,[199] of Davos, Barton,[200] of New York, who still believe in the curative power of this culture-product. But do not these distinguished practitioners also in their private practice insist upon the very best hygiene and diet for their tuberculous patients?

Specialists in cutaneous diseases have reported cases in which tuberculin has favorably modified the growth of lupus, and others in which the injections did not stop the growth.

What has just been said of Koch's first tuberculin as a curative agent we may say of all its modifications. The tuberculocidin and its child, the antiphthisin of Klebs; the tuberculinum purificatum of von Ruck, Whitman's purified tuberculin, Hirschfelder's oxytuberculin, Koch's new tuberculin R,—all, in the hands of some experimenters, have produced satisfactory results. I do not wish to speak of their respective merits, but from what I have seen, heard, and read, I may summarize their reported curative effects by saying of them collectively: Whenever a new culture-product is discovered, and through experiments on the guinea-pigs is shown to have a specific antituberculous action, it is usually recommended with the following restrictions: It is not to be used in advanced cases, in mixed affections, or as an exclusive remedy, but always in connection with the best of hygiene and the best of diet, and the symptomatic treatment must not be neglected. And the results of the treatment read about as follows: A large percentage of incipient cases have been cured; a small percentage of advanced cases have been benefited; a still smaller percentage have remained indifferent to the treatment; and a very small percentage have died.

Cannot any one, private practitioner or sanatorium physician, report just as good and even better results whenever the hygienic, dietetic, symptomatic, and educational treatment has been carried out conscientiously without the aid of any specific or antibacillary remedies?

Of the serums of Maragliano, Paquin, and others, we can only say the same, though I am glad to acknowledge that I have not yet seen any real ill effect from their employment in tuberculosis. I cannot say this of tuberculin.

Whether or not other bacteriotherapeutists will offer us that long-hoped-for remedy which will cure tuberculosis with a degree of certainty, so that the name specific may be justified, I am not prepared to say. But it seems to me difficult to believe that we will ever have a serum or tuberculin which, in a few weeks, even with numerous injections, will be able to produce enough fibrous connective tissue to strangle countless tubercles which it took years to form, or to create enough phagocytic blood-corpuscles to swallow myriads of bacilli. We may employ serum treatment in acute exacerbations, due to an association of microbes, but to heal a tuberculous lesion we must produce new tissue, new and better blood. How this may best be done I have endeavored to outline in the preceding pages. Even should the future give us a bactericidal substance strong enough to annihilate, without hurting the patient, all the tubercle bacilli which may have invaded him, the hygienic and dietetic treatment in sanatoria or under good medical supervision at home, and in a fairly good climate, where the extremes of temperature are not too pronounced, and the air is relatively free from pathogenic organisms or irritating substances, will still remain the only rational method to build up his much-weakened system and to protect him from intercurrent diseases and possible relapses.

Climatotherapy, Health Resorts, and Sports.

There is hardly any subject on which more has been written than on the climatotherapy of pulmonary tuberculosis. There is yet a vast diversity of opinion as to the respective merits of what are still sometimes called specific climates for consumptives; but the number of phthisiotherapeutists who consider even the best and most suitable climate of secondary importance, and the hygienic and dietetic treatment, preferably in a closed establishment, or under constant medical supervision in congenial surroundings, the all-important fact, is constantly increasing. I do not deny the beneficial influence of certain climatic conditions on the various forms of phthisis; but, with all deference to the opinion of others, I do not believe that there exists any climate with a specific curative quality for any form of pulmonary tuberculosis. Climate can be considered only a more or less valuable adjuvant in the treatment of consumption, but not a specific. A tuberculous patient of the irritable pyrexial type, with much tendency to nasal and bronchial catarrhs, will often do better in a warm climate with little elevation, such as Southern California, Southern Arizona, New Mexico, Western Texas, Florida, etc., in the United States; Jersey and Sidmouth in England; Pau and Hyères in France; San Remo in Italy, etc.

To higher altitudes, such, for example, as Davos and St. Moritz-dorf in Switzerland, or the mountains of Colorado, Montana, Utah, and Wyoming in the United States, may safely be sent early cases with no throat complications, those with chests badly developed either by transmission of a phthisical predisposition or fault of development, and all ordinary cases of phthisis. They are most likely to be benefited in such climates.

Sir Hermann Weber, of London, whose vast experience in phthisio- and climatotherapy makes him perhaps the greatest living authority on the question, objects to high altitudes when the patients must be classed with one of the following ten types: (1) Consumptive persons belonging to the erethic class, whether the affection is early or advanced; (2) phthisis in a very advanced stage; (3) phthisis complicated with extensive emphysema; (4) phthisis complicated with albuminuria; (5) phthisis complicated with disease of the heart; (6) phthisis with ulceration of the larynx; (7) phthisis with rapid progress and constant pyrexia; (8) phthisis with great loss of substance; (9) phthisis with considerable empyema; (10) phthisis in persons who cannot sleep or eat at high elevations, or who feel constantly cold.

In his recent address before the Tuberculosis Congress at Berlin,[201] he elaborated his classification, giving the following indications as to choice of climate for pulmonary invalids:

1· In cases with limited disease at one or both apices, without or with only a slight amount of fever, nearly all climates can be made use of, but especially high altitudes and sea voyages, if the constitution is a strong one.

2. Cases with limited local disease and high fever must be at first treated in their houses or immediate neighborhood.

3. In the majority of cases with extensive disease of one or both lungs, without fever or only slight fever, treatment at only a moderate elevation, or at warm seaside localities, deserves the preference.

4. In advanced disease with fever, neighboring sheltered health-resorts, with careful supervision, should be recommended.

5. In cases of progressive tuberculosis, with scattered foci in both lungs and much fever, localities near home, or the home itself, are the best places.

6. In cases of chronic, slowly progressive phthisis better results are obtained from warm winter resorts, or sometimes from sea voyages.

7. Quiescent cases with extensive damage or cicatrization, are generally better off at only slight elevations.

8. Cases with albuminuria, without fever, should avoid high altitudes.

9. The complication of moderate diabetes does not exclude high altitudes, but the latter are injurious in cases with advanced diabetes and emaciation.

10. Chronic cases, with much catarrh, require places with as little wind as possible.

11. High altitudes are contraindicated in chronic cases with extensive emphysema.

12. For the prevention of scrofula and tuberculosis all healthful climates can be used, but high altitudes have advantages against tuberculosis, and marine climates (including sea voyages) more against scrofula.

13. The cure of tuberculosis during the early stages is possible in all climates. But climate itself, without careful medical supervision, is generally insufficient. The patient's blind reliance on the climate often leads to errors, to aggravation of the disease, and to death.

As an intermediate altitude of between two and three thousand feet, Fletcher Ingals recommends some portions of Dakota, Nebraska, Minnesota, the Adirondack Mountains, and those of Virginia, North Carolina, and Tennessee, as especially suitable for phthisical patients in summer. As typical winter climates he mentions Arizona, Southern California (among the foot-hills as far as possible from the ocean), Southern New Mexico, South Carolina, Georgia, and Texas.

Besides this selection of climates to suit the respective forms of pulmonary phthisis, there are to be considered what I should call climatic idiosyncrasies among tuberculous patients. Of two patients with seemingly the same temperament and at about the same stage of the disease, one feels best and makes most rapid road to recovery in one of the Mediterranean places or Southern California; while the other, who had also been sent to such places, apparently would have died had he not left there in time and gone to Davos, or Colorado, or some other resort of high altitude. I know of patients who got well at the Adirondacks and felt badly at Liberty, and *vice versa*; both places are in the State of New York, and their climatic conditions differ very little. Some patients do well in island and coast climates; others improve greatly on a sea-voyage. While it may be safely said that in the majority of cases any climatic change will do good, too much travel should be discouraged. To send a patient away from home in the advanced stage of phthisis has always seemed to me cruel and useless; it nearly always hastens a fatal termination, which is the sadder since it takes place among strangers and away from home. Those desiring to benefit by climatic changes should travel to warmer climates in the fall, and to colder ones in the spring; thus the acclimatization of the consumptive invalid will be more easily accomplished.

As to the choice of a warmer or colder clime for a cure, Fletcher Ingals[202] may be right in saying that patients who feel better in cold weather should be sent to a comparatively cold climate; those feeling better in summer, to warmer regions. But, in spite of excellent works in phthisio-climato-therapy, such as Weber's,[203] de la Harpe's,[204] Lindley's,[205] and Solly's,[206] our present knowledge of the subject is still limited, and opinions as to the best method of classifying climates as to their respective merits in phthisiotherapy differ vastly. If I were asked to express an opinion on the subject, I would say the best climate for a consumptive is the one where the aërotherapeutic portion of the hygienic and dietetic treatment, as understood to-day by the modern phthisiotherapeutists, can be carried out most easily and most persistently; or, in other words, the best climate for a consumptive is the one which permits him to remain out-doors more and longer at a time than anywhere else. But since an ideal climate cannot be obtained everywhere, and will not be within the reach of everybody, the best thing to do is to get as near these conditions as possible, and preferably at not too great a distance from home. Places where pure, dry atmosphere and some elevation, with protection from winds, can be had, abound more or less in all countries. I cannot conclude this short review of the existing opinions on climatotherapy in regard to pulmonary tuberculosis without mentioning a most important fact which has been very little regarded up to this date in our text-books on climatology. I refer to the relative durability of cures obtained in different climes. I know from personal observation of a number of cases that cures of pulmonary tuberculosis effected in our home climates, which are, in general, not considered as especially favorable to this class of suferers, have been more lasting and more assured than cures obtained in more genial climes away from home.   In these observations I do not stand alone, for such men as von Leyden, Gerhardt, von Ziemssen, Dettweiler, Naunyn, Frankel, and Walthers[207] have had the same experience.

There is another point which seems to me well worth considering in choosing a climate for a lengthy sojourn of a pulmonary invalid.   I have observed that the average pulmonary patient, after he has passed the incipient state of tuberculosis, often does better at a moderate elevation below three thousand feet, or even in our lowlands, when under judicious treatment and constant medical supervision, than in regions of very high altitude under the same conditions.   Why this should be so, may perhaps be explained by the fact that in very high altitudes the respiratory act is more frequent.   There is a greater task put upon the muscles of inspiration and expiration, and the additional work must be performed by that portion of the lung tissue which is not yet involved by the solidifying process of tuberculous infiltration.   In patients in whom the infiltration occupies a considerable area, emphysema of the still sound portion of the lungs may result, causing often great discomfort to the patient, and retarding recovery.

In view of the facts that consumption is a disease of all climes, and that the majority of tuberculous patients come from the poorer classes who can ill afford extensive trips to, or long sojourns in, other regions, the experiences relating to the possibility and durability of cures in ordinary climates are certainly reassuring.   But all patients who can afford to seek other climes should be warned that climate alone will never cure.

In health resorts, no matter how beautiful the climate, if the patients are at liberty to do as they please, I affirm that all attempts at an effective cure are an illusion.   In the great health resorts of the Riviera I have seen any number of consumptives promenading in the close, dusty air of the casinos, gambling, smoking, expectorating everywhere. At the *table d'hôte* they usually eat little or that which is not good for them. Now and then they see a physician whose directions they carry out only so far as does not incommode them. Sometimes they do not even go to consult a doctor, but have some of the countless prescriptions filled of which they brought a supply from home. After a while, feeling no better, they leave, disgusted with the climate that has done them no good, and blame the physician who sent them there.

In the next resort the same thing is repeated, or they go to the mountains for a change. In some cases, by the change of climate and out-door life, they really get better. They will then feel themselves privileged to make long excursions, climb mountains, or in winter skate, ride toboggans, or race on snow shoes. How dangerous such sports are for the phthisical patient, even if on the road to recovery, is well known.

In our American resorts, such as Southern California, Florida, etc., the tuberculous invalid is perhaps less bent on pleasure than the consumptive visitor to the European health resorts, but he is more inclined to business. How often (in Southern California) have I observed the newly arrived guest, after a few weeks' sojourn, plunge into business, especially exciting real estate and other speculations. It is self-evident that under such conditions a cure cannot be hoped for in a disease in which the avoidance of mental and physical excitements is of paramount importance. Any occupation or sport which demands of the pulmonary invalid frequent stooping down, should be considered injurious. Bowling should be prohibited for several reasons: first, it demands stooping; second, it demands a considerable one-sided effort; third, it is an in-door occupation; fourth, there is too much dust raised, the inhalation of which must be injurious to the already irritated respiratory organs.

Bicycling is now quite frequently indulged in in health resorts by tuberculous patients in the earlier stages, and especially by persons as yet only predisposed. Many physicians recommend it as the best means of preventing the outbreak of tuberculosis in the predisposed individual. Now, while fully realizing its valuable therapeutic effects in many other diseases, I consider the bicycle ill-adapted either to the cure or the prevention of pulmonary tuberculosis. There are two great dangers connected with the use of the bicycle for any one whose lungs are already affected or in danger of becoming so. One is the tendency to overdo, the other the danger of taking cold. The excess of muscular exertion results in an unhealthful waste of tissue, which, in the tuberculous individual, is replaced with more difficulty than in others. Bouchard, of Paris, has repeatedly demonstrated that an excess of waste products renders an individual more liable to succumb to infectious diseases, especially tuberculosis. Persons predisposed to this disease often have a rather feeble heart action, and such are, of course, in great danger if they put too much strain upon the heart. Mendelsohn[208] cites several cases of sudden death from this cause. The bent-over attitude is especially injurious to pulmonary invalids. Any one who has practised cycling himself must acknowledge how easily and imperceptibly one overtaxes his powers, and how almost unawares one gets in a profuse perspiration. One is then liable to become quickly chilled when stopping to rest or cool off, or if obliged to stop to fix something about the wheel. Herein lies the second danger to persons who have reason to be especially careful to avoid nasal and bronchial catarrhs, which, in the consumptive or the predisposed, have such an unfortunate tendency to descend into the deeper air passages. Lastly, the nervous strain which all novices undergo while learning to ride I cannot help considering injurious to a relatively weakened or weak constitution. If cycling must be done, I consider the tricycle or four-wheeled vehicle propelled by some easily managed motor, as recommended by Gihon,[209] the safer machine for the pulmonary invalid.

As I stated above, the strict supervision of the phthisical patient in an open health resort is very difficult. Unless the patient is exceptionally situated and very prudent, he has little chance to be benefited in such a place. If, on the other hand, the patient is a convalescent, and has been taught by his physician or in the sanatorium how he should live with a view of getting well, the health resort may well offer him an opportunity to complete his cure.

Freny[210] considers these open health resorts also good places for the scrofulous and the predisposed to consumption; but it seems to me essential that any one, even if only predisposed to tuberculosis, should always subject himself to the guidance of a physician in an open resort, as well as at home. Many an intercurrent trouble may thereby be avoided.

Of the importance of rigorous regulations to prevent the promiscuous expectorating of invalids visiting health resorts, we have already spoken in our paragraph on public prophylaxis. In some States of the Union most frequented by tuberculous patients, there exists a popular feeling that with the influx of pulmonary invalids there is a danger of consumption becoming "endemic." In California, for example, an attempt was made to restrict the immigration of consumptives into that State by legislative procedures. This Draconian measure to settle the question of prophylaxis of tuberculosis was fortunately not carried into effect. Education, judicious and strictly enforced laws, and the multiple creation of sanatoria, especially for the poorer classes, will achieve far more towards the protection of the inhabitants from tuberculosis in such regions. With universal sanitary laws, rigorously enforced, the convalescent or incipient tuberculous patient may go to these resorts, place himself under the care of an experienced phthisiotherapeutist (and there are many in most of these places in Europe and in the United States), and complete his cure under the guidance of his new medical adviser.

At the conclusion of the subject on climatology, it might perhaps not be inappropriate to say a word of the value of pine forests in the treatment of pulmonary affections. Pliny the elder (73-23 B.C.) ascribed a most beneficial action to the air of pine forests in the treatment of phthisis; and ever since there have been physicians in all centuries, who have advised their tuberculous patients to live near the pine forests, and frequent them as much as possible. The majority of German sanatoria for consumptives are built in the midst of or near pine woods. There is no doubt that besides being beneficial to pulmonary diseases these woods improve the sanitary condition of any region, and offer resorts of great value for the care of other diseases, such as local tuberculosis, neurasthenia, general debility, gastric disturbances, etc. The wanton destruction of pine forests in many sections of the United States is therefore deeply to be regretted; and statesmen, sanitarians, physicians, and the people at large should unite in an effort to preserve and cultivate pine forests throughout the country.

PROGNOSIS.

Pathological Proofs of the Curability of Pulmonary Tuberculosis.— Carswell[211] wrote in 1838: "Pathological anatomy has perhaps never afforded more conclusive evidence in proof of the curability of a disease than it has in that of tubercular phthisis." These words from one of the foremost pathologists of his time may be recalled to doubters in the profession as an evidence of how wrong they are in their pessimistic conception of a disease which is eminently curable. By personal inquiry, through letters addressed to the leading pathologists of the world, and by looking up the literature on the subject, I have myself compiled some statistics giving the pathological proofs of the curability of pulmonary tuberculosis, from which I have compiled the table on the following page.

Besides the above, Andral, Meckel, Rokitansky, Ulsperger, Virchow, and Werthmüller[213] have reported cases of healed tuberculous lesions in persons who had died of other than tuberculous diseases.

Laennec[214] believed in the curability of pulmonary tuberculosis. Cruveilhier[215] declares tuberculosis a decidedly curable disease, and so does Charcot,[216] saying: "Phthisis is susceptible to be cured completely and definitely even at the period of cavities." Grancher[217] says: "We affirm the curability of the tubercle; we affirm that, instead of being a miserable neoplasm incapable of organization, the tubercle naturally tends to fibrous formation."

Reported by—	Number of autopsies.	Number of cases in which autopsy revealed healed pulmonary tuberculous lesions.
Boudet, of Paris	135	116
Beaux, of Paris	166	157
Bennet, of Mentone	73	28
Baudet, of Paris	197	10
Marsini, of Basle	228	89
Bollinger, of Munich	400	69
Heitler, of Vienna	16,562	789
Chiari, of Prague	701	78
Flint, of New York	670	75
Loomis,[212] of New York	763	71
Letulle, of Paris	189	92
F. P. Weber, of London	....	29
Ormeroth, of London	....	50
Vilbert, of Paris	131	17
Fowler, of London	1,943	177
Martin, of London	445	42
Joseph Coats, of Glasgow	103	25
Rogée, of Paris	....	51 per cent.
Standacher	....	27 "
Thomas Harris, of London	....	39 "
Fürbringer, of Berlin	....	10 "
Renvers, of Berlin	....	30 "
Birch-Hirschfeld	....	12 "
Bugge, of Christiania	....	27 "
Osler, of Baltimore	....	7.5 "
Walker, of Chicago	....	4 "
H. M. Biggs, of New York	....	30 "

Clinical Proofs.—Of eminent men known in history, who in their early youth or manhood were declared to be phthisical and who attained relatively old age, may be mentioned the German poet Goethe, Napoleon I., and our own Peter Cooper. Dr. Hermann Brehmer was a consumptive when he started the first sanatorium for tuberculous patients in 1859, over which he presided for more than thirty years with great success. His most celebrated pupil, Dr. Dettweiler, entered his sanatorium as a consumptive, became Brehmer's assistant, and has since been for twenty-five years active as the medical director of the Falkenstein sanatorium. The late Dr. Péan, of Paris, who died at the age of sixty-five, was declared phthisical when twenty. These are but a few examples of well-known cases.

There is no doubt that every practitioner who has had consumptives under his care can report some successful cures. But there is also no doubt that the clinical evidences of the curability of tuberculosis show a far greater number of cases cured by the hygienic and dietetic treatment in special institutions than by any other method.

I append here the statistics obtained in sanatoria for poor as well as for paying patients. I will first give an interesting table compiled by Manasse,[218] covering 5,032 patients who passed through Brehmer's Sanatorium in Goerbersdorf, Germany, during the years 1876-86.

Stage of the disease.	Number of patients.	Cured.	Almost cured.	Cured and almost cured.
First	1,390 (27.62%)	387 (27.8 %)	430 (31.0%)	817 (58.8 %)
Second	2,225 (44.21%)	152 (6.83%)	325 (14.6%)	477 (21.48%)
Third.......	1,417 (28.17%)	12 (0.48%)	33 (2.3%)	45 (3.14%)
	5,032	551 (11%)	788 (15.6%)	1,339 (26.6 %)

The following statistics, with the exception of the last six numbers, were collected by myself, Nos. 18, 19, and 20 were reported by Dr. Beaulavon[219]; Nos. 21, 22, and 23 I have taken from Hohe's recent statistics.[220]

Name of Sanatorium.	Reported by—	Mortality, per cent.	Cures, per cent.		Improved, per cent.
			Absolute.	Relative.	
1. Falkenstein, Germany.	Dr. Dettweiler..	4–4.5	14	14	45
2. Hohenhonnef, Germany....	Dr. Meissen	....	14.5	28.9	
3. Ruppertshain, Germany...........	Dr. Nahm........	....	13	....	77
4. Muskoka Cottage Sanatorium, Canada......................	Dr. Elliott	15	16	25	33
5. Sharon, Mass., U. S. A , ...	Dr. Bowditch. .	....	Arrested cases. 25		
6. Goerbersdorf Sanatorium, Germany, Brehmer	Dr. Achtermann..	7.51	Cures. 25		50.55
7. Goerbersdorf Sanatorium, Germany, Roempler	Dr. Roempler. .	7.5	25–27		50
8. Goerbersdorf Sanatorium, Germany, Pückler	Dr Weicker	4	....		72
9. Reiboldsgrun, Germany..	Dr. Wolff.........	2.5	....		70.72
10 Davos, Switzerland....	Dr. Turban	4.36	40		40
11. Nordrach, Germany	Dr. Walther .. .	....	30		65
12. Halila, Finland	Dr. Gabrilowitch .	13.5	36.7		33
13. Canigou, France	Dr. Sabourin......	....	43.8		
14. Adirondack Cottage Sanitarium. Saranac, N. Y.....	Dr. Trudeau.....	....	20–25		30–35
15. Loomis Sanitarium, Liberty, N. Y.	Dr. Stubbert	....	25		50
16. Chestnut Hill, Pa	Drs. Cohen a n d Bacon	17.33	8		11.5
17. Winyah, Asheville, N. C............	Dr. von Ruck..	4	26.64		42.47
18. Leysin, Switzerland.	Dr Burnier... ..	17.2	11.3		58.2
19. Rehburg, Germany	Dr. Thornspecken..	28	40		32
20. Ventnor, England	Dr. Coghill..	8.5	16.4		65.4
21. Haufe Sanatorium, St Blasien . .	Dr. Sander	....	Much improved. 17		67
22. Schömberg, Germany	Dr. Baudach......	....	....		82.9
23. Malchow b Berlin, Germany	Dr. Reuter	....	43		40

I will add that the sanatoria at Ruppertshain, Malchow, Chestnut Hill, and Halila are for the poor. In the Adirondack and the Loomis sanatoria, at Sharon, at Muskoka, and at Ventnor the patients pay part of the expense. At the Adirondack, Ruppertshain, and Muskoka sanatoria advanced cases, as a rule, are not admitted. At the Chestnut Hill Hospital for Consumptives (Philadelphia) all cases, no matter how far advanced, are received. To distinguish between the terms absolute and relative cure, I will give Dettweiler's definition. He calls absolutely cured the re-establishment of the normal functions of all the organs and the complete disappearance of the bacillus. He calls a person relatively cured when his general well-being has reappeared in spite of regular coughing-spells with some expectoration in the morning.

We may ask how long these reported cures have lasted. Among 99 patients discharged from Falkenstein as cured 72 were alive and well at the time the inquiry was made, which was after the patients had left the sanatorium from three to nine years. In 15 cases a relapse had occurred, but 12 of these patients had improved again; 12 had died.[221] Dr. von Ruck, of Asheville, has told me that he had written to 605 of his former patients who had left the sanatorium from one to three years before; 457 responded, directly or through friends. Of these, 67 felt absolutely cured; 70 felt relatively cured; 258 felt still improved; 62 were worse or had died.

E. R. Baldwin, of Saranac Lake, reported at a recent meeting of the American Climatological Association[222] that at the Adirondack Cottage Sanitarium they were in constant correspondence with 115 patients who had been discharged in the last ten or twelve years; and while a few had relapsed slightly, the majority of them were well and at their homes.

The clinical evidences of the curability of tuberculosis and of scrofulous diseases in childhood, by the hygienic and dietetic treatment in seaside sanatoria, aided by modern surgical attainments, are equally surprising. The seaside sanatoria for scrofulous and tuberculous children of Belgium and France report from 70 to 80 per cent. of cures; those of Germany 50 per cent., and those of Italy 35 per cent. The less good results in Italy seem to be explained by the fact that rachitic diseases predominate in these institutions.

From the preceding statistics it will be seen that the prognosis of tuberculosis cannot and should not be considered anything but favorable, especially in the pulmonary form, of which we will speak first. Leaving aside cases in the last stages of the disease, the prognosis will always depend upon many factors besides the extent of the lesions,

The question will often arise, especially in somewhat advanced cases, whether a definite opinion should be given to the friends or relatives of the patient, and whether or not he should be told his true condition. There is hardly a disease in the world of which, except in the last stages, it is more difficult to give a definite prognosis than of pulmonary tuberculosis. Any one who has had a number of tuberculous patients under his observation will agree with me when I say that there are cases in which, to judge from a careful physical examination, the best hopes of recovery should be held out to the patient; and still he rapidly declines and sometimes unexpectedly dies. On the other hand, not infrequently patients surprise us. Their extensive pulmonary lesions left us not the least hope, and we may have told the friends of the apparently gloomy aspect of the case; and lo! some years later, one fine day, the patient presents himself at our office, if not cured in the *ad integrum* sense, at least to all outward appearances in perfect health.

Nor can our knowledge of bacteriology aid us much in this respect. On examining sputa from advanced cases one often finds a relatively small number of bacilli in the field of the microscope, while the examination of the expectorated product of a convalescent patient, or one with very limited pulmonary lesions, reveals sometimes enormous quantities of bacilli (No. 10, according to Gaffky's scale). This expectoration may have come from one single cough in days or weeks, and the sudden appearance of countless numbers of bacilli may have been due to the detachment of, perhaps, a very small focus of encysted tuberculous substance. The encystment of larger foci in a strong, fibrinous shell may explain the absence or very small number of bacilli in the sputa of apparently doomed patients. Again, the onset of an exacerbation, due to congestion in an old tuberculous case, is usually accompanied by a bronchorrhœa causing rapid dilution of the expectoration and a consequent diminution of the number of bacilli in the microscopic field.

I have found it good policy to be always most careful in making any positive declaration to the relatives or friends of the patient. A prognosis in a case of pulmonary phthisis does not depend only upon the condition of the patient's lungs, his power of digestion and assimilation, but it depends also upon his temperament, his social condition, and his means. I believe, in many cases Grancher's maxim, "le pronostic de la phtisie pulmonaire commune depend en effet du malade autant et plus que de la maladie" (the prognosis of ordinary pulmonary phthisis depends in reality as much and more on the patient than on the disease), is only too true. So I think the best thing to do is to tell the patient that the chances of his recovery depend upon his obedience in carrying out the treatment prescribed for him. If he is of a particularly melancholy disposition "suggestion therapy" will, of course, form an important factor in the management of the case. This will be especially needful when there is a consumptive family history, for, as I stated in the paragraph on the early diagnosis, I have learned how difficult it is to dissuade a patient from the preconceived idea that he has to die of consumption because some one in his family died of it. A cheerful disposition, a strong will, and a good stomach are essential points in favor of a good prognosis.

It seems to me that a good many physicians attach an unduly great value to early hemorrhage in their prognosis, interpreting it too often as an unfavorable symptom. I cannot enter into the discussion of the various types of hæmoptysis, but I wish to say that I firmly believe with Pidoux,[222] Grancher, Dieulafoy,[224] and others that there are cases of early pulmonary hemorrhages which are actually a benefit to the tuberculous patient, causing an elimination *en masse* of the bacilli, thus finally effecting a cure. All physicians who have treated a number of tuberculous patients have among their recovered cases some in which the first symptom which brought the patient to the physician was a hemorrhage of considerable magnitude. Even the cases in which the patients tell us that they have had several early hemorrhages, and that they felt better after each one, are not rare, and occasionally we have a chance to confirm a betterment in their condition through a physical examination after an attack of hæmoptysis. Of course, frequent hemorrhages, and especially if of considerable magnitude, during the latter course of the disease, must, as a rule, be considered as an unfortunate sign. Equally unfavorable in regard to prognosis should be considered an increased insomnia, dyspnœa, or an œdematous condition, a chronically rapid pulse, even without fever, and secondary complications such as tuberculous laryngitis, pharyngitis, nephritis, pericarditis, or severe intestinal and articular complications.

The return of the menses in a woman, when the suppression was due to the progress of the tuberculous disease, must be considered as a favorable symptom; and increase in weight, when concomitant with an improvement of the local pulmonary condition, is, of course, the most encouraging factor for a good prognosis. But increase in weight alone, and a stationary or even progressive pathological process of the lung tissue, a phenomenon which does occur occasionally, means rather the contrary to a favorable augury.

To the value of the diazo reactions[225] as a positive sign of an unfavorable prognosis, I should not wish to attach infallibility; however, we should resort to it in as many cases as possible and learn to suspend judgment in doubtful cases.

It is often asked how long it will take to cure a curable consumptive. This question is the most difficult to answer. Incipient pulmonary tuberculosis has been cured by hygienic and dietetic treatment under constant medical supervision, in sanatoria and at home, in three months. Moderately advanced cases have been cured in from six to twelve months; with some it has taken two years. The cases which can only be improved must be expected to remain under medical supervision more or less all the time.

The prognosis of primary laryngeal tuberculosis is, of course, a great deal better than that of secondary tuberculous laryngitis. The former, however, as has been stated, is extremely rare, and we must acknowledge the gravity of the majority of cases of tuberculous laryngitis. Still, I think, even in secondary laryngeal tuberculosis one is not justified in being too pessimistic. Grave as this complication is, by judicious hygienic, dietetic, climatic, and local treatment, life certainly has been prolonged and made comfortable in many cases. Even absolute cures become more and more frequent. Schmidt,[226] Besold,[227] Levy,[228] Chappell,[229] and others have reported cases of absolute cure. I myself have observed several apparent recoveries during my visits to the European sanatoria.

More hopeful than any of the serious complications, however, is a tuberculous peritonitis. Statistics recently given by Walter in the Harveian lectures,[230] state 50 per cent. recoveries in adults through laparotomy, and Herzfeld[231] reports 62 per cent. of recoveries (18 out of 29, including 7 children). The most gratifying prognosis of all we have certainly in the scrofulous and tuberculous diseases of childhood, if these little ones can be placed in time under judicious medical and surgical treatment in seaside sanatoria. As mentioned above from 50 to 75 per cent. can be restored to health.

Lastly, a word as to the prognosis in children of tuberculous parents. In view of our knowledge of the rarity of bacillary transmission, and our acquaintance with the means of preventing contamination from tuberculous parents, the prognosis concerning the offspring of tuberculous parentage should not be bad. While this statement should not be considered as an encouragement to the propagation of a race subject to tuberculosis, I must say that I have seen children from tuberculous parents grow up strong and healthy, thanks to the care and wisdom of the family physician and the good common sense of the parents. Of course, it must be stated that these families lived in excellent hygienic surroundings, and could afford for themselves and their children such comfort and care as is essential in the prevention of tuberculosis.

THE SOCIAL ASPECT OF ˙TUBERCULOSIS.

No disease has of late occupied the public mind as much as tuberculosis, especially in its pulmonary form. Physicians, sanitarians, statesmen, and philanthropists, all have contributed to arouse public interest, and to seek thus a co-operation with the people at large. Since 1888 there has convened in Paris every two years a congress devoted to the study of tuberculosis in all its aspects. In May, 1899, a ·most remarkable gathering of physicians, statesmén, and philanthropists took place in Berlin under the patronage of Her Majesty the Empress. All the civilized countries were represented and many interesting contributions were read—all for the same purpose, to combat tuberculosis as the "white plague" of the people (Volkskrankheit). Other congresses of smaller magnitude for the study of tuberculosis have since convened in this country and abroad. The deliberations of all these gatherings have resulted in the almost unanimous opinion that through the multiple creation of sanatoria, especially for the consumptive poor, the mortality from tuberculosis and the spread of the disease could most effectually be reduced.

In England special institutions for the consumptive poor were first inaugurated some fifty years ago. The following figures, which were kindly sent to me by the Registrar-General of London, show the result of these institutions as factors in the reduction of the mortality from tuberculosis in that country.

The death rate per million of the population of England and Wales from pulmonary tuberculosis—

In 1870 was	2,410	In 1893 was		1,468
" 1875 "	2,202	" 1894 "		1,385
" 1880 "	1,869	" 1895 "		1,398
" 1885 "	1,770	" 1896 "		1,307
" 1890 "	1,682			

The objections to the establishment of special institutions for consumptives need still to be overcome in some sections of this and other countries. That from the presence of properly conducted sanatoria for consumptives not the least danger can arise to the employees of the sanatorium, or to persons in the locality where such institutions may be placed, has often been demonstrated. At that excellent American institution, the Adirondack Cottage Sanitarium, at Saranac Lake, under the direction of Dr. E. L. Trudeau, not one of the nurses or medical attendants who have worked in it in the past fifteen years has ever contracted pulmonary tuberculosis. From the official statistics concerning the mortality from tuberculosis for forty and for one hundred years, respectively, before and after the establishment of sanatoria for consumptives in certain villages in Germany,[222] I will only summarize here by saying that in the two villages, Goerbersdorf and Falkenstein, where five of the largest sanatoria are situated, the mortality from tuberculosis has actually decreased among the village people more rapidly and more largely than anywhere else, it being now one-third less than before the establishment of these institutions. Thus we see that properly conducted sanatoria for consumptives not only serve as hygienic educators to individuals and families, but as instructors in hygiene to whole communities. The example in scrupulous cleanliness set by employees and inmates of such sanatoria thus bears its fruits.

The first state institution for the consumptive poor in the United States was inaugurated at Rutland, Mass., in September, 1898. We reproduce here its general plan, which gives an idea of the excellent arrangement to secure sunlight and air for all the rooms. It receives only invalids in the first stage of the disease, but has done most excellent work since its foundation.

General hospitals are ill adapted to the treatment of tuberculous patients. The consumptives in general hospitals must always constitute more or less of a danger to their fellow-patients suffering from other diseases, leaving aside the fact that the tuberculous invalid can hardly receive there the care he needs.

The treatment of a poor consumptive in the average tenement house is out of the question. One must have visited these dark, gloomy apartments, and have studied the hygienic and social conditions of these sufferers and their surroundings, to appreciate the impossibility of such a task.[233]

The social problem of tuberculosis is a stupendous one. To get at the root of the evil, there should be, besides the rigorous enforcement of the regulations and sanitary measures outlined in our chapter on general public prophylaxis, first, the creation of more sanitary tenements for the poor, for even special institutions for the treatment of consumption will be of little avail in solving the tuberculosis problem without a better housing of the laboring class. ‑ So long as the law will permit tenements to exist or be constructed anew which, owing to the lack of air, and light, and want of cleanliness, constitute veritable hotbeds of tuberculosis, so long will sanatoria and special hospitals serve only as recipients of the supply of the tuberculous patients daily created anew. Secondly, provision should be made for educating the poor in hygiene, in practical cooking, in the care and feeding of children, and in temperance. It is not the absolute poverty so much as the ignorance of many of these people which causes them to be insufficiently fed. There is as much waste, or more, among the poor as there is among the rich. Substantial meals can often be prepared with relatively little. cost, but how to do this is not known among the poor. A wide field is open here for the philanthropically inclined woman. The hygiene of the household

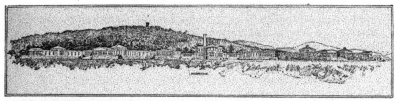

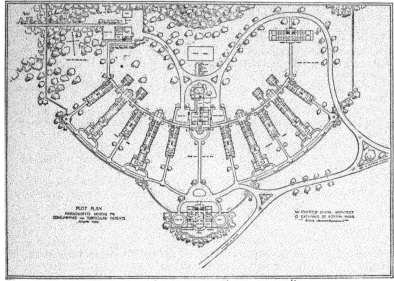

Fig. 50.—Massachusetts State Hospital for Consumptives.

should be taught to girls at schools, and so should the evil of intemperance be impressed upon all school-children.

The question of what is to be done with the numerous consumptive individuals and poor families in whom tuberculosis exists, is a very difficult one to answer, and the State and municipalities will have to combine with the philanthropical institutions in order to solve it.[234] If any government is in earnest in its endeavor to combat tuberculosis effectually, besides its regularly enforced laws against bovine tuberculosis, its thorough hygienic measures against tuberculosis in man through sanitary regulations and public instruction, it must take

upon itself the care and treatment of the curable and incurable tuberculous patients among the poor and among those of limited means.
I mean here by limited means a financial condition which does not
permit a tuberculous patient to enter a private sanatorium, or to
have at home such medical, hygienic, and dietetic care as will assure
him the best possible chance of recovery.[*]

An important point to be considered would be how to recruit the
patients, and how to discriminate between the proper and improper
cases. In previous writings[256] I have made the following suggestions
in regard to these questions, to which I have nothing to add:

"Just as there exists in nearly all States or municipalities a commission or a number of special examiners for the purpose of determining who is a proper subject for state care in an asylum for the
insane, so should there exist a commission for the determination of
admission to a municipal or state institution for consumptives.
Such a commission, composed of a certain number of general practitioners and health officers, should be aided in its work by the charity
organizations. Each case should be investigated by a combined
committee of physicians and laymen, for the following purposes:

"1. To determine the applicant's condition by a medical examination.

"2. To visit his home if he has been found tuberculous, and to
institute such hygienic measures as seem necessary (distribution of
pocket spittoons, disinfectants, etc.).

"3. To examine the other members of the family, in order to
find out if any of them have also contracted the disease, and, if so, to
counsel proper treatment.

"4· To report in full to the sanitary authorities concerning the
condition of the patient's dwelling. Its renovation or even destruction may be imperative when it is evident that tuberculosis has become 'endemic' there, owing to the condition of the soil or to other
sanitary defects.

"5· To determine the financial condition, whether the patient is
or is not able to pay, and whether or not by his being taken to an
institution the family will become destitute.

"If the latter should be the case, it would be necessary for the
municipality to provide for the family. In many cases a letter of
inquiry, sent to the former medical attendant of the patient, would
materially aid the work of the investigation committee.

"Any individual should have the right to present himself for examination, and every physician should be at liberty to recommend
any person for examination to the board of his precinct or district."

The institutions needed to carry out this plan would be:

1. A centrally located reception hospital and dispensary. The
dispensary should treat the ambulant tuberculous patients, whose

---

[*] The system of government in the United States makes a government insurance
against tuberculosis, such as exists in Germany, impracticable.

admission into the sanatorium is impracticable or has to be delayed for want of room. These dispensaries should also serve the patient discharged from the sanatorium as a place to seek counsel, and thus aid in his continued improvement and guard against the possibility of a relapse.

2. One or several city sanatoria, located in the outskirts, and if possible in a somewhat elevated region, where the atmosphere is known to be pure. Here all patients should pass through a preparatory sojourn before being sent to the mountain sanatorium. The more advanced cases would all be retained here.

3. One or several mountain sanatoria at no greater distance from the city than three or five hours by rail, at an altitude, if possible, of between one thousand and two thousand feet, on porous ground, with southern exposure, as nearly as possible protected from the coldest winds by higher mountains, and preferably surrounded by a pine forest. A farm in the vicinity, where the thoroughly convalescent patients could do light work, might make the institution in a measure self-supporting. To this place the selected incipient and the improved cases from the city sanatorium should be sent to complete their cure. To the mountain sanatorium there should also be attached a department for children suffering from pulmonary tuberculosis.

4. Several seaside sanatoria for the treatment of children afflicted with tuberculous diseases of the joints and other tuberculous (scrofulous) manifestations.

5. A maternity sanatorium where tuberculous mothers should be received a few months previous to their confinement, and surrounded by the best hygienic and dietetic care. They should also remain in the sanatorium for some time after childbirth. It is only by taking away these mothers from their unsanitary tenement homes, and placing them under constant medical supervision in such an institution, some time before and after their confinement, that the fearful mortality among tuberculous mothers after childbirth can be reduced.

The beneficial effect on the woman's and child's constitutions through such an arrangement can hardly be overestimated. Leaving aside the physical well-being thus largely assured to mother and child at a period when their organisms need the most tender care, the hygienic training which the mother will have received in such an institution will be of lasting utility to herself and child, to the family, and to the community.

These maternity sanatoria need not be situated at a great distance from the city. All that would be essential is that they should be erected on good porous ground, preferably somewhat elevated, and in a locality where the atmosphere is as pure as possible. The buildings should be constructed according to the principles of modern obstetrical science and modern phthisiotherapy. The physician in charge should be experienced in both these branches of medicine.

From the foregoing it will be seen that I am in favor of treating these tuberculous patients near their homes, and in the same or nearly the same climate as that in which they will have to live and work after their restoration to health. My reasons for advocating such principles are founded on the experiences of all modern phthisiotherapeutists, which have shown that the hygienic and dietetic treatment in special hospitals is feasible and successful in nearly all climates. Furthermore, it is quite evident that for social and economic reasons the majority of tuberculous patients will have to be treated near their homes. Only by adhering to this principle can we expect to cope successfully with tuberculosis—this disease of all climes, but which is most prevalent in large centres of population, where civilization has seemingly attained the highest standard.

To do away with all possible doubts as to the necessity of state and municipal care for the consumptive poor, and to evidence that by doing this the States and municipality must be the moral and financial gainers in the end, even leaving aside the improved sanitary condition by which such a course must be followed, we will take the State of New York, which is the State having the largest population, for an example. It is estimated that there are in this State about 50,000 tuberculous invalids. Of these probably one-fifth belong to that class of patients which sooner or later become a burden to the community. These 10,000 consumptives, absolutely poor, will sooner or later have to be taken care of by the public general hospitals. While they may not stay in one hospital twelve months continuously, they will certainly occupy a bed in one of the public institutions for that length of time before they die. According to the last annual announcement of the public charity hospitals of New York, the average cost per patient per day in the general hospitals was $1.16. Thus the cost to the commonwealth will be $4,234,000 per year for caring for the 10,000 consumptives.

What would be the expense if they were taking care of in a sanatorium? Experience in this country and abroad has demonstrated that the maintenance of incipient cases in well-conducted sanatoria can well be carried out for one dollar per day. If these 10,000 would be sent to a sanatorium in time, at least 6,000 of them could be lastingly cured after a maximum sojourn of 250 days, at an average expense of $250 per capita. Thus for $1,500,000 6,000 individuals would be made again breadwinners and useful citizens. If the remaining 4,000 invalids were kept in the sanatorium one year before they died, it would cost $1,460,000. Thus taking away from the tenement districts 10,000 consumptives, curing more than half of them and caring for the other half, and destroying 10,000 foci of infection will cost $2,960,000. Not taking care of them in the earlier stages of their disease they will probably all die, since this 10,000 represents the absolutely poor who now live under the most unhygienic conditions; but before dying they will have cost the community $4,234,000.

Consumption is a disease which usually attacks the individual at the time of life when he is most productive and most useful to the community. If cured of tuberculosis in a sanatorium, he will not only be unable to communicate his disease any longer to others, but the sanitary training and moral education which such an individual, coming from the poorest and often most ignorant classes of society, will have received, can only be productive of a vast amount of moral good in the sphere of his future activity. The hygienic benefit which the community derives from taking care of even the hopeless cases among its consumptive poor is too obvious to need further demonstration.

Thus, in conclusion, we might say that tuberculosis should to-day be considered a decidedly preventable, and in many of its forms a very curable disease. The necessary factors for its prevention are, first, a better understanding of the infectious character of tuberculosis; secondly, a more rigorous public and private prophylaxis; third, an improvement of the sanitary conditions of the tenements, more public baths, parks and breathing places; fourth, a general improvement of the conditions of the poor, and, above all, a more widespread hygienic education of all classes, which might best be accomplished by instructions in schools for the young, by public lectures for the adult, and by the formation of local and national societies for the prevention of tuberculosis. The factors essential for the cure of tuberculosis are a more thorough knowledge on the part of the practitioner of the methods of modern phthisiotherapy, and the combined efforts of physician, statesman, and philanthropist to further the multiple creation of sanatoria and special hospitals for the treatment among the poor of consumptive adults, and scrofulous and tuberculous children.

Bibliographical References.

Sources of Infection and Prophylaxis.

1. Baillie: Traité d'Anatomie pathologique, Paris, 1803

2. Laennec: Traité de l'auscultation médiate et des maladies du poumon et du cœur, 1re édit, 1819.

3 Villemin. Cause et nature de la tuberculose. Bulletin de l'Académie de Médecine de Paris, December 5, 1865.

4. Robert Koch Die Aetiologie der Tuberkulose. Berliner klinische Wochen-schrift, No. 15, 1882

5. Sawitzky· Zur Frage über die Dauer der infectiösen Eigenschaften des getrockneten Sputums. Centralblatt für Bacteriologie, Bd. xi., 1892.

6. R. Wurtz et Lermoyez. Du Rôle bactéricide du mucus nasal. Comptes rendus de la Société de Biologie, 1893. p. 756.

7. Villemin. De la Prophylaxie de la phtisie pulmonaire Union médicale, 1868, p 150.

8 Hermann Weber: On the Communicability of Consumption from Husband to Wife. Clinical Society Transactions, London, 1874, vol vii.

9. Tappeiner. Ueber eine Methode Tuberkulose zu erzeugen. Virchow's Archiv, 1878, Bd. lxxiv., p. 393.

10. Cornet· Die Verbreitung der Tuberkelbacillen ausserhalb des Körpers. Zeitschrift für Hygiene, 1888, Bd. v., pp. 191–332.

11. Krüger: Einige Untersuchungen des Staubniederschlages der Luft in Bezug auf Tuberkelbacillen. Inaugural Dissertation, Bonn, 1889

12. Straus: La Tuberculose et son Bacille, Paris, 1895.

13. Hance: A Study of the Infectiousness of the Dust in the Adirondack Cot tage Sanitarium. Medical Record, December 28, 1895.

14 Murrell Lancet, April 10, 1897, p 1018.

15 Galtier. Dangers de la viande et du lait tuberculeux. Congrès pour la tuberculose, 1re session, 1888, p. 78.

16. Spillmann et Haushalter: Dissémination du bacille de la tuberculose par mouches. Comptes rendus de l'Académie des Sciences, 1886, vol. cv., p. 352.

17 Hoffmann Die Gefahren der Verbreitung der Tuberculose durch unsere Stubenfliege. Correspondenzblatt der ärztlichen Vereine im Königreich Sachsen, 12, 1888

18 Flügge: Deutsche medicinische Wochenschrift, 1897, No. 42.

19. Goldie: Spread of Tuberculosis. Journal of the American Medical Associa-tion, August 26, 1899.

20. Grancher. Maladies de l'Appareil respiratoire, Paris, 1890.

20 a Yersin: De l'action de quelques antiseptiques et de la chaleur sur le bacille de la tuberculose. Annales de l'Institut Pasteur, 1888. p. 60.

21. Weise: Handkerchiefs for Consumptives. Lancet, November 14, 1891.

22. L. H. Petit· Sur quelques modes peu connus de contagion de la tubercu-lose par la voie buccale. Revue de la Tuberculose, i., ii , 1894.

23. Cornet: Die Tuberculose. Handbuch der speciellen Pathologie und The-rapie, Bd. xiv., 1899.

24 Mosler: Ueber die Infection der Darmschleimhaut beim Verschlucken tuberkulöser Sputa. Deutsche medicinische Wochenschrift, 1883, No. 19.

25. Prudden and Hodenpyl. Studies on the Action of Dead Bacteria in the Living Body. New York Medical Journal, June 6. 1893.

26 Grancher et Ledoux-Lebard: Tuberculose aviaire et humaine. Archives de Médecine expérimentale et pathologique. 1892, p 25

27. Straus, I.. Sur la tuberculose du paroquet. Archives de Médecine expérimentale, January, 1896 Weise, T.. Consumption and Canaries Journal of the American Medical Association, vol xxxii

28. Steinthal: Ueber Hauttuberculose durch Inoculation und Autoinfection. Deutsche medicinische Wochenschrift, 1888, No. 10.

29. Dubreuilh et Auché. La tuberculose primitive. Archives de Médecine expérimentale, 1890, p. 601.

30. Von Eiselsberg· Beitrag zur Impftuberculose beim Menschen. Wiener medizinische Wochenschrift, 1887, No 53, p. 1729.

31. Leloir: Etiologie et pathogénie du lupus. Etude expérimentale et clinique sur la tuberculose par Verneuil, 1892, tome iii., p. 482.

32. Wolters: Ueber Inoculationslupus. Deutsche medicinische Wochen schrift, 1892, No. 36.

33. Lipp: Ein Fall von Lupus des Gesichtes. Wiener medizinische Presse, Bd. vii., 1889, p. 475.

34. Surmont, H.: Article Vaccine, Traité de Médecine et de Thérapeutique. Brouardel, Gilbert, et Gironde, vol. i , 1895, p. 207.

35. Brouardel: Article Vaccina, Twentieth Century Practice, vol. xiii

36. Reclus, P.: Clinique chirurgicale de l'Hôtel Dieu, Paris, 1888, 514–527.

37. Schuchardt, K.: Die Uebertragung der Tuberkulose auf dem Wege des geschlechtlichen Verkehrs. Archiv für klinische Medicin, Berlin, 1892, xliv.

38. Carrera y Miro: Contagio tuberculoso por la via genital. Gaceta médica catalana, Barcelona, 1888, xi., p. 385.

39. Cornet. Die Tuberculose, Wien, 1899, p. 160.

40. Petit, L. H.· Tuberculose et rapports ab ore. Revue de la Tuberculose, vol. ii., p. 234.

41. Lindemann: Deutsche medicinische Wochenschrift, No. 30, 1883.

42. Jacobi, in Knopf's Pulmonary Tuberculosis, Philadelphia, 1899.

43. Maas in König's Lehrbuch der Chirurgie, 4 edit., vol. ii., p. 588.

44. Willy Meyer: Ein Fall von Impftuberculose in Folge ritueller Circumcision. New-Yorker medicinische Presse, June, 1887.

45. Collins and Murray· British Medical Journal, June 1, 1895.

46. Novy and Waik: Medical News, May 21, 1898.

47. Chalmers: The Causation of Tuberculosis and its Prevention by Legislation. Practitioner, London, June, 1898.

48 Cornet: Zeitschrift für Hygiene, vol. vi., part 1, 1889.

49. Biggs: The Action of the Health Department in Relation to Pulmonary Tuberculosis. A Report, 1897.

50. Flick: The Contagiousness of Phthisis, Philadelphia, 1888.

51. Galtier: Congrès pour l'étude de la Tuberculose, Paris, 1893, p 213.

52. Gartner: Congress für innere Medicin, Berlin, 1887.

53. Lichty: Journal of the American Medical Association, November 26, 1898.

54. Emmert: Is Our Public School System Conducive to Tuberculosis? Transactions of the Iowa State Medical Society, 1898.

55. Ravenel. Geographical Distribution of Bovine Tuberculosis. Transactions of the American Medical Association, October, 1897.

56 Pearson: Directions for Inspecting Herds for Tuberculosis, Philadelphia, 1897.

57 Rabinowitsch: Zur Frage des Vorkommens von Tuberkelbacillen in der Marktbutter. Deutsche medicinische Wochenschrift, No. 32, 1897.

58 Brush, E. F.: Human and Bovine Tuberculosis, New York, 1898.

59. Virchow: Nahrungsmittel. Bericht über den Kongress zur Bekämpfung der Tuberkulose als Volkskrankheit, 1899, p 346.

60. Barrier: Société Centrale de Médecine Vetérinaire, 1899, p. 255.

61. Sheldon: Tuberculosis of the Dog. Journal of the American Medical Association, December 9, 1899.

62. Bang: Die Tuberculose unter den Hausthieren in Dänemark. Zeitschrift für Thiermedicin, 1890, p. 409.

63 Birch-Hirschfeld: Beiträge zur pathologischen Anatomie und allgemeinen Pathologie, 1891, p. 429.

64 De Renzi: La Tizichezza polmonare, Napoli, 1889.

65. Nouvelles recherches sur la hérédité de la Tuberculose. Lyon médical, 1891, p. 325.

66. Jacobi, A.: Relation du premier cas connu de Tuberculose chez un fœtus humain. Congrès de la Tuberculose, 1891, p. 327; and in Küss, De l'Hérédité parasitaire de la tuberculose humaine, Paris, 1898.

67. Landouzy: Hérédité de la Tuberculose. Revue de Médecine, 1883, p. 1014.

68. Lannelongue: La tuberculose externe congénitale et précoce, Paris, 1887.

69 Kellogg Experimental Researches Respecting the Relation of Dress to Pelvic Diseases of Women. Transactions of the Michigan State Medical Society, 1888.

70 Barth Deutsche Medicinal-Zeitung, November 15, 1897.

71 Freudenthal· Some Points regarding the Etiology and Treatment of Post-nasal Catarrh, etc. Journal of the American Medical Association, November 9, 1895.

72. Barnes· The Arid Atmosphere of Our Houses in Winter. Transactions of the American Public Health Association, vol. xxiii.

EARLY DIAGNOSIS OF TUBERCULOUS DISEASES

73. Knopf, S. A.: Pulmonary Tuberculosis: Its Modern Prophylaxis and the Treatment in Special Institutions and at Home, Philadelphia, 1899. Early Recognition of Pulmonary Tuberculosis. Journal of the American Medical Association, December 9, 1899.

74. Ambler: The Early Diagnosis of Pulmonary Tuberculosis. New York Medical Journal, February 12, 1898.

75 Goldschmidt: Bericht über 5 mit dem Koch'schen Heilmittel behandelte Fälle von Lepra. Berliner klinische Wochenschrift, 1891, p. 28.

76 Babes und Kalendero: Ueber die Wirkung des Koch'schen Heilmittels bei Lepra Deutsche medicinische Wochenschrift, 1891, p. 115.

77. Guidet: Essay Historique sur les indices du debut de la Tuberculose pulmonaire, Paris, 1898.

78. Straus et Teissier: De l'emploi de la tuberculine comme agent revelateur de la syphilis. Semaine médicale, 1893, p. 364.

79. Whittaker. The Earliest Possible Recognition of Tuberculosis. Medical Record, vol. li., p. 826.

80. Anders, J. M.: The Early Diagnosis and Treatment of Pulmonary Tuberculosis. Pennsylvania Medical Journal, December, 1899.

81. Cornet: Tuberculin als Diagnosticum der Tuberculose, Wien, 1899.

82. Grancher: Bulletin médical, August 28, 1885, p. 817.

83. Cabot and Whorisky: Substitutes for Tuberculin in Diagnosis. Journal of the Boston Society of the Medical Sciences, January 17, 1899.

84. Hippocrates: Epidemies. Book iii.; Littré's translation, 3d section, t. iii., p. 97.

85. Galen: Ed. Kuhn, t. xvii., p. 723.

86. Razes: Helchauy. Ed. Sal. Favent, Venise, 1506, folio 81.

87. Daremberg· Œuvres choisies d'Hippocrate, 2d edition, 1855, pp. 447, 469.

88. Behier et Hardy: Traité élémentaire de pathologie interne, Paris, 1846, tome i , p. 273.

89. Landouzy: Congrès de la Tuberculose, Paris, 1888, p 383.

90. Dewèvre: De la prédisposition des roux de la tuberculose. Thèse de Paris, 1883.

91. Mahoudeau: Article Roux. Erythrisme in Dictionnaire des Sciences Anthropologiques, Paris, 1884-95.

92 Delpeuch: De l'habitus tuberculeux, et en particulier de la prédisposition des roux de la phthisie selon Hippocrate. Presse médicale, No. 57, July 19, 1899.

93. John Beddoe. On the Proclivity of Phthisis Commonly Ascribed to Persons of Xanthous Complexion. Edinburgh Medical Journal, 1858-59, vol. iv., p. 10.

94. Loomis, H P.. Certain Points of Interest in Phthisis. Medical Record, May 14, 1898.

95. Ewald: Trauma und Phthisis. New-Yorker medicinische Monatsschrift, September, 1899.

96. McLean: Personal Observation in Pulmonary Phthisis. Medical Record, May 14, 1898.

97. Murat. Gazette hebdomadaire de Médecine et de Chirurgie, March 5, 1899, p. 221; Un signe nouveau pour le diagnostique précoce de la tuberculose pulmonaire. Revue de la Tuberculose, 1895

98. Ch. Amat. Le diagnostic précoce de la tuberculose pulmonaire pour servir de base à la thérapeutique prophylactique. Bulletin général de Thérapeutique, February 28, 1898, p. 303.

99. Roe, J O.· Early Diagnosis of the Laryngoscopic Picture. Medical Record, vol. lv., p. 690.

100. Straus: Communication à l'Académie de Médecine, sur la presence des bacilles tuberculeux virulents dans les cavités nasales d'individus sains frequentant des locaux habités par les phthisiques, July 3, 1894. La tuberculose et son bacille, 1895.

101. Papillon: Diagnostic précoce de la tuberculose pulmonaire en particulier chez les chlorotiques. Thèse de Paris, 1897.

102. Loomis, H. P.: The Pretuberculous Stage of Phthisis, or the Condition which Antedates Tuberculous Development, and Some Aids to Its Diagnosis. Medical Record, vol. liv., p. 829

103. Osler: American Text-book of Diseases of Children.

104 Meissen: Ueber die frühe Erkennung der Lungentuberkulose. Therapeutische Monatshefte, November, 1898.

105. Katzenbach: Journal of the American Medical Association, December 9, 1899.

106. Grancher: Maladies de l'Appareil respiratoire, Paris, 1890.

107. Turban: Beiträge zur Kenntniss der Lungentuberkulose, Wiesbaden, 1899.

108. Fernet: Sur le diagnostic précoce de la tuberculose pulmonaire. Bulletin de l'Académie de Médecine de Paris, October 11, 1898, p. 253.

109. The Dangers Following the Use of Iodized Preparations in Tuberculous Subjects. New York Medical Journal, March 5, 1898.

110. Bouchard: Application de la radioscopie au diagnostic des maladies du thorax. Revue de la Tuberculose, vol. iv., p. 273.

111. Kelsch: Sur le diagnostic précoce des affections tuberculeuses du thorax par la radioscopie. Bulletin de l'Académie de Médecine, December 21, 1897.

112. Espina y Capo: Revista de Medicina y Cirugia Practicas, November 25, 1898

113. Stubbert: Comparative Diagnosis in Pulmonary Tuberculosis by the Roentgen Rays. Medical Record, May 22, 1897.

114 Williams: Application of X-rays in Diagnosis of Tuberculosis. Medical Record, September 10, 1898.

115. Crane: Skiascopy of the Respiratory Organs. Philadelphia Monthly Medical Journal, March, 1899.

116. Arloing et Courmont: Sur la recherche et la valeur clinique de l'agglutination du bacille de Koch par le sérum de l'homme. Académie des Sciences, séance de September 19, 1898.

117. Bourland: Four Cases of Pulmonary Tuberculosis. Philadelphia Medical Journal, December 23, 1899.

118. Kyle: Text-book of Diseases of the Nose and Throat, 1899.

119. Mayer, E.: Tuberculosis of the Upper Air Passages. Medical News, May 14, 1898.

120. Clavier: Péritonite tuberculeuse. Thèse de Paris, 1895.

121. Kiliani: Zur Diagnose und Therapie chirurgischer Gelenkerkraukungen. New Yorker medicinische Monatschrift, February, 1900.

122. Bulius: Jahrbuch für Kinderheilkunde, 1899, Nos. 2 and 3. Journal of Tuberculosis, No. 2, vol. i.

TREATMENT OF PULMONARY TUBERCULOSIS.

123. Unterberger: Ueber Scrophulose, Tuberculose, und Phthisie und die Behandlung in Haussanatorien, St. Petersburg, 1897.

124. Daremberg: Traitement de la Phtisie pulmonaire, vol. ii , Paris, 1895.

125 Millet: The Night Air of New England in the Treatment of Consumption. Maryland Medical Journal, January, 1900.

126. Bowditch, V. Y.: Boston Medical and Surgical Journal, July 16, 1885; and Journal of the American Medical Association, August 1, 1885.

127. Fox, Sidney A.: A Report of Sixty-nine Cases of Lung Disease Treated with the Pneumatic Cabinet. New York Medical Journal, June 26, 1886.

128. Houghton, A. F.: Journal of the American Medical Association, November 7, 1885.

129. Hudson, Jr., E. Darwin: Present Status of the Pneumatic Treatment of Respiratory Diseases. Medical Record, January 9, 1886.

130. Jensen: Same journal and date as Houghton's article.

131. Ketchum, Joseph: The Physics of Pneumatic Differentiation. Medical Record, January 9, 1886.

132. Westbrook, Benj F.: Pneumatic Differentiation. New York Medical Journal, January 26, 1886.

133. Williams, H. F.: Antiseptic Treatment of Pulmonary Diseases by Means

of Pneumatic Differentiation. Medical Record, January 17, 1885; Pneumatic Differentiation. New York Medical Journal, July 16, 1885.

134. Platt: On the Practical Application of the Pneumatic Cabinet. New York Medical Journal, June 26, 1886.

135. Quimby The Pneumatic Cabinet in the Treatment of Pulmonary Phthisis. International Medical Magazine, January, 1893.

135a. Rubner: Bekleidungsreform und Wollsystem. Zeitschrift für Diätetische und Physicalische Therapie, vol. ii., No. 1.

135b. Ambler: Dress as a Factor in the Causation of Catarrhal Diseases. Charlotte Medical Journal, May, 1899.

136. Knopf: Dress Reform and its Relation to Medicine. Southern California Practitioner, August, 1889.

137. Baruch: Principles and Practice of Hydrotherapy, New York, 1898.

138. Dettweiler: Die Behandlung der Lungenschwindsucht in geschlossenen Heilanstalten, Berlin, 1884.

139. Liebe: Alkohol und Tuberculose, Tübingen, 1899.

140. Finkler: Eiweissnahrung und Nahrungseiweiss. Deutsche medicinische Wochenschrift, 1898, No. 17.

141. Knopf, S. A.: Pulmonary Tuberculosis, etc. Alvarenga Prize Essay, Philadelphia, 1899, and Les Sanatoria; traitement et prophylaxie de la phtisie pulmonaire, 2d edition, Paris, 1900.

142. Flick: A Further Report on the Treatment of Tuberculosis by Iodoform Inunctions. The Medical News, March 2, 1892.

143. Daremberg: Traitement de la Phtisie Pulmonaire, Paris, 18? .

144. Ransom: The Treatment of Phthisis, London, 1896.

145. De Renzi (Naples): The Lancet, December, 1897. .

146. Charité Annalen, xxii., 1897. Jacob's Bericht über Creosotal aus Leyden's Clinic.

147. Cornet: Die Tuberculose. Kapitel Chemische Mittel, Wien, 1899.

148. Stubbert: Sanitarium Treatment of Pulmonary Tuberculosis. St. Louis Medical Gazette, December, 1898.

149. Bouteron: L'Antisepsie pulmonaire par la Voie rectale. Presse médicale, February 15, 1899.

150. Flick in Otis's Some Modern Methods of the Treatment of Phthisis. Pray Prize Essay of the New Hampshire Medical Society for 1897.

151. Alexander: Die Behandlung der Phthisie durch Injectionen von Oleum camphoratum Pharm. Germ. Berliner klinische Wochenschrift, No. 48, 1898.

152. Kobert: Ueber die medicamentose Behandlung der Tuberculose Bericht über den Kongress zur Bekämpfung der Tuberculose als Volkskrankheit, Berlin, 1899.

153. Lafont: Gomenol Thèse de Paris, December, 1899

154. Landerer: Die Behandlung der Tuberculose mit Zimmtsäure, Leipzig, 1898

155. Mann: The Management of Pulmonary Tuberculosis with Special Reference to Treatment by Sodium Cinnamate. Medical Record, February 4, 1899.

156. Flick: The Therapeutics of Tuberculosis Therapeutic Gazette, January 15, 1900.

157. Drozda: Gundzüge einer rationellen Phthisiotherapie. XII. Internationaler Congress, 1897.

158. Whitaker· Canada Lancet, January, 1899.

159. Brunet: Suc pulmonaire; Effets physiologiques et thérapeutiques, Bordeaux, 1898.

160. Organotherapie.　Deutsche medicinische Wochenschrift, 1899, Nos. 87, 88.

161. Débove: Recherches sur l'alimentation artificielle.　Communication faite à la Société des Hôpitaux, séance du 14 Avril, 1882.

162. Manges: The Treatment of Coughs with Heroin.　New York Medical Journal, November 26, 1898.

163. Grancher: Leçons Cliniques sur les Maladies de l'Appareil respiratoire, Paris, 1890.

164. Starke: Phthisis.　Dietetic and Hygienic Gazette, March, 1899.

165 Flick· Nitroglycerin as a Hæmostatic in Hæmoptysis.　Philadelphia Medical Journal, February 19, 1898.

166. Brannan, J. W.: The Treatment of Pulmonary Hemorrhage.　New York Medical Journal, vol. l., p. 218.

167. Andrew. Harveian lectures.　British Medical Journal, 1890, vol. ii., p. 942.

168. Wolff· Die moderne Behandlung der Lungenschwindsucht, Wiesbaden, 1894.

169. Kemp· Intestinal Hydrotherapy.　Transactions of the New York Academy of Medicine, February 3, 1898.

170 Winternitz: Zur Pathologie und Hydrotherapie der Lungenphthisie, Leipzig und Wien, 1887.

171. Daremberg: Traitement de la Phtisie pulmonaire, vol. ii., Paris, 1895.

172. Marmorek· Le Streptocoque et le Sérum Antistreptococcique.　Annales de l'Institut Pasteur, July, 1895.

173. Weaver: Antistreptococcic Serum in the Treatment of Consumption.　Journal of the American Medical Association, September 5, 1896

174 Stubbert: Sanitarium Treatment, etc.　St. Louis Medical Gazette, December, 1898.

175 J. Blake White: Phthisis Treated by Intrapulmonary Injections of Carbolized Iodine.　Medical Record, May 22, 1886.

176 Dettweiler. Die Behandlung der Lungenschwindsucht, etc., Berlin, 1884.

177. Rose: Ueber nicht-medikamentöse Schlafmittel　Zeitschrift für Krankenpflege, vol. xx., No. 7, 1898.

178. Buxbaum: Die Krankenpflege der Schlaflosigkeit, vol. xx., No. 8, 1898.

179. Yonge: Insomnia in Pulmonary Phthisis.　Scalpel, May, 1899.

180. Landon Carter Gray: Neurasthenia: Its Symptoms and Treatment.　Medical News, December 16, 1899.

Treatment of Complications.

181. Schmidt, M.: Die Krankheiten der oberen Luftwege, Berlin, 1894

182. Freudenthal: The Treatment of Dysphagia and Cough, Especially in Tuberculosis.　Philadelphia Medical Journal, March 25, 1899.　-

182a. D. de Darrese: Traitement de la tuberculose laryngée par l'iodoforme. La Tuberculose Infantile, February 15, 1900.

183. Gleitsmann: The Treatment of Laryngeal Tuberculosis.　Medical Record, December 4, 1897.

184. Abrams: The Therapeutic Value of the Solar Rays.　Philadelphia Monthly Medical Journal, March, 1899.

185. Gebhardt: Die Heilkraft des Lichtes, Leipzig, 1898.

186. English: Therapeutic Hints.　Medical Record, January 14, 1899.

187. Gerhardt: Beförderung der Ausathmung.　Zeitschrift für Diät und physikalische Therapie, No. 1, vol. i., 1898.

188. Leyden: Ueber pneumothorax tuberculosis. Deutsche medicinische Wochenschrift, 1888.

189. Byford: Non-Operative Treatment of Tuberculous Peritonitis. Virginia Medical Semi-monthly, July 21, 1899.

190. Bier: Heilwirkung der Hyperämie. Münchener medicinische Wochenschrift, 1897, No. 32.

190a. Millioz: Les bains de soleil prolongés comme traitement des tuberculoses articulaires. Thèse de Lyon, 1900.

191. Hoffa: Behandlung der Tuberculose, etc. Münchener medicinische Wochenschrift, February 28, 1899.

Education, Discipline, and Marriage Relation

192. Tarnier: Grossesse et Tuberculose. Journal de Sages-femmes, October 1, 1894.

193. Gaulard: Rapport sur un cas tuberculeux. Presse médicale, December 8, 1894

194. Knopf: Les Sanatoria, etc. Thèse de Paris, 1895.

195. Hippocrates Foesin's edition, lib. 3 De Morb., p. 493. v. 16.

196. Mendelsohn Die Krankenpflege (Hypurgie) Lehrbuch der allgemeinen Therapie, Bd. 1, Wien und Leipzig, 1897.

197. Pentzoldt-Stintzing: Handbuch der Therapie der Erkrankungen der Atmungs- und Kreislauforgane, Jena, 1898.

Culture Products.

198. Whittaker: General Impressions from Six Years' Use of the Old Tuberculin. Journal of the American Medical Association, November 6, 1897.

199. Spengler: Deutsche medicinische Wochenschrift, No. 36, 1897.

200. Barton: The Scientific Treatment of Tuberculosis. Medical Record, September, 1897.

Climatotherapy, Health Resorts, and Sports.

201. Weber: Klima und Seereisen in der Behandlung der Tuberkulose. Bericht über den Kongress zur Bekämpfung des Tuberculose als Volkskrankheit, Berlin, 1899.

202. Ingals: Diseases of the Chest, Throat, and Nasal Cavities, 1897.

203. Weber, Hermann· Climatherapie, 1886.

204. De la Harpe: Formulaire des Stations d'Hiver et des Stations d'Été.

205. Lindley and Widney: California of the South, 1888

206. Solly: A Handbook of Medical Climatology, Philadelphia, 1897.

207. Walters. Sanatoria for Consumptive Patients. Practitioner, June, 1898.

208. Mendelsohn: Deutsche medicinische Wochenschrift, April 30 and June 18, 1896.

209. Gihon: The Bicycle in its Sanitary Aspect. Medical Record, October 3, 1896.

210. Franz: Communication au Congrès de la Tuberculose, Paris, 1888.

PROGNOSIS.

211. Carswell· Pathological Anatomy, London, 1838.

212. Loomis, H. P.: A Study of the Processes which Result in the Arrest or Cure of Phthisis. Medical Record, January 9, 1892.

213. Werdmüller in Manasse's Heilung der Lungentuberkulose, Berlin, 1892.

214. Laennec: Traité de l'Auscultation médiate Edition de la Faculté, 1879.

215. Cruveilhier: Traité d'Anatomie générale, vol. iv., p. 538, Paris.

216. Charcot: Traité de Médecine, Article, Phtisie pulmonaire.

217. Grancher: Maladies de l'Appareil respiratoire, Paris, 1880.

218. Manasse: Die Heilung der Lungentuberkulose in Anstalten und Kurorten, 1892.

219. Beaulavon: Contributions à l'étude du traitement de la tuberculose pulmonaire, etc. Thèse de Paris, 1896.

220 Hohe· Die Bekämpfung und Heilung der Lungenschwindsucht, etc., München, 1897.

221. Dettweiler: Bericht über 72 seit 3-9 Jahren in Falkenstein völlig geheilte Fälle von Lungenschwindsucht, 1886. Medical Record, vol. lv., No. 19

222. Baldwin: In discussion on Subsequent Histories of "Arrested Cures" of Phthisis Treated at the Sharon Sanatorium Medical Record, May 13, 1899

223. Pidoux: Evacuation éliminatrice. Étude générale et pratique sur la Phthisie, Paris, 1874.

224. Diculafoy: Hemoptysie de Defence Cours à la Faculté, Paris, 1894. ·

225. Flamand: Werth de Diazoreaction. Inaugural Thesis, Berlin, 1899, and Schröder von Nagelbasch: Ueber die Bedeutung der Diazoreaction im Harne für die Prognose der Phthisie Münchener medicinische Wochenschrift, 1899, No. 44.

226. Schmidt· Die Krankheiten der oberen Luftwege, Berlin, 1894.

227. Besold: Ueber die Miterkrankung des Kehlkopfs bei Lungentuberculose. Münchener medicinische Wochenschrift, No. 26, 1898.

228. Levy, Robert. Prognosis of Laryngeal Tuberculosis. Journal of the American Medical Association, September 16, 1899.

229. Chappell: Laryngeal Tuberculosis at the Loomis Sanitarium. New York Medical Journal, September, 1898.

230. Walter: Harveian lectures on the Surgical Diseases of Tuberculosis, London, 1900.

231. Herzfeld: Chirurgische Behandlung der tuberkulösen Peritonitis. Mittheilungen aus den Grenzgebieten der Medicin und Chirurgie, Jena, V. 1-23, 1899.

PUBLIC CARE OF THE CONSUMPTIVE POOR.

232. Knopf: Are Sanatoria for Consumptives a Danger to the Neighborhood? Revue de la Tuberculose, vol. iii., pp. 311-319, Medical Record, October 3, 1896.

233 Knopf: Tenements and Tuberculosis. Address delivered before Tenement House Exhibition, February 20. Journal of Medicine and Science, Portland, Maine, April, 1900. Journal of the American Medical Association, May 12, 1900.

234 Leyden: Ueber den gegenwärtigen Stand der Behandlung Tuberculoser und die Staatliche Fürsorge fur dieselben, Berlin, 1898. Moscow Address, 1897.

235. Knopf: The Tuberculosis Problem in the United States. North American Review, February, 1899.

TUBERCULOSIS OF THE SKIN.

BY

JOHN T. BOWEN,

BOSTON.

TUBERCULOSIS OF THE SKIN.

Introduction.

SINCE the discovery of the tubercle bacillus and its general recognition as the cause of tuberculosis, it has been found that several forms of cutaneous lesions, that had previously received a different interpretation or had been regarded as obscure in their pathology, are due to the action of this bacillus on the tissues of the skin, and are to be classified as forms of cutaneous tuberculosis. Many cases of obscure "ulcers" belong in this class, as well as a considerable proportion of cases that had been called simply papillomata, for it has been shown that the histological appearances that are seen in many of these papillomata are the indirect result of the action of the tubercle bacillus.

The tubercle bacillus has been found to be constantly present in four distinct clinical types of cutaneous lesions—tuberculosis cutis or miliary cutaneous tuberculosis, lupus vulgaris, tuberculosis verrucosa cutis, and scrofuloderma. The claim of these types to a place in the class of cutaneous tuberculoses has been, therefore, firmly established. Besides these types there are other affections, which are regarded by a certain number of authorities as caused by the toxins produced by the bacilli, as the "tuberculides" of the French writers, lupus erythematosus, etc. No one has demonstrated the presence of the tubercle bacillus in these lesions, however, and their relationship to tuberculosis is very far from proved. They are enumerated at the end of this article, with a short discussion of the reasons that have been offered for including them among the tuberculoses.

Symptomatology.

TUBERCULOSIS CUTIS.

Synonyms.—Miliary tuberculosis; ulcère des phthisiques.

This is the rarest of the forms of cutaneous tuberculosis, and has been found only in subjects affected with tuberculosis of the internal organs. It was first recognized upon the skin by Cornil and Ranvier, although its existence upon the mucous membranes had been known previously. Chiari was the first to publish a careful histological description of this form, from five cases which he had met with post mortem, in all of which the lesions were seated on the lower lip. Jarisch was the first to describe it clinically.

The lesions are situated almost exclusively at the juncture of the mucous membrane with the skin at the entrance to the mouth, nose, anus, or vagina, although they have been occasionally described on other parts of the skin. Sometimes the cutaneous ulcer is accompanied by a similar affection of the adjoining mucous membrane, and sometimes the skin alone is affected. The ulcer is shallow, and rarely attains a considerable size. The edges are characteristic, being made up of numerous jagged indentations which give them a serrated appearance, and the ulcer looks as if "gnawed out." The indentations are caused by the degeneration of miliary tubercles. The floor is not as a rule crusted, but is covered by a viscid secretion, and sometimes miliary tubercles in the form of yellowish elevations are seen on its surface. Sometimes these miliary tubercles are seen at the edges, before the degeneration that gives rise to the indented, serrated appearance has taken place. No other variety of cutaneous tuberculosis has these features, but there is a close analogy with miliary tuberculosis of internal organs and with tuberculous ulcers of the tongue. Another attribute of these ulcers is that they are extremely painful. This may be due in a measure to their situation at a point where they are constantly exposed to irritation from the secretions.

Of twenty-two cases of this affection observed at the Vienna Clinic, Kaposi states that eighteen were in men and only four in women, while the age varied from twenty-eight to sixty years. More than one-half of these cases died in the hospital, and internal tuberculosis was found at the autopsy. The course of these lesions varies somewhat, as they may increase quite rapidly or pursue a steady chronic course. They are usually single, but may be multiple. The fact that when on the lips they are often associated with tuberculosis of the lungs, and when on the anus with tuberculosis of the intestinal tract, points to the conclusion that they are produced by autoinoculation from the sputum and from the intestinal discharges. In like manner, when seated on the penis they follow a tuberculosis of the urinary tract, and when on the vulva a tuberculosis of the uterus or tubes is present. As a rule, this form of tuberculous ulcer makes its appearance when the internal disease is pretty far advanced, but Kaposi lays stress upon the fact that this is not always so, and that the internal lesions may be slight or wanting.

Some instances of ulcers caused by the tuberculous infection of wounds have been recorded, in which the lesion is described as having the clinical characteristics of this form of miliary tuberculosis. A secondary infection of the glandular system and of the internal organs sometimes follows. In many of these instances the clinical description is not sufficiently clear to warrant us in placing the affection in the type now under discussion; in other cases, as in those published by Doutrelepont, a transitional form between tuberculosis cutis and lupus is suggested. Another class of cases has been described, in which an infection with tuberculosis was produced by the practice of sucking the wound by the operator in the Jewish rite of circumcision. Syphilis has in this way been transmitted from mucous patches in the mouth of the operator, and in some countries the method has been abandoned on that account. Well-marked cases of tuberculosis have undoubtedly arisen in this way, when the operator was affected with pulmonary tuberculosis. An ulcer forms at the site of the wound, and this may be followed by tuberculous infection of the inguinal glands, the lungs, or the meninges, and the death of the infant may follow speedily. In a case reported by Lehmann ten children were infected from the same operator, three of whom died. Other instances of the infection of a number of children from one operator are recorded. The place of these tuberculous ulcers among the varieties of cutaneous tuberculosis has not been definitely settled, but they approach more nearly to tuberculosis cutis than to the other forms.

An important characteristic of this miliary form of cutaneous tuberculosis is that it often contains tubercle bacilli in large numbers, such as we never meet with in lupus or scrofuloderma. Further allusions to this will be made in the section on pathological anatomy. The ulcers are to be differentiated from epithelioma by the absence of a hard, glistening edge and a hard floor; and from lupus by their painfulness, by the absence of a bright-red, easily bleeding floor, and by the absence of lupous nodules.

LUPUS VULGARIS.

Lupus vulgaris is distinguished from the other forms of tuberculosis of the skin chiefly and in the first instance by the presence of the so-called lupous nodules. These lupous nodules are small at the outset, and may either remain so or increase considerably in size. They are of a dark, reddish-brown color, and of soft consistency, as are all the infiltrations of tuberculosis. They become paler, but do not disappear, on pressure. They are situated in the corium, and by their development, involution, or degeneration cause most of the appearances that are to be seen in various stages of the lupous process. These lupous nodules tend to recur constantly during the course of the affection, both in the places where they have occurred before and in the adjoining tissue. They can scarcely be felt with the finger when the skin is put upon the stretch, but when perceptible they give a decidedly soft impression. This softness it is that distinguishes them from the infiltrations of syphilis and leprosy. When we have simply the presence of these lupous nodules without further evolution, the name *lupus maculosus* has been used for this stage of the process by certain writers.

This type may persist throughout the course of the disease, or, more frequently, the individual lupous nodule undergoes various changes which give rise to a number of different clinical forms. To these forms many different and for the most part useless names have been given. A *lupus élevé* is produced when single nodules slowly enlarge and form elevations appreciable to the touch. *Lupus tumidus* is a term applied to areas of infiltration of considerable size, formed from the coalescence of lupous nodules, and this form is apt to be slow in its course. The tendency, however, of all tuberculous lesions is to instability, and sooner or later either absorption or breaking down occurs. In the former case the nodules sink in and disappear gradually, leaving the epidermis shrunken and scaling—*lupus exfoliativus*. The loss of tissue caused by the absorption of the lupous infiltration is replaced by a cicatricial depression. *Lupus serpiginosus* is a name which has been applied to a special form or arrangement of the lupous infiltration; new nodules group themselves at the border of a patch of lupus, and the central part undergoing involution, while new lesions appear at the periphery, a serpiginous form is produced. When the nodules are scattered about without order, the term *lupus disseminatus* has been used.

The nodules of lupus, instead of disappearing by absorption, may break down and ulcerate—*lupus exulcerans*. The tuberculous neoplasm becomes cheesy degenerated, which causes it to break down with involvement of the overlying, thinned epidermis, so that an ulcerated surface is the result. The lupous ulcer is covered with crusts when not deep in extent, and these crusts are partly masses of cheesy material from the breaking down of the nodules, and partly the results of a secondary septic infection, which is common to all ulcerative processes. When the crusts are removed, the lupous ulcer is found to be more or less rounded, with soft reddish edges, and with a red floor covered usually with granulations. The ulcers are not painful. It is very seldom that tubercle bacilli can be found in the secretion from these ulcers, which consists of a granular detritus, pus cells, and large numbers of the pyogenic microorganisms. The edges and floor of the ulcers are very soft to the feel, and readily permit the entrance of a blunt instrument.

Secondary changes may occur in the lupous ulcer, not wholly peculiar to tuberculosis. It may take on a papillary, fungous character, as happens upon the nose especially, which may become greatly hypertrophied and covered with fungus-like vegetations, which leave, when removed surgically, a very small stump, the only healthy remnant of the nasal tissues. Lupus is very apt to follow the lymph channels when it extends downwards, and in this way it may attack the deeper structures, sparing neither muscle, cartilage, nor bone. *Lupus vorax* is the name that has been given to the process when it progresses both superficially and deeply. When it extends very rapidly over large surfaces, it is called *lupus phagédénique*. In this latter rare variety there is probably a secondary infection besides the tuberculous process.

Lupus of the Face.—In a very large proportion of cases lupus is absolutely limited to the face, and in a majority of cases the face is one of the regions attacked. Here we find almost all the various clinical forms. The anterior portion of the face is most frequently involved, and the nose is its special seat of predilection. It is probable that the mucous membrane of the nose is very often the starting-point of the process, and that the lupous nodules that are seen first on the alæ are secondary to an unrecognized affection of the mucous passages. Cartilage is a tissue that is rapidly invaded by tuberculosis, and the cartilaginous septum may be completely destroyed, so that the nose looks as if it had been hacked off. In syphilis, on the other hand, the bony skeleton is chiefly affected, so that in this disease there is a sunken-in appearance of the upper part of the nose, while the tip remains intact and seems to project upwards. Lupus may attack the cheeks, lips, and ears, and sometimes the whole face is the seat of lupous lesions. The ears may become enormously hypertrophied from the extent of infiltration with the tuberculous process and from secondary papillary, fungous outgrowths. In this case, when the diseased tissue has been removed, the outer ear may be reduced to a mere stump. It is very seldom that we find a primary lupus of the forehead or scalp. When in these places it is usually from extension from adjacent foci. Lupus of the scalp does not ulcerate until the process has been present for some time. When it ulcerates it is usually covered with greasy crusts, and the hairs may remain unaltered for a considerable time. In advanced cases, where the whole face has been invaded, the most frightful disfigurement may result. The skin may be so atrophied and cicatrized that the mouth can scarcely be opened for speaking or for the reception of food. The nose may be reduced to a mere stump, with two small apertures for the nostrils, or the latter may be entirely obliterated. The eyelids may be almost totally destroyed, and the ears reduced to a formless remnant.

Lupus of the Genitals.—It is very seldom that we find lupus seated upon the genital organs, and in most cases it is consecutive to a lupus of the groins and thighs. It may, however, appear primarily on the penis and scrotum. Hebra stated that he had met with but one case on the penis. It is very rarely found upon the vulva, and many cases described as lupus in this situation are undoubtedly entirely different affections.

Lupus of the Extremities.—Next to the face, the extremities are the most common seat of lupus. In 312 cases collected by Leloir, the extremities were affected in 52. In 30 of these 52 cases there were other tuberculous lesions on the integument. It is more frequent in men than in women, while the reverse is true when it is situated upon other parts. The forearms and lower legs are the parts of the extremities most affected, and the process is very apt to extend from above downwards. The region of the joints is very frequently affected, and there are often present deep, scrofulous lesions and caries of the bones. It is usually seated upon the extensor surface of the extremities, although it may occur on the flexor aspect. Cases of lupus developing primarily upon the palms and soles are on record, but they are very rare. Lupus in this situation is much more apt to pursue a serpiginous course than in other places.

In subjects of twelve years and over, very great mutilation may result from lupus of the extremities, where it has attacked the deeper structures, including tendons, fasciæ, bones, and articulations. When it is seated in the skin over the joints it may, by the resulting cicatrices, cause a pseudo-ankylosis, or parts or the whole of fingers and toes may be totally destroyed. The appearances are often much like those of lepra mutilans, or sarcoma and mycosis fungoides may be simulated. It may often be difficult to recognize the nature of the process when it has produced these great mutilations, without taking into account the antecedents of the patient or finding some signs of tuberculosis in other portions of the body.

Another deformity may be added to those that result from the contraction of scars, and from the caries, necrosis, and fistulæ in the deeper structures, and that is a great thickening and induration of the cutaneous tissues, so that a condition of elephantiasis is produced. The causes of this are somewhat varied, and include the venous and lymphatic stasis produced by the contraction of the cicatrices, the dermatitis set up by the lupous process, and frequently recurring attacks of lymphangitis and sometimes of phlebitis. The successive outbreaks of lymphangitis are perhaps the most important factor, leaving the skin in a state of chronic œdema. When this has persisted for a long time, there begins to be a new formation of connective tissue. The connective tissue of the skin and the subcutaneous tissue become greatly hypertrophied, and the periosteum and bones are thickened and enlarged, so that the whole member may be greatly increased in size—a so-called pseudo-elephantiasis. Very often in these cases there is a condition of chronic dermatitis, with papillomatous and frambœsioid projections from the surface of the skin. These papillomatous masses are commonest on the back of the foot, and may extend upwards towards the knee. They may be red and may bleed easily, or they may be covered with thickened, dry incrustations of epidermis. They may contain small abscesses, and superficial or deep fungous ulcers may follow, penetrating sometimes to the necrosed bones. Fresh eruptions of lupus commonly appear from time to time on these hypertrophied arms or legs, or the lupus may disappear and be completely masked by the pseudo-elephantiasis. In this latter case the diagnosis, without other data, may be a matter of extreme difficulty. The attacks of lymphangitis are of a similar nature to those that occur in true elephantiasis, but they are not so frequent, nor do they lead, as a rule, to so great an enlargement of the part. These cases of pseudo-elephantiasis are not common, and when they occur it is usually on the lower limbs. Leloir and Doutrelepont have stated that they have never met with a case on the arms. Although extremely rare, it is occasionally seen on the arms, and the writer has met with a well-marked example in the case of a girl of seventeen, where the left forearm was enormously enlarged and in a state of chronic œdema, the surface of the skin presenting numerous foci of lupus.

Lupus of the Mucous Membranes.—The mucous membranes are in the larger number of instances affected secondarily to the skin, yet primary lupus here is probably more common than has been supposed. Lupus of the mucous membranes is more difficult of diagnosis than that of the skin, as the characteristic signs are masked and removed by the thinness of the epithelium, which offers little resistance to the process and easily becomes macerated by the secretions. No typical lupous nodules are present, but we see papillary elevations, which, according to Chiari and Riehl, are the primary lesions. They coalesce to form plaques, more or less denuded of epithelium, and may either be absorbed or break down to form ulcers. These ulcers may offer great difficulties to the diagnostician, and it

is often impossible to distinguish them by their clinical appearances
from the tuberculous ulcers of the mucous membranes that sometimes
accompany an internal or general tuberculosis. This, however, is of
minor importance, since both are forms of the tuberculous process.

We are often called upon to differentiate these lupous ulcers from
those of syphilis, and this is of extreme importance. Chiari and
Riehl consider the reappearance of the primary lesions in the cicatrices an important aid to diagnosis. In this case they appear as
reddish-brown nodules seated in the scar tissue, and bear much
resemblance to the primary lupous nodules of the skin. The absorption of these nodules in some places and their breaking down and
ulceration in other places afford a help to their recognition. Ulceration is more likely to affect the larger infiltrations.

Lupus of the Nasal Mucous Membrane.—Of late years the belief
has been rapidly gaining ground that primary lupus of the nose is
of far more common occurrence than has been previously supposed,
and that a large proportion of the cases of lupus of the external integument that occur upon the face are produced by its extension
from the mucous membranes. Recent observations on leprosy have
tended to show that in this disease also the mucous membrane of the
nose is a favorite starting-point, so that an analogy between the two
diseases may perhaps be traced in this way. One reason why the
frequency of nasal lupus has been underestimated is that it has often
been taken for a chronic eczema, coryza, or impetigo. Lupus of the
nasal mucous membrane always has a slow course, and is usually
first indicated by a chronic coryza. Leloir has noted epistaxis as
one of the first symptoms in a number of cases. Lupus in this situation rarely attacks the bones, while exerting a most destructive
action on the cartilaginous parts.

Lupus of the Conjunctival Mucous Membrane.—In this situation
lupus is rarely primary. There is great hyperæmia of the mucous
membrane, which is covered with soft, reddish-gray, painless infiltrations, which resemble granulations somewhat, and are usually dry.
Sometimes exuberant and vegetative appearances are seen. The disease is usually unilateral, developing upon the lower lid and sometimes extending to the bulbar conjunctiva and to the cornea.

Lupus of the Mucous Membrane of the Mouth and Pharynx.—A
lupus of the face is sometimes complicated by the presence of the
process in the mouth and pharynx. In this situation it is rarely
primary. It may develop upon the gums, which are greatly swollen,
softened, and boggy, easily bleeding, and covered with bright-red
elevations. The writer has seen a case in which the entire gum of
both jaws was affected in this way. On the mucous membrane of

the cheeks and lips, grayish, rounded elevations, resembling mucous patches, are sometimes seen. On the hard palate we may find an appearance of tumefaction with granular elevations, or a simple exaggeration of the folds of the mucous membranes. Instances of perforation of the bony palate are on record.

Lupus of the tongue is so rare that its existence has been denied by a certain number of dermatologists. Leloir has, however, recorded a case observed at the Saint Sauveur Hospital, where the diagnosis was confirmed by bacteriological and histological proofs, and a few other cases have been reported. It seems to be always secondary, and is usually accompanied by lupus of the mouth, pharynx, or larynx. In a case of extensive lupus seen by the writer, in which almost the whole face, together with the gums and soft palate, was affected, the central portion of the dorsum of the tongue was occupied by a deep chronic ulcer, its floor made up of uneven and exuberant granulations, which were covered with a grayish exudation. The edges were soft and slightly raised. The ulcer was sensitive to pressure, and very rebellious to treatment. A microscopical examination was not possible, but there can be little doubt that this was a lupus ulcer. In the cases reported by Leloir and others, the lesions consisted of tubercles and sclerous elevations, and there was little ulceration.

Lupus of the larynx is also rare. It is usually secondary, although three or four cases of its primary occurrence have been reported. It occurred in two cases out of one hundred examined laryngoscopically by Leloir. It is said to be more common in women than in men. It usually arises from the extension of a lesion of the pharynx or nasal cavity, and it is sometimes associated with lesions of the skin. It is almost always found upon the epiglottis, and may spread to the vocal cords. Cough and expectoration are not prominent symptoms, but there is an increasing hoarseness which may be succeeded by complete aphonia. Chiari and Riehl, who have made the most complete study of this form, assert that the first appearances are small papillary elevations, which may be single or in groups, and which after a time are either absorbed or break down to form ulcers of an irregular or round shape, with soft, flat edges, and covered with purulent secretion. They closely resemble in many respects the lupous nodules of the skin, and like the latter they tend to recur in the cicatrices. The mucous membrane is anæmic in appearance, except at the very beginning of the affection. The course is eminently slow, and dangerous complications—such as chondritis, perichondritis, necrosis, and œdema of the larynx—rarely occur. There is apt to be marked enlargement of the cervical glands. The diagnosis of lupous ulcers from the appearances is often a matter of great difficulty. There may, as has been claimed, be some points of distinction between lupous ulcers and tuberculous ulcers associated with tuberculosis of the lungs. The appearance of lesions similar to the nodules of lupus of the skin, and the tendency to a recurrence in the cicatrices, are to be emphasized especially. As the two processes are etiologically the same, these points of distinction are of minor importance, and may be due simply to a greater or less acuteness in the course of the tuberculous process. Leloir and Michelson have both laid stress on the fact that it is very difficult to distinguish between lupus of the mucous membranes and other forms of tuberculosis of these structures.

TUBERCULOSIS VERRUCOSA.

This form of tuberculosis is identical with the anatomical tubercle or wart—verruca necrogenica—that has long been recognized as affecting those working at dissections or autopsies, ward tenders, etc. It was first pointed out by French writers, Besnier and Vidal in particular, that this growth occurred on the hands of people who had performed autopsies on the bodies of consumptives, and they further called attention to its resemblance to certain forms of lupus. In 1882 this form was described by Leloir and Vidal as a variety of sclerous lupus, and in 1884-85 tubercle bacilli were found in the tissue. The name tuberculosis verrucosa cutis was given to it by Riehl and Paltauf in 1886. They pointed out that it was not uncommonly found on the hands of butchers, cooks, and those who had to do with animals or animal products, and that it had a close relationship with verruca necrogenica. Further investigations have proved beyond doubt that the so-called anatomical wart is a verrucous tuberculosis, at least in a great majority of instances. It may be, as is suggested by Leloir, that the pyogenic microorganisms in certain instances give rise to clinical appearances that may resemble this form, but the microscope would always settle the diagnosis.

There is more diversity in the clinical characteristics of this form than was indicated in the original description of Riehl and Paltauf. This is owing chiefly to the existence or not of secondary inflammation. If there is much inflammation, we have at the outer edge of a growing plaque a bright-red, erythematous band, while the next zone towards the centre is made up of pustules. The centre of the plaque is covered with crusts and a warty outgrowth. Between the elongated papillary excrescences there are fissures from which pus may be squeezed out. If the secondary inflammation is slight or wanting, there are no erythematous and pustular zones, but we may have only a tubercle of rather soft consistence, with a tendency to papillary **hypertrophy of its surface.** The warty tendency may in some instances be very slight, but it is a marked characteristic of this form. The patches may be small or large, in some instances occupying the whole back of the hand. The affection is most commonly met with on the hands and exposed portions of the body. Many years ago McCall Anderson described a form of lupus verrucosus, or scrofuloderma verrucosum, in which warty outgrowths were found in children on the backs of the hands, on the elbows, and on the knees. The writer has observed a number of these cases, and is convinced that they are examples of tuberculosis verrucosa. In some instances they have been associated with tuberculosis of other tissues. Tuberculosis verrucosa rarely ulcerates, but it may disappear by absorption, leaving a cicatrix, and this is especially true of the cases observed in children.

This form of tuberculosis is very chronic in its course, and the patch or patches may remain for years without undergoing any marked alteration. In some cases, however, it has been followed by tuberculous infiltration of the adjoining lymphatic glands and by foci of lupus in the vicinity, and cases are on record in which tuberculosis of the internal organs has led to a fatal result. As a rule, however, it progresses very slowly and does not in the least affect the health of the individuals. Now that this form is well recognized, it is shown to be more frequent on the hands of pathologists and those who handle morbid material than had been imagined. It is also known that in a great many instances the affection has been acquired from nursing a consumptive patient or relative. From the frequency with which we can show that there has been a direct exposure by contact to tuberculous tissue, it is now believed that this form represents the results of a direct inoculation of tuberculosis upon the skin in the parts where it is commonly found. Those parts are, as has been said, the backs of the fingers and hands, the elbows, and knees. It is very probable that the clinical appearances of this form are determined somewhat by the structure of the skin in these, its favorite localities.

SCROFULODERMA.

When tuberculosis is seated in the deeper structures, in the subcutaneous tissues, and the skin also is involved, we call the condition scrofuloderma. As a rule, these lesions have their starting-point in a lymph gland or in a lymphatic trunk, since it is through the lymphatic system that the poison is carried; but oftentimes no association with a lymphatic structure can be detected clinically, and the process seems to originate in the subcutaneous tissue. They may arise from nodules formed around a lymph channel, perilymphangitic nodes, and a series of scrofulous lesions and ulcers may be seen along the course of a lymphatic trunk. As a rule, the skin is involved only secondarily and by extension of the process upwards from the deeper structures. Leloir has occasionally observed a more or less extended plaque of lupus become transformed directly into a scrofulous ulcer, but this is very exceptional. Not infrequently, however, lupous nodules are seen in the cicatrix of a scrofuloderma.

When observed at the outset these lesions appear as soft, circumscribed infiltrations of the deeper tissues, over which the skin is freely movable. They are neither tender nor painful, and are usually chronic in their course. After a time the skin becomes involved by the extension of the process upwards, and appears thinned, hyperæmic, and of a bluish color. The nodule softens perceptibly, and finally breaks down; the contents, which consist of necrotic tissue, serum, and pus cells, are evacuated, and the so-called scrofulous ulcer is the result. These ulcers vary much in size and in depth. If the process has arisen in the deep-lying lymph glands and channels, a deep ulcer is produced, which may send fistulous passages and openings down to the cartilage and bone. If, however, the affection had its origin in the more superficial tissues immediately below the skin, we find a more or less extensive superficial ulceration, with reddish, soft edges. In general, the soft consistence of these nodules and the edges of the ulcers afford an important aid in differentiating them from syphilis and other affections with which they may be confounded. Another diagnostic sign of some importance is the fact that the edges are apt to be undermined, since the extent of the breaking down is greater than the original point of opening. Several openings may be present, separated by small bridges of skin. These ulcers have a soft, easily bleeding floor, made up of pale granulations and covered usually with a purulent secretion. They may occur on any part of the body, but are commonest about the face and neck. As in the case of lupous ulcers, scrofulous ulcers, especially those of the extremities, may take on a papillary hypertrophy, so that vegetating and fungous forms arise.

The course of scrofuloderma is very slow, especially in the case of children, in whom the infiltrations are situated deep in the skin and remain hard and unchanged for a long time. Sometimes a fibrous capsule is formed about the infiltration, which shuts it off and interferes with its farther progress, and very rarely absorption of the lesion may take place before it has become broken down and opening has taken place. Occasionally an acute inflammation may occur, in which the tuberculous tissue may become merged, and as a result the whole mass may be eliminated and healing may occur with the formation of cicatrices. As a general thing, after remaining hard for a longer or shorter period, the nodule softens and breaks through the epidermis, and the ulcer which results pursues a chronic course and increases in extent from the constant breaking down of the infiltrated edges. The scars that are left from these scrofulous ulcers are not distinctive in form or in appearance, except possibly as regards their irregularity, bridges and bands of cicatricial tissue being often seen ramifying between areas of sound skin, in a net-like way.

Pathology and Morbid Anatomy.

The histological appearances of the forms of cutaneous tuberculosis that have been described vary to a considerable extent, in connection with the clinical type. Essentially, however, they present many features common to one another and to the process of tuberculosis wherever found. It is not intended in this place to enter into a full discussion of the histogenesis of tubercle. The best modern belief, however, regards the large cells, resembling epithelial cells that have been called *epithelioid* cells, as the ones chiefly concerned in the process. These cells are the first to appear, and are derived from the fixed connective-tissue cells, as has been proved by Baumgarten's karyokinetic figures in the cornea of animals inoculated experimentally with tuberculosis. The epithelioid cells form the centre of the tubercle or nodule of granulation tissue, which is produced in some way by the action of the tubercle bacillus. Besides these central epithelioid cells, other cells are present that go to make up the nodule. We soon begin to find large cellular elements with nuclei arranged more or less peripherally and a homogeneous centre—the so-called Langhans giant cells. These cells, of very varying size, are produced from the epithelioid cells, by the process of nuclear division taking place at a much more rapid rate than that of the cell itself.

The other cells that are chiefly concerned in the tuberculous process are the lymphoid cells or lymphocytes and the so-called "plasma" cells of Unna. These varieties of cells make up almost entirely the inflammatory infiltration, which surrounds the central zone of epithelioid and giant cells. The epithelioid and giant cells are to be regarded as forming the true tuberculous neoplasm, and the lymphoid and plasma cells as more or less secondary. The lymphoid cells are very small, mononuclear cells, deeply staining, with a small amount of protoplasm surrounding the nucleus. Larger mononuclear leucocytes are also seen, but they are few in number. Together with the lymphoid cells we find also, sometimes in great numbers, the plasma cells, to which so much importance has been attached by Unna. These are large mononuclear cells, with protoplasm that takes the stain from nuclear coloring reagents, and with a nucleus situated usually at one end of the cell. Unna has named these cells plasma cells, and considers that they are derived from the connective-tissue cells, and that they play an important part in the pathology of skin diseases, so that he has named the various neoplasms in which they occur plasmomata. He has modified his earliest opinion that they are peculiar to the tuberculous process. He lays stress upon their coloring properties, as that their protoplasm is stained deeply by polychromic methylene blue, and that they do not decolorize like other cells. Marschalko, who has published an excellent article on this subject, lays more stress on the eccentric position of the nucleus and the character of the protoplasm than on their staining properties. Marschalko and others have shown conclusively that these "plasma" cells are not derived from the normal connective-tissue cells of the part, but that they are produced from the lymphoid cells. Councilman, in his studies of acute interstitial nephritis, has shown that they exist in this process in large numbers, and that they enter into the interstitial tissue of the kidney by emigration from the blood-vessels. He has observed them emigrating from the vessels as full-formed plasma cells, and has also seen them formed from emigrated lymphoid cells by mitotic division. It has also been shown that these cells are not peculiar to pathological processes. They are formed normally in the mucous membrane of the intestine, and some observers have stated that they occur in the spleen, lymph glands, and bone marrow. It may be confidently asserted that lymphoid and · plasma cells have the same origin, and that both are derived from the blood-vessels.

Polynuclear leucocytes may also be seen in tuberculosis of the skin, but these do not appear as a rule until a later stage of the process, when the tissue has become degenerated and breaks down. Mast cells are also seen as in other chronic inflammatory processes, sometimes with extended branched processes, and filled with granules deeply stained with aniline coloring agents. Their origin and destiny are unknown.

A characteristic of the epithelioid and giant cells that form the centre of the tuberculous neoplasm is that they are unstable and sooner or later begin to degenerate. The cell protoplasm becomes coagulated, and the nuclei lose their capacity for receiving stains. The intercellular substance is included in the degeneration, and the result is a coagulation necrosis or cheesy degeneration. This cheesy degeneration, as well as the presence of the Langhans giant cells, was considered at one time as pathognomonic of tuberculosis. But cheesy degeneration has been shown to occur in numerous other conditions, and the typical Langhans giant cells may occur in the tissue about vessel ligatures, and in the gummatous and lichenoid forms of syphilis. Although, therefore, a pretty typical histological picture is found in cutaneous tuberculosis, there are no pathognomonic features. It is to the presence of the tubercle bacillus that we must look for a positive sign. This bacillus has been found to be constantly present in all forms of cutaneous tuberculosis, although often so sparingly that its detection is a matter of extreme difficulty.

TUBERCULOSIS CUTIS.

In this form the structure of the pathological infiltration offers a close similarity to that of the miliary tuberculosis of internal organs. There are numerous foci of tuberculous tissue, usually superficial, but sometimes extending to a considerable depth. These foci are made up of epithelioid and giant cells surrounded by a zone of lymphocytes and probably plasma cells. An early necrosis is a marked feature of this form, and the microscope shows an early degeneration and softening of the centre. The tuberculous foci form by their coalition masses of softened, cheesy-degenerated tissue, and oftentimes the unaltered granulations can be found only at the edges of the necrotic masses. The epidermis is therefore broken through quite · early in the process, leaving the ulcerated surface so characteristic of this form. In an ulcer of this type examined by the writer, the upper part of the corium was transformed into a necrotic mass, in which very few of the cells retained the stain. Below and at either side, however, typical, small, tuberculous foci with the characteristic cell structure were to be seen. The necrocis had involved the overlying epidermis, which had disappeared in the ulcerative process. Tubercle bacilli were present in large numbers, both in the necrotic area and in and about the miliary nodules, so that each field showed them in enormous numbers. The large number of bacilli found in this form has been noted by almost all who have studied it, and this may be asserted to be one of its chief characteristics, in distinction from the other varieties of cutaneous tuberculosis in which they are always few. In this respect we find a further analogy with the miliary tuberculosis of the internal organs. For this reason this form has been classed as a true tuberculosis of the skin, and its existence has been offered as an argument against the tuberculous nature of lupus, in that we have here a form that corresponds completely with tuberculosis in other situations, and that differs markedly from lupus. While it is true that there are some pathological distinctions from lupus, it is also true that these differences are those that distinguish an acute from a more chronic and sluggish tuberculosis of other parts. The process of necrosis is much more speedily accomplished, owing in all probability to the large number of tubercle bacilli that are present in this form, and these same phenomena occur in acute tuberculosis of other tissues.

LUPUS.

When a section from a lesion of lupus that has not been present a very long time is examined under the microscope, one sees, with a low power, masses of cells arranged in nodules or foci, and scattered through the middle and lower layers of the corium. The papillary layer is rarely affected primarily, and is involved only later by the extension upwards of the lower foci. The nodule is made up of the characteristic central giant cells of the Langhans type and of epithelioid elements, while around them we find with more or less regularity masses of plasma cells and lymphoid cells. The normal connective tissue has disappeared within the affected area, as have the blood vessels and lymphatic channels. At the edge of the nodule there is usually some proliferation of the connective tissue, which may form a sort of wall about the neoplasm. The central epithelioid and giant cells soon begin to suffer degeneration; their protoplasm becomes homogeneous, and the nuclei do not readily stain. This degeneration has been considered by Weigert and others to be a coagulation necrosis. A true cheesy degeneration does not occur in lupus, as the necrobiosis does not, on account of the chronic character of the process, usually progress to that degree. The absence of this cheesy degeneration was formerly advanced as an argument against the tuberculous nature of lupus, but its slow progress and the small number of bacilli present are sufficient to account for this difference. The large number of giant cells and the smaller proportion of epithelioid cells present in lupus, as compared with tuberculosis of many other tissues, may also be explained by the slow development of this form, as has been experimentally shown by feeding animals with attenuated cultures of tubercle bacilli.

The nodules of tuberculous new formation continue to appear and to follow oftentimes the blood and lymph channels, and larger areas of infiltration are produced by their coalescence. After the mass of partially degenerated new formation has increased in size and the epidermis has become thinned by the pressure, the outer skin is broken through and a lupous ulcer is the result. Properly speaking, there is no suppuration in uncomplicated lupus. That which has been called suppuration is usually this softening and breaking down of the granulation tissue. A true suppuration occurs only when a septic process has been grafted on the tuberculous tissue.

Besides this process of degeneration that is going on in the epithelioid cells, we have also a regenerative process. When the cells are not so far affected as to undergo an advanced necrosis, they may proliferate, and new connective tissue may be formed. This process is seen at the edges of the nodule, and the lupous scar tissue that replaces the nodules when they disappear by degeneration is formed in this way. This lupous scar tissue is regarded by Unna as still possessing many of the characteristics of lupus.

When this process of regeneration occurs to an extreme degree, we see the forms of elephantiasis that have been described in the section on symptomatology. Large portions of the body are converted into dense masses of fibrous tissue, in the midst of which nodular foci of degeneration are found to a varying extent. It is to the varying degree of connective-tissue new formation, as compared with the degeneration of the neoplasm, that is due in some measure the great variety of clinical forms that we meet with in lupus.

Another phenomenon that we meet with in lupus is a proliferation of the epithelium. The epidermis is generally thickened above the infiltration in the corium, and the horny layer may be greatly hypertrophied in the papillary verrucous forms. In these latter cases the rete may send its interpapillary prolongations deep into the corium, and this, together with the outgrowth of the papillæ that accompanies the epithelial proliferation, produces the warty form that we refer to. In some instances the appearances of epithelioma are simulated, and it is necessary to cut sections with the greatest care and absolutely perpendicularly to the surface, to decide this question. The glandular epithelium may also proliferate, as was pointed out many years ago by Lang. These changes in the epithelial elements are to be regarded, so far as our present knowledge allows us to determine, as secondary phenomena caused by the irritation produced by the tuberculous neoplasm, and not a direct result of the presence of the bacilli. It is probably analogous to the epithelial proliferation that is sometimes seen in syphilis and in other chronic inflammatory affections.

Colloid lupus and myxomatous lupus have been described by Leloir. In colloid lupus the centre of the nodules is stained a yellowish-orange color by picrocarmine, and presents other appearances similar to the colloid tuberculosis of the lung. It is not a virulent form. Myxomatous lupus is another rare form, in which the connective tissue, and to some extent the neoplasm itself, has undergone a mucoid degeneration. The bacilli in this form are very few in number and are enclosed in the giant cells.

A complication that should be spoken of in this place is that with carcinoma. Malignant epitheliomata may occasionally develop in the territory covered by lupous infiltrations or scars. When this occurs the course of the malignant growth is apt to be more rapid than usual, and when the face is the seat of the disease a large portion of the tissues may be destroyed before death occurs.

Lupus is not rich in tubercle bacilli, but still they may be found in all the forms, if a long enough search is made. The time required for their detection renders their diagnostic value rather small. When seen they are very frequently enclosed in Langhans giant cells, but they may be anywhere in the tuberculous tissue. The small number of bacilli in lupus is in striking contrast to what is found in the miliary form, in which large masses are present.

TUBERCULOSIS VERRUCOSA CUTIS.

In this form of tuberculosis the tuberculous neoplasm is seated essentially in the upper papillary layers of the corium. In their description of typical cases in which the warty element is much accentuated, Riehl and Paltauf state that the horny layer is much increased in thickness over the elongated papillæ, and also dips down into crypt-like depressions at the base of the papilloma. Between the horny scales, dried masses of exudation are found, with nuclei that have not wholly lost their capacity for being stained, and also a granular detritus. The stratum granulosum is occasionally wanting in certain places. The prickle-cell layer is increased in size, and the interpapillary prolongations penetrate deeply into the corium in many places.

The most important changes are in the upper layers of the corium, as has been said. It is only occasionally that the lower and subcutaneous layers are affected. The papillæ are enlarged in all dimensions. In the subpapillary layer are seen numerous isolated or irregularly confluent foci of cell infiltration, which are mostly extended in a horizontal direction. These foci have all the characteristic histological features of tuberculous deposit in other situations. The centre is occupied by epithelioid and giant cells, which in some instances have lost their characteristics and have become merged into a cheesy-degenerated mass. At the periphery are masses of lymphocytes and their derivatives, the plasma cells.

Besides these tuberculous foci that have been mentioned, there are also foci of inflammation and suppuration. These occur chiefly where the epidermis dips down very deeply, and often result in a breaking through of the epidermis and a sloughing of the superficial tissues. Tubercle bacilli are found in the giant and epithelioid cells, and also free in the granulation tissue. Micrococci are found in the foci of acute inflammation and suppuration.

Since the original description of this form by Riehl and Paltauf, it has been established that these miliary subepidermal abscesses that were regarded by them as a secondary infection, but as a characteristic of this form, are by no means a constant feature. Certainly they are not present often enough to render their absence a point of any consequence. In the cases of this form examined by the writer, in which the lesions were seated upon the elbows, knees, and hands of children, the suppurating foci were almost entirely wanting. There is also a great difference in the extent to which the papillary outgrowth is developed. It is true, however, that the papillary hypertrophy usually occurs at the outset of the process, while in lupus it comes at a later period, after ulceration has taken place. The most important anatomical feature of this form is the situation of the tuberculous neoplasm in the upper papillary layers. Many transitional forms may occur between a verrucous tuberculosis and lupus, and it may often be difficult to say from a microscopical examination alone which of the two varieties we are dealing with. As to the number of bacilli that are present, Riehl and Paltauf found them more numerous than in lupus, but far less so than in miliary tuberculosis. The writer's own studies have found them to be very sparingly present in the cases examined, quite as much so as in lupus.

SCROFULODERMA.

Scrofuloderma, or tuberculosis of the subcutaneous tissues, offers the well-marked characteristics of tuberculosis in other parts. We find foci of granulation tissue, composed of epithelioid and giant cells, surrounded by lymphoid cells, in the subcutaneous tissue and in the glands, which may become confluent, undergo a cheesy degeneration beginning at the centre, and break through the thinned layers of overlying epidermis, so that a characteristic ulcer is produced. The death of the tissue usually occurs to a greater extent and in a more marked degree than in lupus, and large areas of softened, cheesy-degenerated tissue are often produced. The resulting ulcer has the characteristic soft, undermined edges. All these scrofulous glands and ulcers have been shown by inoculation experiments to be a true tuberculosis in this situation. A careful search will always reveal the presence of tubercle bacilli, sometimes in considerable numbers. At other times they are sparingly represented, and on the whole are less numerous than in tuberculosis cutis, but more so than in lupus.

Etiology.

There can now be no question that the four forms of cutaneous lesions that have been described are caused by the inoculation of the skin with the tubercle bacillus. This has been proved by finding the bacilli present in all cases, although sometimes in small numbers, and by the production of tuberculosis in the lower animals by the inoculation of pure cultures obtained from these several types of lesion. It remains to consider in what way the inoculation takes place. The older theories, such as the existence of a diathesis in the case of scrofulodermata—the "scrofulous diathesis"—have been generally abandoned. Nor is it necessary to assume the existence of an hereditary or acquired predisposition for tuberculosis more than for any other infectious disease.

Heredity.—Much less importance is now attached to the part that heredity may play in the etiology of tuberculosis than formerly, when it was not known that the disease was caused by a specific microorganism, which could be proved in many instances to produce the disease by direct inoculation. It must be conceded, however, that in the case of the typical clinical form of lupus the predisposition at least may be transmitted to the descendants. At all events, we are not yet in a position to deny this possibility absolutely. Of three hundred and twelve cases of lupus observed by Leloir, a similar affection occurred in the parents or in a brother or sister in twenty-six instances. It has not, however, been shown that lupus, or cutaneous tuberculosis in general, is especially common in the descendants of people who have had tuberculosis. It is always difficult to say in a given case that the tuberculosis may not have been acquired during the early months of infancy, inasmuch as unquestionable cases of congenital tuberculosis must be extremely rare, if they occur at all. The fact that mother and child are in such intimate association at this time renders the probability of infection a plausible one. Certain statistics have shown that when the mother has tuberculosis the proportion of children affected with the disease is larger than when the father is the one affected; and the reason for this has been thought to lie in the greater chance of infection that the intimate contact with the mother offers. Upon the whole, there is little absolute proof that heredity plays any considerable part in the etiology of cutaneous tuberculosis. We have no absolute knowledge that the disease is ever, strictly speaking, inherited, although there are certain facts that should make us cautious about disputing this possibility. On the other hand, we know that infection after birth is an undoubted fact, and that almost all of the cases that have been ascribed to heredity may be equally well explained on the theory of an infection.

Direct Inoculation.—The form of tuberculosis in which a direct inoculation can be demonstrated with the greatest frequency is the verrucous form—tuberculosis verrucosa cutis. As has been stated, this affection was first noticed on the hands of those engaged in the performance of autopsies or of dissections, and was called anatomical wart. It is the result of a direct inoculation of the virus of tuberculosis upon a previous cut or abrasion of the skin. It is a question whether the unbroken skin may be invaded by the bacilli through the hair follicles. Some observations on the lesions acquired by pathologists render the latter supposition at least tenable.

It is found also upon inquiry that these warty tuberculous lesions occur with great frequency, as was pointed out by Riehl and Paltauf, on the hands of cooks, butchers, and people who are in the habit of handling animal products, which are liable to infection from tuberculosis. A number of instances have been noted in Boston of cattle men who had charge of the live stock on trans-Atlantic steamships becoming infected. In the case of women, it can be shown in a surprisingly large proportion of cases that the patient was nursing or was in intimate contact with a relative or friend who had tuberculosis of the lungs at the time when the lesion made its appearance.

In these cases an opportunity of infection is offered by the soiled linen and handkerchiefs which the subject of the tuberculous lesion was in the habit of washing. A direct infection from the sputum and from the sputa cups is also a probability. An instance has been recorded by Dubreuilh of a woman who had cleaned the sputa cups of a tuberculous relative and who developed warty nodules upon her fingers, which were followed by scrofulous lesions upon the arm and suppurating glands in the axilla. The presence of tubercle bacilli was detected in all of these lesions, and inoculation experiments upon animals proved successful. A number of instances of scrofuloderma consecutive to these warty lesions have been observed at the Massachusetts General Hospital, and have been recorded by White. The infection is carried from the verrucous lesions through the lymphatic channels, and the scrofulous ulcers are produced through the breaking down of tuberculous nodules along the course of the lymphatic trunks, or from the infected lymphatic glands. Several instances are on record of general tuberculosis and death resulting from these warty lesions. We not infrequently see typical patches of lupus in connection with these warty and scrofulous lesions, showing the close relationship of the various forms of this disease.

The occurrence of tuberculosis upon the penis as the result of inoculation during the rite of circumcision has already been referred to. Stab wounds and bites may also afford an entrance to the poison, as well as the holes in the ears that are made for earrings.

Autoinoculation is seen in its most typical form in the miliary ulcers that occur at the outlets of the mouth, nose, anus, and vagina, in subjects affected with tuberculosis of the internal organs. In these instances bacilli in large numbers are given off with the secretions, and a crack or fissure offers an opportunity for autoinoculation at the edge of the skin. Not infrequently tuberculosis verrucosa is found upon the hands of consumptives, and in these cases it is fair to assume an autoinoculation from the sputum.

The verrucous form is the one in which the evidence of a direct inoculation can most frequently be obtained. With regard to lupus, it is much more difficult to trace an inoculation. Still a sufficient number of cases are on record to render it certain that this form also is produced, at least in some instances, in this way. Leloir relates a number of instances in which there seemed to be good evidence of a direct inoculation of lupus from tuberculous secretions. Lipp and Jadassohn have also published similar cases. In Jadassohn's case a typical lupus developed upon the forearm of a woman of thirty, at the point where she had been tattooed by a person who had at the time tuberculosis of the lungs and had used his saliva for moistening the pigments. In one of Leloir's cases a young child developed a plaque of lupus at the centre of the cheek, at a spot which had previously been the seat of a chronic eczema, and which the mother, well advanced in pulmonary tuberculosis, had been in the habit of dressing with a poultice of bread crumbs moistened by her own saliva. Leloir believed that a large proportion of cases of lupus were due to direct inoculation. He pointed out that lupus occurs most often on regions that are exposed to an infection from an external agency, as the nose, cheeks, lips, ears, and hands, and that this form develops as a rule at a time when the child is brought much into contact with other people, in the process of dressing, feeding, fondling, etc. The writer has seen an instance in which a woman of thirty-five developed a small but typical patch of lupus of the chin. For over a year previous to the appearance of this lesion, she had been in the habit of paying frequent visits to a woman who suffered from an advanced lupus of the face, and whom she had kissed on several occasions.

Indirect Inoculation.—By this we mean a secondary inoculation of the skin from subcutaneous or deep-seated foci of tuberculosis. We not infrequently see nodules of lupus appearing at or near the edges of a scrofulous ulcer, or in the cicatrix which has replaced such a lesion. Occasionally cases of lupus are met with which have arisen from tuberculous fistulæ, and the writer has seen a case in which the buttocks were covered with patches of lupus, which began to appear soon after an operation for anal fistula. Sometimes deep-seated glands may become tuberculous, and from them a typical lupus develop in the vicinity, and this is also true of bone lesions. The lupous patches usually develop at the free cutaneous border of the fistula over which the tuberculous virus is poured. They sometimes appear at or soon after the establishment of the fistula, and sometimes are not developed until several years later (Leloir).

It is an interesting fact, as shown by the studies of a number of observers, that a cutaneous tuberculosis secondary to deep-seated foci of disease almost always presents itself in the form of typical lupus. This is contrary to what we see in cases of direct implantation of the virus, in which the papillary verrucous form usually results. Exceptionally, however, a verrucous tuberculosis may develop from distant foci by indirect inoculation, as shown in cases published by Leloir, Besnier, and others.

Lupus from indirect inoculation is more common than might be supposed, since Leloir's statistics show that it occurred 104 times in 312 cases of lupus. In these cases it followed a glandular tuberculosis in 32 instances, a tuberculosis of the subcutaneous tissues in 41, and tuberculosis of the bones or joints in 29. Sometimes a lupus is produced by transmission of the tuberculous virus to the skin by means of the lymphatic channels, without any implication of the intervening structures. Or scrofulodermatous lesions may arise in this way, and lesions may be found at various points along the course of the lymphatic vessels.

Sex.—Tuberculosis verrucosa, which as we have seen is usually the result of direct, demonstrable inoculation, occurs more frequently in men than in women, but this discrepancy may be satisfactorily explained by the greater opportunity for infection that the occupation and habits of the former sex offer. Lupus, on the contrary, is more frequent in women than in men. Of Leloir's 312 cases of lupus, 201 were in women and 111 in men.

With regard to *age*, it has been regarded as almost pathognomonic of lupus. It begins usually between the ages of two and nineteen years, and Hebra has asserted that it very rarely begins after the age of twenty. Of late it has been claimed that instances of its appearance later in life are more common than has been supposed, and the writer's experience accords with this view. It is an undoubted fact, however, that by far the larger number of all cases begin in childhood, and this may be owing to the greater susceptibility of the skin at that age, as well as to the greater opportunity offered for inoculation on the face through kissing, fondling, etc.

As to *climate,* although tuberculosis of the skin is met with everywhere, it seems to be more prevalent in temperate, moist, and cold regions. It is more common in Germany, Austria, and France than in Great Britain or the United States. Racial habits and characteristics must also be taken into account in this connection.

Association with Tuberculosis of the Lungs.—There has been much difference of opinion as to the frequency with which cutaneous tuberculosis is associated with, or followed by, pulmonary tuberculosis. The best statistics, however, show that this association occurs so frequently that we have no right to regard it as the result of a coincidence. Besnier, Neisser, Lailler, Leloir, and others have established this fact indisputably. Renouard's statistics gave 15 cases of pulmonary tuberculosis in 137 patients affected with lupus. Haslund, of Copenhagen, found that 60 per cent. of his cases had, or developed later, pulmonary tuberculosis also. Of Leloir's 312 collected cases, 98 had signs of tuberculosis in the lungs. It is noted that lupous patients develop pulmonary tuberculosis very slowly and in a latent manner. In certain instances it has been possible to trace the spread of the disease from a lupous focus on the hand to a tuberculous lymphangitis of the arm, with scrofulous ulcers developing along the lymphatic trunks, and with finally a pulmonary tuberculosis upon the same side as the affected hand.

Diagnosis.

The rare form of *miliary cutaneous tuberculosis*—l'ulcère des phthisiques—should be easy of recognition to any one who is on the lookout for it. A syphilitic ulcer might be thought of, but it differs from this by the presence at the edges of miliary tubercles, by the punched-out, serrated borders caused by their breaking down, and by the soft consistence of the neoplasm, which is common to all tuberculous infiltrations. Besides these points of distinction, we have the situation of these ulcers almost solely at the outlets of the mucous cavities and their association with tuberculosis of the internal organs. Epithelioma may be ruled out by the absence of hardness of the edges and of the epithelial pearls. Epithelioma is more apt to appear in people advanced in years. Tuberculosis verrucosa is most likely to be confounded with a simple warty or papillomatous lesion, as was the case in former times before the tuberculous nature of these growths was understood. It may also be confounded with the papillomatous lesions that arise from other chronic inflammatory processes. The mode of origin, its course, and the different characteristics that have been enumerated must all be taken into account. The possibility of verrucous tuberculosis should always be entertained in any long-standing, circumscribed, verrucous lesion of the exposed portions of the body. It might also in certain instances be taken for lichen planus or for a chronic eczema. Eczema, when present as a chronic circumscribed plaque, is hard and firm, does not ulcerate or heal by cicatrization, and spreads uniformly if at all. There is usually much less infiltration at the base of a plaque of eczema.

Lupus is more often confounded with syphilis than with any other affection. Lupus is apt to begin in early childhood, and to pursue a much slower, more chronic course than syphilis. It is, as a rule, a much more local affection than syphilis. Before a lupus has broken down, its tubercles, which may be confounded with syphilitic papules, are much softer than the latter; their color is usually more yellow, somewhat transparent; they are less apt to arrange themselves in circinate and serpiginous forms. After ulceration has occurred, it may at times be a matter of extreme difficulty to decide between lupus and syphilis from the clinical appearances alone. The clinical history is not to be relied on in the case of syphilis, as the infection may be denied or unknown, and in any event probably took place at a remote period. The edges of a lupous ulceration are much softer, more friable, and less deeply infiltrated than those of a syphilitic ulcer; its floor bleeds more readily and is more granular. Lupus does not often assume the circinate and serpiginous shape that syphilis does. We may find typical lupus nodules at the border of the lesion, which will render the diagnosis certain. A lupous ulcer is more likely to have begun in early childhood and to have pursued a slow, chronic course. When situated on the nose, lupus seldom attacks the cartilage and bone until a late period, while in syphilis the bony framework may sink in before the skin has become sensibly affected. Oftentimes it may be necessary to hold the case under observation for a certain period, watching for the possible development of lupus nodules or other conclusive signs before the diagnosis is determined. In some instances the iodide of potassium may settle the question. A rapid improvement under its use would point to syphilis.

Epithelioma may be excluded by the lack of its well-known characteristics, as enumerated above under the miliary form of tuberculosis, viz., its occurrence usually in people advanced in life, the great induration of its borders, and the presence of epithelial pearls. Other affections which may be embarrassing possibilities are chronic farcy and leprosy.

The microscope may be a decided aid. In a question as to the possibility of epithelioma it would be conclusive as establishing or rejecting such a diagnosis. Tubercle bacilli, if found, are of course pathognomonic. They are found in such small numbers in the more chronic forms, however, that practically a search for them is not of great value, unless much time is given to it. The histological structure is not convincing proof, as much the same microscopic appearances may be found in certain forms of syphilis, especially in the gummatous and lichenoid varieties.

We have a positive method of proof in successful inoculation experiments, but unfortunately these are rarely practicable.

Prognosis.

With regard to the miliary form—tuberculosis cutis—Kaposi states that the prognosis is not hopeless, as it may heal spontaneously. The larger number of cases, however, have been seen towards the end of life in patients who had serious internal tuberculosis.

The verrucous form yields, in a majority of instances, pretty readily to treatment, if it is attacked before it has been present a long time. Without treatment it may remain stationary for many years. In rarer instances, the virus may be propagated from this focus to other parts or may invade the general system. Lupous nodules may sometimes appear in the cicatrices left after surgical removal of these verrucous lesions.

Lupus may be much benefited or even wholly removed by proper treatment; but as the tendency of the lupus nodule is to recur, the prognosis cannot be said to be favorable, and we must always be prepared for fresh outbreaks. Spontaneous healing may occur in rare instances, but may then be only temporary, and lupous nodules may make their appearance in the cicatrix at any time. In all cases a cicatrix is left as the result of treatment or of absorption. Certain forms of lupus, such as the serpiginous variety, or when lupous nodules are scattered about in thickened sclerous tissue, are especially rebellious to treatment.

Scrofuloderma may in many instances be permanently healed, and a scar, which the patient carries through life, be the only result.

Treatment.

Despite the great advances that have been made of late years in our knowledge of the pathology and probable methods of infection in cutaneous tuberculosis, no important therapeutic discoveries can be recorded. We have no specific drugs, as is the case with the iodide of potassium and mercury in syphilis, which have the effect of causing the absorption of the neoplasm. Koch's tuberculin was hailed at the outset as likely to offer us a sure specific, but further trial has proved that its therapeutic value is of the slightest, and its use has been practically abandoned. It certainly has a remarkable action on tuberculous infiltrations, and as a matter of experiment or of diagnosis it may still have a place. Its injection sometimes causes an intense general reaction, which has, in some instances, endangered the life of the patient. Koch's new tuberculin, so-called tuberculin R, has of late been the subject of some experimentation. The local action upon the diseased tissue is much less pronounced and is longer delayed than in the case of the old tuberculin. Some favorable results from its use have been reported, but while it may be too soon to judge of its value, on the whole its claims of superiority over the old preparation have not been substantiated. The injection of thiosinamin has been recommended by H. von Hebra. It is capable of producing a certain amount of impression on the tuberculous neoplasm, and in particular upon the scar tissue.

PROPHYLACTIC TREATMENT.

Too much stress cannot be laid on the importance of preventive medicine, and tuberculosis of the skin is an affection in which prophylaxis may do much good. Leloir's rules, laid down some years ago, are pertinent and applicable to-day. They are:

1. The avoidance, so far as may be practicable, of bringing the virus of tuberculosis into contact with the skin.

2. The antiseptic treatment of every wound or abrasion that may have been contaminated by the virus.

3. The speedy and complete destruction of all deep tuberculous lesions that may be the source of a secondary inoculation of the skin.

4. The antiseptic treatment of every part of the skin that has been in contact with fæcal matter, sputum, uterine discharges, or other secretions from a tuberculous subject.

5. The greatest possible care of the skin of tuberculous patients.

6. The careful attention to the general health and hygiene of people descended from tuberculous subjects.

INTERNAL TREATMENT.

Modern therapeutics have offered us no advances in the treatment of cutaneous tuberculosis by internal remedies. We know of no drugs that have the power by themselves of healing this malady. A strict attention to hygiene and to the patient's mode of life may often, however, be of great service. A change of climate may aid much by improving the general nutrition. Tonics should be given freely if the system is below par. Cod-liver oil in debilitated subjects will often be of great value. The iodides and iodoform have been recommended by some writers, who claim for them a positive value. Quinine, iron, and the ferruginous mineral waters are oftentimes of great service in improving the general nutrition. Internal treatment, in a word, may be a useful adjuvant of other methods, but cannot of itself produce a cure.

EXTERNAL TREATMENT.

The external treatment of cutaneous tuberculosis is that upon which we must rely in the larger number of cases, and this is chiefly mechanical and surgical. There are numerous methods of external treatment, and almost all have their value in special cases. It is best to rely upon no one method in all cases, but to vary the procedure according to the size and position of the lesion, the age and general condition of the patient, and the complications of the disorder. Most dermatologists have their individual preferences for one or more methods of treatment, and their success usually lies in the facility that they have acquired by constant practice with the favorite method. But the best treatment is to vary the procedure according to the individual case.

SURGICAL TREATMENT.

Excision.—If a patch of tuberculoos tissue is of moderate extent, it may sometimes be excised with good result, and the edges of the wound brought together to heal by first intention. This method is not, however, of very wide application, contrary to what one might suppose. When the lesion is of considerable extent, or when it occurs upon the face, excision will usually cause too great a loss of tissue, as compared with that obtained by other methods of treatment, to justify its selection. It is also not so radical a method as might appear. Oftentimes, when a considerable margin of healthy tissue, both in depth and on the surface, has been included in the excision, we still find new foci of tuberculosis appearing in the cicatrix, which is often hypertrophied and deforming. Excision may often be practised with success in the case of isolated lesions of verrucous tuberculosis. Thiersch's method of skin grafting has been much used and praised by Lang, Jarisch, and others.

Curetting.—Volkmann was the first to employ and bring into notice this method, and it has since been widely used and is a great favorite with many dermatologists. The diseased tuberculous area is thoroughly scraped with the sharp spoon, and in this way the diseased portion is removed while the healthy tissue is not attacked to any extent. The verrucous and sclerous forms are especially adapted to this method, as well as large confluent areas. It is not an advantageous method where there are numerous isolated foci. The hemorrhage may be readily controlled by compression with tampons of absorbent cotton. The curetted surface may then be touched with the thermocautery, or various caustic agents applied. Subsequently Leloir advises the application of parasiticidal and caustic substances, as a recurrence of tuberculous foci in the cicatrix is more than a possibility. Scarification following curetting has not proved sufficient.

Linear Scarification.—Vidal's name is more closely associated with this method than any other, as he elaborated it and worked out the details to a point of great perfection. It was first suggested by Volkmann and modified by Balmanno Squire. Vidal's method consists in the employment of a scarifier in the form of a small, flattened blade, between 2 and 3 cm. long and 2 mm. wide. There are two cutting edges at a distance of about 1 cm. from the triangular point, which is from 1.5 to 2 mm. in length. In scarifying, this instrument is manipulated like a pen by the fingers alone, the outer edge of the palm resting upon some firm support. The incisions are always perpendicular to the surface, and are in parallel lines at a short distance from one another, and are then crossed by another series, so that the second series forms, with the first, angles of from 30° to 60°. The second series of incisions can then be crossed obliquely by a third and fourth series. The depth to which the incision is made is to be regulated according to the degree of resistance that is encountered. Hemorrhage is quite excessive during the first operations, but is readily controlled by tampons of absorbent cotton. The incisions are usually found to have healed in the course of four or five days, and it was Vidal's custom to repeat the procedure at intervals of eight days. He did not recommend the employment of local anæsthesia, as the appearance of the skin is so changed by the freezing mixtures used that it is impossible to see the diseased points.

This method of linear scarification is of great value in cases of rapidly progressive ulcerative lupus, as the spreading may be checked in two or three sittings. It is not of so much value in the fibrous or sclerous varieties, where there is a diminished blood supply. As the blood-vessels at the edge of the lupous neoplasm are probably affected, it is well to extend the incisions well into the sound skin. After the treatment has been pursued for some time, we have only a cicatrix in which small recurrent lupous nodules are scattered, and these have to be destroyed by a different means. They may be touched with the galvanocautery or thermocautery, or bored into with the solid crayon of nitrate of silver. In this way beautiful results are obtained, for the resulting cicatrix is smoother and less disfiguring than that from any other method. In cases of lupus of the face in which it is advisable that the smallest possible amount of scar tissue be left, the method is especially to be recommended.

There are, however, certain definite objections to this method. In the first place, it is of very long duration, requiring many sittings. In a case in Vidal's service referred to by Leloir, one hundred and eighty-eight sittings were held during a period of twenty-two months. For this reason it is often difficult to persuade people to undertake it. It is also painful and attended with considerable hemorrhage.

The greatest objection, however, that has been raised against it is that by opening the blood-vessels and lymphatic channels in the vicinity of tuberculoes foci we run a risk of dispersing the bacilli to other parts of the system. It is a matter of dispute how great this risk is. Besnier considers it a most important objection, and asserts that he has seen an autoinoculation take place with considerable frequency in such cases. Inasmuch, therefore, as some good observers are inclined to regard the danger of a dissemination of the disease as a factor not to be disregarded, this point of view should be taken into consideration in deciding upon the method of treatment to be followed.

Cauterization.—The actual cautery may be used in certain selected cases, but it is not a favorite mode of treatment. It is not possible, by this method, to gauge accurately the amount of destruction, so that as little as possible of the healthy tissue may be included in the destructive process. In cases of isolated, sharply bounded lesions of the trunk or extremities, when the amount of cicatrix resulting is not of great importance, it may be properly used, or it may be used in conjunction with curetting.

The first regular application of the galvanocautery was made by Hebra, who considered it an important aid to the therapeutics of this disease, but rarely practicable except in a hospital. Besnier prefers it to all other methods, and has invented different points and blades with which he cauterizes the diseased points. The small recurrent lupous nodules that appear in the cicatrix are especially well treated by this method, as well as lupus of the mucous membranes. It is important that the platinum point used should not be brought to a white heat, so that bleeding may be avoided. This method has the disadvantage of causing great terror and apprehension in many patients, and it is also very slow in its results. It has been used with much advantage in the verrucous form of tuberculosis.

Treatment by Chemical Caustics.—This is one of the older methods of treatment that has been supplanted in great measure by surgical procedures. Although causing a great deal of pain and destroying a large amount of tissue, it may be used to advantage in certain cases.

The solid stick of nitrate of silver is still largely used. By boring into the tissues vigorously a mechanical effect is added to the chemical action. It has the advantage of not attacking the sound tissue, and one who has had a slight experience in its use can determine at once by the resistance whether or not the portion touched is diseased. Large masses of tuberculous tissue may be removed by the nitrate-of-silver stick, but its chief use consists in its application to recurrent lupous nodules in cicatrices.

Another advantage of this method is that, although the pain caused is considerable, patients do not fear it and will assent to it when surgical methods are rejected. Nitrate of silver is also sometimes used in solution with equal parts of water, especially upon the ulcerated forms. This will not penetrate the epidermis when intact, and in such cases strong solutions of caustic potash have been used as a preliminary treatment.

Arsenical paste—composed of white arsenic 1, cinnabar 2, unguent. emollient 24—has been a favorite application, especially in Austria. It is spread upon linen and applied for three days, renewing the paste each day. It does not attack the sound skin, and poisoning is said not to occur, although it should not be used on a surface larger than the palm of the hand at one time. It is a very painful method, but quick in its action.

Vienna paste, Landolfi's paste, carbolic, pyrogallic, and lactic acids are among the other caustics that have been used. Pyrogallic acid is often employed, and has the advantage of attacking only diseased tissue. Canquoin's paste, which is composed of chloride of zinc, has a very deep and destructive action on the healthy as well as the diseased tissue. It is seldom used at present.

A strong salicylic-acid plaster, from twenty-five to fifty per cent., has been much advocated by Unna. Creosote is added to lessen the pain. This dissolves the epidermis, so that the lupous nodules are laid bare, and they must then be destroyed by other and stronger agents.

Electrolysis.—Gärtner and Lustgarten destroyed lupous nodules by means of a silver plate surrounded by a hard-rubber ring and connected with the negative pole of an electric battery. It is an almost painless method, but the results have hardly justified its adoption. Small nodules, especially when they are of a sclerous nature, may often be removed advantageously by boring into them in various directions with the electric needle.

Affections of Possible Tuberculous Origin.

There are, in addition to the diseases above described, certain affections in which the tubercle bacillus has not been demonstrated, but which are believed by many to bear a close relationship to tuberculosis.

These affections have been described by Darier under the name "tuberculides," and by Boeck as the exanthemata of tuberculosis. The view most generally accepted by those who consider that this group is related to tuberculosis etiologically is that they are produced by the action of toxins engendered by the bacillus. There is as yet no unanimity of opinion as to the forms that should be allowed admission into this class, nor as to the justification of such a class.

Lupus Erythematosus.—For many years there have been strong advocates of the tuberculous nature of lupus erythematosus, Besnier and Boeck being among the foremost advocates of this view. It is maintained that lupus erythematosus is often associated with or followed by long-standing glandular enlargements, and that tuberculosis of internal organs is a frequent sequel. Besnier speaks also of tuberculosis of the joints as a frequent complication. The writer has met with but two instances in which lupus erythematosus was associated with tuberculosis of other parts, in both cases the lungs being the organ affected. Besnier remarks that very few of the subjects of lupus erythematosus live to old age, and that is why the disease is not seen in old people. He thinks that if they lived as long as the majority, we should observe the scars left by it in old people.

Much stress has also been laid on the argument that transitional forms are often seen between lupus erythematosus and lupus vulgaris, but this position is in need of vigorous defence. It may be that in certain cases a slight clinical similarity between the two affections can be traced, but in general a far greater difficulty is experienced in differentiating lupus erythematosus from some other dermatoses than from tuberculosis.

Boeck has endeavored to explain the relationship that he maintains exists between lupus erythematosus and tuberculosis, by the action of the toxins of the tubercle bacillus upon certain nerve centres of the skin, especially the vasomotor-trophic centres. He declares that in a series of thirty-six patients affected with lupus erythematosus, two-thirds showed signs of tuberculosis.

Lichen scrofulosorum (Hebra) is a dermatosis that is regarded by some as a typical example of a tuberculous exanthem or tuberculide. While it is true that the histological structure of this eruption is quite similar to that of tuberculous lesions, it is also true that no one to-day claims that the histological character of tuberculosis is pathognomonic taken by itself. Langhans giant cells and a tubercular structure may occur in other affections, as in the small, papular, so-called lichenoid syphilide. Moreover, experimental inoculation upon animals has failed, and observers have repeatedly failed to find the tubercle bacillus in the papule. Only one observer has recorded the discovery of a single bacillus. Neisser and Jadassohn, however, report a local reaction about the lichen papules after the injection of tuberculin. It is certainly true that this eruption is found most frequently in tuberculous subjects or in those who present extensive glandular enlargement. There is no proof that we have here a true tuberculosis of the skin, and the rôle that tuberculosis may play in the etiology is an interesting but as yet obscure question.

Lupus Erythematosus Disseminatus.—A form of eruption has been described under the name of "folliclis" (Barthélemy), "folliculites disséminées à tendances cicatricielle" (Brocq), "hydradenitis destruens suppurativa," lupus erythematosus disseminatus (Boeck), etc., which has also been regarded as belonging among the tuberculides. This eruption appears in the form of erythematous spots or papules, frequently arising from a deeper-seated nodule, and sometimes showing a small, vesicular formation in the centre. Involution may then occur or there may be suppuration in the centre, resulting in a small, sharply defined scar, which is quite characteristic. The favorite seats of this eruption are the ulnar side of the forearms, the wrists, hands, and ears, although it may affect any part of the body. Sometimes these lesions are grouped and bear a resemblance to lupus erythematosus. These cases have been said to be associated with tuberculosis in many instances, as well as with lichen scrofulosorum. In the cases examined histologically, there is no similarity with a tubercular structure.

Eczema scrofulosorum is described by Boeck as occurring especially in older children or in young adults, and as allied to lichen scrofulosorum, since the affected individuals have in many instances been affected with the latter eruption at some time. It appears as reddish, infiltrated spots, that are often simply scaling, but that may be oozing and crusted, and form circinate and gyrate figures. There are often also small papules about the hairs that resemble lichen scrofulosorum. The thorax and the extensor surfaces of the extremities are the parts most frequently affected. It is apt to be symmetrical, and is frequently recurrent.

Acne cachecticorum and Bazin's erythème induré des scrofuleux have also been included in this class of tuberculides by some writers. Their frequent association with tuberculosis is an undoubted fact, but their etiological relationship with this disease is as yet purely speculative.

YELLOW FEVER.

BY

WOLFRED NELSON,

NEW YORK.

YELLOW FEVER.

Introduction.

THE tropical centres in which yellow fever is endemic are the foci in which there are repeated explosions of the disease in epidemic form. Between epidemics there are sporadic cases. They are the connecting links when a new epidemic is in order.

A particularly hot, dry season, such as Buenos Ayres and Paraguay are experiencing at this writing, February, 1900, a persistent thermometric range between 90° and 102° F., with many deaths from sunstroke, also means cases of yellow fever. Under these circumstances one can quite imagine a tidal wave of the poison of the disease extending outward from the epidemic centre—a wave extending to Brazil, Venezuela, Colombia, the Republics of Central America and Mexico, and radiating as well to the ever susceptible islands of the West Indies; in brief, a mere repetition of its old-time course. Later the peril knocks at all the portals of the Southern United States.

Let us recall the ten-years' war in Cuba—the war extending from 1868 to 1878—a revolution that cost Spain the admitted loss of one hundred and eighty thousand men, of whom less than nineteen thousand were killed in action, or died subsequently of wounds. That appalling death rate, averaging eighteen thousand a year, was due to the action of what the Cuban rebels facetiously styled the efforts of their· best revolutionary generals, Generales Junio, Julio, y Agosto, or Generals June, July, and August, the months when yellow fever yearly takes on its epidemic form. Of the one hundred and eighty thousand lost, yellow and pernicious malarial fevers, diarrhœa, and dysentery killed the majority. The rebels knew of their·climatic allies, and Spain frankly published the total death rate. That war closed in 1878, when the yellow-fever poison had reached a maximum intensity, when, lo! it appeared in New Orleans. Later a severe epidemic appeared in that city and extended outward to Tennessee and elsewhere.

Again, during the last rebellion in Cuba, Spain sent thousands of troops to the island. Yellow fever awaited them. It was absolutely faithful to its history. The men were swept away as they were in the ten-years' war. The poison again reached a maximum intensity, and again it appeared in New Orleans.

The endemic centres are the ones to watch; they are constant sources of peril to the unsuspicious. To-day they are brought nearer susceptible places by rapid express steamers, particularly by the ever-increasing fleet of rapid fruit steamers. Bills of health from such centres in many instances are mere bits of paper. The only and safe rule is that observed at the Holt Quarantine Station, on the Mississippi, that all vessels from ports within the yellow-fever zone must be treated as suspicious vessels. The old French proverb holds in such matters with mathematical accuracy—"Suspicion is the mother of safety."

In what follows I have essayed to transmit an idea of the every-day state of affairs in parts of Spanish America, South and Central, on the Pacific coast of Mexico, and in certain islands in the West Indies. My tropical experience extended over eight years. Five of them were passed on the Isthmus of Panama when canal affairs were at their zenith, and three years subsequently in Spanish America and the West Indies. The study of yellow fever to me was very interesting. I attempted to make the most of my opportunities. The study included the diseases of hot climates, death rates where obtainable, climatology, and, in fine, all matters germane to the theme.

The stamping out of yellow fever, in many of the centres named, seems to me an almost hopeless task. The filthy conditions nourish and assist in maintaining the disease. Such places are, and no doubt will remain, poison centres. Quite apart from any attempt to bring about a better state of affairs in the infected centres, the Spanish American peoples on the old Spanish Main and in the West Indies should cease their unholy practices of evicting their dead, either from their *bóvedas* system or from the earth. Their constant practices lead to the liberation of billions upon billions of death-dealing germs of yellow fever. Panama is one of the world's great commercial arteries, and Nicaragua soon will be an interoceanic transit of the first order; Cuba and other old-time Spanish possessions, all export disease as regularly as they do their India rubber, coffee, dyewoods, and tobacco. The remedy to check new crops of such poisons no doubt is cremation on the one hand, and the Holt quarantine system on the other.

If my descriptive articles are deemed lengthy, I earnestly crave both pardon and patience at the hands of my readers. My sole excuse lies in my wish to place before them the mental methods and daily practices of the peoples specifically named—peoples who either through familiarity with disease of a preventable character, or through lack of knowledge, traditional carelessness, or some other equally potent cause, to-day, as in the past, are profoundly indifferent to anything not personally relating to their own welfare, and even to their own welfare in that respect.

The spread of yellow fever in Central and South America and Mexico, as well as in the West Indies, is a repetition of the history of ship-borne diseases, such as cholera, smallpox, and plague. Previous to the trans-isthmian travel to California, in the forty-nine days, yellow fever seems to have been an unknown disease on the Pacific Ocean. If it existed there previously I have not been able to find any authentic record of it. That trans-isthmian traffic led to the construction of the Panama railway. Then, indeed, yellow fever commenced to travel with and among the passengers to the Pacific coast. Its first station was in Panama City; having found a congenial soil it located itself there. Once well intrenched within the old walled city, it gradually extended its travels up and down the Pacific coasts of South and Central America, and within our own times, say within twenty-five years, has obtained a permanent settlement on the Pacific coast of Mexico.

The case is presented in the sketches that follow. Next in order is the remedy—that is, the protection of uninfected centres. It will be found in the Holt system of maritime sanitation or quarantine—a system that absolutely excludes the poison of yellow fever, smallpox, cholera, and plague; an ideal system by which the populous centres of the South are protected; one that absolutely protects without offering any real impediment to trade.

At the Pan-American Medical Congress in Washington in 1893, I read two papers covering the question of the spread of disease by Isthmian and Cuban practices. I expressed the hope that some day such practices may be suppressed by a council of nations. The records of war, with all their horrors and appalling death rate, sink into insignificance when compared with the march of preventable diseases and their mortality. That such matters should require discussion to-day on the very threshold of the twentieth century is a lasting reproach to our times with their boasted advances in science, arts, and medicine. The responsibility centres along two lines: First, the apathy of those responsible for it; secondly, the indifference of the better informed peoples who have not attempted to suppress such death-dealing practices.

Definition.—Yellow fever is an acute infectious disease of the tropics, properly so called; an infection due to the presence in the bodies of its victims of a specific germ or microorganism. That the disease was due to such an agent had long been suspected. It remained for the late Dr. Domingo Freire, of Rio de Janeiro, to discover the germ, thus solving in part a vexatious problem.

The microorganisms in their own life rôles within the human body produce certain toxic principles of great virulence. The absorption of the toxins leads to a classical train of symptoms easily recognized and grouped together under the name of yellow fever—a name, by the way, associated with a symptom of this disease by the early Spanish discoverers under Columbus.

Yellow fever, as a disease, stands wholly apart. The conditions necessarily are peculiar to itself. It begins with a slow hard pulse, associated as a rule in the tropics with high temperature—104° to 105° F., and occasionally higher. Its symptoms and course are wholly unlike any other disease known to the physician within the tropics. In certain cases there is an almost instant invasion after exposure in an infected port or city.

Some cases are characterized by profound physical prostration, others by a comatose condition, and again others by violent convulsions—cases ending fatally on the fourth, fifth, or sixth day. Cases of the above types best indicate the very marked virulence of the toxic elements generated by the germs in the bodies of their hosts.

The many and conflicting descriptions of yellow fever in some of the text-books in Spanish, French, Portuguese, and English preclude any definition of it, if one accepts the views laid down in the books referred to. As an evidence of the old-time conflict of statements, some authors associate the disease with a malarial cause or element and advise quinine. Yellow fever is wholly unlike tropical malaria in any of its multiple manifestations. Quinine is wholly useless in this disease, and its administration in large doses is contraindicated. Large doses have been tried time and again, and have no effect on the patient's temperature or the course of his disease.

Nomenclature.—The nomenclature is extensive. The Spanish discoverers were the first to make its acquaintance. They named it fiebre amarilla—Anglice, yellow fever. They also called it vomito prieto, or black vomit; the latter a symptom in many fatal cases. They gave the disease its name after noting the deep canary-yellow color of the bodies of its early-day victims—a tint or color always present in severe cases, an indescribably rich yellow after death.

Next in order the French had their experience with it. They gave it three names—fièvre jaune, or yellow fever; also fièvre d'Amérique, and fièvre bilieuse d'Amérique, respectively American fever and American bilious fever.

In due course the English followed the French. Their experience was the exact counterpart of the French and Spanish in the West Indies. They gave the disease several names—febris flava, the Latin equivalent for yellow fever. They reasoned and named the disease as the Spaniards had done. Among the every-day common English names used in the tropics are putrid fever, black vomit, and yellow jack; the latter being used by seafaring people.

The Portuguese had their own experience, and called it febre amarella, or yellow fever. The names almost without exception centred around the first or Spanish name—a name that will, no doubt, cling to the disease for all time.

While the Spaniards discovered the disease, a Portuguese, Dr. Freire, initiated and conducted the investigations that have placed yellow fever in a wholly new light. Nineteen years of his life were devoted to studying this ancient and death-dealing disease. He published his results. In turn he was followed by other highly intelligent and thoughtful investigators, Dr. Carlos Findlay in Havana and Dr. Gererd at Panama. To-day much satisfactory evidence exists that the hitherto dense obscurity surrounding this fever may before long be dissipated and that mankind may inherit the legacy left to it by Dr. Domingo Freire.

History.

It would afford the student of this disease a great deal of satisfaction if he could locate its first habitat, but that privilege is denied him. As far as we moderns are concerned, we date the disease from the time of Columbus and his followers. The disease no doubt existed in prehistoric times, and is buried in that nebulous past that envelops so many infectious and contagious diseases.

In historic times the disease ever has presented the same characteristics in the tropics, in Central and South America, on the east and west coasts of Mexico, and in the West Indies.

Of the many and death-dealing epidemics of disease that have prevailed in the West Indies from 1635 to the present time, none has more constant or notable features than this inveterate foe of the human family. A Spanish historian traces it back to 1493, when Columbus landed in the island of Hispaniola, or Santo Domingo and Hayti of to-day. He states that Columbus lost the greater part of his crew within a year of arrival of a disease ending in death, and that the seamen became as yellow as saffron.

A French writer refers to it in the French island of Guadeloupe in 1635, in 1640, and again in 1648. A neighboring island, an English possession, St. Kitts, suffered from the disease in 1648, and later in 1652. In the year 1655 it had travelled by sea in a northerly direction and appeared at Port Royal, the naval station in the island of Jamaica. Bridgetown, then and now the capital of Barbadoes, British West Indies, was visited by the disease in 1647. It was a novelty to the islands. It was believed to be due to disease that came to the islands in ships after long voyages.

It will be germane to this part of my theme to state that filthy ships and the slave trade have been associated with the disease in the minds of many early writers. An early-day fleet of England's in the West Indies lost between three and four thousand men within a twelvemonth after its arrival in tropical waters.

Judging from the writings of the earliest Spaniards—and they carefully noted their surroundings and the peoples visited by them—it seems wholly fair to assume that the pre-Columbian races bordering on the Spanish main suffered from the same disease. The writings to which reference is made state that the Indian tribes living at sea level suffered from epidemics that swept them away. The natives informed the Spaniards that they lived in camps, and that after a short residence at coast level their camps became foul, when epidemic disease killed them. As soon as possible they moved to a new locality, but a year or more of residence seemed to develop the same conditions, when a new epidemic and a heavy mortality obtained.

To one who has lived and travelled in the countries referred to by the early-day Spanish writers it seems a fair assumption that the disease was yellow fever. Their very primitive camps must have become foul. Human filth and crowding amid such heat and moisture, such rapid vegetable growth, and a corresponding decay necessarily engendered poisons that caused disease and death.

This is pure speculation, but it seems logical. Like produces like. Given a specific infection, a contagium vivum, the filth conditions no doubt kept it alive. In the following pages I shall show that when the Indians of the altas or highlands of South and Central America and Mexico reach coast level, where filth and fever exist, yellow fever sweeps them away.

The Home of Yellow Fever.

With a view of placing a word sketch before my readers I shall give a series of brief descriptions of the several habitats of yellow fever that I have visited, such as Havana, Santiago de Cuba, Colon, Panama City, other places on the west coast of Mexico, and Puerto Rico. Jamaica and the Danish Island of Saint Thomas will be mentioned as illustrating what may be done in stamping out the disease.

I may preface what will follow by stating that to-day the question of yellow fever has an importance to the people of the United States, with its population of seventy-five millions of people, that it lacked earlier. The coast towns of Puerto Rico and of Cuba, with their well-known history of yellow fever, are to all intents and purposes from a scientific and medical standpoint American domestic ports, and as such are in daily communication with the many ever-receptive Southern and other ports of this Republic.

The geographical and other climatic conditions must be described, as necessary to a full and clear understanding of the yellow-fever question. The importance of the whole theme, I believe, cannot be overestimated, particularly when we recall the death-dealing rôle played by Yellow Jack in many ports and cities of this country. We will first consider that nearby hot-bed of pestilence and yellow fever,

CUBA.

Havana.—The city of Havana is within ninety-six miles of Key West, and about three hundred miles from Tampa. That city by a railroad connects with all parts of Florida and the other Southern and Southeastern States. Beyond Key West are many rocky islands and islets, known as the "Thousand Islands." They deserve mention, not as inhabited centres, but as islets used in the past by smugglers engaged in the Cuban-American trade, who have had much to do with introducing exotic disease. It is reported that the smuggling so common under the Spanish *régime* in Cuba still exists.

The streets of the lower part of the city are very narrow and flanked by houses built of a soft and porous stone. The constantly foul-smelling atmosphere there, bad by day and doubly foul by night, tells of ages of unsanitary conditions—subsoil contamination and fecal fermentation. The walls of the houses there give the ocular proof in the lower parts. They are damp for quite a distance up from the street level. One may safely compare their porous foundations and walls to the wick of a lamp. Both transfer from below upwards; one oil, the other foul and pestilential humidity.

Havana of to-day is more than three hundred years old. The early-day Havana was on the south coast, near the present pueblo or town of Batabano, in an air line directly across the island from Havana. The early-day Havana soon became unhealthy and pestilential, and then the present site was selected. The geographical location of the city is of the best. It evidently was built from the shores of the harbor upward. The very narrow streets remind one of the older cities of Spain, narrow streets from which the direct rays of the sun are largely excluded. In the hot and humid tropics the direct rays of the sun play a most important rôle in drying and burning up morbific elements—no sunlight, no oxidation, no drying, hence the constant exhalation from the contaminated soil below.

Leaving the lower part of the city, where one naturally finds much illness, let me very briefly refer to the upper part. The chief plaza or square of the modern part of the city is known as *El Parque Central*. The streets there are wider. It is the residential part for the better classes. The park is large and broad and flanked by wide avenues, on which one finds the chief hotels. Many of them are fine and palatial buildings. During one of my visits to the city I put up at a hotel facing the Central Park. I was given an inside room. Its walls were damp. The bedding was likewise damp, and the atmosphere close. Not far from it, on the main hallway, was a large open grating, fully eighteen inches across. It was in the floor and connected with a very large pipe leading to the common sewer without. Fancy the atmosphere in a hotel that practically was a ventilating shaft for a tropical sewer! Barring damp walls and the atmosphere, the rest was satisfactory. The dining-room was very elaborate; the service excellent.

When what I have described obtains in a modern hotel, what may be expected in the old-time part of the city? Cesspools and houses, with the whole subsoil contaminated by three centuries of indifference, the whole producing a pestilential condition generally. It will take a vast sanitary reform to make Havana a safe or healthful place, either for occasional visits or for residence.

While in Havana I had the privileges of the Government Hospital. I wanted to see its yellow-fever cases, the building, its patio or court, its post-mortem room, etc. The military surgeon in charge was most courteous. Yellow fever was seen and studied; the hospital and its multiple workings were also carefully noted. The building was a large quadrangle. It had over one thousand beds. It admitted soldiers from the army and sailors from the naval vessels. The patients were not separated, the yellow-fever cases being in a ward with others. No restrictions whatever obtained. Ward attendants and others came and went as they pleased. The freedom was absolute and perfect.

I visited the court, the post-mortem room, and stepped from the latter into a narrow alley adjoining the shipping. The hospital is on an arm of the bay. The immediate vicinity of the shipping was instructive. Beyond was a vast slaughter house; its offal and blood were thrown into the bay. It is needless to state that the tideless waters were foul. The admixture of salt and fresh water, slaughter-house offal, and hospital filth made a lasting impression on me. One can fancy the effects on the crews of the shipping anchored near such a pestiferous place. No fact is better known to the student of yellow fever than that a crew may be exposed and may escape while in port. The ship is laden and proceeds on her voyage; cases develop, men die; a new port is made where the climatic and other conditions are favorable and the dread disease appears. The common carriers, ships with sugar cargoes in Manila hemp sacks, are very dangerous.

While the city of Havana has been the habitat of yellow fever for more than one hundred successive years, the season when the endemic disease takes on the proportions of an epidemic is during June, July, and August. When the yellow fever is active in Havana and the western end of the island the eastern end is free from it. During our northern winter Havana has only sporadic cases among foreigners, while the city of Santiago has it frequently as a limited epidemic.

Some years ago a vessel sailing from Regla, in the harbor of Havana, took on ballast exclusively of earth from near the shore. She then sailed for a port in the Southern United States, and there discharged her ballast. Later yellow fever appeared in that Southern port. An official investigation was in order, and the disease was traced to the germ-laden soil from the harbor of Havana. Ballast of whatever kind from any yellow-fever port is always dangerous.

Years ago water taken at a depth of several fathoms from the harbor of Havana was found full of organic matter. That such should be the case need cause no surprise. American steamships plying between Key West and Tampa enter the harbor of Havana after sunrise and leave that day before sunset. They anchor in a central spot in the harbor. This wise precaution is excellent as far as it goes, but it does not go far enough. Such ships, their cargoes and passengers are safe only when disinfection by the full Holt system follows their arrival in any portion of Florida.

Key West had an epidemic of yellow fever. It was traced to infected bedding brought from Havana by a woman. She did not have the disease, but her bedding from that infected city introduced it.

Steerage passengers are particularly prone to bring with them old bedding and blankets.

Santiago de Cuba has had a corporate existence for three hundred and seventy-eight years. It was the former capital of the island of Cuba. It is on the south coast of the island, in the eastern province of the same name, Santiago. The place requires extended mention, chiefly in that it bears on the matter in hand, the study of the habitats of yellow fever. The condition there is largely due to lack of ordinary precautions in dealing with filth and fecal matter. The result is soil and subsoil contamination, that has obtained for more than three centuries. What will be done with the death-dealing inheritance remains to be seen.

The harbor connects by a winding and narrow entrance with the Atlantic Ocean without. The inner harbor is over two miles long and nearly as wide. It is practically landlocked and tideless, owing to the geographical formation there of hills and mountains. It receives a great deal of fresh water. The vegetation along its shores is luxuriant and of rapid growth and rapid decay. This, with the admixture of fresh and salt water, plus contamination from the city, creates a body of water that is almost quiescent and charged with organic matter. If the city was drained into the bay by a modern system of drains and flushing, the harbor in time would become as foul and pestilential as that of Havana.

The city with its wide-spreading suburbs extends from the low and muddy shores of the harbor inland and upland for more than a mile. The incline in that mile from the crest of the city to the street facing the water is one hundred and fifty feet. For purposes of natural drainage that incline is of the best, provided the drainage was taken out by sewers to the sea front and discharged into the open sea, well away from the narrow entrance.

The lower part of the city is badly paved. The streets are narrow. The houses are largely of stone, one and two stories high. Many of the houses have a central court or *patio*. At some point in the premises is a cesspool or privy with no outlet. The odors can be imagined. The people for generations and generations have lived side by side with the cesspools. Theirs indeed is the familiarity that breeds both indifference to smells and contempt for disease.

There is a vast hospital there, built all of forty years ago. It occupies a commanding site on the top of the hillside, completely overlooking the city and harbor. The front of the hospital faces the upper inland section. There is an avenue along that front. Centrally placed between the avenue and the main building was another fair-sized building. It covered a vast cesspool or old-fashioned privy. By day the atmosphere was bad, by night it was vile—that fecal odor so familiar to all students of yellow fever in tropical centres.

People long resident near such poison factories do in a measure become accustomed to them, and escape in non-epidemic times; but when an epidemic of maximum intensity obtains, they in turn pay the penalty, and many of them die of yellow fever.

Just beyond the hospital is the Avenida Concha, or Shell Avenue. It extends at a right angle with the avenue facing the hospital, through the outskirts of the city down the incline to the water front of the bay in the business section. The location of the hospital and its vast cesspool at the top of the incline necessarily means that all the subsoil water drains from the upper level down that incline, impregnating the whole soil with filth in solution or pure fecal contamination. When we further recall the fact that that hospital has been used in treating hundreds—nay, thousands—of cases of yellow fever among the Spanish troops, and that their motions were not disinfected ere being thrown into the cesspool, enough has been stated to emphasize the peril to which I have drawn attention. In fine, that city on the hillside for centuries has been but little better than an inhabited cesspool. During the dry season the endemic yellow fever takes on the usual epidemic tendency, providing of course that the unacclimated material is there. It has done so for many decades.

My visits to Santiago de Cuba, two in number, extended over four months. Its climatic and geographical conditions had my close attention. I also saw cases of yellow fever. Descriptions of this kind necessarily have to assume the personal type. While there, some time was passed at a hotel; it was about midway between the water front and the upper part of the city. The place was deemed first-class. Military and naval officers of high rank made it their headquarters. The rooms were plainly furnished, tropical fashion. The table was excellent. Marvellous to relate, that hotel had a bathroom. The building had a court. As it was on the incline the court was in part below and in part above. A stone stairway led from the lower to the upper part. There were two stories below and two above. My room was on the upper part. In one corner of the upper building was what was facetiously called "the garden." In a large room at one end of that upper part was a vault-privy or cesspool, a huge pit for the use of all the guests of the hotel. An American traveller had a room just over it. I was three doors from him. The atmosphere of that room or privy was vile beyond any description. The vault with its ever-fermenting contents had no outlet, and at times its atmosphere was almost stifling, particularly when the ammoniacal odors were in the ascendency. People hastened to it and hastened away. The poison engendered by that pit, like the vast cesspool on the hilltop, could gravitate only down towards the lower levels and upwards towards the air by means of the porous stone walls. The stone foundations in such soils ever continue their wicklike function of transferring from below upwards the poisons generated in the soil and subsoil.

The prison of Santiago also requires special mention. It was a large two-story building of the usual quadrangle type, with the usual patio. It was on a main thoroughfare, just above the public market. It was filled with criminals of the lowest type, largely the very dregs of the black population, with an occasional white man. Its conveniences so called were in absolute harmony with the conditions described, save an added feature. During the day the urine of the prisoners, dirty water, etc., were kept, and when night was well advanced they were emptied on the street in front of the prison—a main thoroughfare—and allowed to run down hill to the lower and damp levels below, in whose streets foul and stagnant water was to be found at all seasons. Of course such work was done under the cover of night. The people were accustomed to it, and the authorities did not care; and there it ended. If the yellow fever killed the Spanish soldiers and smallpox the blacks, the better classes escaped; and from their utterly selfish standpoint there the matter ended.

HAITI.

Haiti forms a part of the Hispaniola of the time of Columbus. Its capital is Port-au-Prince. It lies about one hundred miles from the eastern end of Cuba. The population of Haiti consists of negroes and their descendants. In a land of such license as prevails in Haiti sanitation is of no moment. The people are accustomed to their own methods. Any taxation for drainage would be an invasion of their popular rights. The general conditions are very repulsive to one who respects law and order. The filth is indescribable.

The capital, or Port-au-Prince, has been purified by fire. It has been all but destroyed repeatedly by that element. Temporarily it did purify the surface at a large cost, but the soil contamination remained.

Dr. Hamilton, when surgeon-general of the Marine Hospital Service, once expressed his surprise to me that no reports on yellow fever came into his possession from the island of Haiti. The explanation was instant. As a negro possession very few whites visited it, and an occasional death from yellow fever would excite no comment there.

A few years later a number of white men visited Haiti, when yellow fever appeared and killed as it usually kills in the West Indies— the majority of those attacked.

To expect any reliable information relative to disease and death rates from such a centre naturally was to expect the impossible. Haiti as an infected centre demands our attention. Its smallpox and yellow fever are preventable diseases.

Puerto Rico.

My trips to Puerto Rico were two in number. During my first visit I was at Mayaguez, a small city on the coast, just across the island from San Juan. Mayaguez is a fairly clean city, but it has the old-time privy or cesspool system. Its surface was clean and in very marked contrast with the city of Santiago de Cuba. My second visit was to San Juan. I was at the leading hotel. Its privy was indoors. The vault or cesspool was built within the foundations of the hotel; in other words, that hotel was built over and around its privy, quite a common condition in many of the West Indian islands and on the Spanish Main. It goes without saying that the soil in the capital is contaminated, and has been for nearly three centuries.

Yellow fever has played an important rôle in the island. The hotel people and steamship people there, as in Havana and other infected centres, will not admit that the disease exists. They want trade for the hotels and passengers for the steamships, and business for the city and island generally.

While Puerto Rico is unhealthy and unsafe for newcomers, the Danish island of St. Thomas, within twelve hours of it by steam, is clean, wholesome, and safe. The contrast between it, while a Spanish possession, and nearby St. Thomas was of the most marked character. An indifference to public health and to the safety of ports trading with it made its neglect all but criminal. It was worthy of the seventeenth century. The contrast was the more apparent and real after one had visited St. Thomas.

St. Thomas.

Fifty years ago this island was the chief centre for trade and shipping. Its importance was due to the fact that it received the products and produce from the greater part of South and Central America on the Atlantic side, and from nearly all the islands of the West Indies. St. Thomas stored the goods and held them for the many vessels, steam and sail, then plying to England and the Continent. The island then was the main portal, so to speak, to Mexico and the

Atlantic coast of all Central and South America.   For a time it enjoyed a flood tide of prosperity.   Soon it obtained an evil name for its yellow fever and cholera.   In time its reputation was of the worst; it was known as a sink of disease and death.   Its evil reputation increased until it, like the Isthmus of Panama, became known in England and on the Continent as the "grave of the European."

· Gradually its vast trade commenced to fall away.   Purchasers from Spanish America and the West Indies proceeded direct to England and the Continent.   The island ceased to be the storehouse for that part of the Western ocean, and the place returned to its early-day quietude.   The experience, however, had been very valuable.   The government had had enough of disease, and the authorities met the situation in the right spirit.   Sanitary measures were enforced and a good working quarantine law followed.   From being an island famed the world over for pestilential diseases, the place became healthy and pleasant; not only fair to one's vision but safe to visit.   The whole has been a timely and most useful lesson in demonstrating what can be done even in the hot and humid tropics, where both soil and climatic conditions foster disease.   .

The capital of the island is Charlotte Amalie; to the world it is known as St. Thomas.   In its harbor lies its chief importance to-day.   It is reached by way of a very narrow entrance.   Within it is almost oval in shape.   The city rises from the sea front, terrace upon terrace, to the upper levels.   The whole place is neat, clean, and very attractive.   It has the usual mixed population of the West Indies, but the island authorities make the careless elements orderly and careful.   The administration of the law is fair and absolutely impartial.   The net result is a quiet and orderly city.

I mention the island as I knew it.   The scrutiny of incoming and outgoing passengers was of the best.   Nothing was taken for granted.   The outgoing passengers took health certificates issued by the authorities.   The sanitary work there undertaken was on a large scale, but between its inception and completion there was no pause.   It was a forward movement from start to finish.   What the Government of Denmark has accomplished in St. Thomas can be repeated elsewhere in stamping out preventable disease.

JAMAICA.

Jamaica, like the island of St. Thomas, has rehabilitated itself.   In the long past both were lands of pestilential disease with an appalling mortality.

We must recall the early history of the island.   It was discovered by Columbus on his second voyage in 1493. It was a Spanish possession for about a century and a half; then England dispossessed Spain. In taking possession, the army of occupation was swept by tropical diseases and what was called pestilence. The old-time fortifications left by Spain were garrisoned by the British. They were at coast level; some near marshes and tropical swamps. Bad water, no drainage, dense crowding, with many unsanitary conditions, produced the usual results—a vast deal of sickness and death. They were the early days when sanitary precautions were unknown.

England's methods of learning have been slow, but experience once acquired has not been forgotten. The persistent and truly appalling mortality among her troops led to the abandonment of part of the coast-level fortifications. The forts at Port Royal only were garrisoned. Many epidemics of yellow fever swept the garrison. After a time barracks were built in the Port Royal Mountains inland and upland from Kingston, the capital. Newcastle, at an elevation of four thousand feet, became a mountain garrison for newly arriving troops. At coast level tropical disease held some sway, but the chief mortality was obviated by the mountain barracks at Newcastle.

The Island of Jamaica has the three climates of mountainous countries in the tropics. In general terms the hotter coast climates extend from coast level to two thousand feet upland; the temperate climate from two thousand to four thousand feet. Newcastle, at four thousand feet, is just at the lower edge of the cold climate. The cold climate extends from four thousand feet upwards to the tops of the loftiest mountains.

I have a special object in referring to lofty parts of Jamaica and of South America. There seems to be a common belief in the United States that yellow fever has no climbing power. In this country, so far as I can ascertain, it never has been traced beyond six hundred feet above sea level. Certain it is, no belief of that sort obtains among the close students of yellow fever in the tropics. In Jamaica, during a season of epidemic of yellow fever, the disease reached the camp at Newcastle and created havoc. In the Republic of Peru, yellow fever followed the line of the Oroyo railway, up into the mountains, and appeared at ten thousand feet above sea level. We must measure the disease by what it has done and what it may do again.

Port Royal is at the extreme point of the Palisades, an arm of sand extending into the ocean about nine miles. That vast sand bar makes the outer shore of the harbor of Kingston. Port Royal and Fort Augusta have been the seats of much mortality among the British soldiers and sailors. Bad as Port Royal was for health in the early days, it at least was surrounded by salt water only. Fort

Augusta on the inner side of the harbor faced the latter, while back of it was a tropical swamp with rank vegetation. The Rio Cobre has its outlet near Fort Augusta. The swamps or marshes have the usual admixture of salt and fresh water. Space does not admit of citing the experience of individual regiments there in the early days. Their combined experience can be written of as simply appalling. The sickness and dying there were the educational factors that led to the abandonment of the fort.

Kingston is a city of about sixty thousand inhabitants, lying about opposite Port Royal. Back of it are the Port Royal Mountains. In its early history Kingston used well water. The city was foul and offensive. Dr. A. N. Bell, who was there about forty years since, when a surgeon in the navy of the United States, has told me that it was an indescribably filthy place. British troops then were swept away by all kinds of disease, yellow fever being the chief killing factor. Reforms were in order. A supply of excellent and pure water was given the city, and with its advent there was an almost instantaneous betterment, particularly regarding diarrhœa and dysentery. Other sanitary measures were introduced step by step. The laws were enforced. Streets and lanes were kept clean. The drains on the surface were flushed. Later a system of drainage was introduced. To have drained the city into the harbor would have converted it in time into the condition of the harbor of Havana, a vast cesspool, but the drains of Kingston empty into the ocean several miles from the city. By no possible chance can any part of the sewage get into the harbor, as the long sand bar is the barrier that excludes it. The beautiful harbor of Kingston thus remains practically pure. It teems with fish.

Kingston, like Charlotte Amalie in St. Thomas, does not offend either the sense of smell or that of vision. Both cities are pleasant and safe to visit. I cite both as illustrations of what experience teaches individuals as well as governments. Genius, we are told, is common sense in working attire. The Governments of Great Britain and Denmark have been among the first to illustrate what modern methods can do in matters of such truly vital importance, the health of their own subjects and the health and safety of the nations trading with them.

Now concerning another theme germane to this question of yellow fever. The unburial of the dead is not permitted. That practice in the past had led to fresh outbreaks of disease and limited epidemics of yellow fever. Once buried in Jamaica, the bodies remain buried. The great danger in unburying the victims of smallpox and yellow fever, the turning out of clothing and the partly decayed wood of the coffins is too obvious to need any comment. Along that line particularly, England in the West Indies has had her experience; it keeps her ever mindful, ever cautious, and ever vigilant.

"Jamaica at the Columbian Exposition of 1893" is the title of a Government blue book. Among its many interesting articles is one on the climate and health conditions of Jamaica. I quote from this article the following extract from a paper read before the Jamaica Branch of the British Medical Association by the late Brigade-Surgeon S. E. Maunsell:

"Beginning at 1817, about the time when a first attempt was made to compile statistics of disease and to classify under various heads the causes of non-efficiency among soldiers, Dr. Maunsell, in a statistical summary, shows, among others, the following remarkable figures:

| Years. | ─RATIO PER 1,000.─ | |
	Admissions to hospital.	Fatal cases.
1817–1836......................	1812.55	121.3
1838–1847...............................	1526.66	63.07
1848–1859...............................	1141.69	32.70
1860–1869..........	994.76	21.25

"During the first of the above-mentioned four periods the soldiers were overcrowded in the enervating heat of the plains; sanitation was almost unknown, ventilation was unheeded, water was collected from the roofs of the barracks whence it drained into tanks, it was never filtered and was too deficient in quantity to admit of ordinary cleanliness. And the other accompaniments of barrack-life were of the same type.

"During the second period the strength of the military forces stationed in Jamaica was much reduced; hence there was more barrack-room accommodation and consequently a decreased mortality.

"The reduction in the years 1848–59 may largely be accounted for by the removal, first started indeed in 1842, of the European troops to Newcastle, four thousand feet above the unhealthy stations and encampments on the plains.

"The improvement in the decade, 1860–69, would possibly have been more marked but for an outbreak of fever in 1867. This is a convenient place in which to pause briefly in our statistics, because one result of the 1867 epidemic was a War Office Commission, the giving effect to the recommendations of which has almost revolutionized the reputation of Jamaica as an unhealthy military station. This Commission plainly showed that in the zone where yellow fever is endemic, an entire dependence on elevation as an absolute and certain safeguard was utterly insufficient, if it were accompanied by a neglect of other reasonable precautions which should be taken in every climate.

"The above-quoted figures show that half a century ago three soldiers out of four stationed in Jamaica were twice a year in the hospital, and that twelve per cent. died every year. Other statistics, which need not be tabulated here, show that more than five-sixths of these fatal cases were caused by fevers, that on an average every soldier had twenty-three days of sickness during each year, each attack lasting on an average thirteen and one-half days.

"We now turn to the military figures for the next two decades and we find:

Years.	Average annual deaths.	Ratio of deaths per 1,000 admissions to hospital.
1870–1879	5	13.77
1880–1889	4	11.36

"In the last-named of these years, 1889, the deaths from all causes were eight per thousand and from fevers *nil*.

"Statistics such as these can have but one meaning, which is that, when proper sanitary precautions are taken and due care is paid to personal hygiene, whether among military men or among civilians, the climate of Jamaica is as healthy as that of any part of the world."

BERMUDA.

The Bermudas, or Somers Islands, are a group of coralline islands, said to number just three hundred and sixty-five, about seven hundred miles from New York. The capital is Hamilton. In times past it had the same experiences that punished Kingston and Charlotte Amalie—epidemics of yellow fever with great mortality.

When in the islands, now just about twenty years ago, I was told of the marvellous rapidity with which yellow fever spread there in the early days. Once landed, a case would be heard of at one point. Almost immediately other cases would be reported, then others, when a grand explosion of the disease followed. Its rapid spread to the unprotected seems magical. The condition exists when there is a certain receptivity in the atmospheric and telluric conditions. Just what the exact condition is remains to be explained. A cosmo-telluric condition is the learned name assigned to it. It obtains in seasons of epidemic yellow fever.

To-day Bermuda is as safe as Jamaica or St. Thomas. These three form the satisfactory side of the yellow-fever problem. They indeed point a moral, and illustrate what cleanliness and common sense can accomplish in stamping out preventable disease. General cleanliness is the keynote to the situation, together with the avoidance of subsoil contamination.

TRINIDAD.

The capital of Trinidad, Spanish Town, is well kept and cleanly. The health authorities there are alive to their responsibilities. But despite precautions yellow fever has invaded that island, as it has all parts of that South American sea coast.

During the last epidemic, in the summer of 1894, Dr. Bevan Rake, the physician in charge of the Lepers' Asylum there, contracted the disease and died. He had passed nearly ten years in the island. The acclimation theory, so-called, has no believers among tropical students of yellow fever. An attack of the disease and recovery constitute the only protection against it.

VENEZUELA.

The coastal cities of Puerto Cabello, La Guayra, and Carupano are of the usual Spanish-American type. The buildings are of stone. Old-time privies and cesspools exist. Time and again that coast has been swept by yellow fever.

An Englishman, who had charge of an engineering work there at sea level, told me of his experience in handling large bodies of mechanics and laborers. The men were nearly all foreigners and whites. Soon after arrival tropical disease appeared among them, such as diarrhœa, dysentery, pernicious malarial fever, and yellow fever. Frequently he read the burial service over three and five of them at a time, and for days together the mortality was simply appalling. Yellow and malarial fevers were the leading killing agencies.

It is the old, old story of engineering works in the parts of the tropics now under consideration. Such enterprises always have meant the wholesale dying of imported labor. History will repeat itself in the future and along the same lines. The black and Indian laborers from the lowlands are swept away by pernicious malarial fever, while the Indian laborers from the *altas* or highlands die of yellow fever like the whites.

UNITED STATES OF COLOMBIA.

Carthagena.—The walled city of Carthagena must be mentioned as a locality in which yellow fever has played a rôle. The mere fact of its being over three centuries old means much to all acquainted with the history of yellow fever.

Carthagena has much in common with other Spanish-American cities on the Spanish Main. Their general insanitary conditions are almost identical. Much of their history is blended with a his-. tory of yellow fever, and for the reason already set forth. The paved streets are narrow. Many of the houses, while two and three stories high, have projecting balconies. The walls in places have been broken down near the sea front and in another place to give admittance to a new railroad. In Carthagena old-time methods and old-time privy vaults exist.

Savanilla.—The port of Savanilla or Sabanilla is Puerta Colombia. A line of railway connects the port with the city of Barranquilla, on the banks of the Magdalena River. It lies in the Tierra Caliente, or tropical belt. It has all of the many features of a coast climate— heat and moisture, profuse vegetation, etc., as well as the usual coastal fevers. It has had its experience with yellow fever.

When in Savanilla I became acquainted with a highly educated Colombian, a graduate in medicine of the University of Paris. The next time that I had any news of him was of his death. Yellow fever had reached that inland city, and the native-born physician was one of its victims. Another illustration, if necessary, to prove the well-known fact that in times of epidemic yellow fever natives do not escape. It is true that the mortality among them is not so great, but they contract the disease. As a general statement the children born between seasons of epidemic grow up and in time become men and women; an epidemic reaches them, when they in turn become part of the victims. This observation holds good for Cuba, Brazil, Colombia, and other places within the tropics, now seats of endemic yellow fever.

PANAMA AND THE ISTHMUS.

To the world the Isthmus of Panama is merely the narrow strip of land, thirty-five miles in width, stretching across the northern part of South America, from the city of Panama on the Pacific Ocean to the city of Colon on the Atlantic.

Modern Panama was founded in 1673 on Villa Corta, a narrow, rocky, volcanic ledge extending into the Bay of Panama. It projects into the ocean from a piece of *mesa* or tableland at the foot of Mount Ancon. Originally it was a walled city. The site was an excellent one. It was selected so as to be safe against the fate that destroyed the original Panama, about three miles to the southwest of the new city.

When I arrived in the city in May, 1880, there was but one principal hotel facing on the main plaza. It was a large and well-built edifice of three stories, with a Mansard roof. As Panama has no water system, the closets of the hotel were connected by piping with a large privy vault within its own foundation. In that land of high temperature and moisture the constant fermenting of fecal matter and the decomposing urine made the atmosphere within the hotel closets simply stifling. When such a condition obtained in the chief of the modern buildings, one can fancy what the old-time buildings were like, the old-time vaults below and within their own foundations in many of them.

Yellow fever had appeared in epidemic form just previous to my arrival. An American official had died in that hotel, and I was the next to fall ill with yellow fever. My illness with its tedious convalescence was to me a whole book on yellow fever—a personal experience of lasting value. The part of the city herein dealt with is within the walls or limits proper of the old city.

Another practice also obtains there, and it is a very objectionable one. Many of the upper and middle classes keep in their houses fecal matter, and it is sent at night by servants and thrown over the walls to the rocky ledges below. Stale urine is thrown into the streets, generally after nightfall. There are certain parts of the city walls easiest of access. In some of these places the full tide washes just below; in others the fecal and other matters are above the influence of the tides. In such cases the refuse simply festers in the sun by day, and emits vile odors by night.

Another objectionable practice is that of dumping household refuse in and among the many old ruins in the city. That work also is done after nightfall. The dangers of such practices need not be dwelt upon. They engender and foster disease. When a poison like yellow fever reaches such centres it becomes endemic; and from the endemic conditions epidemics arise, when the disease spreads and is transported by shipping to other ports near and distant. Such were the methods between 1880 and 1885, and when I again visited the isthmus in 1886 and 1888. No doubt they continue.

Regarding the poison of yellow fever there, as formerly in Havana, Santiago de Cuba, and on the west coast of Mexico, no precautions are taken. People insist on visiting the sick, and no disinfecting is done. I tried to introduce it ashore and afloat, for I had opportunities of seeing the disease amid the shipping, but I think I am quite safe in stating that I was the only practitioner there who attempted the disinfection of infected premises and clothing. The general apathy is simply beyond belief in regard to both smallpox and yellow fever.

The old-time Hospital for Strangers was situated on the Plaza San Francisco. It was an old ruin—an ecclesiastical building. It had been roofed in and made fairly inhabitable. Therein the Sisters of Charity had commenced their work in treating the sick poor. Deaths by the score occurred there from yellow fever. The patients were all in one large room, between the bare walls. It became a thoroughly infected building. Later, when the magnificent system of canal hospitals was completed at Huerta Galla, the Hospital for Strangers was transferred to a new building on the same site. The old building was abandoned, and was used as a storehouse for marine supplies for the Panama Canal Company. Disinfection was not thought of.

At the Military Hospital, on the way to La Boca and the cemeteries, the yellow-fever patients were placed in a large ward amid the other cases. No isolation in that building was attempted; no separate building was thought of. It had had endless cases. An army officer told me of the Colombian Government's experience in bringing in troops from the high and healthy levels of the Republic. A regiment would arrive at Panama in full strength from a military standpoint and in full health. Almost at once the men as a body became indisposed more or less: there was the usual loss of flesh so noticeable among newcomers in the tropics, and many cases of diarrhœa and dysentery occurred. Yellow and pernicious (malarial) fevers soon began. One regiment lost nearly three hundred men by death in a single year. At that rate three and a third years would have exterminated a full regiment. However, such results are not peculiar to the Isthmus of Panama. They obtained in Jamaica in the early days, and are referred to in the section on that now healthy and well-kept island. During the zenith of work on the Panama Canal yellow fever had a constant supply of new victims, a constant carnival of disease and death.

During the fall of 1884 the Panama Canal Company, in the month of September, buried six hundred and fifty-four officers and men, the majority victims of yellow and pernicious fever. As many as seventeen died in a single day in the Panama Canal hospitals. That was an exceptional day, however.

The hospitals were on a most extensive scale, a vast and well-regulated system. Colon also had a full hospital system. The workings of the Panama Canal hospitals were very well known to me, as my brother, the late Dr. George W. Nelson, was the resident medical officer. In that system there was a special building for yellow-fever patients, under the physician-in-chief, Dr. Simon Didier, a graduate of the University of Paris. Elsewhere I have referred to forty-one admissions of yellow-fever cases to the Hospital for Strangers, one patient only surviving. Of twenty-seven cases admitted to the yellow-fever building of the Canal Hospital likewise one only escaped.

The general practitioner had cases of yellow fever first in one hotel, then in another; in this house and in that house. I have had two cases in the same lodging within a few weeks of each other. They were everywhere, ashore and afloat. Anterior to the Canal Company's time epidemic after epidemic had swept Panama and the shipping. The poison of the disease ever awaited the newcomers. It has been so in all infected centres.

In the Gulf of Panama, within three miles of the city, there are two islands: one called Isla de Naos, or the Isle of Ships, and the other named Flamenco. One is the island occupied by the workshops and quarters for the men of the Pacific Mail Steamship Company. Yellow fever has played its sad rôle in one and has created a fat burying-ground in the other. Dead Man's Island is the Island of Flamenco. Owing to the great rise and fall of the tides at Panama, eighteen to twenty-two feet, the ships in the harbor anchor just off the islands in the Gulf, on their Panama side. In 1858 an epidemic of yellow fever got into the shipping at that anchorage. It duly appeared on the United States steamship *Jamestown*, on which as many as eighty officers and men died. They are buried at Flamenco, in the cemetery. A monument marks the site. That ship was almost emptied. A crew took her north to San Francisco. She was kept in the North Pacific for two years when she was ordered to the Hawaiian Islands. Upon getting into the warm belt yellow fever reappeared. Had she been sent to a yellow-fever port and had the disease appeared, the claim might have been made, and with great propriety, that the vessel had been infected *de novo*. But this is clear and emphatic evidence to the student of yellow fever of the vitality of the poison of the disease. In Hawaii yellow fever is unknown.

When yellow fever gets into a wooden ship in the tropics, particularly if she is in any degree foul, that vessel instantly becomes a source of deadly peril to all on board who are susceptible to the disease.

I will cite another case, illustrating the vitality of the poison of the disease. A small vessel in the tropics had had yellow fever on board. She was sent north in the fall of the year, and sunk in a northern river. When winter came on the vessel was frozen in, or submerged in icy cold water all winter. In the spring she was pumped out and raised, after a time put in commission, and sent again to a warm climate. Upon getting into the warm belt, and before making a port, the disease reappeared.

Great Britain, I think, has had one of the largest, if not the largest experience with yellow fever among the vessels of her navy and her merchant marine. When any ship of the Royal Navy of Great Britain develops a case or two of yellow fever, she instantly is ordered

north. If on the West Indian station, she sails instantly for the
coast of Canada, making Halifax harbor.

Colombia to-day controls one of the world's chief highways, and
will control it until the building of the Nicaragua Canal. Meanwhile
it depends wholly upon the traffic of other countries, yet Colombia
remains a disease producer and distributer, and wholly indifferent
to her international obligations.

To emphasize this statement I beg to refer my readers to the
report of the Board of Health of the State of Louisiana for 1882 and
1883. In it one will find a three-page letter from Dr. Quijano Wallis, then president of the Board of Health of the State of Panama.
His letter is a reply to a letter from Dr. Joseph Jones, then president
of the Board of Health of the State of Louisiana; in it Dr. Wallis
regrets the deficient organization of the sanitary service of the State
of Panama. In the eighth paragraph of that long letter Dr. Wallis
writes as follows: " It is sad to confess that of the thirty-three powers
represented at the Sanitary Conference in Washington, Colombia was
the only nation that had not a sanitary service properly organized,
and that did not officially register and publish the prevailing diseases,
the death rate, and information relative to public health." At the
close of paragraph two is the following: "I communicate that the
actual sanitary condition of the ports of Panama and Colon is good,
as at present no epidemic disease reigns, it being well known that
smallpox, yellow fever, and the paludal fevers, in their infinite varieties
and forms, are never absent in these intertropical regions where they
are truly endemic."

The Panama Canal.—The interest of the student of public health
extends in all directions. It embraces engineering works in the tropics and elsewhere. The idea of an interoceanic canal dates back to
1520. In May, 1879, Count Ferdinand de Lesseps convened a meeting of scientists in Paris. Later the Panama Canal Company was
organized. On the 28th of February, 1881, the first detachment of
canal engineers and employees reached Colon and proceeded to Panama. Surveys were made, camps created, buildings erected, etc.

M. Leblanc made himself famous during the first visit of Count
Ferdinand de Lesseps by telling him that if he attempted the construction of a canal across the Isthmus of Panama, there would not
be trees enough there from which crosses could be made to place over
the graves of his laborers. M. Leblanc was an old-timer and knew
whereof he spoke. Thousands and thousands of canal men fell victims to tropical disease, many of whose graves were marked by
crosses, while the graves of hundreds are without crosses. Officers
and men were swept away. The disease respected neither male nor

female, officers nor laborers. They certainly were à niveau—to use one of de Lesseps' historic quotations—"on a level." The influx of thousands of people kept up a constant death roll by yellow fever. There was an epidemic in the shipping at Colon in 1884. In September of that year the Canal Company buried six hundred and fifty-four officers and men. During two seasons of epidemic in Colon, during the time referred to, the burials at Monkey Hill, Colon, averaged thirty to forty a day, it was said, and that for weeks together. The real cost of engineering projects in the tropics, when reckoned by lives alone, is truly appalling.

The Panama Railroad.—Within our times Costa Rica, Venezuela, Guatemala, and the United States of Colombia have had experiences in vast engineering enterprises, conducted within their own borders. The history of the enterprises may be said to have been written in the blood of the engineers and laborers. The history of the building of the Panama Railroad, 1850 to 1855, is of thrilling interest to the general reader, and particularly to the student of climatic disease.

Tomes gives a graphic and truthful sketch of the swamps and jungle on the isthmus, and feelingly treats of the climate. Regarding it he says: "When to this was added a climate which disposes from its prostrating heat to indolence, and an atmosphere the malignant breathing of which is poison, the result which has been accomplished seems almost superhuman." After dealing with the climatic and engineering obstacles he adds: "The unhealthiness of the climate has been one of the most serious obstacles against which the enterprise has struggled. I need not dwell upon the causes which produce those diseases which are endemic on the isthmus. The alternation of the wet and dry season, a perpetual summer heat, and the decomposition of the profuse tropical vegetation must of course generate an intense miasmatic poison; and I was not surprised when the oldest and most experienced of the physicians employed on the railway declared to me that no one, of whatever race or country, who becomes a resident of the isthmus, escapes disease. I am indebted to the same gentleman for some interesting facts. From him I learned that those who were exposed to the miasmatic poison of the country were generally taken ill in four or five weeks, although sometimes, but rarely, not for four or five months after exposure; that the first attack was generally severe, and took the form of yellow, bilious, remittent, or malignant intermittent fever; that although none were exempt, the miasmatic poison affected the various races with different degrees of rapidity; that the African races resisted the longest, next the Coolie, then the European, and last in order the Chinese, who gave in at once."

He then proceeds thus: "A terrible fatality attended the efforts of the railroad company to avail themselves of the assistance of Chinese laborers." Then follows a harrowing word-picture dealing with disease and death among them. "Thus in a few weeks of their arrival there were scarce two hundred Chinese left of the whole number. (Eight hundred had landed direct from Hong Kong.) This miserable remnant of poor, heartsick exiles, prostrate from the effects of the climate and bent upon death, being useless for labor, were sent to Jamaica." Again Tomes writes: "A cargo of Irish laborers from Cork reached Aspinwall [Colon], and so rapidly did they yield to the malignant effects of the climate, that not a good day's labor was obtained from a single one; and so great was the mortality that it was found necessary to ship the survivors to New York, where most died from the fever of the isthmus, which was fermenting in their blood."

Colon.—The city of Colon is the Atlantic terminus of the Panama railroad. Generally one writes or speaks of Colon as a part of the Isthmus of Panama. As a matter of fact, Colon is an island, just off the Spanish mainland. The island connects with the low and marshy mainland by a narrow earthwork, or bed for the railroad. The island is about one mile long and half a mile wide. It is best described by stating that it is quite flat, and in places intersected by mangrove swamps; in short, it has no drainage, natural or artificial. Its formation in part is rocky and in part coralline. Its level above the ocean is but a few feet.

The city of Colon is built largely of wood, and extends along two sides of the water front. The Panama Railroad has its chief offices and machine shops there. The railroad runs along the main business street of the city, over an earthen embankment to the main land. The main street constitutes the chief business section of the city. It is, or was, a very busy thoroughfare. The better class of shops and hotels are to be found on it. The back part of the city, towards the mainland, was chiefly occupied by the negroes. Their habitations were largely of two kinds—wooden houses and ranchos or native huts. That part of the city was unclean.

The deep water front of the place is occupied by the piers of the various transatlantic lines and general shipping, their agency buildings, and near them also the chief offices of the Panama Railway. The inward shipping feeds the railway, and the railway feeds the outward shipping, the whole being interdependent. Above the piers and along the Atlantic front lies the beach, as it is called. There the residences of railway and steamship officials will be found. That sea front is the one redeeming feature in Colon.

In my time on the isthmus, the centre of the city, or a part of it, consisted of a large lagoon. The lagoon had a very narrow exit to the open ocean. It may have measured say fifteen feet across. The rise and fall of the tides there is of no moment so far as it effects any important change in the waters of the lagoon, the variation in the tides (spring and neap tides) being but twelve to sixteen inches. That lagoon in part was just back of a section of the main business street. It was almost enclosed by wooden buildings. It received filth and fecal matter. The level of the privies or cesspools was its level. Owing to the soft and porous coralline formation the contents of that inland sheet of water were foul, frequently quite green, a result of the several conditions named. A part of the lagoon was filled in just before I left the isthmus, but that would in nowise affect the subsoil conditions; they have existed for forty-five years, or since 1855.

Colon, Panama, and the Panama Railway owe their importance to the geographical position of the Isthmus of Panama, the latter a narrow neck of land connecting South and Central America. That trans-isthmian railway connects the Atlantic and Pacific oceans. All students of disease and public health know that cholera, smallpox, plague, and yellow fever follow the lines of commerce. This remark applies to the Panama Railway. It has developed commerce, and it has been the means of carrying disease from the Atlantic to the Pacific and from the Pacific to the Atlantic. I particularly refer to such diseases as yellow fever and cholera. Yellow fever was unknown on the Pacific coast of Central and South America previous to the isthmian traffic. To-day yellow fever has a permanent habitat in both Colon and Panama. From time to time it crops out in the ports of Central America. It is endemic in some parts of the west coast of Mexico. It is a permanent and death-dealing poison in Guayaquil, in Ecuador, and time and again has swept important seaports south of Ecuador, in Peru, etc.

During the summer and fall of 1884, Colon saw its palmiest days. Its multicolored population may have numbered eighteen to twenty thousand. Eight or nine modern languages were spoken there, including modern Greek. In fine, "all sorts and conditions of men" were there. Then another local endemic took on the alarming proportions of an epidemic. Then there was a revolution, which ended in the destruction of the city by fire. During that flood tide of isthmian prosperity the refuse of Colon was collected by the local authorities and carted away out of sight and dumped on the southern end of the island, near the wooden powder and dynamite magazine of the Panama Canal Company. A red flag indicated the location of the powder magazine. The vast poison heap had no danger signal. The idea of burning it was ignored. In getting it out of sight the authorities thought that they had accomplished their duty nobly. The many bodies of poor human wrecks found in the open streets and under the buildings, built on piles, were buried at Monkey Hill Cemetery. As many as two to four would be found in a single day. The real history of that carnival of death in the canal days has yet to be written.

The revolution destroyed isthmian prosperity so far as it depended on the canal works. At that time fully twenty thousand laborers were at work. The natives killed the goose that was laying the golden eggs. It was the beginning of the end of the Panama Canal.

Some may say, What has this to do with yellow fever? I beg to reply by stating that all the several conditions referred to have a direct bearing on the whole theme, and to that end and purpose I have attempted to interweave them as wholly germane to my subject.

The geographical importance of the isthmus will be best shown by mentioning the steamship lines making the port of Colon on their regular all-the-year-around itineraries. The Royal Mail Steam Packet Company, an English line, maintains a service between Southampton, Barbadoes, Haiti, and Jamaica, thence to Colon, and back to Jamaica, returning to England by the same route. The Royal Mail also has an intercolonial service between St. Thomas, the English West Indies, to the island of Trinidad, thence to La Guayra and Puerto Cabello in Venezuela, returning by way of Trinidad, St. Vincent, etc., to the Island of Barbadoes, there connecting with the regular fortnightly packet to and from England. Apart from the regular passenger ships the Royal Mail has a cargo steamer service between Colon, Carthagena, and the port of Sabanilla, all in the United States of Colombia; also from Colon to Port Limon in Costa Rica, thence to Greytown, Nicaragua, and back.

Next in importance is the French Transatlantic Company, sailing from Saint Nazaire in France, touching at Corunna and Santander in Spain, thence to the French West Indian islands of Guadeloupe and Martinique, thence to Colon, etc. Another branch makes Havana, and Haiti ports of call. The homeward trip is via Corunna and Santander in Spain, to Saint Nazaire.

The Hamburg-American Packet Company has an extensive fleet. The home port is Hamburg, thence to St. Thomas, Colon, Colombian and West Indian ports, including Porto Rico, and back to Germany.

The Panama Railway Line plies between Colon and New York. This service is better known as the Pacific Mail Steamship Company; that was its old designation.

The Liverpool and West Indian Line, an English corporation,

maintain a large and excellent fleet, a regular service between Liverpool, Colon, and certain West Indian islands. On the home trip many of the steamers stop at New Orleans, or other important American cotton ports.

The Atlas Steamship Company maintains a regular service between New York, Jamaica, Haiti, Nicaragua, Costa Rica, Carthagena, and the port of Savanilla in the United States of Colombia, thence back to New York, by way of either Haiti or Jamaica.

The Spanish Transatlantic Steamship Company has vessels running from Vigo and Corunna in Spain to Porto Rico, Cuba, and other islands, to Colon, thence back to Spain.

A very considerable steam service is that of English and other vessels trading with St. Thomas and Santa Cruz, Curaçao, Porto Rico and Havana, as well as that of the Cuban lines of Spanish steamers to Haiti, Santo Domingo, Porto Rico, Havana, and New Orleans. I have attempted to set forth the network of steamship lines on the Atlantic side of the isthmus that directly or indirectly are connected with Colon. Sailing ships in that trade are very few, for the winds are not suitable, the Isthmus of Panama being in the belt of calms, or " doldrums."

I deem this very necessary to a clear understanding of the means by which yellow fever has travelled on the Atlantic seaboard; how it has reached England, France, Spain, and elsewhere, in a number of instances to develop into death-dealing epidemics.

The Distribution of Disease by Way of the Isthmus of Panama.

I have attempted to make my observations and deductions regarding yellow fever, its fostering and propagation, clear.

When I reached the Isthmus of Panama in May, 1880, an epidemic of yellow fever was prevailing. The death rate was very high. Of forty-one admissions to the Hospital for Strangers in Panama City all but one died. There, indeed, yellow fever is a death-dealing disease. Nearly all who died in that hospital were waifs from all parts of the earth—the flotsam and jetsam of humanity.

The burial of such unfortunates took place in the then Campo Santo. The cemetery was in a suburb of the city, on the main road to La Boca, or the mouth of the Rio Grande, a river of considerable size emptying into the Bay of Panama, about three miles from the city. If the remains of the victims of yellow fever and smallpox had been allowed to rest in the earth, this part of my article would be unnecessary. The dead in that small God's acre were buried and remained undisturbed for twelve months or less, all depending upon the number of deaths. As a general statement, they were disinterred about once in twelve months. For fully forty years previous to my arrival, most of the dead were buried in that small enclosure, less than an acre in size. The graves had to pay an annual rental, and occasionally the rent was renewed for a year or two, but as a rule they were emptied about once in twelve months or less, all depending on the mortality in the city of Panama. Occasionally a slab of wood or a simple cross marked the grave.

Coffins were not used in the final act. A coffin, even a deal one, at Panama, was a luxury to the masses. The practice then, and no doubt now, consisted in renting a coffin—a custom called by the French in happy phrase a *cercueil d'occasion*. The coffin, with the dead man, woman, or child, was carried by friends to the Campo Santo. The body was taken out, wrapped in a winding sheet, and lowered into the grave. The coffin, having served its purpose as well as having earned its fee, was taken back to the undertaker's shop, to spread new disease and death.

The soil of that cemetery had my close attention. It was largely argillaceous or clayey—a soil whose absorbent powers were of the poorest. For fully forty years that practice of disinterring the remains of the dead had obtained. Bones, clothing, hair, and at times partly decomposed remains, with the occasional remains of a wooden coffin, were thrown out into the open.

Panama had among its residents at that time Mr. John Stiven, a Scotchman. After facing an epidemic of smallpox and one of yellow fever, we joined forces in denouncing the practice of disinterring the dead. A lengthy article in English was published in the *Star and Herald*. It bore our names. The same, carefully translated into Spanish, duly appeared in *La Estrella de Panamá*. The whole question was handled in the plainest of English and in equally emphatic Spanish. The publication of our views created a profound impression. Our handling of the matter did not admit of any contradiction, nor was any attempted. The then President of the State of Panama promised the State Board of Health that the practice of disinterring the dead should cease.

Later there was a huge influx of newcomers—men who came to the isthmus to work on the Panama Canal. The mortality was so large that a new cemetery had to be opened. The new Campo Santo was within two hundred feet of a glen or valley, in which were two Spanish wells dug down for forty or fifty feet below the level of the five cemeteries in that immediate neighborhood. Everything connected with this truly startling theme requires explanation. Why mention the wells? Incredible as it may seem, the water, largely surface seepage and cemetery drainage, was taken from the two wells, and sold by the aquadores, or watermen, in the city of Panama for drinking-purposes.

In our articles denouncing the cemeteries we denounced the wells. The President of the State of Panama promised that the selling of water from the wells should cease. His official statement pleased the public. Tropical apathy followed. The sale of the water continued. Diarrhœa, dysentery, and typhoid fever also continued. For a time the disinterment of the dead in the new Campo Santo did not recom-

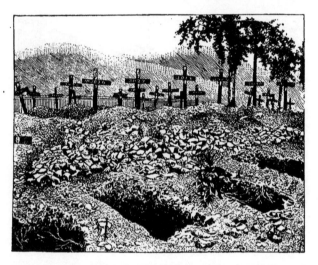

Fig. 51.—Panama Cemetery ; ready-made graves, after the eviction of the former tenants, in the foreground.

mence. It was laid out on an ample scale, and despite the appalling death rate all was well for a time. The old Campo Santo, after its four decades of fertilization by thousands of bodies, became green with grass, and as far as the public was concerned was forgotten.

Soon the new cemetery, in spite of its large size, was wholly filled from fence to fence. Row after row of graves crossed it in almost mathematical lines. Each was marked by a plain cross bearing a number, as shown in the accompanying illustration.

The concessionaire was the owner of the wells and had an undertaking establishment also.

When the cemetery was filled an opening was made in the fence, and he had his men bury in the field adjoining. Then the old plan again came into vogue. The dead, or what was left of them,

were disinterred row by row, save in the new cemetery, and in cases
in which the rent was renewed or a perpetual tenant was laid.   There
were two or three of that class.   I photographed the grave of a perpetual.   All of the dead from the many hospitals were buried in the
new Campo Santo.   The canal authorities buried the dead in plain
wooden coffins.   The coffins, as a rule, were broken up and thrown
out with bones and clothing.   Many of the coffins were in the earth
for less than a year; when a fairly good one was found, the far-seeing
attendants set them up on end against the rear wall of the bóvedas.

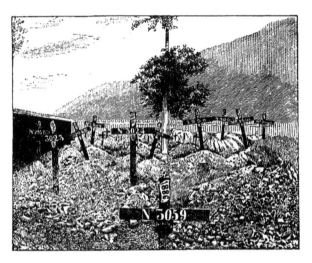

Fig. 52.—Temporary Graves in the Panama Cemetery ; in the foreground is seen the cross of a permanent tenant.

I shall describe that system later.   And they were for sale.   The
vast majority had no coffins.

Now for a general explanation of the grave system.   The first
grave in the first row had 1 on its cross, the next 2, and so on,
until the whole row from the road front to the rear was filled, when
the first grave in the new row was numbered, let us say, 1, 1884.
The crosses bore no names.   A ledger gave the name of the tenant of
No. 1, date 1884.

I left Panama after the Colon rebellion of 1885, but was on the
isthmus again in 1886, and again in 1888.   My last visit was during
March, 1888.   I went out to my field of observation, the Campo
Santo, as that gave me figures relative to the mortality that I could not
obtain elsewhere.   My readers can fancy my astonishment at finding

that all the numbers on the crosses had been doubled. Each grave had a simple wooden cross at its head. I have referred to No. 1, 1884. The number was a permanent designation. The illustration shows the grave "3059, 1886, Perpetual," in the foreground; then we see 3023 and 3024 in the same illustration. The grave 3023 had its first occupant in 1886. He had been evicted and a new body placed therein in 1888, as shown by 1888 below the arms of the cross. So much by way of explanation.

In 1893, just previous to the meeting of the Pan-American Medical Congress in Washington, I had information from Panama that

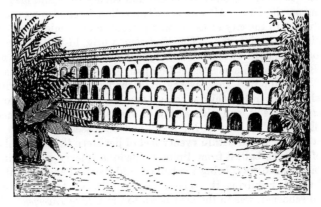

Fig. 53.—Bóvedas in the Panama Cemetery.

the old method continued. I brought the matter before the Congress in one of its sections. My report was buried in the voluminous proceedings. Hitherto, unlike the bodies in Panama, it has "rested in peace."

The bóveda system obtains in nearly all parts of Spanish America. It is a venerable system. To explain the method: The bóveda is as a rule a large quadrangle. In its centre, facing the road, there is a doorway. One steps within, where the four sides are made of solid masonry in its outer parts. On its front one sees, at Panama, three rows or tiers of apertures, into which the coffins are thrust. That done, the external part of the opening is closed by brick work, or at times with a slab of marble set in cement over the brick work. It bears the usual inscription. Rent for the niches, or "ovens," as a foreigner named them, had to be paid in advance for eighteen months. Failing a prompt renewal of the rent the niche is opened, and the coffin is taken out and thrown out on a general dumping-ground at the back. The gateway in the rear wall is just opposite the main entrance. The stately frontal entrance is the way in; the general exit is by way of the humble gateway in the rear. Occasionally the coffins in the rear, when the pile became too large, were burned by the men employed by the individual or individuals holding the concession. In a few instances the rent was renewed, and the bodies were left undisturbed. Again, in a few instances, certain individuals of special prominence were buried within the enclosure in the earth, some of these graves being marked by monuments.

Yellow Fever Afloat.—In September, 1884, the harbor of Colon was full of shipping; the work on the Panama Canal then was at its height. Between eighteen thousand and twenty thousand men were digging on the line. All was activity; yellow fever also was active. The disease in the city of Colon was present in epidemic form. The shipping became infected. The *Effetechia*, a brig, lost all of her crew save one; the cook escaped. Two French steamers lost twenty men. The Royal Mail Steam Packet Company's steamers also lost a few men. One hundred and seventy cases had occurred there, with a mortality of over two-thirds (cases afloat). I visited Colon to see matters for myself, and with a view of verifying certain statements. The English ship, *City of Liverpool*, had six cases on board. She was at her dock, and within twenty feet of her stern there was a large pile of the rock ballast from Bohio Soldado, a quarry on the line of the Panama Railway, being the ballast sold by the Panama Railroad to all vessels requiring it. The *Grace Bradley*, an American three-masted schooner, was in the next berth to the *City of Liverpool*. She had discharged her cargo of ice and was taking in the ballast. Two of her crew sickened with yellow fever and died. She sailed for a Southern port in the United States, with a foul bill of health from the United States Consul.

Another vessel lost her captain and nine or ten of her crew. They wished to clear her, and applied to a physician at Colon, personally known to me, and he issued a foul bill of health. The steamship company would not accept it, but referred the matter to the general agent on the isthmus; he in turn approached the Government. The then acting President issued a clean bill of health, and the infected vessel went to sea from a veritable hotbed of the disease.

My plain statement in the introductory section, in which I referred to bills of health in some cases being but bits of paper, is borne out by the above. The State Board of Health of Louisiana, under the able presidency of Dr. Joseph Holt, so treated them. Mendacity, like yellow fever and smallpox, is endemic in some ports.

Ballast.—In the preceding I have dealt with one phase of callous or criminal indifference, as shown in the sale of rock ballast. I learned subsequently that the *Grace Bradley* proceeded to a Southern port, discharged her ballast in flat cars that dumped it into the sea. She took on cargo and proceeded direct to the port of Philadelphia. In such cases the only safety lies in having such vessels and their ballast disinfected, as that measure of safety is enforced at New Orleans. Some day, ballast of that kind, quarried in an infected centre, transported to an infected city, and there laden on vessels for Southern ports, will speak to the people of the South louder than any caution of mine can. Three cases of yellow fever in New Orleans in 1882 were directly traced to infection from ballast of this kind. The ballast was brought from a yellow-fever port and was thrown on a street in New Orleans.

The Canal Company at the time referred to had a wooden coal hulk in the harbor of Colon. Her name was *La Reine des Anges*, the Queen of the Angels. A hospital ship was necessary. She proceeded to a dock, discharged her coals, was moored off the piers, and did duty during that epidemic afloat as a yellow-fever hulk. She subsequently resumed her peaceful function as a collier. This best illustrates what tropical indifference means. In this case the local authorities were not to blame, but officials of the Panama Canal Company. A permanently infected ship, of wood, selling coal to purchasers at Colon! Of a verity, "Truth is stranger than fiction."

ECUADOR.

The first port in Ecuador south of Panama is Esmeraldas, the port of Guayaquil, the chief city near the coast. It lies almost under the equator. The city of Guayaquil has almost the same relation to that part of the coast that the city of Panama has to the State of that name, in that both have identical old-time conditions. Yellow fever there, as at Panama, is an endemic disease, with constantly recurring explosions in epidemic form. Practically they are annual.

To the credit of the Republic of Ecuador, be it stated, she calls yellow fever yellow fever, and annually gives some data of value to the student of the disease. The death rate of the city of Guayaquil averages from three to four hundred cases annually. The robust honesty of Ecuador is almost startling when measured by the chronic mendacity of the health authorities of many infected centres there away. Especially does Ecuador's truthfulness stand out in a pure white light when contrasted with the absolute darkness of many of the Spanish-American Republics in deliberately suppressing the truth regarding their endemic diseases, such as smallpox and yellow fever.

Costa Rica.

The chief port on the Pacific coast of Costa Rica is Punta Arenas. It is the receiving and shipping centre for the Pacific slope of the Republic. It has a railway extending part of the way to San José.

The chief port on the Atlantic side is Port Limon. It lies on an open roadstead. A small island affords the long pier some protection. From Port Limon a railway extends to San José.

The Republic, owing to its lofty mountains, has three climates. The climate at coast level on the Atlantic side is the counterpart of that at Colon. The climate of the Pacific coast practically is identical with that of the State of Panama on that coast.

Costa Rica, in common with Colombia and Guatemala, has had an extended experience in railway construction. Owing to the great difficulty in getting the Indian natives of the Republic to work at coast level, foreigners were imported by the ship load, nearly all Italians. Almost upon landing the men sickened and were swept away like chaff before a tropical wind. Yellow and malarial fevers, as usual, were the chief factors in piling up a truly appalling death rate. Sporadic cases of yellow fever had appeared from time to time ere the advent of the Italians. The poison awaited them, and when they came the usual explosion followed. Along that hot and humid coast no newcomer from a temperate or northern climate can expect to escape a fever of some kind. Malaria invariably makes its mark in some of its multiple phases, while epidemic yellow fever kills nearly all attacked.

Nicaragua.

Nicaragua has three climates, but only one so far as the student of yellow fever is concerned. Its towns and cities practically are at sea level, or in the "hot lands." Nicaragua has been visited by yellow fever repeatedly. It appeared at Corinto, a Pacific port, some years ago; it extended thence to an old-time city at coast level, the city of Chinendaga. One very naturally looks for yellow fever on the Atlantic coast of the Republic. It has appeared there also. The central plateau in Nicaragua is the well-known lake region, about two hundred feet above sea level. The disease has also appeared there.

The coast climate of Spanish America is merciless, even to the natives. Washington Irving states that Columbus ascertained from the natives of the country that, where many lived in one location at sea level, after a time epidemic disease appeared among them and swept them away. Such is the earliest history of the natives in the pre-Columbian times. What the early epidemics were, we know not.

Certainly the disease was not malaria. Whether it was a form of cholera or pestilence we cannot tell. The one fact that remains, and must appeal to the thoughtful, is this: a crowded hamlet and soil contamination no doubt were the chief factors. The lives and insanitary methods of the people led to the diseases that killed them. When such epidemics appeared, they moved on to a new location. Fecal fermentation and subsoil contamination will occur to many minds. Dense obscurity veils that past, but much has been left to

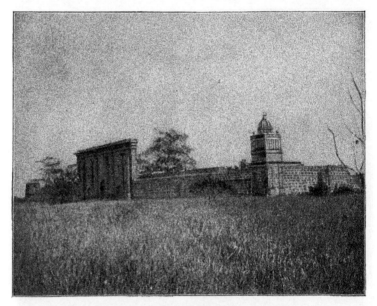

FIG. 54.—The Cemetery at Leon, Nicaragua ; external view.

ponder upon. Greytown, or San Juan del Norte as it is called to-day, is the chief Atlantic town. It lies inside a bar of sand. The shipping anchors well off shore.

The *bóvedas* system of Spanish America, as illustrated in Nicaragua, calls for specific mention. On the outskirts of the historic old city of Leon (a former capital of the Republic) there is a large walled-in system of arches or vaults, seen in the accompanying illustrations. Externally that city of the dead looks like a substantial fortress. The whole quadrangle is built in the most substantial manner. Within, between the blocks of stone, there are spaces or *bóvedas*, admitting the coffin of an adult. Once the coffin is within, the external aperture is closed by brick work, stone, or a marble slab.

Now as to the exact duty or function of the vault system. By looking at the illustration (Fig. 55), just to the immediate left òf the cross in the foreground, one will note five vaults, one above the other, or tier upon tier. The four upper ones have tenants. Failing the renewal of the rent they will be evicted. The ground tier *bóveda*, or vault, is empty. What became of its tenant? The long bones of the body of such a transient may rest in some church, buried under its floor, with an appropriate tablet, or they may have been thrown with

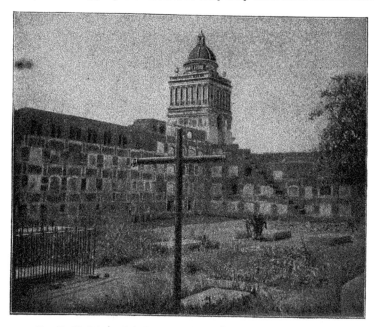

Fig. 55.—The Interior of the Cemetery at Leon, Nicaragua, Showing the Bóvedas.

the skull into the well or final receptacle, to which reference will be made.

Within that dreary and suggestive enclosure there are a few graves. The cross seen in the picture marks one.

Midway between the right and the cross a flight of stone steps will be seen; they lead to the top of the wall. That ornate Moorish tower in the centre of the field has a dual purpose; while being ornamental it has a *post-mortem* function. It covers a deep, dry well. I use that word for want of a better one. Away below the observer may see skulls and long bones; but no small bones, pieces of coffin, or other material, are visible. That receptacle or well presumably is the last resting-place of the remains, but even that statement needs qualification. Once full, that osseous storehouse necessarily would have to be emptied.

What does such a mass of stone work represent in that hot and humid climate? It can represent one thing only—a mass of infected masonry. Within such ovens the changes due to decomposition go on.

To me it seems wholly reasonable to assume that such masses of vaults, be they at Panama, at Santiago de Cuba, or in Nicaragua, must become surcharged with disease. The wood of the coffins, the clothing of the dead, can be but media for transferring to the external air billions of germs of smallpox and yellow fever.

If such centres simply killed their own people, we who live without might bear it with considerable complacency; but the fact must be borne in mind that a completed canal will place that Atlantic coast of Nicaragua within three or four days by express steamers of New Orleans, of Mobile, and of the gulf cities of Florida.

The long and very fertile Mosquito Coast produces an abundance of excellent tropical fruits; the greater part of them reach New Orleans. Many people seem to overlook the fact that New Orleans is the natural port for the Atlantic coast of Mexico and the whole coast of Central America. Fortunately that port is amply guarded by the Holt maritime quarantine system; otherwise it would be in constant peril.

The city of Mobile has many of the old-time conditions of New Orleans—a semi-tropical summer climate, privies and closets, the subsoil contamination, also the fecal odor in parts of the city—conditions constantly inviting yellow fever. If the South is to be kept clear of its old enemy, perpetual vigilance will be the price of safety. That safety lies in efficient quarantine. On the other hand, an open door and no restrictions will mean the planting of yellow fever in the South, or that part of it, as an endemic disease.

SALVADOR.

The Republic of Salvador is on the Pacific side of Central America. It lies between Nicaragua and Guatemala. It is the most densely populated part of Central America. It is exceedingly rich and fertile. Salvador has three climates. Two only interest us—that of the coast and the temperate climate. Its coast has a history identical with that of Nicaragua and Costa Rica. Yellow fever has visited it. Railways connect parts of the Republic with the coast. San Salvador, the capital, and Santa Ana are the chief inland cities. The usual Spanish-American indifference to public health obtains. To expect any anxiety about endemic diseases, such as smallpox or yellow fever, is useless. Such matters are left for enthusiastic foreigners. To the natives the foreigners are an embodiment of pernicious activity. I mention the Republic merely as a link in the extension of yellow fever.

GUATEMALA.

The Republic of Guatemala is the largest of the Republics of Central America, and has the largest population. It extends from the Atlantic to the Pacific, and has the three climates. Its ports on the Pacific Ocean are San José de Guatemala and Champerico. The first connects with the capital, Guatemala City, in the highlands, four thousand feet above sea level. That is in the temperate climate. The Pacific coast ports are backed by swamps and bodies of brackish water, amid profuse tropical vegetation. At coast level the usual fevers obtain: malarial fevers at all times, and yellow fever occasionally.

Champerico is the usual typical Spanish-American city, with the usual privies and the like. A main road extends from it to Quezaltenango, in the upper highlands of the Republic. The elevation of Quezaltenango is just eight thousand feet. Its climate is said to be quite that of a northern centre.

Apropos of the three climates of the tropics, we should make no mistakes regarding the matter. The mountain climate of Guatemala is not the counterpart of a mountain climate in either the United States or Canada. All the mountain climates in South and Central America and the West Indies are wholly deficient in the pure, dry, crisp air so familiar to us.

Livingstone is the Atlantic port of Guatemala. From Guatemala City a cart road extends to the port. Yellow fever frequently has appeared at Puerto Barrios and Livingstone. The coastal conditions there are practically the same as at San Juan del Norte. Livingstone is important to us, owing to its fruit trade with New Orleans and the South; mail steamers run between it and New Orleans. It is an infected port.

The creation of a railway and new port in these countries means a town with old-fashioned privies. Yellow fever comes along in a steamer, which lands a passenger. The new location duly becomes an infected centre. It is a natural sequence.

Railway construction in Costa Rica has been described, simply as dealing with the massing of strangers—I mean whites—and what follows. Railway construction in Guatemala illustrates what yellow fever will do among the natives when they leave the highlands and remain for a brief time at sea level. Guatemalan experience was the same as that of Colombia, when sending her Indian troops from the upper lands of that Republic to Panama at coast level.

Sanitary measures are not taken seriously in Guatemala. Their discussion by the native press is deemed ample. It was that way at Panama. What has been said regarding the absolute lack of sanitary measures in Colombia applies with equal force to Guatemala. There, as in Colombia, smallpox and yellow fever are endemic.

MEXICO.

In 1885 I was in Mazatlan for three weeks. The city is a receiving and shipping centre of importance, on the west coast of Mexico. If it were properly drained it could be made a desirable place. My visit enabled me to make full and extended inquiry as to its epidemic of yellow fever that swept that coast in 1883, and that reappeared in places in 1884 and 1885.

Municipal authorities in Mexico, as well as elsewhere, are very prone to cast blame on some one or some other place. The local authorities promptly disclaimed all responsibility for the epidemic of 1883, and said that it was due to the landing of the body of the purser of a steamship in 1883. He had fallen a victim to the disease while en route from the Isthmus of Panama. That the disease originally reached the Pacific coast of South and Central America and Mexico by way of the isthmus is an historic fact; but in connection with the true history of the Mexican epidemic of 1883, it will be well to state that for several years previous to that date sporadic cases of yellow fever had appeared on the Pacific coast of Mexico. The Spanish-American indifference had obtained. No precautions were taken. The rude experience of others with the disease had made no impression. That coast is very hot. General carelessness is the rule. The poison was kept alive. The usual filth of Spanish-American cities was there—old-time privies, subsoil pollution by fecal and other products. In August, 1883, the fifth and atmospheric conditions being present, they and the necessary food for all epidemics of yellow fever, the presence of many strangers, the people of the coast as a whole being susceptible, there was the usual explosion of the disease, or what we call an epidemic.

By way of illustrating what yellow fever does with newcomers, I shall cite the experience of the Peralta Opera Company, then recently arrived from Spain. They had landed and had taken up their quarters in the Hotel Iturbide, in the centre of the city, near its chief plaza. Soon some members of the company were stricken with the disease; next the prima donna was seized. In a few weeks as many as seventeen of the members of the company were dead. The rapidity with which yellow fever kills newcomers is appalling.

A scientific expedition, en route from the city of Mexico, the latter at an elevation of eight thousand feet above sea level, reached Mazatlan. There was the usual first case; then several among its members; and all died save two.

Remarkable as the statement may appear, I was told that in 1883, and again in 1884, when the disease reappeared, no attempt was made to disinfect premises or bedding. An American was at the hotel while I was there. In a good-natured way he joked me about having the very room in which Peralta died. That did not worry me. I rejoined by stating that I had taken, to my mind, all the upper degrees in yellow fever at Panama. His room was near mine. Within a week he had the disease in a mild form. He never made any further attempts at wit connected with yellow fever. It is wholly needless to state that despite my caution to the proprietor of the hotel no disinfection was practised. After the American's departure his room was ready for the next new and unsuspicious comer.

The epidemic in Mazatlan lasted from August to December, 1883. It killed fully five hundred. It reappeared in 1884, and again in July and August, 1885, killing many.

Previous to the appearance of the disease in 1883, the city had an estimated population of fifteen thousand. At first the townspeople were dazed; then terror seized them, and they fled from the pestilential spot. Thousands left for the nearby interior; others for the mountains beyond, seeking the temperate climate.

The disease to the medical men of Mazatlan was a new experience. What they learned was a mere repetition of what has obtained from time to time in Spanish America—to wit, that the natives of the highlands, upon reaching the coast, contract yellow fever almost at once, and that the whites and they of Indian descent die in about the same numbers.

Following the heavy death-rate in Mazatlan, with a change in the season from wet to dry, the people who had fled returned to their homes. The conditions were all familiar to them save one. The poison of yellow fever had been domiciled and awaited them. Many of them contracted the disease and died. The sickness and death were inevitable, and a result of the lack of precautions in the way of disinfecting, etc.

I proceeded inland by diligence, seventy miles, to a mining town called Rosario. This is a hot inland town on a tableland in the

Tierra Caliente. All the usual conditions there obtained—old-time privies and the like. While there I learned that while the epidemic of yellow fever was at its height in Mazatlan, refugees arrived in the town by stage. They, like the people to whom reference will be made, who landed in Lower California, arrived in Rosario when well, but the poison was carried by them in infected clothing. Such people do not require to be personally infected. Rosario's experience was the counterpart of that of Key West where the disease was introduced in infected bedding from Havana. The course of the disease in Rosario was the old one; not a single variation. It killed many and was left there as an endemic disease. There and elsewhere heat, filth, and moisture are all that is necessary, given the introduction of the poison.

In 1883 the city of Mazatlan became headquarters for the disease. It was taken thence by a Mexican schooner to the port of San Blas, the first port south of Mazatlan. It was the same old story: a first case, then several, then an explosion of the disease. The first case appeared in San Blas, September 23d, and the epidemic lasted until November. While there I traced its history with care. The town is built on a narrow neck of sand. In front is the sea, and back are lagoons. Owing to the great heat and constant moisture the vegetation is rank and luxuriant—rapid in growth and rapid in decay. The place is low, very hot, and notoriously unhealthy. Yellow fever was new to the ignorant lower classes, the bulk of the population in such places. During that awful epidemic the sick were deserted by their relatives, died, and were left unburied for days. Terror seized the people and they fled inland, the majority fleeing for very life to the interior, well inland and upland. It is wholly needless to add that the poison has effected a lodgment at San Blas. Given the necessary soil—new material—it will repeat its former course.

The next Mexican port to the south of San Blas is Manzanillo. Its reputation as a pestilential centre surpasses that of San Blas. The town faces the sea. Back of it there are some woodlands and an immense lagoon, covering several miles. Facing the sea, somewhat beyond the town, there is a bold, rocky cliff. An opening at sea level admits of the entrance of sea water at spring tides. During the long, hot, dry season the water of the lagoon evaporates and leaves it nearly dry. The exhalations from that vast swamp or lagoon are borne far out to sea. I wanted to see the place, and I preferred to see it when the sun was at its highest, and visited it at high noon. A cloud of vapor rose from its surface. A hot, dense, nauseating odor was its chief characteristic, no doubt due to decaying vegetation. The atmosphere was that of a vapor bath.

Yellow fever reached Manzanillo in 1883. It simply repeated its history in one way, and opened a new record in Mexico in another. After ravaging the coast it spread back inland and upland, reaching the city of Colima, on a distant and lofty tableland. Colima for several centuries had had a reputation for healthfulness. It was considered the place of places of the west coast of Mexico and Central America for consumptives. The yellow fever was carried to it in goods and effects from Manzanillo. A case here and a case there, then an explosion of the disease. Its reaching such a lofty inland city was a surprise to the Mexicans; but, as we know to-day, yellow fever does climb, reaching spots many thousands of feet above sea level. The Peruvian experience, when it reached a point on the Oroyo railroad ten thousand feet above sea level, is a case in point.

While the yellow fever was doing its work in Mazatlan, steamships and sailing-vessels were spreading the disease all along the coasts of Mexico and both coasts of the Gulf of Lower California. The chief Mexican ports on that side are Mazatlan and Acapulco; the smaller ports are San Blas, Manzanillo, Guaymas, and La Paz in Lower California. Steamships en route to Central and South American ports from San Francisco and from Panama to the latter city all stop at the chief coast ports of Mexico.

Now, to continue the history of the spread of yellow fever in 1883. While in La Paz I learned that late in August, 1883, the steamship *Newbern* landed many passengers direct from Mazatlan. To all outward appearance they landed in full health. Then a case developed at a hotel in the city of La Paz. The proprietor became alarmed and had the man removed. The patient died. There was an interval of quiet of a few days, when several cases were reported. They established the usual foci, and then the explosion followed and the disease was epidemic. The priest at La Paz told me that at one time, when the epidemic was at its height, fully one-half of the population of two thousand had the disease.

La Paz is a charming little *pueblo* by the sea. The soil is dry, largely sandy. The place fortunately has pure drinking-water. The situation of the town on a sand bank had much to do with its escape from a heavy mortality. There were only seventy-one deaths—a very unusually small death-rate. The conditions there and in Tampa, Fla., are much alike.

Diagonally across the Gulf of California from La Paz is the city of Guaymas. The disease was taken to it by a steamship. She cleared from La Paz and landed her passengers in Guaymas, when the disease appeared. The city lies on an almost landlocked harbor. The usual conditions obtain, together with the old-time indifference. Many of the inhabitants had the disease and many died. Its chief prevalence there was in 1883, but it appeared again in the following year. In detail, it acted as it generally does. In Mexico, as in Florida, it seems to hibernate; in other words, the germ has its season of activity and its period of quiet. This is a matter of common knowledge in all centres that have been invaded by it.

From Guaymas it spread inland and travelled by rail from the city to Hermosillo. In Hermosillo the disease was true to its history. Yellow fever never belies itself. Its fidelity to itself is a fixed and certain quantity; in short, mathematical in accuracy. In Guaymas the greatest mortality was among foreigners. In August, 1885, the disease appeared again. The geographical situation of Guaymas has many features in common with Havana. It is a city practically without drainage, situated on an arm of the sea, the harbor being practically tideless. Much filth is thrown into the bay. That the city is infected goes without saying. A tropical city like Guaymas, unless it is properly drained, like the city of Kingston, Jamaica, bids fair to become a second Havana.

When the disease was epidemic in Hermosillo many Mexicans fled to Arizona. My brother, the late Dr. George W. Nelson, was in Tucson, Arizona, in 1884, and while there learned that several cases of the disease had reached it from Mexico. They were promptly quarantined, and the disease did not spread.

The ways and methods of some individual places and countries are peculiar. While I was in one of the coast towns mentioned, a remarkable bit of information was given me. Just previous to the outbreak of the yellow fever in 1883, the chief medical officer of the Board of Health left for a long holiday in California. Ere sailing he signed many bills of health and left them for his deputy. When the epidemic appeared, the clean bills of health were furnished to all who wanted them. This is not a hearsay statement, but a plain fact. I knew the health officer who signed them. In strict justice to him, I must add that there was no yellow fever when he left. I make no comment of the value of such bills of health. Why the deputy issued clean bills of health when the port was a hotbed of the disease never has been explained.

What precedes relates to matters of truly vital interest to the American States adjoining Mexico. The Republic of Mexico joins California about twenty miles south of San Diego, Cal. The boundary line passes from that point to Yuma in Arizona. About half way between San Diego and Yuma it passes within twenty miles of the head of the Gulf of California.

The city of Guaymas, in the State of Sonora, Mexico, is connected by the Sonora Railroad with Nogales, Arizona. Practically the Sonora Railroad is a part of the Southern Pacific System. The time from San Francisco, Cal., to Guaymas is about fifty hours by railroad; from the city of Guaymas to the hot plains of Arizona but a few hours. The city of Mazatlan is but six days by sea from San Francisco. Protection against so subtle and fatal a disease is imperative. In this, as in other matters, eternal vigilance is the price of safety. The recital of the facts concerning a large number of clean bills of health signed by the chief of the Board of Health should be borne in mind as to what may be expected.

Le Courrier de San Francisco in 1883 or 1884 published an account of a coroner's inquest on a body in that city. The evidence brought out that the dead man and a sick passenger had been landed by a steamship just in from Mexico, and that the body before the jury was that of a victim of yellow fever. I cite this case to show that the security that San Francisco is supposed to have is fancied rather than real. Steamship captains and passengers anxious to get ashore will deceive quarantine authorities. Many of the so-called clean bills of health are worthless, and the only safety during the hot summer months lies in the enforcement of thorough inspection and thorough disinfection of all vessels from suspected ports. We must remember that yellow fever is a portable disease in the broadest sense of the word.

ENGLAND.

Twice the disease has been taken to England, there to spread and cause great alarm. Of the two outbreaks in England, both were late in the season—one in September and one in November.

The appearance of yellow fever at Swansea, in Wales, may be referred to as showing the constant danger attaching to all ships from any port where yellow fever is endemic or epidemic. In September, 1865, the *Hecla*, a copper-laden vessel, returned to Swansea from the infected port of Santiago de Cuba. Upon arrival she had a case of yellow fever on board, and there had been three deaths during the voyage. The sick man and two convalescents were sent on shore. In a few days the crew was paid off, and went on shore also. Two passengers with their luggage were landed. As the barque entered the dock a good many people went on board. An outbreak of yellow fever thus originated ashore. In a carefully prepared table of the cases, Dr. Buchanan showed their invariable connection with the source of the disease, thus adding further proof of the infectious nature of this disease, if perchance badly informed people need it (Quain's "Dictionary of Medicine," 1885).

Southampton, England, was the other place where it appeared. The disease here was introduced by Royal Mail steamers in 1852, steamships that had cleared from St. Thomas, Danish West Indies. The vessels had had one hundred and twenty-four cases en route, with a mortality of just fifty (*The Lancet*, April, 1853).

UNITED STATES.

During the last epidemic of yellow fever in Tampa in 1887, I proceeded there to study the disease and the local conditions. I wanted to compare it with the death-dealing disease that I knew so well on the Isthmus of Panama and in Cuba.

The city of Tampa, Florida, is built on dry, sandy soil, on the edge of the Gulf of Mexico. In location it reminded me of La Paz, in Lower California. The Tampa epidemic killed about ten per cent. of those attacked, while the epidemic at La Paz killed seven per cent.

While in Tampa, under the guidance of the late Dr. John Wall, I saw many cases. The yellow fever seen by me there was not the severe death-dealing disease of the tropics. The small mortality I believed to be due to a lessened intensity of the specific poison of the disease, a modification of the poison due to geographical and climatic conditions, namely, less heat and less moisture, a sandy soil, and less luxuriant vegetable life. The modification of disease by geographical conditions is a well-known fact. The typhoid fever of the tropics is not the typhoid fever of New York or Montreal. In the tropics its mortality is far less. Measles hereaway we do not deem a serious disease. In the tropics measles with pulmonary complication prevails as an epidemic among adult negroes and kills great numbers. Such was the experience of the medical officers of the Panama Canal Company with the able-bodied, broad-chested negroes of Jamaica. I mention this by way of contrast, one poison lessened within the tropics and another intensified.

The solving of many questions anent disease, including yellow fever, must be left to future work. Regarding yellow fever, many faithful and conscientious workers have the problem on their mental anvils. A satisfying solution may come when least expected; when that day arrives, it will be for the betterment of mankind. While yellow fever has no national features, its present habitats are among the Latin races of Central and South America and Mexico. The conditions in Cuba and Porto Rico are hereditary. I cannot say that yellow fever is a filth disease properly so called, but I am quite prepared to state that it is fostered by filth and always has been. Also, that endemic yellow fever and filth conditions are inseparably linked together, a statement amply proven by history and common knowledge.

Etiology.

Where doubt and lack of knowledge have obtained for more than four centuries, the exact etiology of this disease is, like all matters relating to it, surrounded by haze and darkness.

PREDISPOSING CAUSES.

The human mind is so educated that causes and events have to be arranged in a certain chronological order, that such causes and such events may be in general harmony with the reasoning and teaching of the day. I shall try and defer to this time-honored custom, but only in a measurable way, as the subject is peculiar to itself. The exact predisposing cause seems to be the presence of susceptible people within the yellow-fever zone, particularly in spots where the neglect of ages has fostered the disease.

To consult some of the text-books, to which I have referred in passing, adds to one's perplexities. Many conditions have been named as predisposing causes, such as being plethoric, coming from a cold or northern climate, being of the dark-skinned races; and other general causes are cited, such as excesses of all kinds, exposure to the direct rays of the tropical sun, the dampness at night, excessive exercise, fatigue, fear, and the like.

Now, what are the facts as contrasted with the theories advanced? To consider a few of them, the evidence seems to be in conflict with the theoretical views. I ask my readers to remember that my views are based upon the yellow fever of the Isthmus of Panama. A Scotchman (a physician) arrived at Panama. He had passed a part of his life in Peru. He was of large build and well up in years—aged nearly sixty. He sickened and died. Next a Sister of Charity died in the hospital. She was a new arrival, a large, healthy woman, aged over fifty—so much by way of advanced age, and of males and females of full habit.

The case of a French consul and his wife at Panama illustrates another class. There were newcomers. He was tall and slight, an active man, thirty years old. His wife was a dark-skinned Portuguese, quite petite, aged twenty-two. Both had the disease at the same time and died within twenty hours of each other. Here are two contrasts, two elderly people, in full flesh, and two young people of slight build; all had the disease and all died.

If it is necessary to establish an intermediate class, I can cite the cases of a brother and sister, aged twenty and twenty-four. They arrived from France in robust health. They were rather heavy for their ages, their parents were large-framed and heavily built. They had the disease at intervals of a few months and both died. They were in the first bloom of womanhood and manhood. They were the only children of the then director-general of the Panama Canal Company—people whose home was luxurious, people to whom care and anxiety were wholly unknown. Later, their mother, aged about fifty, sickened and died of yellow fever. Of that family of four the father only returned to France.

Race, we are told, is supposed to have an influence, that the dark-skinned and olive-skinned races are more susceptible than the blondes. I shall cite but three cases along this line. I was called to visit a New Bedford whaler at anchor in the Bay of Panama, off Isla de Naos. The chief harpooner, a Cape Cod Indian, had the disease. He was a tall man, over six feet, of a very slight build. His previous health and habits were good. He was brought on shore and died. A Russian Jew, a well-made, well-nourished man, also a new arrival, sickened a few days after arrival, and died. He had a rich olive skin, black hair, moustache, beard, and eyes. Finally, a sailor, a Finn, a very fine specimen of manhood, who was a typical blonde, in skin, hair, and complexion, died in hospital, where I had him under observation, and where I made the post-mortem examination. With such evidence, based upon actual experience in hospital and private practice, the element of racial predisposing causes to me seems to have but small influence. When nearly all attacked die, the predisposing cause in a marked measure seems to rest upon them for having lived and having visited such a centre.

Evidence, medical and legal, is supposed to be based upon facts, and well-attested facts at that. For a moment, let us consider the new arrivals in the tropics. They land from an ocean steamship. At sea they have had a quiet and peaceful life. They land in a wholly new and frequently perplexing environment. The slightest exertion leads to profuse perspiration; the atmospheric conditions to them resemble a vapor bath. As a class, they have no knowledge of the perils that surround them; they are not properly clad for such climates; their warm clothing is wholly unsuited, and that adds very markedly to their general discomfort. On shipboard they have eaten heartily, as a rule, and have had no exercise; the liver is torpid and the bowels are constipated. They move about, visiting places of interest, eat anything and all things, particularly ripe tropical fruits. They perspire freely; in fact, they cannot keep their bodies dry during the daytime. When wet with perspiration, they fail to change and get into dry clothing. Acclimated foreigners resident in such places have a daily bath and change the underwear twice daily. Strangers, when wearied and bathed in perspiration, generally sit by an open window, naturally in a draught. Then follows the classic chill, more or less marked. Then other symptoms, when a physician is sent for, or the patient is sent into a hospital, when the rest of the symptoms appear in order. To repeat an earlier statement, they have placed themselves in grave peril by visiting such 'places.

As a final general statement along this line of experience, the many cases of yellow fever seen by me were associated with constipation, more or less marked. In five years at Panama I noted but a single exception, that of a man who had been in hot climates for several years, who had had malarial diarrhœa previous to sickening with yellow fever.

Race.—First to deal with the white races. The whites of both sexes and of all ages have a remarkable susceptibility to this dread disease. While this remark is made having the tropics in view, it has a general application to all the places visited by yellow fever in its travels.

For a long time, according to some authors, negroes were supposed to be wholly immune. That view, as well as many others, has not been sustained by experience. To-day we know that negroes born between epidemics have the disease, and that their susceptibility is exhausted by an attack and recovery. They in common with the children of natives properly so called, born between epidemics, have a susceptibility; but the negroes and their descendants do not, as a rule, experience the disease in its severest forms. The nearer the negro of mixed descent approaches the white standard the greater is his susceptibility and danger.

It seems fair to assume that the early-day habitats of the black man in Africa, largely along the coasts, that are pestilential, owing to constant heat and constant moisture, may have in some unexplained manner made them less susceptible. Blacks and whites suffer equally from malarial poisoning.

Now for a very brief reference to the natives of such places within the tropics. Men and women of white descent, long resident or born within the tropics, are, both themselves and their children, susceptible. I can best traverse this part of my theme by dealing with Cuban and Brazilian experience, countries where the disease is endemic at coast level and epidemic yearly—I refer particularly to Havana and Santiago de Cuba, to Rio de Janeiro and Santos in Brazil. It is a well-known fact that the children born of such parents have the disease. Indeed, they are deemed more susceptible to it while they are young, and when it appears in epidemic form. In off years—between epidemics—but few cases appear among them; but when the poison becomes intensified, as it does from time to time, the usual explosion follows. Its virulence seems to increase if there is a new and large foreign element, and then the native children have the disease. It is quite true that the death rate among them is less, but they do not escape. This statement explains much to a close student of the disease. During such epidemics an unthinking man might express surprise that the middle-aged and elderly natives es-.cape, but the explanation seems to rest upon the statement that in youth they had the disease in some form or another: in a mild or modified form, an attack of a single paroxysm, with the usual symptoms in part, including albumin in the urine, etc. Hence their after and complete immunity.

Long residence within the infected centres seems in some way to modify the action of the disease among the natives and their children. If perchance they leave the yellow-fever belt very early in life, before they have had the disease, and proceed abroad to be educated, say in England or on the Continent, when later they return to the land of their birth they seem to be equally susceptible with newcomers. In many known cases they have contracted the disease and died. Their having been born in yellow-fever centres, and of native parents or those long resident in such places, has not afforded them protection.

Among the many thousands living in and near the city of Panama, when work on the canal was at its zenith, was a large and prosperous Chinese colony, largely merchants and their employees. I had a large practice among them. While they were very susceptible to malarial diseases, cases that yielded readily to full doses of sulphate of sodium and quinine, given in one solution, they did not seem to be susceptible to yellow fever. During my five years of active work there I failed to see a case of yellow fever among the Chinese, nor did my confrères report any. There may have been cases among them; if so, they were not reported. I cannot offer any explanation for this observation. Some future writer on yellow fever may be able to explain this seeming exception to universal susceptibility to the disease.

Age.—Regarding the element of age. In many diseases well known to us age seems to exert some influence. In yellow fever this law does not hold. I have shown that the children of natives are susceptible. Among newcomers of pure white blood, hailing from cold or northern climates of the United States, Canada, and

Europe, all seem to be equally endangered by the specific poison of yellow fever. I have seen the disease at all ages, from sixty downwards. Necessarily one sees more of it among young and middle-aged men, as they are the ones who start out to make careers for themselves in the tropics, or who travel for European merchants or others.

Sex.—The element of sex among native children or newcomers seems to exert no appreciable influence. Such is my personal experience in private practice and hospital work. The disease strikes equally at all. Given an equal number of males and females, all being newcomers, the disease kills both in about equal numbers. In short, yellow fever respects neither sex, age, nor station in life; it kills with equal impartiality.

What precedes recalls multiple experience at Panama and Colon, also the experiences of others on the Isthmus. Seven brothers (Belgians) arrived on the Isthmus, to put together machinery for the Canal Company. Within four months six of them were killed by yellow fever; the remaining brother, terror-stricken, fled the country.

A wealthy merchant at Panama, a creole by birth, had two sons educated in England. One, after several years of absence, came to Panama. He sickened with yellow fever within a fortnight of arrival and died on the fourth day. Experience failed to teach that wealthy merchant; another son came out from England. Like his brother he was a fine specimen of youthful manhood. He sickened with yellow fever two days after leaving the steamship, and died on the fifth day.

To illustrate an earlier statement apropos of creoles (or the children of white residents in the tropics): An Englishman arrived at Panama. He was a native of Barbadoes, but had been out of the tropics for many years. After a few weeks he contracted the disease and died. He was a man of excellent life and habits.

Personal Habits.—The only individuals attacked by yellow fever in the tropics who seem to have a chance to escape are the total abstainers. A wholly abstemious life regarding the use of malt liquors and spirits stands such in good stead. Of several desperate cases among total abstainers I have three in memory; two were my patients, one a vice-consul general of the United States, and the other a port surgeon of the Pacific Mail. One, in early life, had resided in Rio de Janeiro, and the latter had been a steamship surgeon with the Pacific Mail ere settling at Panama. While both were delirious for days, both recovered. The third case was my own.

The moderate drinker, as a rule, is lost from the start. The liver in such cases plays a most important rôle. The use of alcohol in any form by newcomers within the tropics is a very pernicious habit.

The climate alone taxes the liver, and alcohol adds to the trouble. If one must live in the tropics, or try to live there, let total abstinence be made a rule of life.

Mental Characteristics.—Why certain classes of whites should succumb to yellow fever and die almost to a man is difficult to explain, except upon racial lines. But there is a difference, and a very marked one at that. Let me cite from experience at Panama. When the Panama Canal was under construction, the men who were in practice had to do with several classes of whites. Among the latter the Latin race were in the majority. The Frenchman who is cheerful and sunny when well, is another man when ill. The death-dealing climate of the Isthmus, the alarming death rate, and constant attendance at funerals had made a lasting mental impress. When such men sickened with yellow fever, they lost all hope, and would exclaim, "*Je suis perdu!*"—"I am lost!" Their morale deserted them and they died almost to a man. Among my early experiences at Panama, I recall twenty-seven patients admitted to the yellow-fever ward of the Canal Hospital. Of them, twenty-six died, the twenty-seventh man escaped; he expected to recover, and his case was not of the usual fatal type. He sickened at the Grand Hotel, at Panama, where I attended him up to the time he went into the hospital. Just what that racial peculiarity consists of in the Latin races I cannot explain. The Italians, in the same way, abandoned hope. The physicians at Panama who were in constant contact with yellow fever knew full well that such a loss of will power generally meant death.

In turn, let us consider the Anglo-Saxon races, and by this term I mean Americans and Englishmen and their descendants. Among such I recall several cases. The men had wills and strong ones; they expected to recover, and they did recover. That national characteristics should have an influence on such a disease may seem a novel statement, but experience and the facts both point to such a conclusion.

A man had been told by his physician that his case was hopeless. "Well," said the patient, "if I am going to die, I shall have my own way; I want some champagne." He had it and recovered. Another case of a wilful man. He had just turned the danger point; he insisted on being shaved; he would not listen to his physician; he died while the barber was shaving. A will may save, but badly used the will may destroy a man—as in the latter case.

Season.—Some diseases are known to recur at seasons more or less well defined. This general statement applies equally well to yellow fever, when it takes on an epidemic character in the tropics. Upon the regularity in advent of the "seasons" depends the quiescence or the activity of the germ or poison of this disease.

The seasons within the tropics are two, the wet and dry seasons, or the summer and winter of the tropics. While the term winter is used, such lands are strangers to cold, the average temperature being 80° or thereabouts.

The general health of such centres, tropical cities at sea or coast level, depends on "regular seasons." The prompt coming of the "wet season" with its torrential rains, thunder, and lightning, purifies the atmosphere by washing it, and cleanses the filthy surface by flooding it with water. If the "seasons" are regular, a fairly healthy "wet season" or summer may be predicted. All things are comparative. A fairly healthy season thereaway would be deemed an unhealthy one in a Northern or temperate climate. In healthy seasons the death rate of Panama is fully threefold that of New York.

If the rains are late, scanty, and alternated by very hot days, the general terrestrial and atmospheric conditions are favorable to great activity of the poison of the disease. In short, given the food, newcomers, an epidemic more or less limited may safely be forecast. The duration of the epidemic and the mortality being in absolute harmony with the number of strangers, and the continued arriving of new blood or new fuel, such poisons or diseases are not stamped out. They consume the available fuel, and become quiescent only when the pabulum is exhausted.

A typical irregular season means late rains, three weeks and a month late, with days of great heat. The heat generates a vapor-like atmosphere, a species of hot vapor bath, that is very trying and exhausting to all alike, old residents or newcomers. Such heat and moisture naturally favor great and irregular activity in vegetable life. While Dame Nature is stimulating vegetable life, she also intensifies putrefactive and fermentative changes, when the contents of the old-time privies and pest heaps are in a state of active fermentation. Personally, I am of opinion that too much stress cannot be placed on such filth conditions in the tropics. Given a clean city, *above and below the surface*, yellow fever kills but few people.

The hot-houses of yellow fever are within the tropics. In them, as the veriest tyro knows, it is fostered and kept alive by the filth conditions already described at length. The callous indifference of the Latin races within the tropics is exasperating. The people in many tropical cities live in literal hotbeds of filth and disease. A day may dawn when such practices will be dealt with by the enlightened nations of the earth. May the day be hastened when such criminal and death-dealing methods will be arraigned at the bar of public opinion.

That the masses of the people in such centres know full well the dangers to foreigners I have shown in the boasts of the Cuban revolutionists and their famous death-dealing generals—June, July, and August.

In attempting any forecast of what yellow fever may be expected to do in any given locality, tropical or extratropical, all of the conditions of such cities or towns must be known. Any filthy town or city whose subsoil is impregnated with fecal matters having a sufficient temperature, is a spot in which yellow fever will be true to itself and cause havoc and death.

ACCLIMATION.

Just what acclimation is is indeed a mystery. If an attempt is made to apply it to any supposed immunity from yellow fever, the word conveys nothing to the mind of the student of that disease. Acclimation by many is supposed to be a synonym for immunity. I am firmly of opinion that no immunity from yellow fever exists, save as a direct result of having had the disease. A person who has had the disease and who has made a perfect recovery I deem wholly immune, and that immunity lasts for life if he or she continues to reside within the tropics. Having had the disease means the tissue change that protects once for all.

A sufficient residence—say five to ten years—formerly was supposed to be sufficient for the purposes of acclimation. A man living on the Isthmus of Panama died there after residence of thirty-six years. He had passed through epidemic after epidemic of yellow fever, but the disease killed him after more than a third of a century. Another case, one occurring in my practice at Panama, was in the person of an American who had lived in or near the city of Panama for sixteen years, a well-built, hardy man of good life and habits, but he sickened with the disease and died.

Second Attacks.—One hears a great deal about second attacks of yellow fever. I have never seen one, and being anxious for information I made diligent inquiry among medical men and others during my travels in Spanish America and the West Indies, and there was but one reply, never had they seen or heard of an authenticated case, nor did any layman know of a case.

We know from experience that second attacks of some diseases do obtain, but common experience regarding second attacks of other diseases have no application to tropical yellow fever. That as a disease seems to stand wholly apart. One attack exhausts the individual's susceptibility.

Bacteriology.

This and all succeeding ages will remain indebted to Louis Pasteur for his researches in chemistry, pathology, and bacteriology. A very brief reference to his work and methods will assist in a clearer understanding of much that follows. Pasteur, while investigating one of the tartrates of lime, discovered a living ferment, a microorganism resembling the yeast plant. The latter had been discovered by Cagniard-Latour and by Schwann. Having located a fact other processes in fermentation were studied, such as acetic, lactic, and butyric fermentation. He proved conclusively that they were due to organisms. He verified Schwann's studies and researches anent putrefaction, and proved that the latter process likewise is due to organisms. He then began investigations regarding splenic fever. Davaine had discovered its bacillus in 1863. Following Davaine, Koch took up the work initiated by the former and traced the disease step by step, concluding his personal work in 1876. Pasteur, in turn, verified Koch's work, grafting on much originality and masterly thinking. Next, Pasteur commenced investigating chicken cholera.

He demonstrated that the virulence of pathogenic organisms could be "calmed" or "attenuated" by a variety of methods, as well as by transmission through animals. In that way he attenuated the bacillus of splenic fever. That done, he proceeded to "vaccinate" sheep and cows, and so made them wholly immune to subsequent inoculations of virulent virus.

The published accounts of Pasteur's work led my friend Dr. Domingo Freire, of Rio de Janeiro, to new thoughts and active research in connection with the yellow-fever endemic in the city of his birth.

FREIRE'S MICROCOCCUS.

As far back as 1883, Freire duly stated in print that he had discovered the specific germ or cause of yellow fever, an agent that introduces itself into the bodies of its victims in a variety of ways. The microorganism, to which he gave the name cryptococcus xanthogenicus, is a micrococcus. He constantly found it in the blood and tissues, in all well-defined cases of yellow fever.

The microbe of yellow fever may be cultivated in a variety of media. It thrives well on peptonized jelly at a temperature of 30°

C. When the mass in tubes is pierced by a long needle, the usual nail-like colonies are formed; the top or head of the nail being on the surface, while the growth extends along the whole line of the puncture. The colonies at first are white. Later they produce a pigment of the color of yellow ochre, then a brown pigment, and finally a black one.

Freire's fluid cultures were made in bouillon, after the methods of Miquel and Loeffler. The cultures became turbid at the end of a few days. The primary deposit was white; then a dark deposit was noted at the bottom of the tubes, and at a later period the liquid became yellow. Upon longer keeping the yellow color was intensified.

Apropos of the action of the germ upon gelatin, Freire found that it liquefied it, forming a round depression in the tubes. In the bottom of the cup-like cavity a heavy brown sediment was seen. After an interval of fifteen days the colonies increased, taking on a dark yellow color with a black central kernel, resembling the kernel or point of a smallpox pustule.

With culture experiments conducted on agar-agar, the colonies developed a marked tendency to grow to one side. In the course of a few days they became quite yellow.

The micrococcus was reproduced on potato cultures. When the Esmarch tubes or plate cultures were made at the end of the first week, small colonies of a pure milk-white color were seen. The cultures exhaled an odor, due to the toxic substances elaborated by the germs.

Heat and cold exerted the usual influences. The room temperature accelerated the growth of the colonies, while cold checked growth. In short, laboratory work simply confirmed what obtains in yellow-fever centres—to wit, the alternation of periods of activity and periods of quiescence.

Microscopic Appearances and Morphology.—Regarding the general microscopic appearance and morphology of the cryptococcus zanthogenicus, Freire describes it as being in the form of a round cell with regular edges. The cell measures from one to two micromillimetres. The micrococci are found in a variety of groups. Sometimes they form chains, sometimes clusters. Again, they are seen in isolated masses. The cells present a clear refracting and very characteristic central point. They are rapidly stained by fuchsin violet and methylene blue.

Reproduction.—The cryptococcus zanthogenicus is reproduced by spores. The spores seem to be wellnigh indestructible, as they successfully resist a temperature of 200° C. The fact that these cells are spore-producing explains much, according to Freire, that has hitherto been buried in speculation and theory. It fully explains the remarkable vitality of this death-dealing germ and emphasizes the imperative necessity of a general sanitary reform in all the habitats of yellow fever.

Freire, in his several publications in Portuguese and French, gives the full details of his experimental work with animals. He used blood from yellow-fever patients and cultures of his yellow-fever microbe. The animals used by him in his experiments were rabbits, guinea-pigs, chickens, pigeons, dogs, monkeys, and frogs. Several of the animals named were suitable agents to demonstrate the inoculability of yellow fever. Chickens and pigeons were not susceptible to the poison, but they served to regenerate its virulence.

In using cultures of the first strength in animals, he found that a small dose injected with a suitable hypodermic syringe produced fatal results. Cultures of the third attenuation did not cause death, except when large doses were used. Cultures of the fifth and sixth attenuation killed guinea-pigs when administered in large doses. Freire's first direct transmission of yellow fever from man to animals was made on the 14th of April, 1883. Using all possible care from a scientific standpoint, a gram of blood was taken from the heart of a person, who was dead less than an hour, a victim of yellow fever. He injected it into the saphenous vein of a rabbit. Five minutes later the animal became restless and breathing became very difficult. In fifteen minutes tetanic convulsions were noted. The animal died in just twenty minutes, stricken, Freire believed, by the virus introduced directly into the circulation. He attributed the animal's death to the ptomains of the germs actively expending their force on the nerve centres.

He proceeded to verify this first experiment by taking a gram of blood from the dead animal and injecting it into a guinea-pig. The animal died several hours later. In its blood he found a great quantity of micrococci. In the body he found lesions resembling those occurring in man with yellow fever.

Continuing his experiments he injected a gram of the blood of the animal last mentioned into another guinea-pig. In a few hours there were signs of depression; the ears and feet became cold, and there were evacuations of a black color. A drop of its blood revealed a large quantity of micrococci. The animal died on the third day.

At the hospital in Jurujuba, blood was taken from a patient with yellow fever and injected subcutaneously into a hen. Before the experiment the animal's temperature was 41° C.; the following day it was 42.2° C. No appreciable symptoms were observed apart from the increased temperature. The hen lived. In pigeons the same negative results were obtained.

Dogs were promptly killed by strong cultures of the microbes, but they resisted considerable doses of the ptomains resulting from such cultures.

In his many experiments in inoculating guinea-pigs and dogs with pure cultures of the cryptococcus zanthogenicus, Freire succeeded in producing the most characteristic symptoms of the disease, such as jaundice, nasal, gastric, and intestinal hemorrhages, and he found post mortem black vomit in the stomach.

Freire states that while he was conducting his early experiments, the profession was still imbued with the opinion held by Pasteur that the microbes themselves were the poisonous agents. At that time it was not known that the microbes could elaborate poisons which expended themselves on the body, thereby producing disease and death. Freire seems to have been the first to express such an opinion.

The Attenuated Virus.—Attenuations of the virulence of his microbe were brought about in a variety of ways. The easiest and best method consisted in repeating successive transplantings to the fourth, fifth, or sixth attenuation. The activity of the cultures diminished according to the number of attenuations. The first culture was virulent, the second less so, and the third still less. Upon reaching the seventh and eighth transplantings he had cultures whose energy was almost lost.

Freire never dared to inject in man cultures of the first or second degree. During severe epidemics he occasionally used cultures of the third attenuation, the reactions being so intense as to resemble an attack of yellow fever, but without any fatal results.

For general vaccinal inoculations he used both the fourth and fifth transplantings. They produced sufficiently energetic reactions (quite enough to impress on the receiving organism a specific effect) from which resulted individual resistance, or the condition known to us under the name of immunity.

The *modus faciendi* of Freire's vaccinations or inoculations was as follows: The deltoid region was the one chosen. The same precautions were observed as in making an ordinary vaccination under modern conditions. The part was carefully washed with soap and water, then carefully rinsed or bathed with cold water, finally bathed with a 1:1,000 solution of mercuric chloride.

The quantity of fluid injected under the skin varied according to the age of the patient. For adults 1 to 2 gm. was used, the quantity depending upon physique. For robust, full-blooded men and women,

2 gm. For children from three months to two years the quantity injected did not exceed 0.25 gm.; between the ages of two and five years, 0.333 gm.; between the ages of nine and sixteen, 0.5 to 1 gm. Better results were obtained with the smaller than the larger quantity if the children were under the standard of full health.

Results.—The inoculations of the attenuated cultures were followed by local as well as general symptoms of reaction. The arm, in part or as a whole, was affected. The superficial redness was not accompanied by any pain. Freire states that the general reaction consisted of the symptoms of yellow fever, but in a modified form; to wit, those of the first stage of the disease, frontal headache, suffused conjunctivæ, epigastric tenderness, pain over the kidneys and back, malaise, pains in the limbs, tongue clammy and reddish at the end, nausea, and sometimes vomiting. The temperature rose to 38° or 39° C., rarely as high as 40° (100.4°, 102.2°, 104° F.).

As a general statement all the symptoms disappeared suddenly after an average duration of twenty-four hours. Occasionally the general disturbance lasted three days. At times, a slight jaundice, partial or general, was observed. In all cases the inoculation puncture was surrounded by a large or small zone of a beautiful yellow color. During the febrile reaction the urine contained a small quantity of albumin. In a few instances epistaxis occurred.

The following results were obtained in 734 cases personally conducted by Freire. He classified them under four divisions. First, strong reaction; second, ordinary reaction; third, feeble reaction; fourth, no appreciable results—briefly classed as *nil*. Of the above number 360 were strong reactions; 195 ordinary reactions; 148 feeble reactions; 31 *nil*—total 734.

An interesting and confirmatory statement made by Freire relates to thirty-four persons in whom the reactions had been strong, or of his first class. They submitted to a second vaccination. No appreciable result followed. He accepted this as proof that they had been thoroughly protected by the first vaccination.

Freire's work received state-aid recognition as early as November 9th, 1883, when a grant was made to further the investigation. Year after year following that date grants were made. In December, 1890, the Government of Brazil, by a special·act, created and equipped a bacteriological institute in the city of Rio de Janeiro.

Statistical Results of Freire's Preventive Vaccinations.

In 1883–84 418 vaccinations were made—307 among strangers and 111 among Brazilians; nearly all were made by using the lancet; seven were not successful. Freire's published statements show that in the houses where the vaccinated and unvaccinated resided, there was a large mortality from yellow fever among the latter, while the disease was of a very mild character among the vaccinated, or they escaped altogether. In the same interval, 1883–84, there were 653 deaths among the non-vaccinated, whose general receptive conditions were identical with the 418 who had been vaccinated. Among the 653 fatal cases of the disease 577 were strangers and 73 Brazilians—nearly all new arrivals in Rio de Janeiro.

In 1885 the lancet was abandoned and a graduated Pravaz hypodermic syringe was used. With it the bouillon cultures were injected under the skin of the arm. Three thousand and fifty-one inoculations were made in the infected centres of the city of Rio de Janeiro, 865 being in strangers and 2,186 in Brazilians. The majority of the strangers were new arrivals. The immunity of the vaccinated was absolute, while 278 non-vaccinated died of yellow fever, of whom 200 were strangers and 78 Brazilians.

In 1885–86 the number vaccinated was 3,473, as follows: strangers 710, Brazilians 2,763. Among the Brazilians were 222 who came to coast level, or the city of Rio de Janeiro, from the interior of the republic; consequently their receptivity was the same as if they had been strangers from abroad. Among the Brazilians were 489 children, who, because of their youth, have an increased susceptibility. The majority of the vaccinations were made in localities where the disease had developed its greatest intensity. During the year 1885 only 1 of the vaccinated died; 7 died in 1886. The death rate was scarcely 0.2 of one per cent. The deaths among the non-vaccinated numbered 1,667.

In 1888–89 3,525 were vaccinated, of whom 988 were strangers and 2,537 Brazilians. The vaccinations were made in different cities where the disease was epidemic—to wit: Rio de Janeiro, 2,087; Campinas, 651; Vassunras, 199; Nicteroy, 163; Santos, 133; Densengano, 102; Serraria, 80; Rezende, 54; and Cataguazes, 56. The death rate per centum among the inoculated was 0.79. In Santos, Serraria, Rezende, and Cataguazes the immunity of the vaccinated was absolute. The mortality from yellow fever among the non-vaccinated was 4,135, of whom 2,800 were strangers. Among the Brazilians inoculated there were 1,740, who could be added to the total of strangers from the point of view of receptivity, as they came from the interior. Freire's experience with the natives from the interior was the counterpart of the experience at Panama with the natives of Colombia, who came from the lofty tablelands of that republic to coast level. Their receptivity was identical with that of strangers from Europe or elsewhere.

In 1889-90 363 vaccinations were made, divided as follows: Rio de Janeiro, 97; Campinas, 215; Miracema, 51. Among the vaccinated in Rio de Janeiro 41 were strangers recently arrived. Among the 215 vaccinated in the city of Campinas, the greater number were not acclimated. The death rate among the vaccinated was 1 per cent., while the deaths among the non-vaccinated were 1,086, of whom 724 died in Rio de Janeiro, 350 at Campinas, and 12 at Miracema.

In 1891-92 39 were vaccinated at Rezende, 81 at Nicteroy, 34 at Parahyba, 28 at Barra Mansa, and 818 at Rio de Janeiro—total, 1,000, of whom 377 were strangers. Nearly all of the vaccinated lived under conditions most favorable for contracting the disease. The death rate among the vaccinated was eight-tenths of one per cent. On the other hand, the deaths among the non-vaccinated were 3,830. At Parahyba, Rezende, and Barra Mansa the immunity of the vaccinated was absolute. The deaths among the non-vaccinated in the places named numbered 139.

In 1892-93, from the standpoint of public health, the interval was a satisfactory one. The tendency to an epidemic was small. The death rate relatively was small in comparison with preceding years. Total vaccinations, 183; 158 at Rio de Janeiro, 25 at Santos, 8 at St. Paulo. Foreigners 122, Brazilians 61. The mortality among the vaccinated was 1 per cent. Indifference among the people replaced the panic observable when the disease was epidemic. While such was the case the influence of the Bacteriological Institute was very small.

In 1893-94 290 were vaccinated, 107 being foreigners and 183 Brazilians. Of these 274 were from one to three years of age; 90 of them had been in the city of Rio de Janeiro for from several days to three years. Those vaccinated as a class lived in the most infected parts of the city, locations in which the official statements registered the largest number of deaths. The epidemic of 1893-94 was one of the most fatal. There were 4,900 deaths, of which 4,506 were among strangers. The mortality was greatest between the ages of eleven and forty years. Among the vaccinated the death rate was 2 per cent. If the rule of Jemble (see below) had been applied to the vaccinated, the death rate among them should have been 35 instead of 2 per cent., counting those who had resided in Rio de Janeiro from one to three years.

It was during this period that the city of Rio de Janeiro was bombarded by the insurgent navy. This explains the increased unhealthiness of the city and the truly appalling death rate. The intensity of the poison was well marked and very instructive along two lines: first, the general mortality, and secondly, its increased death rate among the vaccinated.

In 1895, 1896, 1897 there was but little fever, and only 336 vaccinations were made, distributed as follows: 153 foreigners, 183 Brazilians. In the total of the foreigners 110 had been in Brazil from a few days to three years at the maximum. Among the 336, 227 returned to the institute in order to allow Dr. Freire to note the results. There were 103 strong reactions, 72 ordinary, 41 weak, 11 *nil.* This gives a percentage of 45 of strong reaction and 4.8 of vaccinations that failed. In other words, the figures indicate that nearly all of the individuals vaccinated were in a state of receptivity.

TABLE OF VACCINATIONS FROM 1883-1897, 12,665 DIVIDED AS UNDER:

Years.	Brazilians	Strangers.	Years.	Brazilians.	Strangers.
1883–1884........	111	307	1890–1891........	623	377
1884–1885.......	2,186	865	1892–1893........	97	61
1885–1886........	2,763	710	1893–1894........	183	107
1888–1889........	2,588	988	1895–1897........	163	173
1889–1890........	263	100			
			Total.........	8,977	3,688

If one estimates the total number of failures, the death rate among the vaccinated was scarcely three-tenths of one per cent.

M. Jemble, in Senegal, French Africa, undertook an investigation to determine the existing relation between individual receptivity for yellow fever and the length of residence of foreigners in that colony. As the result of a long and crucial inquiry, he ascertained that after from one to three years of residence three individuals out of four were stricken by yellow fever, and that the disease was fatal in two out of three cases. Freire reduced this statement to the following formula in which m represents the disease and M the mortality among those who have had from one to three years' residence:

$$m = 0\ 75\ \times 4 = \tfrac{3}{4} \text{ per } 100 \text{ (1)}.$$
$$M = 0.666 \times 2 = \tfrac{2}{3} \text{ per } 100 \text{ (2)}.$$

The total of persons having had from one to three years' residence in infected localities, including Brazilians from the interior, who for this purpose were under identical conditions as to receptivity, with new arrivals (foreigners properly so called) in Brazil, may be calculated as a minimum at about 4,407, dating from 1883 to 1897.

If the formula No. 1 is applied to the 4,407, the calculation shows that 3,300 should have had the disease, and that 2,930 should have died, whereas Freire, in that class, had a mortality of 0.5 per centum. Assuming that the figures are correct and the formula accurate, the inoculations by Freire's method saved 2,908 lives in a total of 4,407, among people who had had from one to three years' residence in or near the city of Rio de Janeiro.

Freire's Serum Treatment.

Having reviewed Freire's figures regarding vaccination it will be well to cite a few cases in which his cultures were used by him as a therapeutic agent. On the 8th of March, 1885, he commenced the use of his cultures in cases of yellow fever. The first experiments were made upon two women, who had entered the ward under his care in the Hospital of the Saude.

First Observation.—March 6th: Maria Joaquina Videira, aged 21; Portuguese; married. She presented all the characteristic symptoms of yellow fever at the end of the first period. The frontal headache was intense, the conjunctivæ were suffused. General pain and malaise. Temperature, 39.5° C. Urine albuminous.

March 8th: The ordinary treatment had been used. Result nearly negative. Freire gave a hypodermic injection composed of 1 gm. of a liquid culture. The injection was made in the arm. All treatment was discontinued, save an acid lemonade to quench thirst.

March 9th: An improvement was noted. The patient had slept well. The headache was less intense. Temperature, 36°; pulse, 68. Complained of being weak and feeble. Lemonade continued.

March 10th: Patient markedly better; fever gone.

March 14th: She entered upon convalescence.

April 6th, or one month after she entered the hospital, she was discharged.

Second Observation.—Maria Angelique, aged 47. Entered hospital March 6th. Mother of the patient just referred to. She entered Freire's ward on the same day as her daughter, and presented all the symptoms of the first period of the disease. Temperature, 40° C.

March 8th: An injection of 1 gm. of the attenuated culture was given. The improvement, as in the preceding case, went on gradually as the result of a single injection. She was discharged on April 6th, the day her daughter went out of hospital.

Third Observation.—Genoveva de Jesus, Portuguese, aged 22, a widow, resident in Rio de Janeiro one year. She had been treated at her residence until May 10th. She had severe pain in various parts of the body, particularly in the joints and across the kidneys. Intense frontal headache. Temperature, 39° C.; pulse, 140. Albumin in the urine. Face and eyes suffused.

Treatment: Application of sinapisms to the extremities. At four o'clock on the day of admission she received an injection of 1 gm. of the attenuated culture.

May 11th: The temperature had fallen to 37.8°. There was still albumin in the urine, but the improvement was marked. Her temperature at midnight had fallen to 37.3°.

May 12th: The patient got up without permission, went out and took a small glass of rum. There was a violent return of the symptoms. The extremities became cold, there was persistent hiccough, and the patient was in a state of collapse.

A second injection of a gram of the attenuated culture was given. Half an hour later the patient received an injection of sulphuric ether. At midnight the patient was better. Temperature, 36.9°. Urine scanty.

May 13th: Temperature, 36.8°. The patient had urinated twice and abundantly.

May 14th: Temperature, 37.1°; pulse, 86. There was some appetite. Free secretion of urine. No albumin. Slight perspiration about the head and neck.

May 15th: Patient better. Convalescence had set in.

Fourth Observation.—Ricardo Maria de Aranjo, aged 23, single, servant, a native of the province of S. Paulo, Brazil. He had the symptoms of the third period of the disease. Temperature, 36.4°. Scanty urine containing albumin. Marked general jaundice, the conjunctivæ being the color of saffron. There was epistaxis, and the gums were bleeding.

May 5th: At 9 A.M. an injection of 1 gm. of the attenuated culture was given. The mouth was rinsed with sweetened lemonade to detach the clots of blood adherent to the gums and lips.

May 6th at 9:30 P.M: Temperature, 36.8° or four-tenths of a degree higher than the preceding day. Pulse, 96. Urine abundant.

May 7th: Marked improvement. Free flow of urine. The hemorrhage from the gums had ceased. The patient slept quietly. Placed upon bouillon and wine, and later, a tonic mixture for the general weakness.

May 8th and 9th: The temperature varied between 36.9° and 37°. Pulse, 81 to 98. The patient was allowed to sit up.

May 10th and 11th: Convalescence had set in and a few days later he was discharged.

Apart from the four cases above given, all treated in 1885, Freire had in all, seventeen cases of yellow fever—in all of which recovery took place. The treatment in the seventeen cases was identical.

Freire was of the opinion that yellow-fever patients should be inoculated as speedily as possible with a view of aborting the disease. He wrote in 1898: "What interpretation can be given to the action of this attenuated culture on the morbid evolution? Is it an exaggerated phagocytosis, producing new hosts that are introduced into the economy? Is it the influence of some antitoxin made by the microbes in the bouillon culture which, acting as an antidote, destroys the deadly effects of its natural toxin?" He then proceeds to answer the last question by saying that "this hypothesis is in harmony with the present view."

GERERD'S EXPERIMENTS.

During my residence at Panama, Dr. L. Gererd, surgeon-in-chief to the Canal Company, became greatly interested in the work then being done in Rio de Janeiro by Freire, and decided to institute work along the same line. His cultures were largely made in Esmarch tubes. At that date (1881–82) bouillon cultures were chiefly used. He made them of all intensities or attenuations. It is needless to say that the starting-point was a drop or two of blood from a patient having well-defined yellow fever.

After a time, having made many experiments, he gave himself a weak injection of one of his cultures—one intended to produce but a very slight reaction. That done, he proceeded to inoculate himself with the blood of a patient suffering from yellow fever. The transmitting agent was the mosquito. He proceeded to the yellow-fever building in the Canal Hospital grounds at Huerta Galla with some hungry captive mosquitos. One of them was allowed to settle on the body of a man having yellow fever in the fourth day of the disease. After the insect had been sucking the blood for a few seconds, she was disturbed, and then allowed to bite Gererd on his hand. She was not disturbed then until she had filled herself to repletion.

What he anticipated followed. The next day he had a well-marked frontal headache, with pain in the limbs and across the back. The temperature was characteristic and there were the usual slow pulse, flushed face, suffused eyes, furred tongue, and constipated bowels. On the second day the symptoms were more intense, with a trace of albumin in the urine. The third day the symptoms reached their height, when the albumin in the urine was markedly increased. The fourth day the symptoms commenced to disappear, when the usual weakness followed. In short, he had had a mild attack of yellow fever. He escaped serious results, and that he attributed solely to a partial protective influence exercised by his inoculation of the attenuated culture of the microbe of the disease.

In June, 1882, he felt that he was justified in announcing his personal results. The following translation of his report was made by me and published in the *Canada Medical Record*. "In the month of June, of 1882, in a report to the superior agent of the Interoceanic Canal Company, resident in the city of Panama, South America, I had the honor to inform him that I had found in the blood of yellow-fever patients some microscopic organisms, some filiform, others resembling a string of beads (chaplets), and lastly brilliant little bodies; that the organisms were constant in appearance and could thus serve as elements of diagnosis. After some trials and a great many failures I succeeded in isolating the microbes, and obtained them in great quantity without the human body by artificial cultivation, in liquids suitable for their nutrition and reproduction. I was then enabled to study the mode of existence of the microbes. If one observes the filiform bodies attentively for a given time, he perceives in their transparent and homogeneous substance a series of small corpuscles, that reflect light more than the other parts of the microbe. Little by little these corpuscles arrange themselves around a central axis or cone, giving the organisms the appearance of a rosary. Soon other changes follow, the string-like formation separates, and in place thereof nothing remains but a mass of brilliant little points. The size of these little points is about one micromillimetre. These corpuscle germs have great resistance. They do not perish by drying, and can, after many years, serve to propagate the disease by regenerating the filiform bodies when placed under favorable circumstances." Gererd, who made a close study of some preparations sent to him, was of the opinion that Jones, of New Orleans, had found the organism during his work in Havana.

Sanarelli's Bacillus.

In 1897, Dr. Giuseppe Sanarelli announced that he had discovered the specific germ of yellow fever. It was found by him in a patient, in a hospital in the island of Flores, opposite the city of Montevideo. Dr. Sanarelli had but recently arrived there from Europe and found the bacillus in the second patient examined.

Its morphology, as described by him, is as follows: "It presents itself under the form of little rods. Generally they are found in pairs. They vary in length from two to four micromillimetres, and, as a general statement, are twice as long as they are broad." This bacillus he named the Bacillus icteroides. "The form of the bacillus does not remain constant, and, like many other microbes, it varies within certain limits, according to the culture media used. . . . It is easily stained by the ordinary reagents. The bacillus has several vibratile cilia—four to eight. It is a facultative anaërobic microbe."

Cultures on Solid Media.—"If the cultures are maintained at a temperature of 20° C., one finds at the end of twenty-four hours small punctiform colonies, having the aspect and dimensions of leucocytes. They are in effect rounded, transparent, and colorless. They are finely granular and brilliant. They never liquefy gelatin. If the colonies are developed by plate cultures, they are very abundant, and form near each other. Their development is quickly arrested. However, they do not keep their initial appearance, and at the sixth or seventh day at the latest they commence to lose their transparency and end by changing into so many black points, later becoming absolutely opaque. If the colonies, on the contrary, develop on the surface and they are sufficiently removed one from another, they continue to increase in size and become spherical, and that while maintaining their brilliant and granular character. Soon a small dark area appears, that is more or less dark and more or less large. It appears in the centre or on the periphery. It is surrounded by a small clear circle from which fine granulations emerge that grow towards the periphery, when they are habitually lost in a delicate network.

"Having arrived at this point, that is to say, the fifth day, the colony presents such a characteristic aspect that once observed, it is difficult to be mistaken. From the fifth to the sixth day, and thereafter, the colony assumes a dark tint of brilliant aspect. The granulations become opaque, then dark and finally completely black, presenting only a little round and transparent zone, in the centre of which the kernel forms with perfect clearness. This particular tendency of the colonies developed on gelatin to become more or less opaque constitutes a diagnostic element of value in distinguishing the icteroid bacillus from other microbes that might be formed near it. It is necessary, however, to declare that the colonies developed on gelatin do not always take on the morphological type that I have described. On certain gelatin cultures, where for causes yet unknown the colonies develop slowly and with difficulty, I have frequently observed those which from the start were completely atypical in aspect and color. These atypical forms may also be observed in cultures normally developed when they commence to age. My later studies have shown that the life of a colony in the laboratory produces sometimes very marked modifications in the aspect of the icteroid colonies on gelatin. Further investigations are necessary to determine to what point this pleomorphism of the laboratory will tend. Meanwhile, I believe that this morphological description applies rigorously to microbes recently isolated from a yellow-fever patient or a cadaver.

"In the latter case, after eight, ten, or twenty days of the life of the colonies, they commence to undergo a slow and gradual transformation. They take on a dark yellow tint. On the surface they are found in layers or concentric rings assuming the form of stars, almonds, lozenges, etc. In a word, they assume such a variety of figures that they cannot be distinguished in detail.

"These morphological characters of the icteroid bacillus are so typical that they may be used in practice as a sure and rapid method of bacteriological diagnosis. The bacteriological diagnosis of yellow fever may thus be made in from twenty-four to thirty-six hours at the outside. It has this advantage over that of diphtheria, that once the characteristic cushion has appeared, the microscopic examination of the colonies becomes superfluous. The bacteriological diagnosis of yellow fever thus can be made without the aid of the microscope. The only difficulty lies in the fact that one frequently cannot obtain from the patients or from a cadaver the material containing the specific microbe.

"During my latest researches I have observed that when the cultures have undergone several passages through animals the colonies lose their property of regularity, not giving the formation on agar-agar of the characteristic cushion. With a view of maintaining the characteristics of the early colonies, I have employed for successive passages those only which have conserved their typical aspect in a complete form.

"This still further proves that the icteroid bacillus shows a great tendency to pleomorphism in all the artificial media. This pleomorphism thus indicates that we cannot as yet consider the morphological study of the microbes of yellow fever as terminated."

Experimental Yellow Fever.—Sanarelli's experiments on man were five in number. He did not use a living culture, but simply a culture in bouillon, fifteen or twenty days old, filtered and sterilized with a few drops of formic aldehyde. In two cases he employed subcutaneous injections; in the three others intravenous injections.

The following is a description of one of these experiments:

"*Observation III.*—N. Q——, aged 35 years, Spaniard; weight, 61 kgm.

"November 12th: At 3:30 in the afternoon, axillary temperature, 37.3° C. Intravenous injection (cephalic vein of the left arm) of 5 c.c. of a filtered culture, sterilized with formic aldehyde. Soon after the injection the patient complained of general malaise. He felt faint and took to his bed. A cup of milk was given to him. The gastric irritability showed itself at once, the milk was vomited. The nausea and vomiting continued. At eight o'clock in the evening the temperature reached its maximum, 41° C. The patient complained of an intense headache, particularly across the forehead, and irritability of the stomach. There were pains in the muscles and in the joints, these pains extending to the lower extremities. A violent agitation followed, which drew from the patient plaintive cries. At the same time general congestion of the skin was noticed; it was more intense in the face and the conjunctivæ. The eyes were red, moist, and brilliant; the pupils dilated. There was a vague look, giving the patient the aspect of a drunken man.

"November 13th: At eight o'clock in the morning the temperature was 39.2°. The general phenomena of the preceding evening were somewhat calmed, but the patient had not slept during the night, and diarrhœa had appeared. The stools, while not abundant, were wholly liquid and very fetid; their color was yellowish. The tongue was furred in the centre, and very red on the sides. The pulse was weak although regular. At midday the temperature reached 40° C. The urine was scanty and of a dark color; it was albuminous, but contained no bile pigment. The scantiness was progressive. At five o'clock in the afternoon, by means of a catheter, a small quantity was obtained for uranalysis. It gave a large quantity of albumin; there was an absence of bile pigment. At five o'clock in the afternoon the temperature was 40° C. The general condition became worse. The pains were more intense than at the commencement; the patient had intervals of delirium. He barely answered questions and referred to the stomach, loins, and head as the principal seats of his pain. A light pressure on the regions named drew forth cries. The bilious vomiting had become more frequent. At seven in the evening a violent trembling occurred. There was complete suppression of urine, and the skin commenced to take on a subicteroid tint, most marked on the cheeks. The pupils were contracted, and soon the breathing became hurried—40 respirations a minute. A lack of harmony between the pulse and the temperature was noted. While the latter was 40° C., the pulse was slow and scarcely perceptible. During the night the general condition became worse. The insomnia and suppression of urine were complete. The vomiting and diarrhœa continued almost without interruption.

"November 14th: The patient was prostrated. Temperature, 38.4° C. I bled him to the extent of 30 c.c. I allowed this blood to coagulate in a sterilized vessel to gather the serum. I also made, with all the necessary aseptic precautions, several exploratory punctures in the liver and the kidneys. This enabled me to draw from them a small quantity of juice, which I hastened to examine under the microscope, and which I planted on several kinds of nutritive media. At eight o'clock in the morning the patient was a little better. With a few injections of ether and caffeine, his general condition was bettered. Little by little the patient got better, and recovered at the end of a few days."

Examination of the blood and of fluids obtained by exploratory punctures gave the following results: "The cultures made from the blood on different kinds of nutritive media remained sterile. The coagulation was regular, freeing about 15 c.c. of serum, of a golden yellow color. This serum, when added to a recent culture of the icteroid bacillus in the proportion of one to five, resulted in a partial immobilization and agglutination. After twelve hours I failed to note the total precipitation of the microbes to the bottom of the tube. The small quantities of hepatic juice withdrawn by means of a large cannula, sterilized, proved to be sterile in the cultures, but a microscopic examination of sections stained by osmic acid showed a profound fatty degeneration of all the liver cells where the protoplasm was filled with small fatty globules of various sizes." In the cultures made with the renal juice he found coli bacilli in small quantities.

As a result of these experiments Sanarelli claims that the injection of a filtered culture, in a relatively weak dose, produces in man typical yellow fever accompanied by its imposing array of symptoms and anatomical lesions.

Regarding Sanarelli's alleged discovery of the bacillus, it may be well to state that Havelburg, a bacteriologist of Rio de Janeiro, discovered a bacillus—one said to be identical with the B. icteroides of Sanarelli. Further, Havelburg's bacillus was described in Les Annales de l'Institut Pasteur before the bacillus of Sanarelli. Havelburg made his culture from black vomit.

Finally, we have the bacillus x of Surgeon-General George M. Sternberg—one discovered by him in Havana. It likewise seems to have the same characteristics as Havelburg's and Sanarelli's.

In the fall of 1897 Drs. Eugene Wasdin and H. D. Geddings of the United States Marine Hospital Service were detailed to investigate in Havana the nature of yellow fever. They made a bacteriological study in the laboratory of the Marine Hospital Service in Havana of twenty-two cases of disease diagnosed as yellow fever by the native physicians in attendance, which diagnosis was concurred in by the commission in fourteen of the cases. A bacillus resembling the bacillus icteroides of Sanarelli was isolated from the blood in thirteen of these fourteen cases, while in a number of cases other than yellow fever no such organism was obtained. As a result of these examinations the commission concluded that Sanarelli's bacillus is the true cause of yellow fever.

These conclusions have been rejected, however, by other observers. Thus Dr. Aristide Agramonte, working in the same field in the summer of 1898, states that he found the bacillus icteroides in three cases which were not of yellow fever. He also says that La Cerda and Ramos, in Brazil, failed to isolate this organism in repeated examinations of the cadavers of persons dead of yellow fever. It is not improbable that the bacillus x of Sternberg, the colon bacillus, and Sanarelli's or Havelburg's bacillus may all be found occasionally in yellow-fever sufferers, but evidence is wanting that either of them bears any specific relation to the disease. We may conclude with Agramonte, who says (El Progreso Médico de Habana, March, 1900):

"The work I have been doing for a year and a half regarding the etiology of yellow fever leads me to present the following conclusions:

"1. The pathogenic microorganism of yellow fever remains unknown, notwithstanding the reports of various observers who believe that they have discovered it. New methods and new media must be employed in future cultures and investigations with a view of bringing the question to an issue.

"2. The icteroid bacillus of Sanarelli, lately (1897) described as being the cause of the disease, has no further connection with it than the bacillus coli communis which we find in all cultures from the cadavers.

"3. By employing a suitable technique, the icteroid bacillus will not always be found in cultures made from the blood of yellow-fever patients.

"4. The icteroid bacillus has been found in the tissues of individuals who died from other diseases distinct from yellow fever.

"5. The bacillus of Sanarelli does not agglutinate the serum of patients or of convalescents from yellow fever.

"6. The serum of convalescents from yellow fever does not protect against infection by the icteroid bacillus."

Symptomatology.

The Mild Form.—The cases in this class are rarely met with in the tropics, and when they are the patients are usually newcomers. They present a flushed face, a well-marked frontal headache, some pain in the small of the back, and general malaise, with the usual history of constipation. The pulse is slow and hard—70; temperature, 101° to 102°. The tongue is furred. The urine is high colored. In cases of this class there may or may not be a history of a chill. Nausea and vomiting occur occasionally. Some patients give a history of excellent previous health. They sicken suddenly. On the second day of the fever generally a trace of albumin is found in the urine; the temperature is still above 100°, the face is flushed and malaise continues. On the third day the albumin increases. The presence of albumin is pathognomonic. The fever ceases when the patient enters upon convalescence. In a few cases the weakness is marked and great care must be observed.

French writers describe mild yellow fever under the name of fever of acclimation. Such it is, and the acclimation means a tissue change.

The Severe Form.—The cases under this heading may present the same clinical features as the mild cases if seen at the very outset, save that the flushing of the face may be more marked. Later, the headache is more severe. It may be frontal or occipitofrontal.

The pulse is full, hard, and slow—for a fever, 70 to 80. There is pain in the back, across the kidneys, often of a very severe type; it causes great distress. The tongue is furred; at the outset of the disease the tip and edges are often red; centrally and well back there is a creamy fur. There is the usual history of constipation, frequently extending from three to four or five days, and that in individuals whose bowels have been evacuated daily previous to the constipation. In this, as in the previous class, the patient is generally a newcomer.

The red flush of the face is peculiar. Frequently it is of well-marked boiled-lobster hue, or that noted in severe cases of scarlatina at the outset. Later this red hue extends to the trunk and limbs. At the very outset the eyes may not furnish any information; the conjunctivæ may be quite clear, but later they become suffused; they show the yellow color before it appears in the skin. From the latter symptom the disease takes its name. The heat of the skin is very peculiar. The hand, when placed on the body, tingles as if a gentle current of electricity were playing over its surface. This burning or biting heat has no counterpart in malarial fevers.

In this class one generally gets a history of a chill. The duration and severity of the chill have a significance all their own to the physician. Persistent and severe chills, often of half a day to a day's duration, mean a troublesome and perhaps fatal case.

In a few cases the invasion may be very sudden, as by nausea or sudden faintness, with no history of any chill. Many of the cases of this class are those in which the nervous symptoms are marked, associated with high temperature and delirium.

The gastric symptoms appear early. They have a marked prominence in all severe cases. Complaints are made of the stomach, which is often the seat of a burning sensation. At the very outset pressure over the stomach causes pain; later the gastric symptoms increase.

On the second or third day vomiting appears. The early vomiting is of a white fluid, with abundant mucus. This vomit has been called "white vomit" by Dr. Blair, of British Guiana. As the disease progresses any pressure over the stomach causes intense pain.

The urine during the first day or two is high colored and excreted in fair quantity. Generally on the second day a trace of albumin may be found in it. This albuminuria is pathognomonic. Its appearance, with the several symptoms cited, indicates a severe case of tropical yellow fever.

In this type of case the temperature runs up and keeps high—102°, 103°, 104° on the second or third day. The higher temperature means an increase in all the symptoms and the early appearance of albumin. As noted above, the high temperature is associated with a slow pulse—a slow, hard pulse. This pulse likewise is pathognomonic in this class of cases.

The vomiting is almost constant and very distressing. The stomach rejects everything. There is constant restlessness. The pain across the kidneys and in the sacral region is often excruciating and indescribable.

With the persistent elevation of temperature the general condition of the patient becomes worse. The injection of the conjunctivæ increases. Frequently sore throat is complained of, due to desquamation of the mucous membrane of the throat, later of the mouth. Then blood exudes and collects on the teeth and lips (sordes). The odor of the breath becomes very foul and unbearable. The stripping of the mucous surface of throat and mouth is a symptom of very grave import.

To detect the yellow color of the skin early, gradual firm pressure is made by the open hand placed on the chest or the abdomen, and then withdrawn suddenly. On the scarlet or red field the impress of the whole hand will be found mapped out a yellowish-white tint. Soon the superficial congestion returns and obliterates it. This condition is found on the trunk earliest. This is another indication that the case is a severe one.

The urine becomes scanty, the albumin increases steadily. The percentage of albumin present is of prognostic importance, for in proportion as the blood is destroyed, the quantity of albumin increases; as much as ten to twenty-five per cent. may be noted on boiling.

Such are the general symptoms in severe cases. It will be well to remember that the symptoms do not appear in any fixed order. No arbitrary law can be made for such cases. The previous condition of the patient has its influence in this as in other diseases.

In cases in which the first or initial fever is not fatal the patient may enter upon convalescence. The latter phase, however, in this class is exceptional. As a general statement the patient enters upon the "period of calm," when the disease runs a full course of three stages. The period of calm cannot be fixed in any arbitrary way. It may be reached on the third, fourth, or fifth day of the disease. The name is illusive, it is a mere remission. The temperature may fall two or three degrees, the pulse becomes softer, and the patient appears to be better. But this so-called calm is most deceptive. It may last twenty or more hours, when the secondary fever comes on. A few hours after the appearance of the secondary fever the maximum temperature of the initial fever has been reached. The symptoms are intensified, the vomiting is renewed. There may be suppression of urine. If any urine is procurable, it will be found laden with albumin. Pulse, 70 to 90; respiration, 30 to 40. Black vomit returns and the stools are black; dyspnœa is marked, and hiccough distresses the patient. The gravity of cases needs no further description.

In some cases the patients seem dull and wholly indifferent. In others the nervous symptoms are marked, and delirium may cause much trouble. Sometimes two and three attendants are necessary to keep the patient in bed.

When the patient survives the secondary fever, the crisis frequently is marked by a profuse sweating. Then a little sleep follows. The pulse loses its wiry hardness; the temperature falls. The hitherto inactive kidneys resume their function, and a little highly albuminous urine is passed. Convalescence is, however, slow and tedious.

The Malignant Form.—In malignant cases the patients die during the initial fever. While the symptoms in the severe form are grave, in the malignant type they are violent from the very beginning. The patient is struck down by the intensity of the poison. It is the foudroyant type of the French. Nothing checks the vomiting or eases the pain. The temperature reaches 105°, 106°, or even 107° F.; the latter is the maximum noted by me. Such cases always end fatally. Even when wholly unconscious, any pressure over the stomach, particularly if made just below the xiphoid appendix, will make the patient fairly writhe. The vomiting is per saltem. Often a torrent of it comes just before death. Extreme nervous symptoms, quiet or violent delirium, may or may not be present at the close.

In some of the severe and in all of the malignant cases the yellow tinge of the skin becomes marked before death closes the scene. Black vomit and black stools are met with in nearly all fatal cases. Occasionally a man with black vomit in severe cases may recover, but it is always a symptom of dire import.

• Such, briefly told, are the symptoms of yellow fever as observed at Panama and Colon. On the isthmus of Panama the mild cases are very few in number. To repeat, the cases of mild yellow fever consist of a single paroxysm or access of fever. The patients promptly enter on convalescence, although frequently it is slow. The weakness seems to be out of all proportion to the previous illness. Occasionally a severe case will expend itself in a single paroxysm, when the patient enters on convalescence. The malignant cases are fatal.

Some of the severe cases run through all the stages and enter on convalescence anywhere from the seventh to the ninth day. There

are, however, no fixed rules in such cases, the order of symptoms is
not regular, much depending upon the man, his previous health and
habits.   While many young men of excellent life and habits fall victims, occasionally one escapes, thanks to his having been abstemious.
I recall recoveries in four desperate cases; all had been in grave
peril, one had black vomit.   The total abstainer may escape where
the ordinary drinker is lost from the beginning.

Yellow fever should be seen and studied in its own habitat, for
when it invades extra-tropical countries it is not nearly so fatal a disease.   Nevertheless, it remains one of man's most inveterate foes.

CONVALESCENCE.

In this connection one must not forget malaria.   Its rôle in the
tropics is a constant quantity; no one living in them escapes.   Gererd, at Panama, a specially equipped and enthusiastic worker, devoted a great deal of time to examining the blood of those who
came to the Isthmus, while work was in progress on the line of the
Panama Canal.   Upon arrival the blood of newcomers was found to
be normal.   Among the men exposed to the influences named after
one month's residence he examined the blood a second time, and
found that malaria had made its impress in every case.   I recall cases
of yellow fever in men who had been on the Isthmus of Panama some
months, a year or more, ere contracting yellow fever.   During convalescence well-marked malarial manifestations appeared.

As a general statement the malarial symptoms appeared during
the early days of convalescence, when the patients were profoundly
weak.   A weak quinine mixture acted like a charm in such cases.

Another condition met with in convalescents, especially in patients who have just escaped death, is a very slow pulse.   Its slowness while the fever is at its zenith has been dwelt upon.   Its
slowness during convalescence, when associated with the profound
weakness, is most pronounced; at times it is as low as 35 and 40, and
that perhaps for days together.   Gradually it gets back to the normal rate in proportion as rebuilding of the wasted tissues goes on.

I may state that my own case was a critical one.   Experienced
physicians had given me up as lost.   After the delirium, when I
came to myself, I did not know the nature of my illness.   I had been
on the Isthmus about a month ere I was stricken with the disease.
One day, when in my room at the Grand Hotel, I took my pulse.
Great indeed was my astonishment, not unmixed with some alarm,
to find it but 36, again 40.   Such a pulse in a convalescent was
wholly new to me.

Another feature to be noted during convalescence is the subnormal temperature, at times 97.5° to 98° F. In some cases it will be observable for several days. The subnormal temperature generally precedes the manifestations of malaria.

During the early days of convalescence the motions very often are of an almost waxen-white color; there is no elimination of bile. Gradually as the liver resumes its normal function a little color will be noted in the motions. As the standard of health re-obtains, the motions assume a normal color.

The very rich yellow of the skin may last for weeks, or it may be for a month or two. In my own case it lasted for all of six weeks. The convalescent looks like a man with an attack of jaundice. As the yellow color fades in some cases it is replaced by a deep hue of bronze. Some attribute the pigmentation of the skin to the liver, others, again, to blood changes properly so called.

Pathological Anatomy.

My experience under this heading simply confirms what an able and clear-headed writer on this disease, Dr. Grenville Dowell, has stated, that "yellow fever has no pathology"—the conditions found are so variable.

The bodies inspected at autopsy, as a rule, are of well-nourished people. The majority have been in robust health previous to the attack. The color of the body is of a very rich canary yellow. Soon after death a mottling of purple appears in the dependent parts. The purple and yellow make a marked contrast of colors. Rigor mortis sets in at once, and is of the most marked type. When cold, the bodies are as inflexible as a deal plank. The bodies are, however, a long time in cooling. It is possible that this high temperature post mortem is due, as has been suggested by Dr. A. J. Reese, of Mobile, to the action of the microbes still growing in the infected body.

Yellow fever is a blood disease, and the poison expends itself on the blood, ending in its destruction or death. If this view is accepted, any marked pathological changes, except in the blood, need not be expected, save changes in certain organs, such as the liver, kidneys, etc., due to the imperfect nutrition.

The Liver.—Many writers on yellow fever dwell at great length on the appearance of this organ. That so large and so important an organ should suffer will not cause any surprise to one familiar with malaria and tropical disease. The yellow, or chamois-skin liver is supposed to be the characteristic liver in yellow fever post-mortem examinations. I never saw but one, and that was the net result of upward of one hundred post-mortem examinations made by Dr. Simon Didier, physician-in-chief to the Panama hospitals of the Canal company. In my own work I have found it presenting a normal appearance microscopically. Sometimes it is fatty with an easily detached capsule, and on section showing many tiny oil globules.

The Kidneys.—No constant lesions are found in these organs, and many are normal to the naked eye. Others are large and show degeneration changes similar to those in the liver. In many cases the kidneys appear to be smaller than normal.

The Stomach.—In view of the great burning pain and constant vomiting, including black vomit, one naturally would expect to find here marked pathological changes. The stomach always presented signs of marked inflammation, the coats being decidedly thickened. It contained more or less black vomit. In one case I found all of a pint in it. Frequently the inner surface showed many foci or well-marked points of extravasation of blood, points of a deep carmine hue; again, tiny patches of blood adherent to the walls of the organ.

Dr. Castellaños, then a general practitioner at Panama, and a physician to the military hospital there, had had a very large hospital experience both at Panama and in his native island, Cuba. He told me that the only constant condition found by him in yellow fever was a state of acute inflammation of the stomach and thickening of its walls.

The Intestines.—Frequently they contained the black tarry matter known as the "black vomit stools," a dark pitch-like substance, or altered blood.

The Bladder.—As a rule it was practically empty. We must recall the clinical fact of suppression of urine. I have secured as much as a drachm or two of urine from it. This, when tested, was found to be highly albuminous.

Black Vomit.—Regarding black vomit, nearly all of the cases in which it appeared ended fatally. The French writers on yellow fever happily name·it *marc de café*, or coffee-ground vomit._ The name is clear and very expressive. While at Panama I sent a specimen to Dr. William Osler, who found that it contained "altered blood corpuscles, epithelial cells, portions of food, and various fungi." The vomited fluid, when warm, has a peculiar odor, one very difficult to describe. Confusion may arise in the minds of students of this disease when they first come in contact with it. The question to such a one will be, Are the vomited matters bilious in character, or do they consist of altered blood? Of course I know full well what my microscope told me as to its appearance. I have referred to its odor. It reddened litmus, hence it was acid. To solve the question of a bilious element I decided to taste some of it and found it faintly acid. As I had had the disease, I did not deem the trial as in any sense dangerous to me. I wanted to dissipate a doubt, and that was the only way to do it.

Several decades ago Rees, of Philadelphia, found vibrios in the vomit. This, and Hassel's finding "a hitherto unknown microscopic vegetation in the blood" in the cases that occurred in Southampton, England, to me seem to link two interesting facts, noted and reported by independent students of the disease.

When "black vomit" is allowed to settle, the granular matter, or débris, goes to the bottom of the vessel, while the upper fluid resembles in color weak black tea.

I have referred to blood from the stomach, altered blood, and blood in the stools. When the blood changes appear in a woman, her friends will report that her courses have returned, blood coming from the vagina. This is, however, merely an expression of the profound blood change. In this connection it will be well to state that in fatal cases, as the end approaches, the tongue is stripped of its mucous membrane and presents a fiery-red appearance. In short, the whole mucous tract suffers and the blood exudes anywhere.

Regarding the *blood* found post mortem, it was fluid in the vessels, with scarcely any tendency to coagulation. Its fluidity is remarkable. If the autopsies are conducted a few hours after death, this will be impressed upon one. I recall an instance in which an incision made by me across the forehead, previous to removing the calvarium to examine the brain, was followed by such a quantity of blood that I was startled. The great heat of the body and fluidity of the blood were marked. The patient was, however, dead without any question.

Treatment.

At times a physician may have doubts as to the exact nature of the case that confronts him. I am assuming that he has just been called in and sees the patient for the first time. Is it the invasion of malaria in a newcomer, or is it yellow fever? As the result of a large experience, personally, I am of opinion that much truly invaluable time may be saved by using quinine and sodium sulphate as diagnostic agents. My plan was simple—instant action to clear up the doubt. I gave fifteen grains of quinine with two drachms of sulphate of sodium in a mixture of dilute sulphuric acid and water. I gave it largely diluted. It was given every three hours until two or three doses were administered. In my experience it did not disagree with patients. If the disease was malaria, the joint action of the sodium sulphate and quinine had the usual effect. If no effect was obtained, then I knew that I had to deal with yellow fever. Time, a matter of truly vital importance, had been saved. That mixture was born of tropical experience. It was made as follows:

R Quin. sulph., ... ʒ i.
Ac. sulph. dil., ... q.s.
Sod. sulph., ... ʒ i.
Tr. card. co., ... ʒ ss.
Aq. . . . . ad ʒ viij.
M.

While the mixture is bitter, it is not unpleasant, as the compound cardamom tincture masks the salty taste of the sodium sulphate. A fourth (ʒ ii.) was given in a half tumblerful of water. Two or three doses led to large and free evacuations. When they had been obtained, if the fever, flushed face, and frontal headache remained the case was yellow fever.

The rest of the procedure likewise was born of experience; it was as follows: The patient is first prepared for a vapor bath. It can be given anywhere and in this wise: A chair with a wooden seat is secured. The patient is stripped and seated upon it. His feet are placed in a bucket or tub of hot water, as hot as it can be borne without burning. A spirit lamp is lit and placed under the chair. The patient is then covered with blankets, which are carefully tucked in to prevent the escape of any heat or moisture. That done, a pint of hot lemonade is given, as hot as possible. Soon, in cases so treated, the perspiration would show itself, rolling down the face, arms, and body. The patient was wholly enveloped in the blankets, head only outside. In a few minutes the hot, dry skin lost its angry scarlet hue. The pulse became softer and the headache less. The baths lasted ten or fifteen minutes. They never were pushed to faintness. General improvement followed to the great relief of the patient and his anxious friends. The patient next was lifted and placed on a bed, there to be enveloped in fresh blankets. Frequently the perspiration kept on for one or two hours.

. Later, when the skin again became dry, and the pulse hard, and the face red, the vapor bath was repeated in all its details, once or twice if necessary.

Next in order, as drugs are valueless, I gave patients an acid drink, one to be used freely—any of the mineral acids largely diluted. It was a very grateful mixture. I let them take a half tumblerful of it, hourly or half-hourly, if the thirst was great.

By this very simple treatment, two great and, to my mind, most important indications are met: the loaded intestines are emptied, and the hot and burning skin is forced to act and eliminate its secretions. In the great majority of the cases the patients, generally men, have been eating heartily up to the very time of their chill—always sudden, this—and marked constipation has existed for several days. By this treatment the patient is placed in the best position to fight the disease—his system is not surcharged with effete and fæcal matters.

I learned of the vapor-bath treatment from a patient who came to Panama from Peru. It was introduced there by a Dr. Wilson, an Englishman, and in Peru was known as "Wilson's treatment." The idea of a long hot drink was a Jamaican idea—quantities of hot lemonade. I increased the effect by means of the footbath.

Regarding general treatment, a mustard plaster applied over the stomach at times gives some relief, but only in the less severe cases. The thirst is incessant; water in abundance, or, better still, small pieces of ice, and the acidulated drink should therefore be given. The old-time practice withheld water. The vomiting continued just the same without it or with it. It is a most valuable flushing agent, to say nothing of the relief afforded to the fever-stricken patient.

The above meets the general indications, as yellow fever is a self-limited disease; there is no specific remedy. The treatment of yellow fever as laid down in many text-books is vague, and a general confession that we are as much in the dark to-day as the early Spaniards were. Not that the books are lacking in advising remedies and suggestions, but there are so many of them that wholly fail to convince, and when faithfully tried prove absolutely valueless. In my early-day experience I tried a multitude of remedies. They were useless in a specific malady of this class, one in which the blood is attacked and frequently destroyed; at least such is my view.

The symptoms have to be dealt with one by one. In my experience a temperature of 105° F. and upwards in many cases means delirium, sometimes violent delirium. In 1880 I commenced using ice-cold applications in cases of high temperature. Well do I recall the first case when I put this idea of mine in practice. I was in Colon, in consultation there to meet Dr. Charles Williamson, at that time surgeon to the Panama Railroad. The patient was a healthy young man, who had been in that city for years. The case was a desperate one. Temperature, 105.5°. I obtained Dr. Williamson's permission to use the cold cloths. The young man's most intimate friend deemed it a very severe measure; but as the patient's life was in the balance, and the disease was epidemic in Colon, he assented. A tub was brought into the room and filled with large pieces of ice.

Towels were placed on them; as soon as they became wet through and cold they were placed on the patient's body—the arms, legs, and trunk—and were renewed as soon as they became warm. They abstracted heat rapidly; when the temperature fell to 104°–104.5° delirium and restlessness would cease. That was my first case with ice-cold cloths. Black vomit had appeared, and while that generally is a precursor of death, this patient recovered. Later, the patient's friend said that he deemed my treatment at the time an awful expedient, but that it had been successful. This treatment, I believe, was peculiar to myself. In another case, that of a port surgeon to the Pacific Mail Steamship Company, the ice-cloths were used whenever his temperature rose above 105° F., and he became delirious. Instantly they reduced the temperature to 104.5°, when all evidences of delirium ceased. Later, however, the fever increased and ran up to 107°, when the patient died.

Patients of this class should be placed in a well-ventilated room. Good nurses must be selected, reliable ones that will faithfully carry out orders. It is needless to state that more than half the battle depends upon faithful deputies.

Regarding diet, the patients do not want or ask for any form of nourishment. The idea of it seems revolting. If a little broth, free of fat, or milk and vichy is retained, it may be tried. In my experience the stomach fails either to retain or to assimilate any food product, while its presence simply distresses the patient and aggravates the general condition. While spirits and champagne have been advised, I fail to recognize their utility. Common sense and good judgment will best indicate what is needed.

Among many cases one may meet occasionally with one of the severe type, which, after the first fever the period of calm and the secondary fever, enters upon a typhoid condition. Such cases are rare. I recall one in an American physician, who barely escaped. They are obstinate and difficult cases to treat. Convalescence in them is very long and very trying, both to patient and physician.

I have referred to blood changes in this disease. I am of opinion, and have been since my residence at Panama, that the germs and their products expend their poisons in the blood. Gererd proved that the red corpuscles were almost wholly destroyed in fatal cases. In 1888, in a paper read before the State Medical Association of Arkansas, I then (and previously) took the ground that there was a true necræmia or death of the blood. If this view is proven, much of the clinical picture instantly becomes clear, for when the red corpuscles are destroyed necessarily their oxygen-carrying function ceases. Hence the multiple symptoms and delirium, as well as the marked dyspnœa, dwelt upon by French writers on this disease. Gererd pronounced it a veritable disintegration of the blood which became a mere mass of fluid and the débris of red corpuscles.

CONVALESCENCE.

It is needless to state that the management of convalescence requires special care and constant vigilance. While the fever is highest and death is expected the strain on the attending physician is necessarily great and constant. During the convalescence of such cases it is scarcely less so.

Wasting does not obtain during the very few days that the fever is at its zenith. The time is all too short to note any appreciable difference, but with the cessation of the fever proper then indeed the wasting begins and proceeds rapidly. Within a week or ten days after the crisis it is most marked.

As one would infer when the virulence of the poison has been so active in destroying the red corpuscles and tissues, the weakness is, as stated, of a very profound type. As soon as such a patient rallies a little, a ravenous appetite develops. That is a source of great peril, and if the patient or his nurse ignores the advice of the attending physician death may result.

I distinctly recall my own intense longing and desire for food. I lay in a state of constant hunger, thinking of all the things that I wanted as food. Many of them were simply unthinkable as connected with convalescence in this disease. I had an intense longing for meat, pork, or sausage. I mention this as indicating what obtains in a medical man who knew better, but whose body, wasted with disease, incessantly craved food.

The diet must be of the simplest. Beef or chicken broth free from fat; a little jelly or custard, a little vichy or seltzer and milk. Even their administration must be watched. The intense irritability of the stomach must be remembered. Plain water, seltzer, or vichy to allay thirst, as soon as it can be tolerated, may be given freely with marked advantage. It assists in many ways in the process of rebuilding and elimination.

When admissible, the juice of ripe oranges is very grateful. These juices have an excellent effect upon the torpid liver. A few drops of wine and seltzer occasionally will be a grateful change. There must not be any crowding of food. Later, a half of a soft-boiled egg and a little toast may be given.

In due time a mild tonic of iron and strychnine has a marked value.

A case at Panama will emphasize the imperative necessity for
constant caution and constant care. A man on the tenth day of convalescence made a meal of beefsteak. Signs of shock followed and
he died within twenty-four hours. Another case may be mentioned
as indicating the weakness of the heart. A man during convalescence
wished to shave. In spite of a protest a barber was sent for, the man
got out of his bed and sat in a chair. While the barber was shaving
him he died. Cases of this kind sufficiently emphasize what precedes
as to the necessity of constant surveillance.

Sponging of the body with vinegar and water, or cologne and
water, twice a day proves very refreshing. My preference is for the
vinegar and water. The bedding and everything in the patient's
room must be kept fresh and clean. The room must be well ventilated
and pleasant with sunshine, if possible.

Another point, and a very important one, is that all mental excitement must be avoided. No visitors can be admitted and there
must be no excitement of any kind.

For weeks and weeks the patient's stomach will be in a very sensitive state. In convalescence after severe cases I personally do not
think that any meat should be allowed for at least three weeks after
the crisis has been turned. When allowed, it must be carefully
minced and given in small quantity. While this advice applies to
severe cases, it has almost double emphasis in the few cases in which
during convalescence a typhoid tendency is noted. These are cases
in which the disease expends its poison in the usual way, but in which
the debility lasts weeks and weeks, in which the patient is as weak as
an infant.

As soon as the patient is strong enough a bath of tepid water
with a little carbolic acid may be given. At the second bath the
nurse may wash the patient's head and body very carefully with
soap. Four or five baths of this nature may be given on as many
days, their frequency depending upon the patient's condition. A
day or two later the patient may be taken into a nearby room, well
away from any draught, when his room, his clothing, and the effects
that have been in his bedroom can be thoroughly disinfected. As
far as the mattress is concerned, that should be sprinkled with spirits
of turpentine or coal tar and then taken into the open and burned.

The sending of patients to a northern climate to complete convalescence is an excellent measure. Away from the hot and enervating tropics, they pull themselves together much more rapidly.
When fully restored, they can return forever immune.

Frequent reference has been made as to what some of the text-
books say about yellow fever. I recall having read a statement more

than twenty-five years ago, to the effect that a man who had had yellow fever and survived it was damaged for life. I wish to state that there is not a scintilla of truth in this rash statement, not one. Such patients, if previously in good health, duly get back to their former standard. I have had them under observation for months and years afterward, and fail to recall a single instance of any complication or sequel.

Quarantine.

The State of Louisiana is the natural guardian of the mouths of the Mississippi River, which is a great artery extending inland through a vast extent of Southern and Southwestern territory, in the most fertile section of the United States.

For many years previous to Dr. Holt's time, the Mississippi River in summer had been closed. The large and valuable trade between the east coast of Mexico and Central America, the north coast of South America, and the West Indies was diverted and lost to the city of New Orleans. With the advent of the Holt system of maritime sanitation, however, the old conditions passed away, and the city became, as it were, a sentinel on outpost duty.

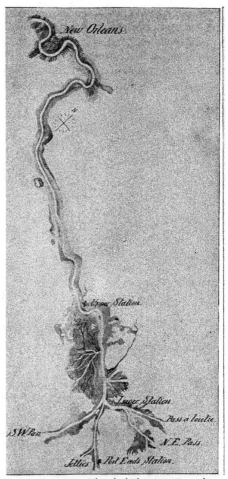

Fig. 56.—Chart of the Mississippi River from New Orleans to the Gulf, showing Location of the Quarantine Stations. Distances: New Orleans to upper station, 70 miles; to lower station, 108 miles; to Port Eads, 110 miles

THE HOLT SYSTEM OF MARITIME SANITATION.

The following is a description of the quarantine station at New Orleans as I saw it in the fall of 1886, while it was still under the personal charge of Dr. Joseph Holt, its originator. The station was located some miles below the city.

In buildings specially erected on the river's edge were the appliances used. First, a building with a large inside wooden chamber.

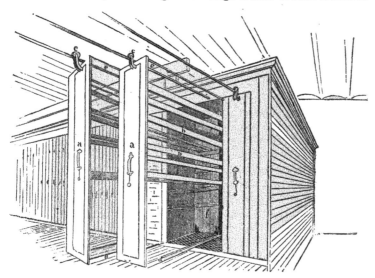

FIG. 57.—Superheating Chamber; Two Panels Drawn Open. *a*, Panels. (Two lower rack bars not shown) *b*, Rack bars; *c*, rollers; *d*, iron bars connecting front and rear panels; *e*, rods upon which panels are suspended and travel ; *f*, rear panel. Galvanized iron half-inch mesh screen in bottom of chamber.

In an adjoining building was the boiler, generating the steam used in the process of disinfection. In front of the building was a pier, at one end of which was a wooden frame supporting a large tank; the latter held the mercuric-chloride solution. A steam tug used for disinfecting at either the lower or upper station was at the pier.

The station practically had three sets or crews of trained men: the men employed at the station proper, the men employed solely on board the tug, and a crew who did work aboard incoming vessels.

The disinfecting-chamber claimed close attention. The chamber then was of wood, as stated, lined by various non-conducting media— five or six layers or coatings. When the chamber was closed, it was an air-tight compartment. Along its floor, under the panels or sections, were the steam pipes connecting with the adjoining boiler house.

Viewed externally it looked like a huge box made up of panels, each with an iron handle without. The panels or upright sections consisted of frames which could be pulled out into the chamber (see Fig. 57). On these frames the passengers' effects were hung. When all were ready or laden, they were pushed home. Then the live moist steam from the boiler played its rôle in destroying germs.

The steam tug had a furnace for generating sulphuric dioxide gas on the main deck aft. The furnace generated the gas, which a

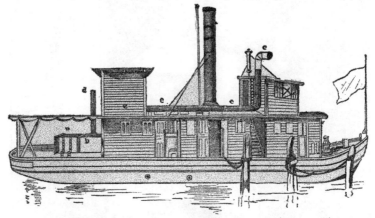

Fig 58 —Tugboat with Fumigating-Apparatus. *a*, Furnace; *b*, reservoir for reception of gas; *c*, discharge pipe, conveying gas to ship's hold ; *d*, escape pipe for gas when fan is at rest and sulphur is burning, closed by a valve when fan is in motion; *e*, house protecting from weather the machinery for driving fan and containing accelerating gearing

steam fan forced into the metallic and asbestos piping, the latter fitting into special openings in one corner of the vessel's hatch-way.

One year later, upon my return from a trip to Cuba, I was a passenger by way of the Mississippi River. A brief *résumé* of our experiences at the quarantine station is as follows: Our loose effects, clothing, etc., were removed from the staterooms by the ship stewards and taken on shore. There the clothing, the contents of handbags, rugs, etc., were hung on the frames making the inner end of the panels or sections; when all was ready, they were pushed into the chamber, all apertures were closed, and the live steam was turned on. The temperature within varied from 190° up to 240° and 300°.

After a time all of the sections were drawn out; in a very few minutes the atmosphere took up the heat and moisture, and the effects were then as dry as when introduced.

While the disinfection of the personal effects of the passengers was being affected, the crew of the tug, aided by the other crew, had been at work disinfecting the steamship.

When all was completed, the ship was given *pratique*, and we proceeded to the city of New Orleans—a clean vessel.

During one of my visits to the station I witnessed the disinfecting of a large British steamship. She was inward bound with a full

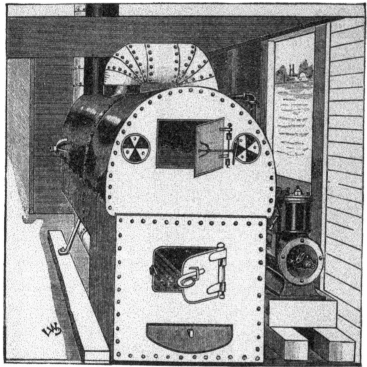

Fig. 59.—Front view of Improved Furnace for the Production of Sulphur Dioxide Gas, showing Sulphur Furnace with Fire Box Underneath, and Curved Pipe Carrying the Gas into reservoir.

cargo of coffee. Her captain, knowing that he was chartered for New Orleans, had prepared his ship by having square wooden boxes placed in one corner of the ship's hatchways. They extended from the combing of the upper hatches to the bottom of her lower holds. The asbestos piping already referred to is fitted into the openings in the wooden boxes. The connections were made and the sulphuric dioxide gas was forced into the after-hold and then forward. The treatment of the vessels naturally depends upon their size or internal

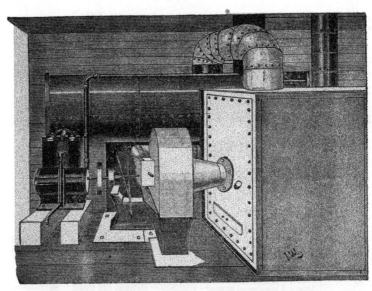

Fɪɢ. 60.—Side view of Improved Furnace for the Production of Sulphur Dioxide Gas, showing Sulphur Furnace, Reservoir, and Exhaust Fan. Curved pipe carrying sulphur gas into reservoir continues on the inside to within six inches of bottom. Section of pipe connecting fan with reservoir curves upward inside of reservoir to within six inches of top.

cubic capacity. The furnace of the tug can generate all of two hundred thousand cubic feet of gas an hour. It is forced in by steam power, and everything alive between decks is killed—tropical cock-

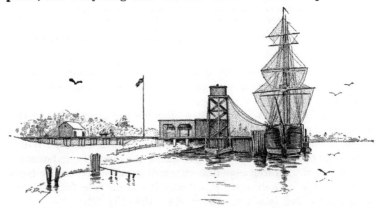

Fɪɢ. 61.—View of Disinfecting Wharf, showing Tug Fumigating vessel ; elevated tank containing eight thousand gallons of bichloride-of-mercury solution, three leads of hose from tank to ship. Gangway leading to building containing superheating chamber.

roaches, rats, and occasionally a stray ship's cat fall victims. The length of the exposure to gas depends upon a vessel's stowage of cargo. The average time for such a ship from a yellow-fever port, arriving during the hot season, is three or four hours. Fig. 61 shows a ship at the pier with the disinfecting-tug alongside. The pipe conducting the gas is seen over the ship's rail port quarter.

In 1889, I again visited the upper quarantine station. It occupied a new site, somewhat above the early one. There were a large

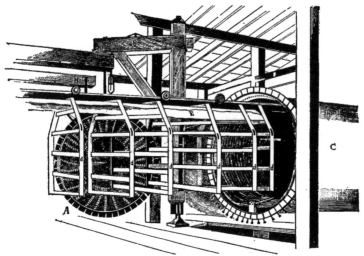

FIG. 62.—End view of Open Heating-Chambers, with Racks Drawn Out. A, Spherical head and heating-cylinder swung back; B, turning-crane from which cylinder head is suspended; C, heating-cylinder; D, travelling racks on which the material to be disinfected is hung; E, canvas over racks to prevent water dripping on racks; H, beams in shed from which tracks are suspended.

brick warehouse, a new dock and buildings, a comfortable residence for the quarantine officer, and suitable quarters for the crews of the station.

The early-day felt-lined modern chamber had given place to iron cylindrical chambers, jacketed with asbetos covering. The end or doors of the cylinder swung back on a crane-like attachment. Within were coils of steam-pipes accurately fitting the inner circumference of the cylinder. An iron cage-like structure replaced the earlier frame of the panels or sections. Practically it was an iron frame or carriage, suspended from overhead tracks. (See Fig. 62.)

THE GROSSE ISLE STATION, CANADA.

Grosse Isle affords an ideal situation for a quarantine establishment. It is in the mouth of the St. Lawrence, with miles of water on either side—hence, well away from any nearby inhabited spot. It lies about centrally in the river. All incoming ocean-going steamships and sailing-vessels have to pass it on their way to Quebec, and to Montreal, one hundred and eighty miles above Quebec. In short, Grosse Isle stands as a sanitary sentinel, on duty at the entrance to

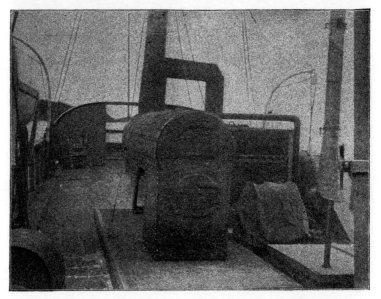

FIG. 63.—Furnace for Generating Sulphur Dioxide on the Grosse Isle Quarantine Boat

the great Canadian artery of commerce. It may be well to remember that the St. Lawrence has a length of two thousand two hundred miles. It is the natural outlet for the great lakes. Hence, this country has a deep and lasting interest in Canada's chief quarantine station.

The station has been there for many years. As far back as 1848 thousands of emigrants were landed there suffering from typhus or ship fever. The station is used in summer only, as the river is closed by ice in winter. There are forty buildings on the island.

The vast system, if necessary, can, upon an emergency, care for an army of newcomers. Over three thousand can be accommodated. The workings can be extended indefinitely by the use of military tents.

The whole system is under the immediate control of Dr. Monti-zambert, who has a staff of highly educated men under him.

As a maritime sanitary station its work is afloat and ashore. The service afloat consists of strong steam tugs, as well as a large iron steam vessel used for transporting supplies and for disinfecting vessels. During the season the tugs are kept under steam and are ready by day or by night to take some of the medical staff off to incoming vessels. The disinfecting-vessel (see Fig. 63) generates the sulphur-

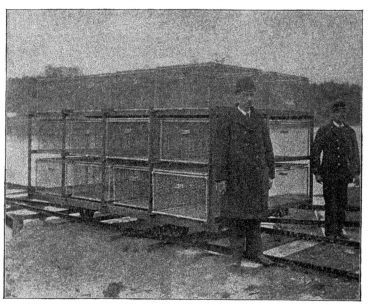

Fig. 64.—Disinfecting-Cages at the Grosse Isle Quarantine Station.

ous-acid gas which is conducted by metal and asbestos piping to the hold of the ship.

The land service. Let us treat a ship and her passengers and crew. A ship on which there may have been a case or several cases of contagious disease arrives at the station. Tugs convey passengers and their luggage, the crew and their effects, to the sea end of the long pier already referred to. There they land, the shore staff of the station awaits them. Steam is up, the disinfecting-room is quite ready. The contents of the trunks and sea-chests are emptied into wire-containers—large box-like affairs (see Fig. 64). They are duly tagged with metal numbers. The wire-containers are placed on metal railway carriages—each carriage can carry three tiers of them. The huge doors (see Fig. 65) of the several disinfecting-chambers are opened, then closed and screwed together. That done, the contents are exposed to dry steam heat, later to live steam, again to dry steam, and when they reach the open air the clothing dries instantly. The trunks, etc., are treated by another process. The temperature of the steam chests is raised to 230° to 240°, or higher, if necessary.

The goods to be disinfected are thrust in on one side of the steam chests and are taken out on the other, when the cars are run into the

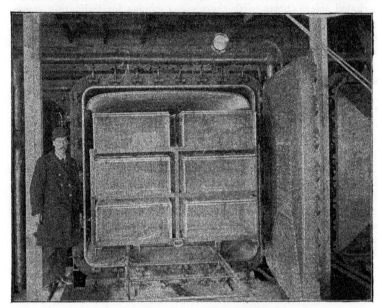

FIG. 65.—Disinfecting-Chamber at the Grosse Isle Quarantine Station.

open air on the pier. There the goods and clothing are delivered to their respective owners. The checking-system prevents any confusion or bother, each individual receiving his own property.

While the effects of the passengers are being disinfected they themselves are conducted to bathrooms in the upper part of the disinfecting-building, each having his room; there they undress and hand all of their underwear and clothing to an attendant. While they are having a thorough bath their clothing passes through the steam chests. After the bath they cross to the opposite side of the building, where they receive their clothing, dress, and are then conducted to the pier.

When the passengers are ready, they enter the detention sheds and remain under observation until such time as may be deemed safe, the interval, of course, depending upon the nature of the disease to which they have been exposed, its period of incubation, etc.

While what we have just described has been going on, the suspected ship has been disinfected and held, if necessary. Ships, crews, and passengers are in the hands of the medical superintendent and his staff until released by him.

The disinfecting-building requires notice. The large asbestos-jacketed steam chests, with their many gauges for indicating steam pressure, etc., are very massive. Work on an extensive scale can be conducted. Two or three vessels can be treated in a single day if necessary.

The detention sheds are comfortably fitted up with good iron bedsteads, wire mattresses, etc.

The long axis of the island is parallel with the long axis of the river. For purposes of administration the island is divided into departments. The health division occupies the upper end, or that nearest Quebec. The sick division contains the hospital. The suspects are in one place and the sick in the other.

.. The suspects are inspected daily. Any passenger who becomes ill is instantly separated from the others in the cabin passengers' building or the steerage sheds, as the case may be. The ill are removed before any disease can reach an infectious stage. Constant supervision under practically military discipline insures safety. The old French proverb, " *La méfiance est la mère de la sûreté*"—suspicion is the mother of safety—has not been forgotten.

POISONING WITH SNAKE-VENOM.

BY

THOMAS R. BROWN,

BALTIMORE, MD.

POISONING WITH SNAKE-VENOM.

WHILE the subject of snake poisoning is one which does not appeal to the great majority of practising physicians, nevertheless a knowledge of the subject is of extreme importance—not only because of the fact that in practically every portion of the tropical and temperate regions of the earth poisonous snakes are found, and therefore every physician should have the requisite knowledge for dealing rapidly and effectively with any case of snake-bite that may fall to his care, but also because of the extremely important rôle that snake-venom and the poisoning by serpents has played in the development of that most interesting and absorbing of modern therapeutic measures, serum-therapy and the establishment of artificial immunity. In fact, within the past few years the journals of experimental medicine, especially those devoted to the subject of natural and acquired immunity, have been crowded with articles on the action of snake-venom upon animals, the preparation of antivenomous sera, and the exact relationship which exists between toxin and antitoxin, while in the more practical journals we find an ever-increasing number of reports of cases in which poisoning by snakes has been successfully treated by means of antivenene.

Also, when one considers that in India alone over twenty thousand lives are sacrificed annually to the poisonous Ophidia, it can at once be seen that the subject is one of sufficient magnitude to appeal to every one interested in the general subject of medicine in its broader sense.

The Poison Apparatus of the Snake, and the Mode of Injecting its Venom.

The great family of snakes, the order Ophidia, has three divisions —the Ophidia colubriformia, which are innocent, the Ophidia colubriformia venenosa, and the Ophidia viperiformia, the last two of which are poisonous and compose the Thanatophidia, a well-merited name when their extreme destructiveness is considered.

Snakes are provided with sharp, recurved teeth, firmly fixed in the maxillary, palatine, and pterygoid bones, but the arrangement of the teeth is different in the different orders, thus furnishing us an easy method of differentiation of the poisonous from the innocent snakes. The harmless snake has two complete rows of small, ungrooved teeth—an outer, maxillary, and an inner, palatine; there are usually twenty to twenty-five teeth in the outer row. In the venomous snakes, on the other hand, the outer row is represented by one or more large tubular fangs, firmly ankylosed to the maxillary bone, which is movable and by its movements causes the erection or reclination of the fangs, this being especially marked in the Viperidæ, where the maxillary bone is reduced to a mere wedge and where the fang is much more formidable than in the cobra or other colubrine snake.

The fangs when reclined are covered by a sheath of mucous membrane, in which lie also several loose reserve fangs in different stages of growth, one of these reserve fangs taking the place of the working fang if it should be lost by accident or shed, becoming fixed to the maxillary bone and being placed in communication with the duct of the poison-gland. The teeth, although described as perforated, are really not so, but, being folded on themselves, give either an open groove, as in Hydrophidæ, a complete canal, as in Cobra, or a more complete tube still, as in Viperidæ. The poison is secreted by a conglobate racemose gland, the analogue of the parotid salivary gland, situated in the temporal region posterior to the orbit; the gland opens by a duct into the capsule of mucous membrane enveloping the base of the fang, the venom thence flowing into the dental canal. At the orifice of the duct a sphincteral arrangement of muscle fibres has been described by Fayrer in the cobra and by Weir Mitchell in the rattlesnake. In the full-sized cobra the poison gland is about the size of an almond. In the injection of the poison, the temporal and masseter muscles, which close the jaw in the act of biting, at the same time compress the poison gland and force the poison through the duct, the whole movement being strikingly analogous to the mode of action of the ordinary hypodermic syringe. The extent and mechanism of the erection of the fangs differ somewhat in different species; in the viperine snakes the erection is brought about by a rotation of the maxillary bone caused by a pushing forward of the ecto-pterygoid bone.

Varieties of Poisonous Snakes and their Distribution.

Poisonous snakes are widely distributed over the temperate and tropical regions of the globe; in fact, with the exception of the Pacific Islands and New Zealand, almost every country in this territory has its representatives of either the colubrine or viperine family, or both. The number and virulence of the snakes, however, differ markedly in different countries; thus in India, Australia, Africa, South and Central America the venomous serpents are much more numerous and far more poisonous than in Europe and North America.

Of the poisonous snakes of North America, so carefully collected and described by Stejneger, the best known are: of the family Elapidæ or coral snakes, Elaps fulvius or harlequin snake, Elaps euryxanthus or Sonoran coral snake; of the family Crotalidæ or pit vipers, of the genus Agkistrodon or Ancistrodon (in which the tail ends in a point and does not possess a rattle), A. contortrix or copperhead, and A. piscivorus or water-moccasin or cotton-mouth; of the genus Sistrurus (in which the tail is provided with a rattle and the top of the head is covered with regular shields), S. catenatus or massasauga, S. catenatus consors or Gulf Coast massasauga, S. catenatus Edwardsii or Edwards' massasauga, S. miliarius or ground rattlesnake; of the genus Crotalus (in which the tail is provided with a rattle and the top of the head is covered with numerous scales), C. molossus or dog-faced rattlesnake, C. horridus or banded rattlesnake, C. adamanteus or diamond rattlesnake, C. atrox or Texas rattlesnake, C. atrox ruber or red diamond rattlesnake, C. confluentus or prairie rattlesnake, C. lucifer or Pacific rattlesnake, C. tigris or tiger rattlesnake, C. cerastes or horned rattlesnake, C. lepidus or green rattlesnake, C. Mitchellii or white rattlesnake, and C. Mitchellii pyrrhus or red rattlesnake.

In South America are found Elaps corallinus or coral snake, Elaps lemniscatus, Lachesis mutus and rhombata, or bushmaster; in Central America, Bothrops lanceolatus or lance snake; in the West Indies, Craspedo-cephalus; in Africa, Naja haje or asp, Naja hæmachates, Naja noir and Cerastes; and in Australia, Hoplocephalus curtus or tiger snake, Pseudechis or black snake, and Acanthophis or deaf-adder.

In Europe, the common adder (Pelias or Vipera berus) is found throughout practically the whole continent except the northernmost countries, while in Dalmatia, Hungary, and Greece we also have Vipera Redii, and in Southern Europe the sand-viper (Vipera ammodytes).

Perhaps the most attention has been paid to the Thanatophidia of India, due to their great abundance and extreme destructiveness and the fact that much of the best recent work has been done with the poison of these snakes, cobra poison being the most commonly employed venom in the experiments of Fraser, Calmette, and others. Our knowledge of Indian venomous snakes is also very great because of the monumental work of Sir Joseph Fayrer on the subject.

The venomous Indian colubrines are: of Elapidæ, Naja tripudians or cobra, Ophiophagus elaps or hamadryad, Bungarus ceruleus or krait and Bungarus fasciatus or sankni; of Xenurelaps, X. bungaroides, and the various species of Callophis; and Hydrophidæ, a very numerous and extremely poisonous family of sea-snakes, but, on account of their habitat, not very harmful. The Indian viperine snakes are represented by: Daboia Russellii or chain-viper and Echis carinata or kuppur or phoorsa snake. These are true vipers, while the Crotalidæ or pit-vipers are but feebly represented by Trimerisuri, Peltopelor, Halys and Hypnale, which are much less poisonous than their American congeners, Crotalus, Lachesis, and Craspedocephalus.

Snake-Venom.

Various methods are employed in procuring the venom for experimental purposes. Obviously, to kill the snake to extract the venom is an extremely wasteful procedure, and therefore various methods of obtaining the venom from the living snake have been devised. The method employed by Calmette and his students at the Pasteur Institute at Lille is as follows: the snake is grasped with catch forceps, about three feet long, and next caught between the thumb and index finger of the left hand; the jaws are then forced apart and the fangs cleared of their sheath of mucous membrane by the thumb and forefinger of the hand grasping the snake, after which the poison is collected in a watch glass which is held beneath the poison fang, pressure being exerted during the time upon the poison gland; after the venom has been collected, a funnel is placed in the snake's mouth and a raw egg introduced, by which means the snakes are kept alive and well. The average yield of venom by this method is from two to three cubic centimetres.

Other investigators have somewhat different methods of collecting the venom, some getting the snake to strike against a stick covered with rubber, others using a wineglass or similar vessel covered with animal membrane or filter paper, the object of these procedures being to prevent the snake from breaking its poison fang.

Venom is a clear limpid or viscous fluid, from pale straw to yellow in color, of an acid reaction and of a specific gravity of from 1.050 to 1.065; most venoms are tasteless, but cobra-venom is said to have quite a bitter taste. Venoms dry rapidly at a temperature of 20° C. in the desiccator, and the dried residue resembles dried egg-albumen, cracking in such a manner as to suggest that it might possess a crystalline structure.

Venoms usually contain from twenty-five to fifty per cent. of solids, but, as Martin has shown, this may be as little as twelve or as much as sixty-seven per cent. in certain cases. This dried venom, if protected from moisture, apparently keeps indefinitely, Mitchell having preserved some for twenty-two years without any deterioration of its qualities. It also seems to keep indefinitely in glycerin or alcohol, but the watery solutions rapidly undergo putrefaction and diminution of toxicity.

Microscopically a few epithelial cells and occasionally micro-organisms are to be found, but the presence of the latter is probably due to contamination from the mouth, and the attempt to grow cobra-venom in gelatin has been utterly unsuccessful.

As to the effect of heat upon snake-venom, this will be gone into at greater length under the "Chemistry of Venom." Suffice it to say here that although a gradual impairment of the venom's toxicity takes place with the increase of temperature, even boiling for a short time does not entirely destroy it. Mitchell has shown this for rattlesnake poison, except for the venom of Crotalus adamanteus (diamond rattlesnake), the toxicity of which is entirely destroyed by heating to 80° C., while Wall has demonstrated that cobra poison resists boiling even better; the latter investigator has shown that a dilute solution is more easily destroyed than a strong one, the former in the case of cobra poison being rendered inert by heating for thirty minutes at a temperature of 106° C.

CHEMISTRY OF VENOM.

Although the composition of venom has been the subject of much speculation and experiment for many centuries, the only work of real chemical value has been done during the past fifty years. In fact, all the investigation done previous to the middle of the nineteenth century necessarily concerned itself with the grosser characteristics of snake poison, as chemistry, and especially organic chemistry, had not arrived at such a state of development that it could hope to cope with such an intricate problem as the chemistry of the complex body —snake poison. Indeed, the only results of all the early so-called chemical work was in the exploiting of large numbers of much vaunted antidotes which "abode their destined hour and went their way," gaining a certain credence among a few, but rapidly sinking into forgetfulness. Fontana seems to have been the only one of the early savants who possessed anything like a true understanding of the subject, and many of his conjectures regarding the nature of venom, made in 1781, have been verified by recent work. The first real chemical analysis of snake poison seems to have been made by Prince Lucien Bonaparte in 1843, who, working with the venom of the European viper, came to the conclusion that it was albuminoid or proteid in nature; he called the supposed active principle echidnine or viperine.   Crotaline, echidnotoxin, and echidnose have been names given to the active principle by other investigators.

In 1860, Weir Mitchell commenced a series of experiments on rattlesnake poison, and his work, together with that of Reichert, has done much to clear up the question of the chemistry of venom, and to prove definitely that the toxic substances are proteid in nature. This is especially interesting because of the fact that many bacterial poisons are toxalbumins, and so snake poisoning and intoxications by various bacteria should bear certain resemblances to each other, a relationship which Mitchell noted in 1860, calling attention to "the singular likeness between the symptoms of rattlesnake poison and those of certain maladies, such as yellow fever," an analogy already noted by S. L. Mitchell, Magendie, and Gaspard, the last of whom also called attention to the resemblance between snake poisoning and poisoning by putrefying substances.

Before the definite establishment of the proteid nature of venom, however, many attempts were made to prove that the toxic principle was not proteid in nature.   Thus Blyth tried to demonstrate that a crystalline substance, cobric acid, was the toxic substance, but this claim was effectually disposed of by Wolfenden.   Other investigators, notably Gautier of Paris, have endeavored to show that a ptomaïn or alkaloid was the active principle, but the experiments of Gibbs, Wolfenden, Pedlar and Armstrong, who made careful chemical analyses of the venom by the most approved modern methods, show beyond any doubt that ptomaïns or leucomaïns play no rôle whatsoever in the poisoning, and that the toxic principle is undoubtedly a substance or substances bearing a close resemblance to the proteids.

Mitchell and Reichert, working on the venoms of the rattlesnake, cobra, copperhead, and water-moccasin, came to the conclusion that there were two or more proteid constituents in venom, and subsequent work seemed to show that there were at least three, two soluble in distilled water, one not; two coagulable at 100° C., one not.   Their method of separating these different constituents was as follows: water was added to the venom and the precipitate obtained was separated from the fluid by filtration.   From the fluid thus obtained a substance was extracted by boiling and dialysis, while a third proteid substance was obtainable from the residue.   A simple method of obtaining the second, dialyzable proteid is to boil the venom, which throws down or destroys all the proteids, and then to filter or dialyze.

The various reactions of this body, its positive reaction with the xanthoproteic, Adamkiewicz, and Millon reagents, the faint reddish tinge with copper sulphate and potassium hydrate, the fact that it formed a precipitate with solutions of mercuric chloride, absolute alcohol, and potassium ferrocyanide in the presence of dilute acetic acid, the absence of a precipitate with carbon dioxide gas, solutions of ferric chloride and copper sulphate, and glacial acetic acid, led Mitchell and Reichert to the conclusion that this constituent of venom belonged to the group of peptones, and to it they gave the name venom-peptone. It showed, however, certain anomalous reactions, such as the formation of a precipitate with dilute acetic acid which redissolved in excess, the formation of a precipitate with large quantities of sodium chloride which redissolved in an excess of glacial acetic acid, and its precipitation by caustic potash and solution in excess of nitric acid with the formation of a yellow color. The precipitate obtained by adding water to the original venom gave the following reactions: soluble in a small quantity of sodium chloride and reprecipitated when this reagent is added in excess; soluble in weak solutions of magnesium sulphate, but entirely reprecipitated if this salt is added to saturation, which precipitate is soluble in weak acids but precipitated by addition of strong nitric acid; and positive reactions with the xanthoproteic and Millon reagents. Because of these reactions the substance was believed to be a globulin, most closely related to paraglobulin, and to it Mitchell and Reichert gave the name venom-globulin. The third substance, which remained after the extraction of the peptone and the globulin, judging by its positive xanthoproteic and Millon reactions, its precipitation by weak acids and alkalies, its solubility in water, and its coagulability at 65.5° C., seemed to be an albumin, probably most closely related to serum albumin, and was called by them venom-albumin.

According to Mitchell and Reichert's experiments, the globulin seems to act more upon the circulation, respiration, and blood, tending to destroy the red blood corpuscles, prevent coagulation, produce ecchymosis, lower blood pressure, and paralyze respiration, while the peptone seems to' act more upon the tissues, tending to cause œdema, putrefaction, and sloughing.

Their venom-albumin they regarded as probably harmless. Wolfenden, from the above-mentioned anomalous reactions of the dialyzable proteid and its precipitation by acetic acid and potassium ferrocyanide, maintains that it cannot be a peptone, but must be an albumose or syntonin.

Martin and Smith, who investigated the poison of the Australian black snake, Pseudechis porphyriacns, separated successfully three proteids, "one an albumin, and the other two albumoses. The albumin is not virulent, but the two albumoses (corresponding to the proto- and hetero-albumoses of Kühne) are extremely poisonous. They each have the same physiological action, and this is the same as is produced by the venom itself."

Martin gives the following table to show the behavior of the venoms of the cobra, the Australian black snake, and the rattlesnake with the usual reagents:

Reagent.	Cobra Venom.	Pseudechis Venom.	Crotalus Venom.
Nitric acid............	Precipitate; solution on heating, reappearing on cooling.	Precipitate; solution on heating, reappearing on cooling.	Precipitate.
Picric acid............	Ditto................	Ditto................	
Millon's reagent	Usual proteid reaction..	Usual proteid reaction..	Usual proteid reaction.
Caustic potash, and trace of copper sulphate.	Pink biuret reaction	Pink biuret reaction.....	Pink reaction.
Saturation with chloride of sodium.	Precipitate.............	Precipitate	Precipitate.
Saturation with sulphate of magnesium.	Precipitate.............	Precipitate	Precipitate.
Saturation with sulphate of ammonium.	Precipitate; filtrate proteid free.	Precipitate; filtrate proteid free.	
Dropping fresh venom into excess of water.	Slight cloud	Cloud.................	Considerable cloud.
Dialysis	Small precipitate; filtrate contains proteid.	Precipitate; filtrate contains proteid.	Considerable precipitate; filtrate contains proteid.
Five-per-cent. solution of sulphide of copper	Precipitate.............	Precipitate	Precipitate.
Alcohol (absolute)....	Precipitate; solution in water.	Precipitate; solution in dilute saline solution.	Precipitate; solution in saline solution.
Ferrocyanide of potassium and acetic acid.	Precipitate	Precipitate	Precipitate.
Boiling solution	Precipitate; solution still contains toxic proteid in large amount.	Precipitate; solution still contains toxic proteid.	Precipitate; solution still contains toxic proteid in small amount.

According to Mitchell, the two chief constituents of venom are present in different proportions in the different varieties of venomous snakes, there being much less globulin, in fact but a minimal amount, in the cobra, while in the crotalid snakes it is present in large amounts; according to his researches, the amount of proteid coagulable by heat is 24.6 per cent. in Crotalus, 7.8 per cent. in Ancistrodon, and only 1.75 per cent. in Cobra; while in Daboia, Wolfenden found beside the globulin a certain amount (percentage not given) of albumose or syntonin, which he found dialyzed with greater difficulty than the corresponding constituent in the case of Crotalus.

According to Martin, " Cobra poison contains proto-albumose, and so does pseudechis poison. Crotalus venom would appear to contain a body which is more accurately placed among the deutero-albumoses."

Calmette regards the non-coagulable, dialyzable constituent of venom as its true toxic principle.

It will thus be seen that while most venoms contain (*a*) a proteid coagulable by heat, and (*b*) a proteid or proteids not thrown out of solution by this means, which are present in widely different proportionate amounts in different species of snakes, it is nevertheless extremely difficult to assign exact positions and names to these bodies, because of the somewhat arbitrary and artificial means of differentiation at present in vogue, and because of the fact that many of the constituents of various venoms give atypical reactions, rendering it impossible to assign them definitely to any special group, so that it is largely a matter of individual opinion whether, for example, the substance under discussion should be considered a globulin, a peptone, or an albumose. Thus the whole question of the exact position of the various constituents of venom in the proteid family must be left *in statu quo* until a more definite and scientific means of differentiation of the various members is possible. Until then the venoms will be regarded by some observers as made up of globulins and peptones, by others as composed of globulins and albumoses, and by still others as albumoses alone.

TOXICITY OF VARIOUS VENOMS, AND CAUSES OF VARIATIONS IN TOXICITY.

We shall discuss later on the question whether the fundamental toxic principle of all venoms is the same or not, but here we shall simply speak of the toxicity of various venoms, and the influence of various agents upon this toxicity.

It has long been known, for instance, that the bite of the snakes of the tropics is far more dangerous than that of the corresponding varieties in Europe; also of the same species of snake, as for example the cobra, the bite is more venomous the hotter its habitat.

There is also a marked difference according to the time of year, the bite being more dangerous in the warmer season; indeed, the toxicity of the venom in the same snake varies from day to day, being more on hotter days, less on cooler days; also the bites of hungry snakes are less severe than those of well-fed ones. The activity of the venom depends also upon the health of the snake at the time. The amount of venom expelled, besides depending somewhat upon the factors just mentioned, also depends upon the variety of the snake and its size. The usual yield from the Indian snakes (at the Pasteur Institute) is from 2 to 3 c.c., and a good-sized cobra will furnish from 30 to 45 mgm. of dried venom.

The poison acts most readily upon warm-blooded animals, especially if injected directly into the veins, when death is often practically instantaneous, but it is deadly to cold-blooded animals as well, and to the lowest forms of invertebrate life.

According to the great majority of observers, a venomous snake ·cannot poison itself or any of its species, and, in fact, only slightly any other species of poisonous snake, while innocent snakes it poisons quickly. Mitchell and Reichert regarded the order of toxicity of the snakes upon which they experimented as cobra, copperhead, water-moccasin, and rattlesnake. Fayrer, from his studies upon the Indian Thanatophidia, places the snakes according to destructiveness in the following order: cobra, krait, echis, daboia; this, however, does not mean the order of toxicity of the various venoms, as Ophiophagus elaps, Bungarus fasciatus, and the various members of Hydrophidæ are nearly if not quite as deadly, but much less destructive quantitatively, either on account of their being less frequent or on account of their habitat. A vigorous cobra can kill several dogs or from twelve to twenty fowls before its bite becomes impotent, and then the immunity is of short duration as the poison is quickly reformed.

Following the line of work instigated by Roux and Vaillard in the case of tetanotoxin, Calmette and Martin, working separately, have investigated the toxic value of some of the venoms, i.e., the number of grams of a susceptible animal (rabbit) killed by one gram of the venom introduced subcutaneously. Calmette's results are:

Cobra,	4,000,000
Hoplocephalus curtus,	3,500,000
Pseudechis,	800,000
Pelias berus,	250,000

while Martin placed the toxic power of the venoms of the Australian snakes somewhat higher, thus:

Hoplocephalus curtus,	4,000,000
Pseudechis,	2,000,000

Effect of Heat, Cold, and Various Reagents upon Venom.

To understand definitely the effect of temperature upon venoms, we must remember that in practically all venoms we have two and perhaps more proteid substances, and that the loss of toxicity which the venom undergoes by heating depends partly upon the relative amounts of those substances present. Besides its power in coagulating one or more constituents of the venom, thus rendering them inert, heat also impairs the toxicity of venom apart from the influence upon its solubility, or in fact upon any changes demonstrable by chemical tests. The temperature at which coagulation of a certain portion of the venom takes place differs in different snakes; thus, according to Martin, it is from 60° to 70° C. in Crotalus; from 70° to 80° C. in Cobra; from 70° to 80° C. in Daboia; and 85° C. in Pseudechis.

The diminution in toxicity brought about by this means depends upon the variety of snake, as we have seen before; thus in Crotalus there is 24.6 per cent. of coagulated proteid; in Ancistrodon 7.8 per cent., and in Cobra 1.75 per cent., demonstrating in the first place how much less cobra venom is affected by heat than crotalus venom, and in the second place suggesting that if there is any difference in the symptomatology of poisoning by the different venoms it may be due to the different proportion of these different toxic proteids, and thus by heating the various venoms to that temperature at which coagulation occurs, the symptoms may be made to harmonize more closely with each other.

As regards this last point, Martin and others have noted that if crotalus venom is heated to from 75° to 80° C. (or pseudechis venom to 85° C.), besides a marked diminution in its toxicity, it has entirely lost the power to produce the characteristic effects of viperine poisons (the "globulin" of Mitchell having been coagulated), and the symptoms which it calls forth are quite comparable to those of cobra poisoning, i.e., slight local reaction, and no hemorrhagic extravasation nor intravascular clotting. Besides this rendering inert of a certain portion of the venom by coagulation, there is a gradual impairment in toxicity brought about by subjecting the venom to high temperatures. Perfectly dry venoms stand a temperature of 100° C. without any diminution of their toxic power, but if the venom is in solution, a diminution of toxicity takes place, depending in the first place upon the length of time during which the heat is applied, and in the second place upon the dilution of the venom, the greater the dilution the greater its susceptibility to the influence of heat; viperine poisons are especially sensitive to heat when in solution. Heating solutions of most venoms to 102° C. for twenty minutes completely destroys their toxicity.

Thus it will be seen that the effects of heat upon the constituents of venom are very analogous to those upon the toxic albumoses of abrus and the proteids produced by the metabolic activities of Bacillus anthracis. Cold, on the other hand, seems to have practically no effect upon venom, freezing not affecting it in the least.

As to the effect of various reagents upon snake venom, this subject will naturally be taken up more in detail under the head of treatment. Obviously, those reagents which form insoluble compounds with proteids or destroy them altogether, will have the same effect upon snake venom. Thus the chlorides of gold and platinum, silver nitrate, nitric acid, permanganate of potassium, and the hypochlorites all render venom inert; as also do carbolic acid, if added to the solution of venom, and the caustic alkalies if allowed to stand in contact with venom for a prolonged time.

Mitchell found that permanganate of potassium, ferric chloride either in the form of the tincture or the liquor, tincture of iodine, bromine, and hydrobromic acid were especially effective in destroying the toxicity of the venom. He and Reichert proved in their long series of experiments upon snake venom that most of the reputed local antidotes of snake poison do not render the venoms inert, *i.e.*, are worthless as antidotes.

According to Calmette, gold chloride in solutions of 1:100 and a one-per-cent. solution of calcium hypochlorite, freshly prepared and containing eighty per cent. of available chlorine, are the most effective chemical reagents to render venom inert, this investigator regarding permanganate of potassium, although exerting the same power *in vitro*, as of no practical value, because of the rapidity with which this power is lost when the permanganate is brought in contact with the tissues. According to Andrews the precipitates formed with venom by ammonia, alcohol, chloroform, and mercuric chloride are all capable of being redissolved in an excess of the reagent or in water, and of being as toxic as the original venom itself. All the reagents which are of use locally in the treatment of snake-bite will be treated of at greater length under that heading.

Effect of Various Digestive Ferments upon Venom.

It has been shown by experiments that the venoms of most snakes are absolutely unaffected by gastric digestion, although rapidly destroyed by the pancreatic juice. Mitchell has thus shown that venom, especially the kind which contains a very large amount of dialyzable constituent, if introduced into the stomach during the intervals of digestion can produce death by absorption of the unchanged venom from the stomach, but that this does not occur when the venom is taken on a full stomach or after it has reached the duodenum. Recently Wehrmann has carried on an elaborate series of experiments upon the action of various ferments upon venom, the results of which, briefly stated, were as follows: The ferments having a very active digestive (and therefore destructive) effect upon venom were ptyalin, papaïn, and pancreatin; the feebly active were pepsin, présure, and amylose, while the inactive were emulsin, sucrase, leucocytic oxydase (oxidizing ferment prepared from leucocytes), and the oxydase of mushrooms.

Thus, according to Wehrmann, venom, if introduced by the mouth, is first partially destroyed by the ptyalin and the destruction is completed by the pancreatin, the pepsin playing but a slight rôle in this process. Of special interest is the energetic action of ptyalin upon venom, as venom in so many ways represents a true saliva. This destructive action by the digestive ferments of the body upon the toxins produced by glandular or bacterial activity has been already noted by Nencki, Sieber, and Schoumow-Simanowski in the case of the toxins of diphtheria and tetanus, while Ransom has given animals enormous doses by the mouth, as much as one hundred thousand times the fatal dose of tetanus poison, without doing them any harm.

RELATION OF VENOM TO VARIOUS OTHER PRODUCTS OF ALBUMIN HYDRATION.

Recently attention has been called to the striking resemblance existing between venom and the digestive ferments on the one hand, and the products of the vital activity of bacteria on the other. In all these processes, i.e., the formation of venom by the cells of the parotid gland, the transformation of the less readily absorbable proteid material into the more readily absorbable by the pepsin and trypsin of the gastric and pancreatic juices respectively, and the digestion of albuminous material by the bacilli of diphtheria, anthrax, and tuberculosis, the albumins are hydrated, forming albumoses, all more or less poisonous if given subcutaneously or intravenously, and other products, usually of somewhat simpler chemical composition, as leucin or tyrosin, or some organic acid. This relationship is made even more striking by the discovery of the fact that in the case of the diphtheria bacillus this transformation is brought about by a ferment, while Lacerda and Wehrmann, working separately, seem to have demonstrated a somewhat analogous property in the case of venom.

Lacerda in 1884 stated that venom emulsifies fats, coagulates milk, dissolves fibrin, and coagulates white of egg, but does not convert starch into sugar; but, as in his experiments no attempt was made to keep the venom sterile, Wehrmann repeated the experiments, taking the greatest precautions to prevent contamination. His conclusions were that venom does peptonize fibrin, but does not convert starch into sugar or invert sugar, thus confirming Lacerda's results.

C. J. Martin gives as his view of the above-mentioned relationship that "the cell (of the venom gland of the snake) by a vital process directly exercises hydrating influence on the albumin supplied to it by the blood, the results of which influence are the albumoses which we find in venom. The difference between this process and the digestion by pepsin or by anthrax bacilli is that in the case of the cells of the venom gland the hydration stops short at the albumose stage and is not continued so as to form peptone, as is the case with the others mentioned."

MODE OF ENTRANCE OF THE VENOM INTO THE BODY.

As will be seen later in discussing the symptomatology of snake-bite, the symptom complex presented to us depends largely upon the mode of entrance of the venom into the body. The usual method is by subcutaneous inoculation, the poison being absorbed from the subcutaneous tissues by the blood-vessels, while if the snake injects its charge of venom directly into a vein, the effects manifest themselves almost immediately. The rapidity of absorption from the serous cavities lies between the two more common methods just mentioned.

Cases have been described in which absorption has taken place from the conjunctiva, while the venom, especially if it contains a large amount of dialyzable proteid, as we have in cobra poison, can be absorbed from the stomach, especially if it is in a fasting condition. Of course, if there are wounds or abrasions of the mucous membrane of the digestive tract, absorption can take place rapidly from these.

The natives of India demonstrate the absorbability of snake poison by the rectal mucosa by the habit they have of inserting rags moistened with venom into the rectum of their enemy's cattle, death usually being promptly brought about by this means.

MODE OF ELIMINATION OF VENOM.

But little is definitely known regarding the mode of elimination of venom, although the subject is undoubtedly of great importance from the therapeutic standpoint. Experiments have shown that small quantities of the poison can be obtained from the liver and kidney, and Feoktistow has called attention to the gross anatomical lesions found in the kidneys of poisoned cats. The extent of these lesions, as we shall see later on, depends largely upon the snake from which the venom was obtained. Mueller in 1893 called attention to the urine as being in all probability one of the eliminating channels of venom, and Richards and Ragotzi have definitely proven this by animal experimentation.

Alt has shown that some, at least, of the venom is eliminated by the stomach, while Wooster has suggested that possibly through the sweat glands some poison may be gotten rid of. Others have thought that the salivary glands might play some part in this process. The facts above mentioned would suggest that, besides the usual treatment, it might be well to wash out the stomach and to administer diaphoretics, diuretics, and purgatives, so as to hasten elimination by all the probable channels.

Symptomatology.

Snake poisoning presents a widely diverse symptomatology, the symptoms in any special case depending in the first place on the variety of snake; in the second place on the quantity of venom injected; in the third place on the method of introduction of the poison, whether intravenous, subcutaneous, or by the mouth; and in the fourth place on the resisting-powers of the person or animal bitten.

In regard to the first point—the variety of snake—we must remember that the venoms of snakes differ markedly not only in their absolute toxicity, but also in the relative amount of the different toxic proteids present. Thus Cobra has a very small amount of non-dialyzable proteid (the globulin of Mitchell and Reichert), while Crotalus has a comparatively large amount of this constituent.

Mitchell and Reichert, using the venoms of the cobra, rattlesnake, copperhead, and water-moccasin, concluded that the symptoms produced by the two constituents of venom, their venom-peptone and venom-globulin, differed markedly from each other. According to them "the globulins produce swelling and blackening of the parts by infiltration of coagulable blood, they are the more potent in producing ecchymosis, in destroying the coagulability of the blood, in modifying the red blood corpuscles, and in the production of molecular changes in the capillary walls; their action on the accelerator centres of the heart is more notable than that of the peptone, hence they are more active in causing the increased pulse rate; they exert, too, a more marked action on the vasomotor centres in producing the primary fall of pressure, and are the greater depressants of the heart; they also act more powerfully on the respiratory centres to paralyze them.

"The *peptones* are more active in the production of œdema, in the breaking down of the tissue, in the production of putrefaction and sloughing; they have little power to produce ecchymosis, to prevent coagulation, or modify the blood corpuscles; they have less tendency to accelerate the pulse; they tend to increase the blood pressure by irritating the capillaries, and are the principal factor in exciting the peripheries of the vagi nerves in the production of the increased respiration rate."

Thus, according to the greater or less proportion present of the first constituent, we have more or less marked local reaction, so marked in crotalus and so slight in cobra. Also snakes differ very markedly as to their absolute toxicity; this, speaking generally, being more marked the more torrid the snake's habitat, and differing also according to the weather, climate, and temperature, the general physical condition of the snake itself and whether it is fed or is fasting.

As to the second point, the amount of venom injected, this depends on the size of the snake, its general condition, and how long previously it has emptied its poison gland.

As to the method of injection of the poison, as we have seen before, the general symptoms appear most rapidly and severely in the case of intravenous injection, as when the fang directly penetrates into a vein, more slowly in the usual method of subcutaneous injection, while if by any chance the poison should have been injected into the mouth, the symptoms are usually wanting, although in a few cases death has taken place from absorption of the poison from the fasting stomach.

The local symptoms are usually more marked in the case of poisoning by the serpents of Europe and North America where the case usually ends favorably, or if the termination is fatal, it is delayed for some time, than in the case of bite by the Indian snakes where death is frequently almost instantaneous or takes place within a few hours. Thus, in the case of a bite by Elaps corallinus or Naja tripudians the symptoms start with unconsciousness and deep coma leading in a few hours to death, while in other cases, especially if the poison is injected directly into a vein, the patient becomes collapsed, vomits, and dies with or without convulsions, and with no local symptoms whatever.

The pain differs within very wide limits, sometimes occurring immediately after the bite, again not until the appearance of the local symptoms, in still other cases not until after the local symptoms are well developed, and sometimes not appearing at all.

Thus, in discussing the symptomatology of snake-bite, we must remember that we are dealing with local and general symptoms, the relative intensity of each of these depending upon the various factors we have already enumerated.

The local symptoms, speaking generally, consist of a rapidly appearing, inflammatory, local œdema of the affected spot, followed later by more or less ecchymosis and gangrene, with or without pain and often with the appearance of lymphangitis and local phlegmons. In the Crotalidæ, where the local lesion is especially severe, besides the œdema we have extensive gangrene of the affected portion of the body; according to Fayrer, Naja (a colubrine) kills without destroying the blood's coagulability while Daboia (a viperine) produces complete permanent fluidity.

The constitutional symptoms are to be ascribed to an intoxication of the cerebral and spinal centres, especially those of the medulla, inducing paralysis, especially of respiration, paræsthesias, and precordial pain. Besides these we often have a marked tendency to hemorrhages from the mucous membranes and organs of the body (hæmoptysis, hæmaturia, etc.), diarrhœa, vomiting, disturbances of vision and amaurosis, headache, dizziness, and violent dyspnœa, these symptoms differing according to the variety of snake; thus, for instance, the hemorrhagic tendency being especially marked in the Crotalidæ.

Perhaps it will be of interest to give here more in detail the symptoms of poisoning by the common varieties of snakes.

Cobra-bite.—After the bite, there is usually a burning pain at the seat of inoculation followed soon by local redness, tenderness, and swelling, the swelling extending thence towards the body if the bite is upon one of the extremities; congestion is marked and usually within half an hour the constitutional symptoms make their appearance, the patient becomes drowsy or faint, and extremely weak in the lower extremities, soon reaching such an extent that he is unable to stand. There is generally profuse salivation, and paralysis of the glossal and laryngeal muscles, rendering speech impossible, although the patient seems to be conscious, nausea and vomiting being also frequently present at this stage. The paralysis then becoming more general, the patient lies prone upon his back, unable to move, while the respirations become more shallow and slower, finally stopping altogether, the pulse becoming progressively feebler and the patient wearing an expression of extreme anxiety. Until respiration ceases, the pupil, although contracted, responds to light. After respiration ceases, convulsions frequently occur (due probably to the asphyxia), and shortly afterwards the heart stops beating.

Rattlesnake-bite.—Here the local symptoms are much more marked, the pain usually being severe and the discoloration about the wound being extremely marked, due to the extravasation of blood from the vessels. The constitutional symptoms, frequently occurring within fifteen minutes, are very striking; they are progressively increasing prostration, rapid feeble pulse, nausea and vomiting, and staggering gait; the pupil is dilated and there is frequently mental disturbance. If death does not occur in this stage the local symptoms play a more important rôle than in cobra poisoning, the tissues becoming swollen and discolored, the swelling and discoloration rapidly spreading, and symptoms of a general infection setting in, often associated with local gangrene. The patient may thus die a considerable length of time after the bite, due to these secondary complications. If recovery takes place, it is in almost every case extremely sudden, the change from an apparently moribund condition to one of apparently good health often taking but a few hours; in cobra poisoning also the return to health is very rapid, these rapid recoveries, which occur without treatment in many cases, undoubtedly being the cause of reputed wonderful cures after certain forms of medication.

In poisoning by the *Indian viperine* snake, the symptoms are much like those of rattlesnake-bite, there being, however, a much greater tendency towards hemorrhage from the various organs and mucous membranes of the body, which may continue for quite a while after the more marked symptoms of the intoxication have disappeared. In contrast to poisoning by the cobra, the pupil is widely dilated and unaffected by light, and albuminuria is an almost constant symptom, in cobra poisoning the urine practically never containing albumin.

In *bite by the European viper*, the symptoms resemble markedly those of rattlesnake poisoning but usually in a minor degree, the prostration is not so marked, recovery is more likely to occur and takes place usually within twenty-four hours, while the local symptoms are as a rule less extensive. We may, however, have secondary gangrene or suppuration which may terminate fatally.

In *bite by the Australian colubrine*, the symptoms resemble in some respects those of cobra poisoning; in others those of viperine poisoning; the pain and local swelling are, however, usually not severe, an irresistible desire to sleep being perhaps the most striking feature of the initial stage. The symptoms of prostration are extremely marked, the respiration is usually at first slightly accelerated, although it becomes slower and more shallow with the increase of the coma. Convulsions are not so common as in cobra poisoning, but extravasation of blood from the mucous surfaces and hæmaturia or albuminuria are more commonly found; the pupil is widely dilated and does not react to light. If recovery occurs, the secondary local symptoms are slight.

According to Martin, the convulsions seen so frequently in poisoning by the viperine snakes are probably due to intravascular clotting of the blood.

We thus see that there is quite a marked difference in symptomatology between the bites of the two great families of snakes, the viperines and the colubrines, especially as regards the local symptoms, the constitutional symptoms being more alike and the cause of death usually being paralysis of respiration. In the patients that recover, besides the secondary local manifestations we have already mentioned, other symptoms may persist for a long period of time, such as local paralyses in the most diverse parts of the body, paræsthesias of various kinds, pemphigoid eruptions and pain often appearing periodically at the seat of inoculation, secondary nephritis, lasting disturbances of vision, and dry gangrene of the limbs.

Morbid Anatomy.

As might be expected, the number of carefully made autopsies upon the victims of snake poisoning is extremely small, and most of our knowledge of the pathological effects of venom upon the organs and tissues of the body has been derived from animal experiments.

The pathological findings differ, of course, according to the nature of the snake and the rapidity with which death ensues; in cases in which death has taken place almost instantaneously very little is to be made out except the local lesion, with sometimes some slight injection, especially of some one of the mucous tracts.

In *cobra-bite* there is ordinarily rigor mortis, the blood is usually fluid, although clots are sometimes to be found in some of the veins, there is often congestion of the lungs and the bronchial mucosa shows marked injection, the veins of the pia mater are engorged with blood, while the only thing to be made out at the seat of the bite is some swelling and a slight effusion of blood-tinged serum into the tissues.

In the case of death from poisoning by the *viperine snakes*, the bitten spot and the tissues thereabout show marked œdema and extravasation of fluid blood and sometimes a disintegration of the muscular tissue nearby, while in many of the organs of the body, especially the kidneys, hemorrhages may be found. Hemorrhage from the mucous surfaces is also to be found, and the blood is fluid, while in the case of the *Australian snakes* the findings are in the main the same as in cobra-bite, although there is a somewhat greater tendency towards hemorrhages, especially of the lungs and mucous tracts.

PHYSIOLOGICAL AND PATHOLOGICAL EFFECTS OF SNAKE VENOM AS SHOWN BY EXPERIMENTS UPON ANIMALS.

Since the early work of Mitchell on the physiology of snake venom, this has proven a subject of much interest to many physiologists, and the valuable discoveries of Mitchell and Reichert, Feoktistow, Kaufmann, Brunton and Fayrer, Martin, Ewing, Ragotzi and Nowak have been the result of this interest. It will be impossible to give more than a brief *résumé* of the results obtained by these investigators, but, before doing so, it will be well again to call attention to the various symptoms of snake poisoning, and how different they may be according to the method of introduction of the poison into the system, and also to call attention to the great value' of these experiments in showing us the exact clinical symptoms of snake poisoning, so impossible to study carefully in the case of human beings owing to the necessity for active and immediate treatment.   Of course we are not justified in concluding that the results obtained upon the lower mammals will prove applicable to man in all respects, but the resemblance between the symptoms in either is probably very close.

Upon the *muscles and subcutaneous tissues* venom induces rapid necrotic changes, especially after viperine poisoning, causing "œdema, swelling attended with darkening of the parts by infiltration of coagulable blood, breaking down of the tissues, putrefaction, and sloughing" (Mitchell).

The *blood*, according to most observers, is rendered incoagulable, although Martin insists that if the poison of viperines and perhaps of cobra is rapidly introduced into the circulation, extensive intravascular clotting takes place.   The same also takes place if small quantities of venom are injected directly into a vein, this being followed in a few minutes by the directly opposite condition, *i.e.*, permanent fluidity.

The *red blood corpuscles* undergo great modifications, first losing their biconcave shape and becoming spherical, then becoming softened and fusing together, while later, as Martin has shown with *pseudechis* poison, the hæmoglobin is entirely dissolved and the cell disintegrates.

The addition of venom to a drop of blood shows that the *leucocytes* first lose their amœboid movements and later become destroyed, although more slowly than the red blood corpuscles, while examination of the blood of animals which have been poisoned with venom experimentally shows an initial marked decrease in the number of leucocytes, followed by a marked increase if the animal recovers (Martin) or succumbs (Halford); Calmette describes the leucocytosis as being *immediately* after the injection of the poison.

Upon the *blood-vessels* the poison has a most striking effect, a rapid dissolution of continuity taking place in the walls of the capillaries with an immediate escape of blood into the tissues.   According to Mitchell, hemorrhages of this nature into various organs of the body probably account for many of the abrupt and unexpected symptoms seen in snake poisoning.   This destructive action of venom upon the blood corpuscles and the vascular tissue seems to be in direct proportion to the amount of proteid, coagulable by heat and non-dialyzable, the venom globulin of Mitchell, that the venom contains; thus it is most marked in Viperidæ, less so in the Australian species of snakes, and very slightly marked in Cobra.

The *germicidal power of the serum* is completely destroyed by venom, as Ewing has shown in Crotalus and Martin in Pseudechis. This accounts for the rapid appearance of bacteria in the tissues of persons or animals dying from snake poisoning, giving rise to the idea a few years ago that there was a "spontaneous generation" of bacteria in this condition. It is because of this also that secondary infections are so likely to arise.

As to the action of venom upon the *nervous system* there is a marked difference of opinion. According to Mitchell, "the direct action of venom upon the nervous system, save as concerns the paralysis of the respiratory centres, is of but little importance," while Feoktistow believes that venom is pre-eminently a nerve poison, paralyzing both vasomotor and respiratory centres, a view with which Kaufmann agrees. According to Kaufmann, we first have a very brief stage of increased primary nervous excitation lasting but a short time, followed by a drowsiness lasting until death, the general sensibility and the ability to perform reflex or voluntary movements being affected much sooner than the intellectual faculties.

Wall believes that the chief effect of cobra poison is in extinguishing the various nerve centres and that the respiratory centre is peculiarly susceptible to this poison, while Brunton and Fayrer conclude from their experiments upon frogs and mammals that besides this paralysis of the reflex activity of the cord, the nerve endings in the muscle are affected by venom as by curare, and Ragotzi, who has confirmed these experiments, thinks that "failure of respiration is mainly brought about by this paralysis of the nerve endings in muscle, and that the direct action of cobra poison on the central nervous system is altogether subsidiary."

The *respirations* are at first increased and deepened, but soon afterwards they become decreased and shallower, the former condition being brought about by an irritation of the peripheries of the pneumogastric nerves, the latter by a depression of the respiratory centres; this latter condition is especially marked in cobra poisoning, as cobra venom seems to have a peculiar elective affinity for the respiratory centres.

The effect on *blood pressure* consists in an enormous lowering of arterial tension, due, according to Kaufmann, to a considerable vascular dilatation, especially in the abdominal viscera, while according to Mitchell the variations in arterial pressure are due to three causes:

depression of the vasomotor centres, depression of the heart, and irritation and consequent constriction of the capillaries.

The increased activity of the accelerator centres and the direct toxic action of the venom upon the heart are the two antagonistic factors in determining the *pulse rate*.

The *temperature* is generally slightly elevated if the absorption is slow, but is almost always lowered when the general state of profound depression has been reached. Feoktistow and others have shown by directly observing the heart in the open thorax, that a marked diminution in *cardiac activity* follows the injection of venom, this being very marked in the case of crotalus and other viperine poisons, and of the poisons of the Australian snakes, but much less so in the case of cobra venom.

The tendency towards hemorrhages into the various organs and cavities of the body and from the mucous membranes is most marked, as we should expect, in the case of viperines and least marked in Cobra. Thus hemorrhages into the *lungs, kidneys,* and *heart,* and bloody effusions into the *pleural* and *pericardial cavities* are most frequently seen in poisoning by Viperidæ, least in poisoning by Cobra, the symptoms in the case of poisoning by the Australian snakes lying between these.

Nowak has called attention to the resemblance between the pathological effects of snake venom and the lesions of yellow fever, laying especial stress upon the steatogenous and necrotic changes and leucocytic infiltration seen in the *liver*, leading in cases of slow poisoning to almost complete destruction of that organ, the acute parenchymatous or hemorrhagic changes in the *kidneys*, and the fatty changes sometimes seen in the *spleen*.

The poison in producing these manifold lesions in the body circulates unchanged and does not congregate in any great amount in any especial organ; it may be obtained in pure condition from any of the organs of the body.

We have seen that in the production of the effects upon the respiratory and circulatory apparatus, antagonistic factors are at work, easily understood when we remember that all venoms contain two or more chemically different proteid substances. Also to a great extent, many of the pathological changes depend directly upon the relative quantities of these proteid constituents in the venom under discussion. Calmette, however, as we shall see later, believes that the fundamental toxic principle of the venoms of all snakes (and also of scorpions) is the same, and that the difference in symptomatology and pathological changes depends upon certain albuminoid substances in the venom which have but little to do with the real cause of death.

Martin and others have recently studied the effects of venom upon cold-blooded vertebrates and invertebrates. These, as a rule, require relatively larger doses to produce death than birds or mammals. According to Martin "snakes, especially the venomous kinds, possess a considerable amount of immunity; but they succumb to large doses in the same manner as other reptilia," while Fayrer states that "a snake cannot poison itself or one of its own species and scarcely any of its congeners and only slightly any other genus of poisonous snakes, but it kills quickly innocent snakes," an opinion with which most observers agree. Venom produces cessation of the heart beats upon the fresh-water mussel and the crayfish, but apparently has a very slight effect upon infusoria or spermatozoa, or the cilia from the frog's mouth or oyster's gill. As we should expect, venom putrefies in the same way as do other proteid substances.

Diagnosis.

The diagnosis of snake-bite is usually easily made from the history that the patient gives and from the symptoms, but the wound should be carefully examined to make sure that the snake was a poisonous one. If the wound consists of one or two isolated punctures, it is almost certain that it was caused by a venomous snake, while the size of the punctures and the distance between them usually furnish us with some criterion as to the size of the snake and the probable amount of poison injected. If possible, the snake should also be obtained, as all the poisonous snakes of this country, with the exception of the harlequin snake, Elaps, can be easily recognized by the pit between the eye and the nostril.

Causes of Death in Snake Poisoning.

The causes of death in snake poisoning may be either primary or secondary. The primary causes of death may be (1) general paralysis, especially of the respiratory centres; (2) paralysis of the heart by tetanic arrest of cardiac action, probably due to the action of the venom upon the cardiac ganglia, this being undoubtedly one of the causes of instantaneous death when a large amount of venom is injected directly into a vein, although, according to Kaufmann, death which follows the direct introduction of the poison into the veins must be regarded as being due to "gastrointestinal apoplexy and the stupefying action exercised directly upon the nervous system"; (3) a combination of these causes; (4) hemorrhages in the medulla; and (5) possibly the inability of the red blood corpuscles to perform their function. It is certainly true that, in the great majority of cases, death is due to paralysis of respiration, as the respiratory centres are the most vulnerable portions of the system to the venom.

According to Ragotzi, however, this "failure of respiration is mainly brought about by the paralysis of the nerve endings in muscle and the direct action of cobra poison on the central nervous system is altogether subsidiary," while according to Feoktistow snake venom is a nerve poison *par excellence*, paralyzing the vasomotor as well as the respiratory centres.

The secondary causes of death may be (1) a secondary local or general infection, due in part to the direct effect of the poison upon the tissues and in part to the destruction by it of the bactericidal effects of the blood serum; (2) a marasmic condition brought about by persistent complications, such as hæmaturia, albuminuria, gangrene, etc., and (3) a hemorrhagic or a toxic nephritis, seen especially in the viperine snakes, the venom of which is extremely detrimental to the renal tissue, producing albuminuria and hæmaturia, while in cobra poisoning the secondary renal complications are extremely rare.

Rapidity of Death.—The rapidity with which death ensues differs within very wide limits, depending in the first place upon whether the cause of death is primary, when a lethal termination occurs comparatively early, or secondary, when the patient may live for days and even weeks before dying; in the second place, on the variety of the snake, the toxicity of its venom, and the quantity injected; in the third place, on the mode of inoculation, whether intravenous or subcutaneous; and, in the fourth, on the size and general physical condition of the victim.

If the quantity of venom is large, the snake very poisonous, and the poison injected directly into a vein, death is almost instantaneous, especially if the victim is in a weak physical condition or of small size.

In 65 cases of death caused by the Indian Thanatophidia, Fayrer found that in 7 death occurred in less than one hour, in 8 between one and two hours after the bite, in 9 between two and three hours, in 35 between three and twenty-four hours, while in the remaining 13 death occurred more than twenty-four hours after the inoculation.

Prognosis.

The prognosis in snake poisoning depends upon a great number of factors, the species of snake, the toxicity of its venom, the quantity of poison injected, the mode of inoculation, the site of the wound (in ninety-five per cent. of Fayrer's tabulated cases the bite was upon the extremities, and here the prognosis is more favorable than in the case of bites upon the face or breast, because in the former case absorption can be lessened by the application of a ligature), upon the treatment employed and the length of time before it is begun, and upon the physical condition and size of the patient. In those cases in which the poison is injected directly into the veins, the prognosis is much more grave than when the bite is subcutaneous, as in the former case local treatment is absolutely useless.

The mortality also differs according to the family to which the snake belongs, being worse in the case of bites of the Elapidæ and Hydrophidæ than in those of Crotalidæ, in which, in turn, the prognosis is worse than in the bites of the European vipers.

According to Fayrer, the result is invariably fatal if one of the Indian snakes, Cobra, Hamadryad, Bungaris, or Daboia has inoculated its full charge of venom into its victim. In America, according to Mitchell's series, the mortality varies usually between twelve and twenty-five per cent., while Ellzey gives fifteen per cent. as the usual proportion of deaths; in Europe Bollinger gives the mortality as about ten per cent., while in Australia it is given as about seven per cent.

In India, where the mortality according to Fayrer is from twenty-five to thirty-five per cent., in 1869 there were 11,416 deaths from snake-bite out of a population of 120,976,263, while in 1898 there were 21,901 deaths from this cause, i.e., about 1 in 12,000. Of course the mortality depends somewhat upon the treatment employed and especially upon the rapidity with which it is used, thus naturally, cœteris paribus the mortality will be less in countries where the average intelligence of the people is higher and treatment will be rapidly inaugurated, as in North America and Australia, than in India where the inhabitants are ignorant and superstitiously opposed to most forms of scientific medication. As to the comparative value of the different therapeutic measures, this will be taken up at length in the portion of the article devoted to treatment.

Prophylaxis.

The poisonous snakes in this country are undoubtedly rapidly decreasing in numbers, due in the main to the advances of civilization, but in some cases without apparent cause. In many cases this destruction has been brought about by hogs, who have an especial fondness for snakes and whose tough hide and thick layer of fat offer a great protection against snake-bite; in other cases by birds and harmless snakes. In the case of the latter, which in some cases seem to possess a certain immunity against snake venom, portions of partly digested poisonous snakes have been found in their stomachs; and in this country the king snake, Lampropeltis getulus, is reputed one of the greatest enemies of the rattlesnake.

Thus, while extermination of poisonous snakes is much to be desired, the indiscriminate destruction of snakes is to be greatly deplored, as the innocent snakes are inimical to the poisonous snakes in many cases, and also are of the greatest importance to the gardener and farmer; and in the killing of snakes a most careful discrimination should be employed.

In certain countries where poisonous snakes are very plentiful a bounty has been offered by the government for each poisonous snake killed, but so far this has seemed to have been of little use in decreasing the cobra of India and the fer-de-lance of Martinique, although Kaufmann thinks that it has done much good in exterminating the viper in certain districts of France. His figures, however, seem rather to prove the inefficiency of this method of prophylaxis due in part to the lack of discrimination between noxious and innocent snakes, and in part to the inevitable venality of those who pay the bounty.

Treatment.

The most interest regarding snake poison has from the beginning centred about the treatment of the condition; in fact, from time immemorial frequent attempts have been made to obtain some substance which would prove effective in this condition. To demonstrate the hopelessness of this search until within the past few years, one has but to glance over the myriad medicaments that have been recommended and used in this condition, drawn from the animal, vegetable, and mineral kingdoms, most of them based upon utterly unscientific and irrational grounds, and many coming directly from the realms of alchemy, witchcraft, and voodooism. And yet in no condition more than in this does the old adage, " bis dat qui cito dat," hold good, as the application of a rational line of treatment within a few moments of the bite is of more value than any drug in the pharmacopœia a few hours afterwards.

In the treatment of snake-bite we have three things to consider: first, to prevent, as far as possible, the absorption of the poison, which of course is to be brought about by local treatment; second, to counteract, and if possible neutralize, the constitutional symptoms; and third, to hasten the elimination of the poison. So many drugs and procedures have been recommended for both local and general treatment that in this article we will speak only of those which have been used to a greater extent than the others, and which have been accompanied by some measure of success in the hands of their adherents.

· LOCAL TREATMENT.

As the prime object is to prevent the absorption of the poison, by proper and prompt local treatment we may get cures in cases in which a few minutes' delay or the wasting of time in useless proceedings would inevitably result in death.

In the first place, a tight ligature should be applied above the bitten spot, if this is upon the extremities which we have seen it is in about ninety-five per cent. of all cases. As much of the poison as possible should then be removed by scarification of the wound, excision in some cases, amputation perhaps if the bite is on a finger or toe and the snake a very poisonous one, tight bandaging from above and below towards the wound, cauterization of the bitten area, and cupping or sucking the wound, although this last procedure is vigorously opposed by Fayrer and others. About and into the wound should then be injected some one of the substances which experiments have shown to be rapidly destructive to the venom, usually by oxidizing it into harmless or less harmful substances. The local reagents, the use of which has been attended with the most success in the hands of those who have used them, are nitric acid, permanganate of potassium, chloride of gold, hypochlorite of calcium, chlorine water, chromic acid, bichloride of mercury, ferric chloride, bromine, and iodine. Besides these local remedies, many others have been used, such as common salt, olive oil, the fat of some animal, sodium and potassium hydrate, sodium bisulphite, tartaric acid, carbolic acid, and ammonia. Fayrer has recommended the use of nitric acid or the cautery locally, while Mitchell and Reichert used ferric chloride, bromine or iodine or their acids. According to Kaufmann, chromic acid in solution of $1:100$ is the most effective local reagent, as, besides producing the greatest precipitate in the venom, it is also an extremely active oxidizing agent. According to Kaufmann's experiments, chromic acid is a potent reagent not only when it is injected with the venom, but also when introduced some time after the poisoning. One of his experiments is very interesting. Four dogs of equal size were inoculated in the thigh with the same amount (two drops) of fresh viper venom. One was left untreated and the others were given hypodermically at the seat of inoculation, and five minutes afterwards, one-per-cent. solutions of chromic acid, permanganate of potassium, and bichloride of mercury respectively, all showing local reddening. Within twenty-four hours the dog that had been untreated died; the other three recovered, but in the case of the dogs in which permanganate of potassium and bichloride of mercury had been used, large, slowly healing ulcers were left, while in the dog in which chromic acid had been injected there was no ulcer.

Permanganate of potassium has been recommended by Blyth, Brunton and Fayrer, Lacerda, Aron and Richards, Lacerda recommending a one-per-cent. solution of this reagent, while Aron thinks stronger solutions (from three to five per cent.) are preferable. Lacerda has saved life experimentally by injecting permanganate into the wound two minutes after the inoculation of a lethal dose of venom, while Richards has been successful four minutes afterwards. Calmette has recommended chloride of gold in one-per-cent. solution, and as it forms an insoluble precipitate *in vitro* with venom there seems to be no reason why it should not be efficacious, although Kanthack did not find it so. Calmette has also recommended freshly prepared solutions of calcium hypochlorite (1 : 60), and has been successful with this thirty minutes after the inoculation of the animal, while Lenz has used chlorine water with success in some cases.

In the southern portion of the United States of America a mixture of bromine, potassium iodide, and bichloride of mercury has been much used. Experiments seem to show that the tight ligature is of the greatest importance, as the absorption is much slower because of the induced anæmia.

The principle of the local treatment is to prevent as far as possible the absorption of the poison, to remove as much as possible by appropriate means, and to neutralize, as far as one is able, the remaining portion by the use of reagents that render the venom inert either by forming insoluble precipitates or by oxidizing it into harmless substances. As absorption even with ligation of the limb is comparatively rapid, it is absolutely essential that the local treatment, to furnish any hope of success, must be used within a few minutes, according to most observers, five to thirty minutes after the bite, as after all the poison has once reached the general circulation local treatment is obviously useless.

HASTENING THE ELIMINATION OF THE POISON.

As it has been definitely shown that the venom is eliminated by the kidneys and stomach, and probably also by the sweat glands and the salivary glands, it is of great importance to use procedures designed to bring about this elimination as rapidly as possible. For this purpose washing out the stomach, free purgation, the drinking of considerable quantities of fluids, and the administration of diuretics and diaphoretics have been used, and in certain cases seem undoubtedly to have proven of value.

GENERAL OR CONSTITUTIONAL TREATMENT.

As we have stated before, the only chance of success that local treatment offers is in its application within a very few minutes of the bite, and as this is obviously impossible in the great majority of cases, our one hope of bringing to a successful termination many cases which would otherwise prove fatal lies in the use of some general remedy given either by mouth, hypodermically, or intravenously, which will neutralize or destroy the venom or counteract its effects, as it is being diffused throughout the system. As, however, the venom itself is proteid in nature, it will obviously be impossible to get any diffusible chemical which will destroy the venom or render it inert, as this reagent must perforce act upon the organs and tissues of the body also, since they contain many proteid constituents. As Mitchell and Reichert said in 1886: "The fact that the active principles of venom are proteids and closely related chemically to elements normally existing in the blood, renders almost hopeless the search for a chemical antidote which can prove available after the poison has reached the general circulation, since it is obvious that we cannot expect to discover any substance which, when placed in the blood, will destroy the deadly principles of venom without inducing a similar destruction of vital components in the circulation. The outlook, then, for an antidote for venom which may be available after the absorption of the poison lies clearly in the direction of a physiological antagonist, or, in other words, of a substance which will oppose the actions of venom upon the most vulnerable parts of the system." The constitutional remedies that have been used in the treatment of snake-bite are legion, due partly, perhaps, to the remarkable and sudden improvement which takes place in some cases without any treatment whatsoever, and thus if *any* remedy should have been used in a case of this kind, to it would undoubtedly be ascribed the most marvellous curative powers. The substances most extensively used in the treatment of snake-bite are alcohol, ammonia by intravenous injection, and strychnine given hypodermically. Among the other remedies recommended and used for combating the constitutional effects of snake poisoning may be mentioned calomel and iodide of potassium, the water of Luce (a volatile alkaline water), strophanthus (advised by Bancroft), caffeine, atropine, jaborandi (recommended by Bosso); and from the vegetable kingdom, Phlomis, Uvularia grandiflora, Aristolochia serpentaria, Dorstenia brasiliensis, and many other plants. In choosing a constitutional remedy, the symptoms to be especially treated are the extreme depression of the functions of respiration and circulation; thus the three remedies most prized are naturally strongly stimulating in nature.

Alcohol has been the most used of all the remedies, partly because of the ease and quickness with which it may be obtained, and partly because of the apparent success of the remedy in certain cases. In fact there seems to be no doubt that in a few cases, when the amount of venom injected was but barely more than the minimal lethal dose, life has been saved by a proper administration of alcohol in some form. It must not be forgotten, however, that undoubtedly in many cases it has done harm, since if given in sufficient quantity to cause intoxication, the vital functions, instead of being stimulated, are depressed and the patient's chances of recovery are diminished rather than increased, as alcohol has no beneficent direct action whatsoever upon the venom.

Ammonia has been given by the mouth for many years in the treatment of snake-bite, but it is only a comparatively few years ago that its intravenous injection was recommended by Halford, although he did not in the least regard it as an antidote. The method employed was the injection of from ten to sixty drops of the "liquor ammoniæ fortior," somewhat diluted with water, into the median or jugular vein. The adherents of this method claimed that it was a true antidote, and it was extensively used in Australia from 1874 to 1876, but investigations and animal experiments carried on by an especially appointed Australian commission, by Richards, and by Brunton, seemed to show that this remedy exerted no beneficial effect whatever.

According to Calmette, the use of either alcohol or ammonia should be discouraged, as each only does harm.

Strychnine, recommended by Pringle in 1868, has come most prominently to the front within recent years as a remedy in snake poisoning, due in the main to the work of Mueller in 1889, who regarded it as a true antidote.

According to Mueller, "strychnine is the exact antithesis of snake poison in its action, snake poison turning off the motor batteries and reducing the volume and force of motor-nerve currents, strychnine, when following it as an antidote, turning them on again, acting with the unerring certainty of a chemical test, *if given in sufficient quantity.*"

Mueller has always insisted that the drug should be pushed until it showed distinct signs of its own physiological action, and has sometimes given as much as one to two grains hypodermically. Richards, however, found that strychnine seemed to have no effect in curing animals artificially inoculated with snake venom, while Kanthack concluded from his investigations that "Nothing is to be expected from this treatment, and no false hopes should be raised or fostered as to a cure by strychnine."

In 1892 Huxtable collected a series of cases of Australian snakebite, some untreated and others treated by the hypodermic injection of strychnine; in the former (313 in all) the mortality was 4.1 per cent., while in the latter (113 in all) the mortality was 13.2 per cent., i.e., the mortality was over three times as great in the cases treated by strychnine injections as in the untreated cases.

This does not mean, however, that strychnine is responsible for the increased mortality, as it was in the more severe cases alone that this remedy would be likely to be used, and too many favorable reports have been received to make it probable that no cases at all have been cured by this method. In fact, strychnine, although not an antidote, is a powerful stimulant and, like alcohol and ammonia, may possibly save life in those cases in which barely more than the minimal lethal dose of poison has been injected, besides being useful in milder cases in lessening the nervous and cardiac depression.

Artificial respiration has been tried on animals in cases of snake poisoning by Fayrer and Brunton, because of the resemblance of the symptoms to those of poisoning by curare, Weir Mitchell having previously suggested this procedure on purely theoretical grounds. These investigators were able to keep animals alive by this means as long as ten hours, and Richards for several days; but no definite cures have been obtained by this method, although a case has been reported from Ceylon in which the life of a man seemed to have been saved by this procedure, the patient dying, however, two days later of pneumonia.

Tracheotomy has been advised and occasionally used in those cases in which the œdema has spread to the glottis and there was danger of suffocation.

TREATMENT WITH ANTIVENOMOUS SERUM AND THE PRODUCTION OF ARTIFICIAL IMMUNITY.

Stimulated by the results obtained in diphtheria, tetanus, poisoning by ricin and abrin, and other forms of intoxication, numerous investigators have turned their attention during the past few years to the establishment of an immunity against snake poisoning and to the preparation of an antivenomous serum. To believe that this establishment of an artificial immunity against snake poisoning was possible, one had but to consider the number of undoubted cases among the natives of India and Africa which were based on too good evidence to leave any room for doubt.

Among the interesting facts in connection with this point, it may be of interest to note that many of the natives of Australia regularly take the poison by mouth; that in India the dried heads, poison , glands, and gall bladders of poisonous snakes are regularly taken as a preventive and cure of snake-bite, generally by the mouth, sometimes by tattooing; that some of the natives of Africa rub themselves with dried venom before going into the places where venomous snakes abound; and that in all these, too many cases have been reported of complete immunity against the bite of poisonous snakes to leave one at all doubtful that an effective method of preventing snake venom from being lethal is known and practised where poisonous snakes abound. In all these examples and in the case of the immunity of poisonous snakes, the production of the artificial immunity is probably due to the absorption from the alimentary canal or from the skin in the case of human beings, and from the alimentary canal or from the poison gland itself in the case of the poisonous snakes, of frequent, small doses of venom, non-lethal but protective.

Fraser in 1869 first showed that an artificial immunity against the minimal lethal dose of cobra venom could be produced by the administration of repeated small doses of cobra venom, but it was Sewall in 1887 who first called especial attention to this subject by proving that pigeons that had repeatedly received small doses of rattlesnake poison could withstand as much as seven times the minimal lethal dose of the poison, while Kaufmann and Phisalix and Bertrand demonstrated the same thing in the case of the European viper, and Kanthack in the case of the cobra. Following this work, which showed conclusively that vaccination against snake poisoning was possible, Calmette, pursuing the line of investigation inaugurated by Tizzoni, Roux, Behring, Kitasato, and others in the case of diphtheria and tetanus, endeavored to obtain from these vaccinated animals a serum possessed of protective and curative properties. In July, 1896, his results had been attended with such success that he presented them to the Royal College of Physicians and Surgeons in London. These experiments were designed to show both the preventive and the curative powers of his serum and were as follows:

1. The lethal dose of cobra venom being found to be 1 mgm. of dried substance (subcutaneously administered), which will kill a rabbit in twelve hours, or 2 mgm. which will kill in sixteen to seventeen minutes, 3 c.c. of the protective serum were injected, and six hours

later 2 mgm. of the dried venom; no symptoms occurred in these immunized rabbits, while control animals died in sixteen or seventeen minutes.

2. A second series was given 5 mgm. of the dried venom subcutaneously, and one hour later 3 c.c. of the antivenomous serum; all remained well.

3. In a third series, 3 c.c. of the antitoxin was injected one-half, one, and one and one-half hours after the injection of a fatal dose of the poison, and only in the last case (*i.e.*, when injected one and one-half hours afterwards) did the rabbits die.

All the animals that recovered in these experiments were perfectly well eight days later.

The first experiment was designed to show the preventive, the second and third to show the curative powers of the serum.

In concluding another article on the same subject, Calmette says: "Animals may be immunized against the venom of serpents either by means of repeated injections of doses at first feeble and becoming progressively stronger, or by means of successive injections of venom mixed with certain chemical substances, among which I may especially mention the chloride of gold and the hypochlorites of lime and soda; the serum of animals thus treated is at the same time preventive, antitoxic, and therapeutic, exactly as is that of animals immunized against diphtheria and tetanus."

Following this report of Calmette, the English commission that was appointed to consider these results advised that they should be put to a practical use, and since then antivenomous serum or antivenene has been used in Europe, Asia, and Africa. Calmette's method of producing his serum is as follows: a watery solution is first made from the dried venom of three different varieties of snakes, viperine and colubrine (Crotalus durissus, Bothrops lanceolatus, and Naja tripudians), so that 1 c.c. of the solution represents 1 mgm. of the dried venom. Healthy horses are then given subcutaneously either gradually increasing doses of this solution alone or gradually increasing doses of this solution mixed with gradually decreasing doses of some neutralizing agent, as calcium hypochlorite. The initial dose is usually 0.5 mgm. (one-half the minimal lethal dose of the horse) and the injection of gradually increasing doses takes place about every two or three weeks; at the end of one year the horse can resist a dose which would kill twenty-five horses not previously immunized, while at the end of two to three years this resisting-power would be again doubled; after reaching this point the immunity is kept up by venom injections every month or two. After about sixteen months the serum is of sufficient immunizing strength to be of practical value, and is withdrawn from the horse in the usual way and sterilized by heating for one hour on three successive days at a temperature of 60° C.

According to Calmette, this serum, if kept in air-tight vessels, can be preserved without impairment of its immunizing power in even the hottest countries, although Hankin and Martin have each found a considerable diminution in this power in serum kept in India and Australia respectively. No serum of less than 1,000 units (or 10,000 units in the vessels of 10 c.c. capacity in which it is preserved) is sent out, while to countries where very venomous snakes abound, serum of 2,000 or 4,000 units (or 20,000 or 40,000 units in 10 c.c. of the serum) is sent. Calmette determines the number of units in any especial serum by dividing the weight of the animal (rabbit) in grams by the quantity of serum in cubic centimetres necessary to be given intravenously five minutes before the injection, in order to protect it against a dose of venom which would otherwise kill the animal in from fifteen to twenty-five minutes, although Martin, Semple, and Lamb insist that the only way to eliminate errors is to give ten or a hundred times the minimal lethal dose and see how much serum it will take to prevent death. As to the amount to be given human beings, this obviously depends upon several factors, chief of which are the resistance of the subject and the quantity and toxicity of the venom. As to the former, it would seem that the larger the animal the greater the resistance, weight for weight. Thus Calmette has shown that it takes twice as much venom to kill 500 gm. of rabbit as to kill 500 gm. of guinea-pig, and the same general rule holds good regarding the dog, the monkey, and the ass. It is therefore fair to suppose that man's resistance is proportionately higher, and this is borne out by a study of the relative mortality of man and animals in cases of snake poisoning. As to the second point, the amount of venom injected, this of course is impossible to determine definitely, but as Fayrer has stated, the cobra never injects less than 0.019 gm., while the average amount is between 0.03 and 0.045 gm. As Fraser has determined that the minimal lethal dose for a man of 60 kgm. would be 0.0317 gm. of dried venom, and as Fayrer has shown that in India the mortality from snake-bite is between twenty-five and thirty-five per cent., and that death usually occurs in from six to twelve hours, it obviously follows that man's resistance to snake venom undoubtedly is greater than that of the lower animals, and that a dose of 10 or at most 20 c.c. of the stronger serum should be sufficient in most cases to prevent death by the most poisonous snake if given very shortly after the bite.

We must also not forget in the first place that the whole amount of poison injected does not have to be neutralized by the serum, but only the excess over the amount that the fluids and tissues of the body can deal with, usually regarded as about 0.03 gm. in a man of 60 kgm.; and in the second place that the usual amount injected by a serpent is probably but slightly more than the minimal lethal dose.

Although the results are based upon experiments *in vitro* and upon animals, the success of the treatment in a number of cases in human beings seems to show that the conclusions are not unwarranted. Fraser, working entirely independently, has been able to confirm the experiments of Calmette in the case of Cobra of India, Crotalus of America, Sepedon hæmachates of Africa, and a serpent of undetermined species of Australia. His experiments were made on both horses and rabbits, and he was able to show experimentally that a serum of considerable antitoxic power could be produced and that it could act both protectively and curatively against snake poisoning, Fraser calling especial attention to the fact that a much larger dose must be given in the latter than in the former case. He was, however, unable to produce serum of the same high degree of immunizing power as Calmette, and computed that it would require 350 c.c. of his serum to cure a man of ordinary size, a quantity utterly impracticable on account of its bulk and the expense necessary to its preparation.

Phisalix and Bertrand have also confirmed Calmette's results in most particulars. It is, however, with Calmette's serum, antivenene, that the practical tests upon human beings have been made.

As we shall see later, various views are held regarding the value of an antivenomous serum prepared with the venom of one variety of snake against poisoning by other varieties of snakes. Calmette believes that the toxic principle of all varieties of poisonous snakes, and also of scorpions and lizards, is the same, and that the other effects are produced by "phlogogenic" substances—albuminoid in nature, which have but little to do with the cause of death; while Cunningham and others believe that an antivenomous serum is only effective against the poison of the same species of snake as that through which the immunization was produced.

It will thus be of interest, both in this connection and also from the practical point of view of "result," to mention more in detail a few of the cases of snake-bite in which cure has been brought about by the use of Calmette's antivenene.

Calmette reports the case of an Ammonite boy working at the Bacteriological Institute at Saigon in Cochin China, who was bitten on the hand by a cobra, and almost immediately the symptoms of violent intoxication set in; 12 c.c. of serum was injected, and imme-

diately the symptoms began to subside, and by the next day the boy
was well; a woman bitten by the same lot of snakes died in two
hours, untreated.

Gould reports the case of a coolie bitten by a full-grown krait
(Bungarus ceruleus), who was cured by 20 c.c. of the serum, local injection of calcium hypochlorite, and ligature.

Rennie reports the case of a Hindoo boy of twelve years, who was
brought to him in a state of collapse, with labored respiration, irregular and intermittent cardiac action, and complete paralysis of the
left side, after having been bitten a short time before by a poisonous
snake about eighteen inches in length, probably a krait; 12 c.c. of
Calmette's antivenene was given and during the administration respiration ceased entirely. Artificial respiration was kept up for twenty
minutes, after which the effect of the serum was noticeable and the
patient rapidly regained consciousness and power over his respiratory
muscles, and in ten days was perfectly well. Two especial points are
of interest in connection with this case: first, that this remedy may be
used with hopes of success in the most severe cases; and second,
that the serum will retain its properties for an indefinite time in any
climate, as the antivenene used in this case had been in Rennie's possession for four years in the plains of India.

Keatinge and Ruffer report a cure in the case of a girl bitten by
the Egyptian cobra, and who, when first seen, was in a comatose condition. A dose of twenty cubic centimetres of the serum was given
in this case.

Prasad Sing treated successfully with antivenene a case of cobra-
bite in a woman who had been bitten one hour previously and brought
to the hospital in an apparently dying condition.

Thus far, reports have been received showing that cures have been
obtained by administration of antivenene in persons who have been
bitten by the following varieties of venomous snakes: (1) Naja tripudians (cobra) of Indo-China, (2) Bungarus ceruleus (krait) of India,
(3) Naja haje (asp) of Egypt, (4) Naja noir of West Africa, and (5)
Bothrops lanceolatus of Central America. Many other cases have
been reported in which it was impossible to identify the species of
snake. Martin has been unable to get good results in those bitten
by the Australian snakes, although he finds that the antivenene has
a definite although slight immunizing power against the uncoagulable
element of the venoms experimented with.

Immunity.

Administration of Venom by the Mouth.—Fraser has carried on a series of experiments in connection with this point. He found that animals (cats and white mice) could be given large doses of venom by the mouth (in the case of the mice one thousand times the dose which would be lethal if subcutaneously administered), and that no toxic effects were to be made out, but that an immunity appeared within two hours of the administration of the venom, lasting five or six days. While the time, two hours, is too long for this method to be of practical value, these experiments are of interest in connection with the immunity which some of the natives of tropical countries seem to have acquired by taking venom by the mouth. In the experiments with the venom, Fraser regarded the results as proof that an antivenomous substance was normally present in the venom, and that this substance alone was absorbed from the stomach.

Effect of Organic Extracts.— Myers and Calmette have carried on a series of experiments upon the value of organotherapy in snake poisoning in connection with Wassermann's theory of "Seitenketten-Immunität," which in turn was based on the theory of Ehrlich that "every antitoxin-producing toxin is specific in the sense that it produces its symptoms by chemical combination of its toxophoric atoms with some cell substance in the body of the susceptible animal," from which Wassermann argued that if the toxin and specific cell substance be mixed *in vitro*, the toxin should be neutralized, as he has found with tetanotoxin and an emulsion of the spinal cord.

Myers, in the case of Cobra, and Calmette in the case of Bothrops lanceolatus found, however, that emulsions of brain or spinal cord had no effect whatsoever upon the toxicity of snake venom. The former investigator found that of all organic emulsions, the one made from the cortical substance of the adrenal body was the only one which invariably influenced cobra poison, either preventing death or prolonging life when injected with a lethal dose of venom.

Protection Afforded by Bile, Biliary Salts, Other Antitoxins, etc.— The facts that in all cases venom is rendered inert shortly after it reaches the duodenum, and that bile is frequently found in the armamentarium of the Hindoo snake charmer, have led some observers to investigate the action of bile, the biliary salts, etc., upon venom, as it is fair to suppose that the bile plays some rôle in the neutralization of the venom in the cases mentioned above.

Fraser has shown that the bile of the African cobra, puff-adder, and rattlesnake, when mixed with the venom of the same variety of snake, prevented lethal doses of the latter from producing death. The amount of bile necessary to produce this result was even less than the amount of venom given; thus, in the cobra, 0.1 mgm. of bile per kilogram of body weight rendered powerless the minimal lethal dose, in the rattlesnake 0.25 mgm., and in the puff-adder 1 mgm.

The bile of innocent snakes was found also to have immunizing power but to a much less extent, while ox bile was still less effective, and the bile of rabbits and guinea-pigs least so. As bile itself is poisonous if introduced hypodermically, Fraser attempted to extract the active principle, and he did so by treatment with alcohol and solution of the residue in water. This was found to be innocuous and could be concentrated, so that Fraser thinks that it may possibly be of value in the treatment of snake-bite.

Besides bile, other substances have been found which increase somewhat the animal's resistance to snake venom. Thus, Phisalix has found that cholesterin, the biliary salts (glycocholate and taurocholate of sodium), tyrosin, and other substances have this power. Besides these substances, various antitoxins have the same effect. Thus Marmorek has shown that animals immunized against anthrax or tetanus furnish a serum antitoxic to snake venom; also that dogs immunized to a high degree against rabies are capable of great resistance to snake poison; while Calmette and others have shown that rabbits vaccinated against snake venom become resistant to poisoning by abrin, while those vaccinated against abrin may in turn acquire a certain degree of immunity against snake venom, diphtheria, ricin, or even sometimes against anthrax, and animals vaccinated against erysipelas or rabies may possess a serum that may be preventive against snake venom.

In some cases the injection of serum from normal dogs or horses or the injection of simple beef bouillon seems to increase the power of resistance. According to Calmette, this antitoxic action of bile, cholesterin, other antitoxins, etc., is no real immunity, but is simply a transitory cell stimulation of non-specific nature, by means of which the resistance of the cells is increased so that they can withstand the toxic effects of the minimal lethal dose.

Duration and Transmissibility of Immunity. — Calmette, Fraser, and others have called attention to the marked difference between the duration of the period of immunity in vaccinated animals and in those that have received the antitoxin. In the former case the immunity is slowly produced but is of long duration, animals losing their immunity the more rapidly the more quickly they have become immunized, while in the former case the immunity is established within a few minutes but lasts only a short period of time. For instance, Calmette found that a rabbit that had been slowly immunized to such a point that it could withstand a dose capable of killing one hundred and twenty non-vaccinated rabbits was able at the end of eight months to resist three times the ordinarily lethal dose, while the immunity after the injection of antivenene lasts from twenty-four hours to ten days, according to the dose.

As to the transmissibility of immunity, Calmette has shown that the female rabbit is able to transmit her immunity to her young, provided the gestation takes place at the height of the immunizing period, and that this transmitted immunity will be retained for about two months, while the immunized male rabbit is absolutely unable to transmit his immunity to his offspring.

Immunity of Snakes and Certain Animals.

The relative immunity which venomous snakes and certain animals, as the mongoose and the eagle, seem to possess against snake poison has long been a subject of discussion, but as yet no entirely satisfactory explanation has been given. According to Calmette, there is always a small amount of antitoxic substance in the serum of the mongoose (Herpestes mungo), while Phisalix and Bertrand, and Wehrmann have demonstrated that the serum of poisonous snakes, although usually toxic, is rendered antitoxic by heating to 60° C. Fraser has shown that venomous serpents possess a definite substance in their own blood serum, which possesses antidotal properties against their own venom and that of other specimens of serpents, which he thinks is probably produced by a slow but constant absorption of poison from their mouths and poison sacs.

Specificity or Non-Specificity of Antivenomous Serum.

The question of the specificity or non-specificity of antivenomous serum is one of both practical and theoretical importance.

Calmette believes that the toxic principle in the venom of all snakes and of scorpions and lizards is the same, and that the difference in symptomatology depends upon the presence or absence of certain "phlogogenic" substances, albuminoid in nature and coagulable by heat (85° C.), which may produce the local hemorrhages and œdema, the hæmaturia, etc., but have little to do with the real cause of death. Thus, after heating, all poisons, both viperine and colubrine, produce the same effects, although differing in the degree of their intoxication of the nerve cells. In preparing his serum, however, after bringing it up to a high immunizing power with the venom of

cobra, or a mixture of two or three venoms, he injects as complex a
mixture of venoms as possible so that these phlogogenic effects will
also be neutralized. Calmette has studied the venom of the following reptiles: Naja tripudians, Crotalus durissus, Bothrops lanceolatus, Naja haje, Cerastes, Bungarus fasciatus, Pseudechis, Hoplocephalus curtus, H. variegatus, Acanthopis antarcticus, Trimeresurus
viridis, and Trigonocephalus contortrix, and concludes "that the venoms of all reptiles of different countries present very close analogies,
and that an animal artificially immunized against a very active venom,
as Naja or Bothrops, is very resistant to all less active venoms."
Cunningham has come to directly opposite conclusions from his experiments, believing that "the blood serum of animals which have
been immunized through repeated treatment with a snake poison is
effective as an antivenene, but only against the poison which comes
from the same species of snake through which the immunization was
produced."

Martin, also, as stated before, has found that Calmette's antivenene is of only slight value in the treatment of Australian snake-bite,
calling attention to the fact that its only neutralizing effect is upon
the non-coagulable element of the venom, but also expressing the
belief that before long the serum will be practicable. According to
Kanthack, most snake poisons are of the same physiological group,
and therefore a successful result could be expected from the same antidote; but serum prepared against cobra venom is ineffective against
daboia venom. It is impossible definitely to decide this question,
but the number of successful cases reported from Africa and India in
which the poisons of very different varieties of snakes were the toxic
agents, the many different varieties of snake poison against which
many investigators have shown the serum to be effective in animal
experiments, as Lepinay's demonstration that animals immunized
with the serum resist the viruses of Bungarus, Trimeresurus, and
Naja, and Calmette's experiment with the long list of snakes already
mentioned as well as with lizards and scorpions, lend much credence
to Calmette's theory.

RELATION BETWEEN SNAKE VENOM AND ANTIVENENE.

Although it would be distinctly out of place in a work of this nature to go deeply into that subject of great present interest, the relation between toxin and antitoxin, this article would be incomplete
without briefly calling attention to some of the views regarding this
relationship in the case under discussion.

Calmette holds the view that the antagonism of the antivenene and venom is indirect, *i.e.*, the antivenene so acts upon the body cells as to enable them to withstand or destroy the venom, bringing about a certain "insensibilization" of the cells, this being the view held by Roux, Metchnikoff, and Buchner as regards the general subject of toxin and antitoxin.   In support of this, he showed by experiment that if a lethal dose of venom and a neutralizing dose of antivenomous serum be mixed in a test tube and injected into an animal, there are no injurious effects; while if the mixture, after standing for a sufficient length of time to bring about any chemical reaction if it should take place, be heated to 70° C. (at which temperature the antitoxic serum loses its efficacy) and then injected, death occurs as if the animal had received no antidote whatever.   He has suggested recently that the rôle of the leucocytes in the fixation of the venom may be very important by a process of intracellular digestion or phagocytosis.   He bases this view upon the leucocytosis "always noted after the injection of venom," and upon the fact that fresh leucocytic extract, if mixed with serum, definitely retards its action.   This view is supported by Wassermann, Delarde, Nikarnarow, and Marenghi.

On the other hand, Kanthack, Fraser, Stephens and Meyers, and Martin and Cherry believe that the venom and antivenene react chemically upon one another, and that they can do so without the assistance of the living organism, *i.e.*, practically the theory of Ehrlich and Behring.   In proof of this they report a number of test-tube experiments in which the power of venom to preserve the fluidity of the blood, etc., is prevented by admixture of antivenomous serum, although Tschistovitch has shown that "the coagulating power of the blood is not directly allied to the antitoxin."

In regard to Calmette's experiments mentioned above, they claim that if the venom and antivenene had been left in contact a longer time, the results would have been different.

Fraser and others believe that the antitoxin is a normal constituent of venom, while Phisalix and Bertrand claim that by heat or filtration a separation of a toxic and a vaccinating substance from normal venom is possible.   This Calmette violently opposes, interpreting the experiments in a very different way and performing the same set of experiments under a somewhat modified technique with opposite results.

Whatever our views regarding the specificity or non-specificity of antivenomous serum or the relation between toxin and antitoxin, the practical results so far obtained are of great promise, and it seems quite possible that a real antidote to snake poison has at last been found.

Calmette suggests that a supply of serum be kept at all the important stations in the countries where poisonous snakes abound, but he also insists that there must be no relaxation whatsoever in the application of local remedies, as these are all of the greatest assistance in preventing the absorption of the venom and increasing the chances of recovery.

Treatment of Other Diseases with Snake Venom and Antivenene.

Dyer has reported five and Woodson one case in which leprosy was treated by injections of antivenene. In four of Dyer's cases a marked improvement was seen, and in one a practical disappearance of the lesions present and of other evidences of the disease. Woodson's case showed marked improvement in every way, which he thinks will prove permanent.

In India, injections of cobra venom in a few cases of bubonic plague appear to have been followed by immediate improvement, and these cases and experiments made upon monkeys, according to the adherents of this method, "seem to give promise of ultimate success." According to them, the *rationale* of the treatment may be that the poisons of plague and snake-bite are antagonistic in their effects upon the nervous system. Venom has also been used in the treatment of tetanus.

MEDICO-LEGAL VALUE OF ANTIVENENE.

Hankin has recently called attention to the possible value of antivenene in the detection of snake poison used for criminal purposes, reporting a case in point; he suggests that by this means the use of snake venom for poisoning cattle in India may be prevented.

Bibliography.

The literature on this subject is so immense that no attempt has been made to give a complete bibliography. The list of titles given consists of all the more important works used in the preparation of the present article. This comprises most of the articles of importance published since 1886. A complete bibliography up to 1886 is to be found in Mitchell and Reichert's "Researches upon the Venom of Poisonous Serpents," Smithsonian Contributions to Knowledge, vol. xxvi.

Alt: Untersuchungen über die Ausscheidung des Schlangengiftes durch den Magen. Münchener medicinische Wochenschrift, 1892, xxxix., p. 724.

Ameden: Serpent Poison as a Remedial Agent in Tetanus. Medical News, 1883, xliii., p. 339.

Andrews: Antivenene. Lancet, 1899, ii., p. 609.

———— On the Preparation and Use of Calmette's Antivenene. British Medical Journal, 1899, ii., p. 661.

Aron Experimentelle Studien über Schlangengift. Zeitschrift für klinische Medicin, 1883, vi.

Baird and Girard. Catalogue of North American Reptiles in the Museum of the Smithsonian Institution, Part I., Serpents, 1853.

Beveridge: A Case of Snake-Bite treated by Dr. Calmette's Antivenene. British Medical Journal, 1899, ii., p. 1732.

Blyth· The Poison of the Cobra de Capello. Analyst, 1877, i., p. 204.

Boulenger: Catalogue of the Snakes in the British Museum, London, 1893.

Brieger: Ueber Ptomaïne, Berlin, 1885.

Brown, Thomas R.: On the Chemistry, Toxicology, and Therapy of Snake-Poisoning. Johns Hopkins Hospital Bulletin, 1899, No. 105.

Brunton: Remarks on Snake Venom and its Antidotes. British Medical Journal, 1891, i., p. 1.

Brunton and Fayrer. On the Nature and Action of the Poison of Naja Tripudians and other Venomous Snakes. Proceedings of the Royal Society, vols. xxi., xxii., xxiii.

Calmette: Étude sur les venins des serpents. 3e mémoire, Annales de l'Institut Pasteur, 1890, ix.; Comptes rendus de l'Académie des Sciences, 1894, 1895, and 1896.

———— Étude expérimentale du venin de Naja tripudians, etc. Annales de l'Institut Pasteur, 1892, vi., p. 160.

———— Étude expérimentale du venin de cobra. Annales de l'Institut Pasteur, 1893, vii.

———— Étude sur le venin des serpents. Annales de l'Institut Pasteur, 1894, viii.; 1895, ix., p. 225.

———— Snake-Venom and Antivenomous Serum. Lancet, 1896, ii., p. 431.

———— Treatment of Animals Poisoned with Snake-Venom by Injection of Antivenomous Serum. Lancet, 1896, ii., p. 449

———— Le Venin des Serpents. Société d'Éditions Scientifiques, Paris, 1896.

———— Sur le venin des serpents et sur l'emploi du sérum antivenimeux. Annales de l'Institut Pasteur, 1897, xi , pp. 214, 238.

———— Appendix on Snake-Poison and Snake-Bite. Allbutt's System of Medicine, 1897, iii., p. 835.

———— Sur le Mécanisme de l'immunisation contre les venins. Annales de l'Institut Pasteur, 1898, xii., p. 343.

Camus et Gley: Nouvelles recherches sur l'immunité contre le sérum d'anguille. Annales de l'Institut Pasteur, 1899, xiii., p. 779.

Cunningham: Experiments on Various Reputed Antidotes to Snake Venom. Scientific Memoirs of Medical Officers of the Army in India, 1897, part x., Calcutta.

Dobbyn: British Medical Journal, 1895, ii , p. 64.

Dürigen· Deutschland's Amphibien und Reptilen, Magdeburg, 1897.

Dyer. New Orleans Medical and Surgical Journal, 1897, October.

Elliott· An Account of some Researches into the Nature and Action of Snake Venom. British Medical Journal, 1900, i , p. 309.

Ellzey: Venomous Snakes of the United States and Treatment of their Bites. Virginia Medical Monthly, xi., p 249.

Ewing: The Action of Rattlesnake Venom upon the Bactericidal Power of the Blood Serum. Medical Record. 1894, May 26th.

Fayrer: The Thanatophidia of India, London, 1872.

———— The Nature of Snake Poison. British Medical Journal, 1884, i., p. 205.

Feoktistow: Ueber die Wirkung des Schlangengiftes auf den thierischen Organismus. Mémoires de l'Académie impériale de Science, S. Petersbourg, 7th series, xxxvi , No. 4.

Frank. Immunität, in Lubarsch und Ostertag, Ergebnisse der allgemeinen Pathologie, 1896, i., p 127.

Fraser The Treatment of Snake Poisoning with Antivenene. British Medical Journal, 1895, ii., p. 416.

———— Immunization against Serpents' Venom and the Treatment of Snake-Bite with Antivenene. Lancet, 1896, i , p. 1156; British Medical Journal, 1896, i., p 957.

———— Antivenomous Properties of the Bile of Serpents and other Animals. British Medical Journal, 1897, No. 1907; Lancet, 1897, ii., p. 119.

Gautier. Sur les alcaloïdes derivés de la destruction bactérienne ou physiologique des tissus animaux. Bulletin de l'Académie de Médecine, 2e series, 1886, xv., p. 65.

Halford: Thoughts, Observations, and Experiments on the Action of Snake Venom on the Blood, Melbourne, 1894.

Hankin: The Medico-legal Value of Antivenene in India. Lancet, 1897, i., p. 262.

von Jaksch: Vergiftung mit Schlangengift. Nothnagel's specielle Pathologie und Therapie, 1897, i., p 525.

Jordan. Manual of the Vertebrates in the Northern United States, 1899.

Josso: Gazette hebdomadaire de Médecine et de Chirurgie. 2e series, 1882, xix., p. 835.

Kanthack: Chloride of Gold as a Remedy for Cobra Poison. Lancet, 1892, i., p. 1296.

———— On the Nature of Cobra Poison. Journal of Physiology, xiii.

Karlinski: Deutsche medicinische Wochenschrift, 1896, xvi , p. 1199

Kauffmann: Du venin de la vipère. Mémoires de l'Académie de Médecine, 1889, xxxvi.

———— Vipères de France, 1893.

Keatinge and Ruffer: Case of Snake Bite Treated with Calmette's Antivenomous Serum. British Medical Journal, 1899, ii., p. 9.

Kelly: The Recognition of the Poisonous Serpents of North America. Johns Hopkins Hospital Bulletin, 1899, No. 105.

Kossel: Berliner klinische Wochenschrift, 1897, No. 7.

Lacerda: Leçons sur le venin des serpents du Brésil, 1884.

Marmorek: Annales de l'Institut Pasteur, 1895, ix., p. 393; 1896, x., p. 47.

Martin: Observations on the Poisonous Constituents of the Venom of the Australian Black Snake. Proceedings of the Linnæan Society, N. S. W., 1892.

———— On Some Effects upon the Blood Produced by the Venom of the Australian Black Snake. Journal of Physiology, 1893, xv.

———— On the Physiological Action of the Venom of the Australian Black Snake. Proceedings of the Royal Society, N. S. W., 1895.

———— Curative Value of Calmette's Antivenomous Serum in the Treatment of Poisoning by Australian Snakes Lancet, 1897, ii., p 1292.

———— Snake Poison and Snake Bite. Allbutt's System of Medicine, 1897, iii., p. 809.

———— Curative Power of Calmette's Serum in Bites by Australian Snakes. British Medical Journal, 1898, ii., p. 1805.

Martin and Cherry: Transactions of the Third Session of the Intercolonial Medical Congress, 1892, p. 152. British Medical Journal, 1898, i., p. 1120.

Martin and Smith: On the Venom of the Australian Black Snake. Proceedings of the Royal Society, N. S. W., 1892.

Mitchell: Researches upon the Venom of the Rattlesnake. Smithsonian Contributions to Knowledge, 1860, xii.

Mitchell and Reichert: Preliminary Report of the Venoms of Serpents. Medical News, 1883, xlii., p. 469.

———— Researches upon the Venom of Poisonous Serpents. Smithsonian Contributions to Knowledge, xxvi.

Mueller· On the Pathology and Cure of Snake Bite. Australasian Medical Gazette, 1888–89, viii., pp. 41, 68, 124, 179, 209.

———— Snake Poison and its Action, Sydney, 1893.

———— On Hematuria in Snake-Bite Poisoning. Australasian Medical Gazette, 1893, xii., p. 247.

Myers: Immunity from Cobra Poison. Lancet, 1898, i., p. 1055.

———— Cobra Poison in Relation to Wassermann's new Theory of Immunity. Lancet, 1898, ii., p. 23.

Nicholson: Indian Snakes, Madras, 1874.

———— British Medical Journal, 1896, ii., p. 1165.

Notes from India British Medical Journal, 1896, ii., p. 444; Lancet, 1899, ii., p. 121.

Nowak: Étude expérimentale des altérations histologiques produites dans l'organisme par les venins des serpents venimeux et des scorpions. Annales de l'Institut Pasteur, 1898, xii., p. 369

Phisalix: Comptes rendus de la Société des Sciences naturelles, 1897.

Phisalix et Bertrand: Toxicité du sang de la vipère, etc. Comptes rendus de l'Académie des Sciences. 1893, cxvii., p 1099, 1894, cxviii., pp. 76, 288, 356.

Porter: British Medical Journal, 1895, ii., p. 571.

Ragotzi Ueber die Wirkung des Naja Tripudians. Virchow's Archiv, cxxii., p. 232.

Rennie: Case of Snake Bite Treated with Calmette's Antivenomous Serum. Lancet, 1899, ii., p 1438; British Medical Journal, 1899, ii., p. 1412.

Sanarelli: Annales de l'Institut Pasteur, 1897, xi . p. 695.

Semple and Lamb: The Neutralizing Power of Calmette's Antivenomous Serum. British Medical Journal, 1899, i., p. 781.

Sewall: Experiments on the Preventive Inoculation of Rattlesnake Venom. Journal of Physiology, 1887, viii., p. 203.

Sing: Pioneer, 1899, August 10th.

Stejneger: The Poisonous Snakes of North America. Smithsonian Reports, United States National Museum, 1893, p. 323.

Stephens and Meyers: Test-tube Reactions between Cobra Poison and its Antitoxin. Lancet, 1898, i., p. 644.

Stone: The Properties of Snake Venom. Boston Medical and Surgical Journal, 1898, cxxxviii., p. 321.

Tschistovitch: Études sur l'immunisation contre le sérum d'anguilles. Annales de l'Institut Pasteur, 1899, xiii., p. 406.

Vollmer: Ueber die Wirkung des Brillenschlangengiftes. Archiv für experimentelle Pathologie und Pharmakologie, 1893, xxxi.

Wall: Poisons of Certain Indian Venomous Snakes.   Proceedings of the R
Society, 1881, xxxii., p. 333.

————— Indian Snake Poisons, their Nature and Effect, London, 1883

Wehrmann: Toxicité du sang et de la bile des serpents.   Annales de l'Inst
Pasteur, 1897, xi., No. 11.

————— Contribution à l'étude du venin des serpents.   Annales de l'Inst
Pasteur, 1898, xii., p. 510.

Wolfenden: On the Nature and Action of the Venom of Poisonous Sna
Journal of Physiology, 1886, vii.

———— On "Cobric Acid," a so-called Constituent of Cobra Venom.   Jou
of Physiology, 1886, vii , p. 365.

Woodson: Treatment of Leprosy by Injection of Calmette's Serum Antiven
Philadelphia Medical Journal, 1899, iv., p. 1231.

Wooster: New Treatment for Snake Bite and other Poisons.   Science, 18
xx., p. 255.

MUSHROOM POISONING.

BY

BEAUMONT SMALL,

OTTAWA.

MUSHROOM POISONING.

THE subject of mushroom poisoning is of much importance to the practising physician, who may at any moment be called upon to care for such a case. In Europe, where fungi are articles of every-day diet, accidents are constantly occurring from the mistaken use of poisonous species. In America this form of food is not utilized to the same extent, and cases of poisoning are not so frequent; but very severe illnesses and deaths do occur from this cause, and an autumn rarely passes without some such case being referred to in our medical publications. In some instances it is due to the gathering of poisonous forms with the common mushroom. At other times it arises from the desire to gather species that are not so well known; and occasionally we find that the attractive appearance of the poisonous forms has tempted a child to gather and eat. In works upon this subject very many cases are reported, and the large percentage of deaths is noticeable. Ziemssen quotes the cases of a mother and daughter, both fatal; of a mother and child, both fatal; of five officers, all of whom died; of a family of seven, with three deaths. Blyth refers to the statistics of fifty-three cases of poisoning by *Amanita phalloides*, of which forty ended in death.

The earlier reports of cases are generally very imperfect and brief, and many of the more recent ones have the same deficiency. Others, however, are very carefully and minutely reported and are valuable contributions to the subject.

Illustrative Cases.

The following are a few illustrative cases:

Two adult males ate, at 8:30 A.M., at breakfast, a quantity of mushrooms supposed to be *Amanita cæsarea*, but in reality *A. muscaria*.

The first man ate about two dozen. At 8:45 he complained of feeling unwell, and at nine was found on his bed in a state of collapse. He complained of a sense of impending death, and there rapidly supervened blindness, trismus, difficulty in swallowing, unconsciousness, and convulsions. Death took place in the evening of the second day. The treatment consisted in the administration of emetics, and apomorphine and atropine hypodermically.

The second man ate about one dozen. After breakfast he rode to his office. At 9:30 he began to complain of diplopia and drowsiness. At ten o'clock he was found sitting in his chair, half stupid, with retraction of the head. He rapidly became unconscious and remained so for five hours, excepting upon two occasions, when he regained consciousness for a brief period. Cold sweats were a prominent symptom. There was no rise in temperature, no pain, nor any nausea. The treatment consisted in the hypodermic administration of apomorphine, which was of no effect. Strychnine and atropine were then given; of the latter, gr. $\frac{1}{50}$ every two hours, about gr. $\frac{1}{10}$ being given in the twenty-four hours. Castor oil and sweet oil were also given. The man recovered.[1]

A boy, aged 12 years, ate, at 11:30 A.M., about one-third of the pileus of an *Amanita phalloides*. No ill effects were felt until 1 A.M., when he awoke complaining of thirst, which was followed by vomiting and purging. These symptoms continued all night, and less severely during the day. Castor oil and citrate of magnesia were given. The following morning he awakened with severe abdominal pain, and when seen by the physician he was feverish and suffering from palpitation, purging, vomiting, and extreme exhaustion. A mixture of chloroform, morphine, and cardamoms was given; also whiskey. The symptoms eased during the day, but the prostration continued. He slept the following night, but about 7 A.M. was seized with convulsions and died in half an hour, on the fourth day after eating the fungus. The post-mortem examination was made thirty-six hours after death. Rigidity was well marked, the face was cyanotic, and dark-brown fluid was issuing from the mouth and nostrils. Upon opening the abdomen, marks of recent peritonitis were seen as bands of lymph gluing the small intestines together. The stomach contained a small amount of dark fluid, the mucous membrane was inflamed, and the walls were softened. The whole of the small intestine was inflamed and there were numerous spots of gangrene. The liver was anæmic, the heart was empty, and the lungs were healthy.[2]

Mrs. N——, aged 55 years, ate a third of a raw mushroom, probably *A. phalloides*, about 10 A.M. No symptoms appeared until 7 P.M., after supper, when abdominal cramps commenced and steadily increased in severity. Vomiting began at 8 P.M., with marked prostration. The patient was found in a condition of collapse, with a temperature of 100.5° F.; pulse small, rapid, weak; respirations shallow; slight tympanites and abdominal tenderness; the pupils were contracted; there were cold perspirations, pallor, and an anxious, drawn expression, with mild delirium, intense retching, and profuse watery stools. Treatment: morphine sulphate gr. $\frac{1}{4}$, atropine nitrate gr. $\frac{1}{100}$, strychnine nitrate gr. $\frac{1}{40}$; and hourly, fluid extract of belladonna gtt. i., fluid extract of nux vomica gtt. ss., bismuth subnitrate gr. ij.; after every emesis, sodium bicarbonate ℥ ss. in half a glass of water; whiskey ad libitum, and hot applications. From 12 P.M. the symptoms gradually subsided. The treatment was continued for two days.[3]

Five persons, aged 13, 22, 29, 40, and 45 years, ate of what was probably *Amanita verna*, prepared as a stew, at nine o'clock in the evening, five hours after the fungi had been gathered. No discomfort was experienced until towards morning, when all were attacked with pain in the stomach, nausea, and a sickening sensation at the epigastrium. Twelve hours after the mushrooms had been eaten all the symptoms had increased in severity, and in addition there were retching and vomiting. In thirty hours there was intense gastro-enteric irritation with relaxed bowels and distressing tenesmus. As these symptoms subsided they were followed by prostration, coldness of the surface, and a tendency to coma. In two of the patients who had eaten more than the others the symptoms advanced to coma and coma vigil, with the features shrunken, skin dusky, and pulse scarcely perceptible. One, aged thirteen years, died in fifty-six hours; another, aged twenty-two years, in sixty-three hours. The treatment consisted in the administration of bismuth and creosote, morphine, stimulants, heat to the surface, and atropine. The atropine was not begun until twenty-four hours had elapsed; it was given in repeated small doses until each patient had had respectively $\frac{1}{30}$, $\frac{1}{25}$, $\frac{1}{25}$, $\frac{1}{20}$, and $\frac{1}{20}$ of a grain. Temporary improvement was noticed after each dose of the antidote.'

Father, mother, and child, aged 5 years, ate twelve, eight, and five mushrooms respectively, supposed to be *Amanita muscaria*, *Amanita phalloides*, and *Amanita verna*. They were gathered during the morning and eaten at dinner.' Nausea and headache were complained of during the afternoon. At six o'clock more were eaten. The same symptoms were noted, but in greater intensity. At midnight purging and vomiting became severe, but there was not much pain, excepting cramps in the legs. The vomiting at first consisted of food; then it became choleraic, as also did the stools, and finally of a pink or purplish color. In twenty-four hours the patients became jaundiced and had a peculiar glazed appearance about the eyes. Muscular twitchings took place, especially in the face, arms, and hands. During the next twelve hours the depression became severe, the heart was irregular, the respirations were jerky, and the pupils were dilated. The urine became saffron-colored, and before death it was purplish. The perspiration and breath smelled of mushrooms. In forty-eight hours the mother and child died within half an hour of one another. The child had convulsions for about four hours, up to two hours before death. The mother was restless and unconscious about five hours before death. The father recovered in about twelve hours after the symptoms had commenced. Treatment consisted of morphine gr. $\frac{1}{6}$, atropine sulphate gr. $\frac{1}{150}$, repeated in two hours; whiskey, ammonia, and nitroglycerin.'

A man, aged 52 years, ate of an omelet prepared from mushrooms, among which were *Amanita phalloides* and *Boletus luridus*. Four hours after eating he was found covered with a cold, clammy perspiration; the breathing was stertorous and of the Cheyne-Stokes type; the pulse was almost imperceptible—28 per minute. The pupils were dilated. Atropine was given; also ether, coffee, and rum; and heat was applied to the surface. The symptoms continued to grow worse until one litre of decinormal saline solution was injected.

Improvement followed immediately; this treatment was continued, and in one hour the pulse was 60 per minute, the respiration became stronger, and the patient rallied from the state of collapse. No diarrhœa or vomiting was present at any time.[a]

The Poisonous Principles in Mushrooms.

The poisonous properties of fungi and the active principles that produce the poisonous effects have received much attention from many careful observers. For many years a principle common to all species was sought for, and various chemists described several poisons under as many titles. Thus we have had *muscarine, bulbosine, amanitin, agaricin, agarythine,* and many others. At present all are resolved into two poisons, *muscarine* and *phallin,* the former characteristic of Amanita muscaria, being an alkaloid; the latter characteristic of Amanita phalloides, and an entirely different poison.

In addition to the action of poisonous species, very many instances of poisonous effects have followed the use of species which are known to be free from any poisonous properties. Most of these were undoubtedly due to gastrointestinal irritation, more or less severe, in some cases leading to peritonitis. All, however, cannot be traced to this condition, and in some cases the poisoning has been popularly explained by the fact that the edible form was gathered from a manure heap or from some other decomposing organic matter, which produced a poisonous action. Another explanation is that the mushroom may have been kept too long, and that decomposition and putrefactive changes had begun which rendered it poisonous in character. In the light of modern bacterial science, this idea of a toxic principle being generated by the decomposing mushroom is of much importance. We know that many cadaveric poisons are produced in this way, and we also know that the mushroom has been termed a "vegetable beefsteak" on account of the very large percentage of nitrogenous matter in its composition. The flesh of the mushroom, in addition to a large percentage of water, about eighty per cent., is made up of a proteid or nitrogenous substance called *fungin,* which contains from 3.2 to 7.2 per cent. of nitrogen. It is to this fungin that the mushroom owes its highly nutritive properties.

Muscarine, $C_5H_{15}NO_3$, the most carefully studied and best known of the poisonous principles, is an alkaloid, first described by Schmiedeberg and Koppe,[1] whose investigations form the foundation for our present knowledge of this subject. Their work has been confirmed by others (I. L. Prevost[2]) and reaffirmed by Schmiedeberg.[3]

It is a colorless, syrupy fluid, tasteless and without odor. It is very soluble in water and alcohol, but insoluble in ether; very slightly soluble in chloroform. It is alkaline in reaction and combines with acids to form salts. The sulphate and nitrate are prepared for commerce. They are very hygroscopic and soluble in water and alcohol.

The quantity of muscarine present in the fungus has not been determined. It has been estimated variously from one-fifth to one per cent. of the dried fungus. The percentage varies greatly according to the season of the year, the locality in which it grows, and many such conditions.

Muscarine was formerly considered to be characteristic of the fly agaric and similar fungi, but in the progress of chemical and bacterial science it has been obtained from other and very different sources. It has been separated as a ptomain from decomposing fish and also from horseflesh undergoing the same change (Vaughan[10]). It is also prepared synthetically from cholin by the oxidizing action of nitric acid. Cholin, neurin, and other ptomains to which it is allied are all of cadaveric origin, and nearly all are powerful poisons. The physiological action of muscarine bears a resemblance to that of pilocarpine, and also of calabar bean. It is primarily an excitant to the nerve centres, the period of excitement rapidly passing into one of depression. Upon the brain it is an intoxicant, causing dizziness, vertigo, confusion of ideas, delirium, disturbed vision, ataxia, and other like symptoms, which may end in convulsions, coma, paralysis, and death. Its depressing action is specially directed to the cardiac and respiratory centres, and its fatal effects are due to paralysis of these organs. The heart remains in a dilated state after death. The vasomotor centres are also depressed, causing a lowering of the blood pressure. It increases the secretion of the sudoriparous, lacrymal, salivary, and all other glands, probably with the exception of the kidney. The muscular system is also irritated and weakened, giving rise to muscular fatigue and cramps of the extremities and of the intestines. The pupils are contracted.

The action of atropine upon the heart is directly antagonistic to muscarine, and furnishes us with the physiological and most valuable antidote. Atropine paralyzes the inhibitory nerves of the heart and increases the rapidity of its action. The effect of muscarine is to produce a slowing and weakening of its action. The opposing effect is frequently demonstrated upon the exposed heart, which, when failing from the presence of muscarine, is at once aroused into action by a drop of atropine solution, or, if the atropine has been first applied, the toxic effect of muscarine is prevented.

No cases of poisoning by pure muscarine have been reported. All our knowledge is derived from experimental work upon animals and man. It has been found that 8 to 12 mgm. (gr. $\frac{1}{8}$ to $\frac{1}{5}$) will cause the death of a cat in about eighteen minutes, and 3 to 4 mgm. (gr. $\frac{1}{20}$ to $\frac{1}{15}$) will have the same result in a few hours. Five milligrams (gr. $\frac{1}{12}$) taken by an adult man causes in a few minutes profuse salivation and lacrymation, increased frequency of pulse, nausea, giddiness, confusion, determination of blood to the head, and perspiration. There is no vomiting or diarrhœa. Fatal doses in cats cause salivation, contraction of pupils, vomiting and purging, rapid breathing, and dyspnœa; as death approaches the respirations grow slower, the pupils become dilated, and convulsions usher in death.

The poisonous principle of *Amanita phalloides* has been frequently investigated, and the poison obtained has been variously named. *Bulbosin, amanitin, phalloidin,* and several others have been described, but no satisfactory result was reached until Kobert[11] published the results of his researches and named the poison *phallin*. Phallin is an entirely different poison from muscarine. It is a toxalbumin, a member of that group to which belongs the specific poison of cheese, meat, rattlesnake poison, as well as the toxic agent of diphtheria and other bacterial poisons.

The action of phallin is directed to the blood corpuscles, causing their destruction and setting free the hæmoglobin. It produces such changes in the plasma that the serum escapes from the vessels into the various tissues and cavities, and a condition resembling that produced by cholera is the result. Its action is slow, and the symptoms of poisoning do not appear for an interval of from three or four to twelve or fourteen hours. They begin as severe abdominal pain, prostration, vomiting, free watery evacuations, and symptoms of collapse. Irritation to the nervous system is shown by muscular cramps, tetanic in character, and convulsions. Consciousness usually remains unaffected. The pulse becomes weak and flabby. The kidneys secrete much less urine, and there are signs of albuminuria and hæmoglobinuria.

The presence of this second poison explains the symptoms of many cases of poisoning that were obscure when muscarine was considered the sole poisonous principle of mushrooms. At present *A. muscaria* and *A. pantheroides* have been studied as the source of muscarine only, and *A. phalloides* alone has furnished phallin, but it is not probable that either poison is limited to these particular species. There is much more reason to believe that each poison is widely distributed. Muscarine is certainly the chief poison of *A. muscaria*, but many of the symptoms that follow poisoning by this fungus can be explained only by the presence of phallin.

Pathological Anatomy.

The post-mortem appearances are not very definite. By some it is stated that rigor mortis is absent. Others have found it to exist, but to disappear early. There are evidences of gastrointestinal irritation, and portions of the fungus may be present. The various organs are congested, especially the kidneys. The abdominal and pleural cavity may contain fluid colored by the transuded hæmoglobin. The heart is dilated. In a series of autopsies, when death probably resulted from phallin poisoning, there were numerous small ecchymoses on the pleural surfaces, and also in the lungs, heart, kidneys, liver, and other organs. The blood, also, was found to be of a dark cherry-red color and fluid. The veins were full. Fatty degeneration of the liver has been found in some cases.

Symptoms.

The symptoms that follow the use of poisonous fungi coincide with the results of the experimental work with these poisons. In the majority of cases the symptoms are distinctly those of one or the other poison, sometimes complicated by the irritation of undigested portions of the fungus. In poisoning by muscarine the diagnostic points are the early onset of symptoms, the signs of intoxication, and the functional weakness of the heart and lungs. In poisoning by phallin the symptoms are delayed; there is an absence of cerebral disturbance, and severe gastroenteric irritation, becoming choleraic in character, is the prominent symptom.

In muscarine poisoning the alkaloid is very stable and is excreted with the urine, which retains the intoxicating properties. This, it is reported, the inhabitants of certain districts of Siberia take advantage of in order to prolong their intoxication. The fly agaric is a common fungus in northern Asia, and furnishes the natives with a substitute for the alcohol, opium, and the narcotics of other countries.

The duration and termination of cases of mushroom poisoning vary greatly according to the quantity of poisonous material taken into the system. They are also influenced by the health and strength of the patient. Cases due to muscarine run a more rapid course than those due to phallin. The symptoms begin almost at once, and death may take place in five or six hours; more frequently a fatal termination does not take place until the second or third day. Convalescence is always slow, more particularly in severe cases. When phallin is the poison, the course is slower. Death may take place on the second day, but four or five days is the more common period. In some instances the patient has lingered seven days. Of five officers poisoned by eating *A. bulbosa*, symptoms did not begin until eleven hours had elapsed; two died on the second day, two on the third, and one on the fifth day. In another case a child died on the second day, the mother on the fifth day. In still another instance, one victim died after forty-eight hours, one at the end of sixty hours, and the third on the seventh day.

Treatment.

The treatment consists of measures to allay the gastrointestinal irritation and overcome the depression, and also the employment of special antidotes to counteract the poison. The stomach should be emptied as rapidly as possible for the purpose of removing all portions of the fungi that may remain undigested. Castor oil and enemata should be used with the same object in view; milk, barley water, and other demulcent drinks, bismuth, magnesia, and antacids are to be given for the double purpose of soothing the irritated mucous membrane and of retarding the absorption of the poison. Muscarine becomes very soluble in the acid fluids, and for this reason acids should not be given. Alcohol and ammonia may be required to stimulate the heart and respiration and lessen the general depression.

As special antidotes, tannin, charcoal, and permanganate of potassium have been recommended. The first two are of value in rendering insoluble the poisons, and the latter for the purpose of decomposing the alkaloid; their value, however, is as yet uncertain.

When the poisoning is due to muscarine, the only antidote to depend upon is atropine, which should be immediately administered in all cases of suspected poisoning from this source. Experiments have proved conclusively that when the inhibitory nerves of the heart are depressed by atropine the effects of muscarine are almost entirely counteracted, and when the heart and respiration are failing from the poison, the atropine helps to restore their tone and force. In the cases in which it has been employed, even when death has finally taken place, its favorable effects have been specially mentioned. It should be administered hypodermically, in gr. $\frac{1}{100}$ to $\frac{1}{50}$ doses, repeated hourly, according to the symptoms and its effect.

When *A. phalloides* has been taken and phallin is the poisonous principle, there is no drug that can be employed with the same feeling of hopefulness, as there is no known antidote to this poison. As soon as the poisoning is suspected the same general treatment is indicated for the purpose of removing any portion of the fungus and preventing further absorption. Stimulants should be freely administered. Nitrite of amyl and nitroglycerin may prove of service to maintain the cutaneous circulation. When the severe symptoms supervene and collapse is threatening, intravenous injections of decinormal saline solution or its subcutaneous use will prove of great service, and upon this procedure will depend the greatest hope of success. Transfusion of blood has also been recommended.

Classification of Mushrooms.

The higher forms of fungi which grow so profusely throughout the whole world are classified into three groups, according to their mode of producing spores. These are—

Hymenomyceteæ, in which the spores are external to the lining membrane, which membrane is on the under surface of the pileus or cap and folded as gills. This comprises all such as are commonly called mushrooms or toadstools.

Discomyceteæ, in which the spores are also formed external to the membrane, but in depressions, or lacunæ, on the upper and outer surface, as in the ordinary morel.

Gastromyceteæ, in which the spores are contained in a cavity formed by the membrane, as in the well-known puff-balls.

Of the many thousand species that are included in these three classes, only a few are known to contain an active poison, and nearly all these are closely allied and form a single genus of the hymenomyceteæ. The most important of the many genera of hymenomyceteæ are *Agaricus* and *Amanita*. The former contains the ordinary edible mushrooms, the latter the poisonous forms.

These genera are variously arranged by different botanists, and this want of uniformity has led to much confusion of names. Formerly all were included in the single genus Agaricus, and we will find the poisonous forms referred to as Agaricus muscaria, etc. It is now more general to regard the Amanita as a sub-genus, or as a separate genus, with its distinctive name.

DISTINCTION BETWEEN EDIBLE AND POISONOUS MUSHROOMS.

The structural and botanical differences between the amanitas and agarics are very slight, and their resemblance is the cause of the many accidents that occur. Between the common mushroom and the fly agaric the difference is very marked, and one should never be mistaken for the other, but there are many other edible mushrooms that bear a close resemblance. The danger is also increased by the fact that certain species of the amanitæ, as *A. cæsarea*, are edible; and unless the collector is a skilled mycologist a mistake may easily occur. Many suggestions have been offered to facilitate the recognition of the poisonous and edible species, but none is sufficiently trustworthy to be depended upon without some knowledge of the distinctive characters of each. The most important sign is the presence of the *volva* which is formed on the poisonous species, but is absent from the others. When young, the growing fungus is enveloped in a membrane, which is ruptured as the plant expands, its traces remaining as a cup-shaped ring, or sheath, around the base of the stem, and as excrescences on the upper surface of the cap. This volva is often below the surface of the soil and is easily overlooked. In gathering the fungus, the stem is generally broken off, and the characteristic base with the volva is left behind. The color of the gills is also suggestive, those of the edible forms being pinkish, while those of the poisonous species, with few exceptions, are white. A disagreeable, noxious odor and sharp, acrid taste also indicate a dangerous species.

The points of difference between the common edible mushroom and the two poisonous forms are very concisely described by Dr. W. G. Farlow of Harvard University, as follows:

"(1) The common mushroom has a pileus which is not covered with wart-like scales; gills which are brownish-purple when mature; a nearly cylindrical stalk, which is not hollow with a ring near the middle, and without a bulbous base sheathed by a membrane or by scales.

"(2) The fly agaric has a pileus marked with prominent warts; gills always white; a stalk, with a large ring around the upper part, and hollow or cottony inside, but solid at the base, where it is bulbous and scaly.

"(3) The death cup has a pileus without distinct warts, gills which are always white, and a hollow stalk, with a large ring, and a prominent bulb at the base, whose upper margin is membranous or bag-like.

"(4) Other points of difference are the different places in which these species grow, and also the colors, which, although they vary in each case, are brilliant yellow or red in the fly agaric, white varying to pale olive in the deadly agaric, and white usually tinged with a little brown in the mushroom.

"(5) In the mushroom the pileus averages from three to four inches in breadth, and the stalk is generally shorter than the breadth of the pileus and comparatively stout. The pileus remains convex for a long time, and does not become quite flat-topped until old,

The substance is firm and solid. In the fly agaric the pileus, at first oval and convex, soon becomes flat and attains a breadth of six to eight inches and sometimes more. The stalk has a length equal to or slightly exceeding the breadth of the pileus, and is comparatively slenderer than in the common mushroom. The pileus of the deadly agaric is thinner than that of the mushroom, and, from being rather bell-shaped when young, becomes gradually flat-topped with the centre a little raised. In breadth it is intermediate. The stalk usually is longer than the breadth of the pileus, and the habit is slenderer than the other two species."

The special characteristics of the amanitas are as follows: "*Pileus* (or cap) at first campanulate, then plane; fleshy towards the centre, attenuated at the margin; gills ventricose, narrow behind, free, numerous, at length denticulate, the imperfect ones few, of a determinate form according to the kind, and, with one exception (A. cæsareus), white. *Stalk* generally enlarged at the base, frequently bulbous, solid, or stuffed with a cotton-like substance, which is at length absorbed; ring descending, imperfect, fugaceous; flesh white, unchanging" (Badham).

POISONOUS MUSHROOMS.

The following species, growing in this country, comprise all that are known constantly to possess active toxic properties. There are others that are probably poisonous, but as yet they have not been properly authenticated, nor have any deaths been attributed to their use. Many of them often produce distressing symptoms, but they are uncertain and may often be eaten with perfect safety.

AMANITA MUSCARIA Grev. *Agaricus muscaria* L. Fly agaric. This is a large showy fungus, very common in some localities, growing in oak and pine woods from June to late in the autumn. The pileus is of an orange or yellow color, sometimes becoming brilliant red, in others it varies almost to a white; it is covered with warty excrescences, generally whitish. The under or spore-producing surface is white. The plant is very free from insects and flies and does not blacken when broken. In early growth the pileus is convex, but becomes flat and sometimes concave. The stem is bulbous, white, and and springs from a volva. It is rough and covered with warty growths on shaving-like shreds. It should be readily distinguished from the edible species by its color and appearance, the color of its gills, and its place of growth, as it is never found in meadows, nor does the mushroom grow in woods. The fly agaric is of sturdy growth, ranging from four to sixteen inches in height. Mistakes are more liable to arise in mistaking the fly agaric for some of the edible amanita, as *Amanita cæsarea* and *Amanita rubescans*.

AMANITA PHALLOIDES (Pers.) Fr. Death cup. This species is not so large nor so brilliant as the A. muscaria. It grows from three to six or eight inches high, and is found in woods, but often extends into meadows and fields. It may be gathered in summer and is very common in the autumn months. The pileus is white or fawn-colored, sometimes becoming yellow or greenish and smooth, and the investing membrane, separating from the cap, remains as a deep cup-like volva, which has given it the name of death cup. The stem is white, or tinged in the darker forms, and smooth, excepting when the investing cap is closely adherent, when it has a bulbous appearance. It also is very free from insects and remains of a clear color. Its odor and taste, when fresh, are not noticeable, but after it has been gathered they become disagreeable. Its gills and spores are white.

This species is likely to be mistaken for the common edible mushroom, but it bears a much greater resemblance to *Lepiota naucina*, another fungus having white gills and spores, but quite free from any poisonous properties. Another source of danger is that in some immature specimens of A. phalloides the gills are of a faintly pink color.

AMANITA VERNA Bull. The vernal or bulbous amanita is considered by many to be simply a variety of A. phalloides, and is one of the most important of the poisonous species on account of its resemblance to the common edible mushroom. It is smaller than A. phalloides, more delicately formed, and of a pure white color. It is found in the early summer months and is very common in many localities. In Europe it appears in the spring, from which it derives its specific name. Its distinctive character is the manner in which the sheath adheres to the stem, giving the stem a very bulbous appearance, and depriving it of its cup-shaped volva.

AMANITA PANTHERINUS Deb. is a common species with many varieties. It is of a yellowish-brown color, over which there are many markings of a darker hue, which give it a mottled appearance. The gills and flesh are white. The following instance of poisoning is quoted by Christison: "A boy, having eaten some of the fungus, became delirious and maniacal and gradually passed into a condition of trance. Recovery took place."

BOLETUS LURIDUS Schœff. This fungus is of a different class from the agarics and amanitas, as its spores are formed in lacunæ on the under surface of the pileus. In its shape it resembles the agarics. The upper surface varies from an amber to a brown color; the under surface and stem are of a bright red or ferruginous brown. The flesh is yellowish; when broken and exposed, it changes to a blue. The pileus is from two to six inches broad. The stem is solid, bulbous, sometimes quite smooth, and more or less mottled. It grows in woods and thickets.

Bibliographical References.

1. Prentiss: Philadelphia Medical Journal, September 24, 1898.
2. Plowright: The Lancet, 1879, ii., p. 941.
3. Norris: Philadelphia Medical Journal, October 22, 1898.
4. Shadle: Therapeutic Gazette, May, 1893.
5. Berry: Philadelphia Medical Journal, September 24, 1898.
6. Delobel: La Presse Médicale, September 30, 1899 and British Medical Journal, Epitome 52, 1900.
7. Schmiedeberg und Koppe: Das Muscarin, das giftige Alkaloid des Fliegenpilzes, Leipsic, 1869.
8. Prevost. Transactions of the International Medical Congress, 1878.
9. Schmiedeberg: Transactions of the International Medical Congress, 1881.
10. Vaughan: Twentieth Century Practice, vol. xiii., p. 16.
11. Kobert: Ueber Pilzvergiftung, Dorpat, 1891.

DISEASES OF THE UVULA, SOFT PALATE, AND FAUCIAL PILLARS.

BY

JAMES E. NEWCOMB,

NEW YORK.

DISEASES OF THE UVULA, SOFT PAL-ATE, AND FAUCIAL PILLARS.

Anatomy.—The soft palate is the musculo-aponeurotic curtain projecting downwards and backwards from the posterior edge of the bony palate, its own posterior edge being free and pendulous. It is covered with mucous membrane continuous with that of the surrounding parts. The epithelial cells on its upper surface resemble those of the nasopharynx in being provided with cilia, while those on its under surface are of the ordinary pavement variety seen in the pharynx proper. From its middle hangs a conical projection called the uvula, composed mainly of the azygos uvulæ muscle, which is formed by the union in the median line of two symmetrical strips or bundles of muscular fibres which arise, one on each side of the median line, from the tendinous structure of the soft, and occasionally from the spine of the hard palate. Each side of the base of the soft palate expands into two muscular bundles which sloping downwards become the faucial pillars. The anterior bundle known as the palatoglossus muscle is lost on the side of the tongue, while the posterior known as the palatopharyngeus muscle spreads out below from the posterior cornu of the hyoid bone to the middle line of the pharynx posteriorly. In the triangular space between the two on each side is located the tonsil.

The soft palate is also the site of insertion of two other symmetrical muscular bundles on each side, viz., the levator palati from the petrous portion of the temporal bone and cartilaginous portion of the Eustachian tube, and the tensor palati from the navicular fossa at the foot of the internal pterygoid plate and adjacent parts, ending in a tendon which plays around the hamular process and terminates in the anterior portion of the aponeurosis of the soft palate.

The mucosa in this situation does not present any special peculiarities. The statement is made by some authorities that at the free border of the palate and on the uvula no glands are found. In general the entire region is covered with muciparous glands and lymph follicles. The bases of the glands are said to penetrate the subjacent muscles, so that the contraction of the latter would directly tend to empty the glands.

Physiology.—The office of the various structures entering into the soft palate and related parts is to shut off the neighboring cavity of the nasopharynx in the act of swallowing. Abolition of this function as seen in various paralyses is followed by regurgitation of ingesta into the nose. In addition, the varying position of the muscular curtain is directly concerned with voice production, its elevation allowing the free flow of sound waves through the nasal passages, and being vitally concerned in the production of overtones in singing. The degree of approximation to the posterior wall of the pharynx is also a factor in both the vocal pitch and quality. The peculiar twang noted when the palatal functions are interfered with is ample confirmation of these views. Moreover, various special functions have been assigned to the uvula proper. It has been called the "drip-stone" for conducting to the mouth the secretions from the parts above and behind; it has been looked upon as analogous to the weight on a drop curtain preventing too long a contact of the moist soft palate with the posterior wall of the pharynx; still another view assigns to the uvula the function (during phonation) of a pillar to support the soft palate, the base of the pillar resting on the tongue. The latter view seems unlikely, for most uvulæ rarely touch the tongue in normal phonation, and the muscular tension of the palate itself is ample for its own support.

Malformations and Anomalies.

In 3,000 throats, C. Berens found 84 cases of anomalies of the *uvula*, classified as follows: hypertrophied, 11; pendulous, 2; fish-tail shaped, 39; attached to other parts, 3; deeply cleft, 14; reduced to a worm-like shred, 8; completely separate, 2; supernumerary, 4; absent, 2. Henke[1] in an elaborate article figures no less than 28 varieties of abnormality, all noted in clinical experience. He finds anomalies in 2.8 per cent. of all cases examined, his proportion exactly tallying with that of Berens.

Farlow has called attention to a condition of the uvula often mistaken for relaxation of the organ—namely, the irregular or uneven development of the two sides of the azygos uvulæ muscle. The organ here hangs down on the side of the greater amount of muscular structure simulating a paretic condition. Watson records a case of varicose veins of the soft palate and uvula, the latter being nearly two inches long and made up of venous knots. Cohen has seen a case in which a uvula of considerable size was entirely enclosed in a fold of mucous membrane continuous with the anterior pillars of the fauces, and extending horizontally from the side of one tonsil to its opposite.

The writer has seen several instances of lesser degrees of this same anomaly. Rarely do any of the foregoing conditions give rise to any disturbances. Of far greater moment, however, are the results of developmental errors. The region being symmetrically developed, it is evident that there may be all degrees of failure of the two approximating sides to coapt, so that we may have tissue gaps running from the tip of the uvula way up even to the edge of and through the hard palate. Grobe ascribes this abnormality to the hypertrophy of the bones at the base of the skull, especially the vomer which by its projection prevents the union of the lateral halves of the palatal plate. The subject of cleft palate is, however, outside the province of the present article. Symptoms in this class of lesions may range from a barely noticeable defect of clearness in speech to early death of the infant from inability to nurse. One case of cleft tongue with entire absence of the soft palate and uvula has been cited by Helsham, the case first coming under observation at the eighth month of life.

A study of the uvula in various forms of degeneracy has been made by C. L. Dana, who found defects in either shape or development in nearly one-half of the cases examined. A marked case under this head is that described by Somers.[2] The latter also calls attention to the well-known fact that defective innervation of the soft palate is frequently associated with chronic nasopharyngeal catarrh as is also a sharply bent or twisted uvula.

Defects in the *faucial pillars* are occasionally met with. These generally present themselves as fenestræ or oval slits in the pillars; sometimes they are situated in the pendulous portion of the soft palate. Various theories have been assumed to account for these tissue gaps. Some of them are undoubtedly the result of incision through the pillars for the evacuation of circumtonsillar pus: others may be due to the destructive ulceration of syphilitic and other dyscrasiæ; there are some, however, which are congenital, and these latter have been referred to the prenatal absorption of tissue once formed or to the incomplete obliteration of the original branchial clefts. Some of them can be explained on the theory of a separate investment by mucosa of the faucial pillars. In 1897, the writer[3] was able to collect records of forty-two of these anomalies, and several additional cases have been reported since that time. As a rule, the condition gives no symptoms, and its existence may even be unsuspected until a sore throat or other untoward incident brings the patient under observation. Frequently the tonsils seem to be rudimentary, and in such cases a pocketing of soft foods between the pillars has been observed.

Inflammatory Conditions.

ACUTE UVULITIS.

Acute uvulitis occurring alone is very uncommon as it is generally one feature of a composite inflammation affecting the entire fauces and pharynx. The mucosa at the tip of the organ is somewhat thicker and less compact in structure than elsewhere in the mouth, and this fact presents most favorable conditions for exudation which is apt to assume the œdematous type.

Causes.—A frequent cause is trauma, or occasionally the condition is a result of prolonged, excessive, or mal-regulated vocal effort. Sepsis is often an exciting factor. Patients with rheumatic and gouty tendencies often suffer from this form of sore throat; and finally the loose tissue may become swollen as a part of the local reaction after operations, particularly ignipuncture, on the tonsils.

Pathology.—The uvula becomes swollen and œdematous. It may bleed from the surface or even be the seat of a small hæmatoma. Ripault has reported one case of spontaneous hemorrhage from the organ. The lesson to be drawn from such an experience would seem to be to look carefully after the state of the kidneys.

Symptoms.—The symptoms are those of a sore throat, varying in severity from a slight feeling of discomfort in the fauces to painful swallowing, fulness in the throat, hacking cough, muffled voice, rarely dyspnœa, and in the more severe cases, a slight febrile movement.

Treatment.—In the milder cases the use of a mercurial followed by a saline will relieve all the annoyance. If the discomfort persists an astringent lozenge may be employed. The action of this class of remedies seems to be more satisfactory than that of gargles, for the muscular action in the throat incident to gargling may itself prove harmful. Hot alkaline gargles are advocated by some when the smarting is excessive. When the œdema is marked, free puncture or scarification followed by frequent rinsing with a hot antiseptic solution should be done. It goes without saying that the lancet used for this purpose should be most carefully sterilized and have a sharp point. It is well also to catch the organ with a pair of fine-toothed forceps, otherwise it may slip away from the sharpest instrument.

CHRONIC UVULITIS: HYPERTROPHIED UVULA.

Simple chronic uvulitis is merely one feature in a chronic inflammation of the entire faucial tract, and is especially associated with chronic pharyngitis due to gastric disturbances. The condition is also present in hypertrophy of the uvula, a term we prefer to "elongation."

Causes.—Very few patients go through a siege of sore throats without the sequel of a more or less enlarged uvula. Other causes are the same as those of acute inflammation of the part.

Pathology.—Bearing in mind the structure of the organ, it is easy to see how the mucosa may prolapse upon the underlying muscular cylinder, and present itself as a pointed tip of a pearly-white color and œdematous consistence. In other cases the muscular cylinder is itself enlarged, but here the enlargement is apt to be an increase in the bulk of the uvula rather than a mere elongation. In simple cases of the latter, the length of the organ may be such that it can be made to reach nearly the dental arch in front, or the entrance of the larynx behind. Hoen[4] has made a careful and interesting study of the degenerative changes which the striated muscular fibres of the azygos uvulæ undergo in these conditions of hypertrophy. While there is marked proliferation of the nuclei of the fibres, Hoen regards the change as essentially degenerative in character, the final change being a nearly or quite total disappearance of the contractile substance of the affected muscular fibres.

Symptoms.—Of these there are all grades of severity. They are not necessarily proportional to the length of the organ, for some patients with very long uvulæ make no complaint whatever. Others constantly complain of a tickling, hacking cough, retching on the slightest provocation, and even vomiting. As special excitants of these latter symptoms may be mentioned, a sudden change from one temperature to another (even the cold bath) and fatigue. During sleep the fauces relax, and the patient may awake with sudden laryngeal spasm. Owing to the mechanical conditions present the constant cough may cause slight hemorrhages from the rupture of superficial vessels on the surface of the uvula itself or in the surrounding structures. It also tends to make the organ still longer. This appearance of blood in the expectoration, together with the exhaustion due to the cough itself, often leads to a suspicion of pulmonary disease, for the debility occasioned is no mere fancy. Patients often lose much flesh and strength from this comparatively trivial ailment. Singers find, as a result of hypertrophied uvula, a loss of vocal range, early fatigue, and sometimes a tremulous character to any forced tone.

Treatment.—The treatment is that of the associated catarrhal conditions together with a removal, if necessary, of a portion of the uvula. Most careful attention must be given to the digestive tract. Astringent troches and mouth washes may relieve in mild cases, and may with profit in any case precede surgical intervention. It must be borne in mind, however, that in a case of any severity, their use offers only transient results, and that the old train of annoyances will supervene upon their discontinuance.

Uvulotomy is an operation which has doubtless been performed many times needlessly, but there are some cases which demand it. The late Harrison Allen once remarked to a colleague that he had never removed a uvula. Most of us will meet cases in which the operation will afford relief, and in which it ought to be done. The first practical question is, How much of the uvula should be removed? In the adult the average organ is about three-eighths of an inch long, and when the mouth is closed hangs free in the fauces without resting on the tongue. In making our estimate of the amount of tissue to be removed, we should be sure that the parts are at rest in a normal position: otherwise the uvula will be raised, and the soft palate along with it, thereby distorting the natural relations.

Local anæsthesia may easily be obtained with cocaine in ten-per-cent. solution, most safely applied on a cotton swab. The patient should be seated in a high-backed chair facing the operator, and holding the tongue depressor in his own hands, so that both of the surgeon's hands may be free. The tip of the organ is drawn forward with a pair of fine-toothed forceps, and then with a pair of long-handled scissors curved on the flat, a cut is made through the uvula, care being taken to bevel the organ at the expense of its posterior surface. By this means the denuded area is behind so that the food does not come in contact with it, and moreover the organ acts as a drain for the mucus from above, which is thereby prevented from dropping into the larynx. Healing is thus hastened. De Blois recommends section by means of the galvanocautery loop which prevents hemorrhage, and also the slipping of the mucosa upon the muscular cylinder. Special uvulotomes have been devised, but they offer no advantages over the forceps and scissors. It must be remembered that the organ will contract somewhat in healing, and allowance must be made for this fact in estimating the amount of tissue to be removed. The latter will consist mainly of mucosa, but there are cases in which it is necessary to remove a part of the muscle itself. Pieces of ice held in the mouth lessen the after-smarting.

Severe bleeding is rare, and can generally be checked by the familiar gargle of gallic and tannic acids. For the literature of this complication, the reader is referred to an exhaustive article by the late E. Carroll Morgan.' The shorter the stump, the more likely is the bleeding to be annnoying.

FAUCIAL CALCULI.

Occasional cases have been reported of calculi in the region under discussion. Goodale has reported one case of calculus in the uvula. C. A. Parker removed several years ago, a calculus from the right side of the palate. The site of the stone resembled an ulcerated surface, while the surrounding tissues were hard and inflamed. Deglutition was extremely painful, the pain radiating to the ear. The stone weighed fifty-five grains, was easily crushed, and was quite soluble in hydrochloric acid. The insoluble parts consisted of epithelial *débris*, various spores, and considerable of the mycelium of the cladothrix. These formations doubtless originate in the accumulation of cheesy matter in the crypts of the mucosa. Symptoms are those of a foreign body embedded in the tissues, and the hardness of the mass may lead to a suspicion of malignancy. Exploration with a sharp probe, or, better, with a needle, will reveal their true nature. An incision should be made over their most prominent part, the calculus turned out of its bed, and the latter lightly cauterized. In one instance Anselmier (quoted by Bosworth') finding calcareous masses in a palatal recess passed into the latter a tampon saturated with weak sulphuric acid, and succeeded in dissolving *in situ* the offending material.

Disturbances of Innervation.

PERVERSE ACTION.

Under this heading have been described certain cases characterized by the apparent inability of the soft palate properly to functionate in the production of certain tones so that the voice has a nasal twang. The condition is not constant, and occurs only with certain vowel sounds. No lesion has been discovered, and the affection is doubtless to be referred to some minor defect of innervation, which we are at the present time unable to demonstrate.

CHOREA OF THE SOFT PALATE.

This consists in the rapid raising and lowering of the palate, which is rarely made tense. It may be attended by a ticking sound which is apparently synchronous with the action of the levatores palati. The affection is frequently of a reflex nature, while the cause is often unassignable. In reported cases, removal of lymphoid hypertrophy from the vault and cauterization of enlarged turbinates have been followed by relief. Legroux refers to one case of lateral spasm. There does not seem to be any relation between chorea in general and this particular affection.

PARALYSIS.

Cases have been reported of complete paralysis with anæsthesia. Lecocq narrates two in which the malady presented itself in healthy young women, the prominent symptoms being the classical ones of nasal voice and dysphagia. There was no preceding inflammation and no diphtheria. The absence of facial paralysis excluded the theory of an affection of the seventh pair. (It will be remembered that this nerve gives off in its passage through the petrous bone twigs distributed to the palatal muscles.) No mesocephalic or bulbar affection could be determined. Lecocq called the clinical condition " essential paralysis of the soft palate" due to neuritis starting in the nerve fibres themselves without any extension from a neighboring organ. Medication and the continuous current were without effect, but the interrupted current led to a surprisingly quick recovery. Anæsthesia, with or without loss of muscular power, is sometimes seen in ordinary cases of hemiplegia. Anæsthesia alone would suggest a lesion situated towards the posterior part of the brain.

There is undoubtedly a palatal paralysis due to non-diphtheritic anginas. This proposition was first submitted by Gubler, and later maintained by Bourges,' who saw a case of angina in a child of seven years in which bacteriological examination of the throat failed to show either Klebs-Loeffler bacilli or streptococci. Two weeks after the throat had cleared, there occurred convergent strabismus, nasal intonation with dysphagia, and finally incomplete paraplegia lasting one month. Recovery finally ensued. Paralysis has also been noted after influenza.

The chief causes of paralysis are diphtheria, degeneration of the nuclei in the medulla, pressure on the nerves of the medulla, and neoplasms pressing on the base of the brain. In all conditions of paralysis, the palate hangs more or less flaccid, and is not raised in either phonation or in breathing. The simplest test is to have the patient utter a vowel sound of high pitch. In normal states, the action of the levatores is strongly marked and clearly visible. Reflex stimulation will also prove of service in determining the amount of loss of muscular power.

In these cases, all the vowel sounds have the twang which only the "n" and "ng" sounds should have. In addition, the failure to shut off the nasopharynx in forcing air through the mouth to pronounce "p" and "b" makes of these "f" and "v" respectively.

In cases of paralysis of one vocal cord, the palate on the same side is apt to be more or less affected, and occasionally there is a partial loss of power on the same side of the tongue with more or less atrophy. This symptom complex is especially to be referred to lesions of the anterior part of the medulla. As the conditions of the cord and tongue are manifestly due to lesions of the higher fibres of the spinal accessory and of the hypoglossal trunk, Hughlings Jackson, who was the first to call attention to the association of these three paralyses, was led to believe that the palate received its innervation through one of these nerves.

A mild form of clonic spasm is sometimes seen in connection with severe but simple inflammation of the parts. Also in the later stages of paralysis agitans there may be in the palate movements similar to those in the limbs.

In cases of diphtheria the paralysis may come on early (second week), but is more often seen from one to three weeks after the throat has become clear. The subject is fully discussed in Vol. XVII. of the "Twentieth Century Practice" in the article on Diphtheria.

As to the *treatment* of all forms of palatal paralysis, it may be said that tonics such as iron, arsenic, strychnine, and phosphorus are indicated, together with the employment of the faradic or, in case of loss of response thereto, the galvanic current. Many cases are due to incurable lesions of the central nerve axis, and these, of course, are but little if at all benefited. Those due to diphtheria generally recover, but long-continued treatment is often necessary. Semi-solid food is to be preferred, and the possibility of foreign-body pneumonia from the passage of ingesta into the air tubes must not be forgotten.

Tumors of the Soft Palate and Uvula.

Some idea of the relative frequency of tumors in the general region of the oropharynx may be obtained from the figures of Moritz Schmidt. Out of 33,997 patients examined in the course of ten years in a general nose and throat practice, he found the following: fibroma, 3; papilloma, 40; cyst, 1; polypus of the tonsil, 5; sarcoma, 3, carcinoma, 1.

Benign Growths.

An enumeration of benign growths of the uvula includes papilloma (the most common), fibroma, lipoma, angioma, and adenoma. All of these may also affect the palate proper. (For a valuable bibliography, the reader may consult a paper by P. Good' in the *Archives Internationales de Laryngologie.*) Many of these growths are so small that their presence is not noted by the patient, and they may only accidentally come under the notice of the physician.

Papillomata commonly spring from the edge of the palate or uvula, and are generally anterior. Their cause is not definitely known, perhaps it may be the constant irritation from food and the attrition of opposing surfaces. One or two instances of apparent papilloma have seemed from their early recurrence, and have been found from later microscopical examination, to be true malignant growths.

Fibromata are far less common, in fact quite unusual. Bosworth notes in his treatise the histories of seven occurring on the tonsils, and the same number in the oropharynx. A few have been reported by other writers. Hardly any have been strictly confined to the soft palate, but have occupied the common ground of the palate and the sides of the pharynx.

Lipomata have been reported by Schmidt and Farlow. Their nature would hardly be suspected from their appearance. According to their consistency they would probably suggest either a cyst or fibrous growth.

Four cases of *angiomata* have been reported. In a case noted by W. C. Phillips, the enlarged vessels extended from the uvula up on to the soft palate, causing sufficient difficulty in swallowing to interfere with the patient's nutrition.

Adenomata of the palate are not uncommon, and quite a list of cases is given in all special treatises. Most of them have occurred between the ages of twenty and fifty, and have been twice as numerous in women as in men. The writer has seen one case of adenofibroma of the left side of the soft palate in a man of fifty years. These tumors grow slowly, and are troublesome mainly in consequence of mechanical interference with the palatal functions.

A case of *cyst* of the base of the right posterior faucial pillar has been reported by Jonathan Wright. Examination showed both outer and inner walls covered with squamous epithelium. No glands or lymphoid tissue were noted. It was regarded as an inclusion cyst.

The *treatment* of all the foregoing is purely a matter of surgery.

Some of the smaller tumors can be readily snipped or snared off. In the case of the angiomata the ideal method would seem to be removal with the galvanocautery snare slowly tightened so as to prevent bleeding. In some of the larger masses an extensive dissection may be necessary in order to enucleate the growth completely.

Malignant Growths.

The two varieties of malignant growths generally met with in the palate are sarcoma and carcinoma. Of *sarcoma* Bosworth cites twenty cases, and a few additional ones have been reported each year since his report. The affection seems to manifest itself at an earlier period of life than when occurring in the pharynx proper. All varieties of sarcoma are included in the published records. Growth is as a rule slow. Symptoms first show themselves in the impairment of palatal function and dysphagia. Unless early ulceration occurs, pain is not a prominent feature. In certain cases the growth has seemed to start from the posterior surface of the soft palate and, as it has increased, has come to overhang the larynx and to cause suffocative attacks. Pharyngeal secretion is increased, and from the ulcerated surface, if such be present, there is added the foul discharge characteristic of such growths elsewhere. Bleeding is not common, though Elliott reports one case in which sudden death occurred from hemorrhage. Until the growth invades neighboring structures adenopathy is generally wanting.

In making the diagnosis of a suspected case, iodide of potassium should always be given to exclude the possibility of syphilis. The iodide will frequently diminish the size of the inflammatory zone which often surrounds the malignant mass without producing any effect upon the latter itself. The tumor may be encapsulated or diffuse. Its usually slow growth in this situation renders the differential diagnosis from fibroma practically impossible without the microscope, but the latter tumor is rare at this site.

In the light of statistics and of modern surgery much is to be hoped for from early or even late operation, for sarcoma of the palate does not seem to be especially malignant, at least so far as rapidity of growth is concerned. This favoring circumstance has been referred to the scanty development of lymphatics in this region. Each case must be attacked along the lines suggested by the individual problem. In those cases so extensively diffused over neighboring parts that removal by surgical methods is impossible, we may obtain benefit, even entire absorption, by the injection of the toxins of the Bacillus prodigiosus and of erysipelas according to the plan worked out by Coley and others. A notable success in this direction was obtained by W. B. Johnson.' Other workers following the same procedures have met with entire failure. The plan is certainly worthy of trial in inoperable cases.

As regards *carcinoma*, Bosworth's statistics given in 1892 comprised thirty cases. Since that time we have noted additional cases published by Katzenstein, Walker Downie, Lennox Browne, Mourie, and Gervaert. As with carcinoma in general, the malady is more common in the later decades of life, and almost without exception the cases have occurred in men. The growth shows an inclination to confine itself to the palate, and begins probably in the epithelial structures of the muciparous follicles, thence infiltrating irregularly and ulcerating early. In the cases of Downie and Browne the growth began in the uvula. Extension of the disease is most frequent in the direction of the faucial pillars. Early symptoms are a loss of flexibility in palatal movements with consequent impairment of swallowing and of clearness of speech. Pain comes on early, and is severe. Later are added foul discharge from the ulceration, hemorrhage, and cachexia. Adenopathy may be absent until a very late period in the disease. Occasionally dyspnœa is present, and in some instances it has been so severe as to require tracheotomy.

A differential diagnosis between sarcoma and carcinoma is not always easy in the absence of microscopical examination. A circumscribed mass, slowly spreading, of soft consistency, and rarely ulcerating, points to the former, while the opposite conditions suggest the latter. As regards glandular involvement some doubt may exist, for in both affections this may or may not appear early, provided the disease remains confined to the palate.

Prognosis is unfavorable, though surgical intervention may prolong life or at least render it more comfortable. The parts should be kept clean with deodorizing antiseptic washes, and anodynes local and general must be employed. Cocaine may be used to render swallowing less painful. Here also the new remedy orthoform is of service. It should be applied previous to the taking of food, preferably in mucilaginous suspension.

Syphilis of the Uvula and Soft Palate.

The general topic of syphilis is fully discussed in Vol. XVII. of the present system. It may not be out of place, however, to enumerate here the several lesions of the disease which may show themselves at this special site. While they are rarely confined thereto, it is here that they can be examined with the greatest ease.

The primary lesion is most frequent on the tonsils, next on the soft palate. Modes of infection are kissing, use of infected pipes and other articles, especially drinking-cups, and unnatural practices. For many unusual modes of infection, the reader may consult L. D. Bulkley's work on syphilis in the innocent.[19]

Faucial erythema is a manifestation of the so-called secondary period, and appears at any time from six to sixteen weeks (more or less) after the initial lesion. The mucosa becomes of a purplish-red color, which seems to be mainly due to passive congestion. The appearance is generally symmetrical, reaching off to both sides, but the congested area is sharply separated from the surrounding surfaces, especially at the junction of the hard and soft palate. Sometimes the median line of the palate is clear, and the erythema is situated on both sides, giving rise to the "Dutch-garden" symmetry mentioned by Jonathan Hutchinson. Such a situation and demarcation of the erythema at once suggest specific disease, but these features alone do not make a positive diagnosis. Coincidently we may have an erythema of the skin, or the dermic lesion may present papular features.

The mucous patch may occur during any stage of specific disease, though it is vastly more common in the earlier weeks. It poisons the saliva so that it is really the most contagious form of the secondary lesions. Unless it is carefully treated, it and a portion of the surrounding membrane may become infiltrated and later may ulcerate.

The gummy tumor is the distinctive feature of the tertiary stage. A favorite site is the posterior surface of the soft palate. Later it breaks down, leaving perforations of the soft palate and various ulcerating surfaces, which when they heal lead to the usual deformities of the oropharynx. Large areas may be destroyed, leaving strings of tissue stretching from one part to another. Bleeding from eroded vessels is possible though not common. As a result of the new physical conditions regurgitation of fluids into the nose is frequent, and the soft palate may become adherent to the posterior wall of the pharynx. This adhesion is generally incomplete, for in the seemingly complete cases careful search will reveal a minute opening into the nasopharynx. Gummata do not develop as a rule until five years after the initial lesion, and those on the posterior surface of the soft palate may for a very long time escape notice.

The *symptoms* of all these specific lesions of the palate at first may closely resemble those of a simple catarrhal inflammation with at times some febrile reaction. Many cases come to light in patients who consult a physican for a supposed simple "sore throat." Swollen glands, thick tenacious secretion, difficulties in speech and in swallowing may all be present. In the tertiary stages swallowing may be very painful. The important point is to regard with suspicion all cases which do not yield to simple remedies for the usual catarrhal lesions, although there may be no history or discoverable lesions of syphilitic disease.

Treatment should consist of the classical use of mercurials and iodides with mouth washes. For active processes in the palate the use of the ordinary black wash or bichloride solutions (1:3,000) has given in the writer's experience as good results as those obtained from some of the more modern combinations. For cleansing ulcerating surfaces of secretion peroxide of hydrogen diluted with lime water may be used, followed by an alkaline gargle, and the application to the surface of some stimulating caustic. Nitrate of silver should be used on each mucous patch, and perforations if recent can sometimes be healed by the persistent use of mono- or trichloracetic acid fused on a probe. All alcohol, tobacco, and irritant foods should be interdicted. In the worst cases cocaine applications may precede taking of food, and orthoform may be dusted upon the painful areas. Various surgical procedures have been suggested to prevent and remove when formed the palatal adhesions, but a discussion of these plans is outside the province of the present article.

Tuberculosis of the Uvula and Soft Palate.

The general subject of tuberculosis is elsewhere considered. The object of the present paragraph is briefly to call attention to the more common manifestations of the disease as it affects the palate and uvula.

Pharyngeal tuberculosis occurs in about one per cent. of all tuberculous cases encountered in general medical practice. In the vast majority of cases it is secondary, although it may not be possible at the time of diagnosis to detect tuberculous deposits in other parts of the body. Gradually accumulating evidence, however, makes it certain that there is such a thing as primary tuberculosis of the throat. The uvula and soft palate are favorite seats of this local process. In fourteen cases of pharyngeal tuberculosis reported by Wroblewski, the faucial pillars were affected in all, and the uvula in ten. For some reason not fully understood, the right side of the throat is the one most frequently involved. This may be due to the peculiarities of lymphatic distribution.

Causes.—The general causes of tuberculosis in this situation are those of the dyscrasia in general. The surprising thing is that we do not more often find the local lesions here developed. The exposed situation would seem to favor infection. The buccal secretions may possess some germicidal power, and, as it has been phrased, render the surface of the mucosa immune. In the majority of cases, as noted above, the attack on the palate is secondary. Here the lymphatics are the channel of infection, but the latter may be by direct inoculation. Any irritation to which the part may be subjected increases liability to infection. Local irritation from diseased teeth may act in this way. The theory that infection occurs from contact with tuberculous sputa brought up from below is not now accepted.

Pathology.—As regards the *macroscopical* appearance of the lesion at this site, Kafeman has distinguished two forms, the miliary tubercle which is universally distributed, and the papular form which may be restricted to one or two patches, and is especially apt to be distributed on the posterior surface of the soft palate. The minute structure of each is essentially a small round-celled infiltration of the connective-tissue elements, followed later by an extension of the same process into the vessel walls. Then ensue in turn lessened calibre from obliterating arteritis, cheesy softening, and ulceration. Tubercle bacilli are, of course, the exciting factor, but it may be difficult to find them in scrapings from ulcerated surfaces, or even in bits of tissue removed for examination. The same may be said of the giant cell. To the eye, the uvula and palate seem to be studded with small whitish points apparently beneath the surface, and showing through the mucosa. In the primary cases, the affection is apt to assume the form of a fringe of small excrescences along the anterior pillars.

Later the deposits break down and form the tuberculous ulcer with its reddish worm-eaten-like edge, and possibly a localized periœdema. These broken-down areas, though individually small, may coalesce so that finally the ulcerating surface becomes quite large. The uvula and palate may escape these changes for a long time after they have appeared in the pharynx proper. When the uvula is involved it is apt to become very œdematous and exquisitely tender and painful. While the typical tuberculous ulcer is a shallow one, it must not be forgotten that the destruction may extend deeply and lead even to perforation of the soft palate. Cases of this nature have been reported by Talamon and Grossard.

Symptoms.—In addition to the general features of tuberculosis the most marked symptom in the condition we are considering is painful swallowing, early and marked. Along with this are alterations of palatal function, cough, etc. The patient complains most of all of the odynphagia. Owing to the distress occasioned by taking food, he is apt to avoid it as long as possible, and emaciation is thus hurried. Cervical adenopathy is a late feature.

Diagnosis.—The coexistence of tuberculosis elsewhere will, of course, direct our attention to the possibly tuberculous nature of any ulceration occurring on the palate, but it must not be forgotten that an additional dyscrasia may at the same time be present. The most common one is syphilis, and when there is an absence of evidence of involvement of other organs, it may be extremely difficult to make an early diagnosis. We are to call to our aid the information furnished by the effects of antisyphilitic treatment, and that offered by the examination of scrapings from the ulcerated surface. Bosworth regards as the principal features of the tuberculous ulcer its flush surface, covering of ropy mucus, and the uniform color of the ulcerated area, and of the surrounding mucosa. He suggests the following differential signs:

Syphilis.	*Tubercle.*
Deep excavation.	No apparent excavation.
Bright red, angry-looking areola.	Areola wanting.
Sharp-cut edges.	No sharply defined edges.
Bright yellow purulent discharge, abundant.	Grayish, thick, semi-opaque mucous discharges scanty.
Rapid destruction.	Slow erosion.
Deep extension.	Lateral extension.
No dyscrasia or fever.	Marked constitutional symptoms with high fever.

Treatment.—In addition to the general tonic and hygienic treatment of tuberculosis, a vigorous effort should be made to keep the patient as comfortable as possible even though he should steadily deteriorate. Climatic changes do not seem to be of much avail in this manifestation of tuberculosis. All sources of buccal irritation should be removed, and while a large variety of food may be allowed, it should all be soft and pultaceous in consistence. In bad cases, it may be necessary to "gulp" the food in order to get as much down as possible with a minimum exercise of the muscles of deglutition. Some patients can swallow more easily when lying on the stomach on a couch and drawing nourishment through a tube from a vessel placed on a lower level.

As soon as a positive diagnosis is made, all diseased tissue should, if possible, be removed. The plan most in vogue at the present time consists in curetting, and then rubbing in lactic acid in increasing strength. We may commence with a ten-per-cent. solution, and gradually run up to full strength. The raw surfaces should be regularly cleansed with hydrogen peroxide, and then some antiseptic dusting-powder applied. Iodoform, aristol, iodol, europhen are all applicable. Menthol in olive oil (twenty per cent.) has its advocates, but is not so much used now as formerly. Applications of morphine with tannic acid are strongly recommended. For the relief of odynphagia we may use cocaine, but its employment should be deferred as long as possible. Orthoform finds here a particularly valuable field. In order to insure its contact with the parts as long as possible, it is well to use the following formula devised by Freudenthal:

℞ Menthol,	. . . .	10.0
Ol. amyg. exp.,	. . . .	30.0
Vitelli ovi.	. . . .	30.0
Orthoform.	. . . .	12.5
Aq. dest.,	. . . . . .	q.s. ad 100.0

If the powder is insufflated it may be combined with zinc stearate or bismuth subcarbonate. It is distinctly analgesic, and seems devoid of poisonous properties. A few cases, however, are on record in which, after its extensive application to wounds, headache has resulted with fever, nausea, and dusky erythematous patches over various areas. Von Leyden has given it internally up to a daily dosage of 1.5 gm. without deleterious effects. For the cough a new remedy called heroin is now much used. It is a derivative of morphine, and is used in doses of gr. $\frac{1}{12}$ every three or four hours. It has all the good effects of morphine with a minimum of its disadvantages.

Lupus of the Uvula and Soft Palate.

The relation between lupus and tuberculosis has been a matter of much discussion. At present, Marty's dictum that the former is an attenuated tuberculosis meets with general consent. Most cases occurring in the area under discussion are met with in the second and third decades of life. The malady generally begins in the skin, and after a very variable period appears in the fauces, the buccal surface of the soft palate being the site first attacked. It may start on the free edge or in the body of the uvula itself.

The disease here presents the usual infiltration, leading to the nodules which cause great thickening of the part. The whole palate becomes changed into a lumpy, irregular curtain with the bulbous uvula projecting from its middle. Later comes the peculiar ulceration or wasting away of the tissue, not attended with purulent discharge or necrotic change, but with a gradual disappearance of the previously existing masses. Healing may occur at some points synchronous with an extension of the disease at others. As long as the disease is confined to the uvula and palate, there are hardly any subjective symptoms except in the later stages when dysphagia may supervene, to disappear when cicatrization has taken place. Naturally the functions of the palate are more or less impaired. Later cicatricial changes may lead to the same annoyances as are mentioned under the head of syphilis.

Treatment includes the use of various caustics, curetting, lactic acid, and possibly the excision of the affected tissue. Remedies of the tuberculin class have helped in some cases, but they are in no wise a specific. General tonic treatment should be systematically carried out.

Bibliographical References.

1. Henke : Monatsschrift für Ohrenheilkunde, July, 1898.

2. Somers : New York Medical Journal, November 21, 1896.

3. Newcomb : The Laryngoscope, April, 1897.

4. Hoen : Journal of Experimental Medicine, vol. iii., p. 551.

5. Morgan : Transactions of the American Laryngological Association, 1886.

6. Bosworth : A Treatise on Diseases of the Nose and Throat, New York, 1892.

7. Bourges : Annales des Maladies de l'Oreille, vol. xxi., 1895.

8. Good : Archives Internationales de Laryngologie, vol. x., 1898.

9. Johnson : Medical Record, November 17, 1894.

10. Bulkley : Syphilis Insontium, New York, 1894.

NEURAL AND MENTAL DEFECTS IN CHILDHOOD.

BY

FRANCIS WARNER,

LONDON.

NEURAL AND MENTAL DEFECTS IN CHILDHOOD.

CHILDREN of school age, *i.e.*, between three and thirteen years of age, form one-fourth part of the population of England, and perhaps a still larger proportion of the clients of medical men in practice. It is not my purpose to add to the classical descriptions of neural diseases, but rather to consider in the light of modern scientific investigation certain types or groups of children as they come before us, classed by certain conditions the signs of which we may observe, while studying their descriptions, together with certain points in neural physiology, diagnosis, pathology, etiology, prognosis, and treatment.

Children and young persons in whom there is no disease come under professional notice, for their parents, guardians, and teachers need advice from the physician as to their mental and physical care and training. Plants to be well grown need some supervision from the scientific horticulturist as well as the care of the gardener and his attendant laborers, and many neural and mental conditions of childhood claim careful study as to management. It will here only be possible to give a sketch of the studies upon which the principles of clinical description of the signs observed and the groups of children are based; for further details and experience the reader is referred to other treatises.* The facts given and the value of the signs described are largely drawn from my observations of one hundred thousand children examined individually in schools (1888-94).

In studying both neural and mental defects we are dealing alike with the brain and its modes of action. After ophthalmoscopic study, the simplest signs observable are the motor acts, and the balance or muscular tone of certain parts of the body—movements and postures or attitudes, spontaneous, imitated, or reflex.

---

* See the Author's "Mental Faculty." Cambridge University Press, England; also "Report on the Scientific Study of the Mental and Physical Conditions of Childhood, with particular reference to Children of Defective Constitutions." Published by a Committee, 72 Margaret Street, London, W.

NERVE SIGNS.

Neural defects may be studied by observation and description of "nerve signs" corresponding to the smallest brain areas clinically observable. They may be spontaneous, or elicited by stimulation through the eye, the ear, or otherwise; and may be normal or abnormal. As regards the smallest brain areas, their action is probably indicated by single movements of the smallest parts of the body, *e.g.*, separate digits, and the muscles of facial expression. Movements may also occur in groups, while the serial succession of movements observed may indicate coördination or incoördination. Mental signs will be discussed later.

The clinical study of movements affords the readiest means, almost the only means, of studying brain action,* which in children who have not yet acquired the faculty of accurate verbal expression must necessarily be conducted independently of their replies to our questions, and must mainly be based upon the signs we see in them. I therefore pass on at once to describe certain "abnormal nerve signs" by which we may judge of any neural defects present and the status of brain action. The face, with its many small muscles acting in various groups, is a most accurate index of the brain action and its nerve centres. It is convenient to divide this region into three zones: the frontal above the line of the eyebrows, and a middle zone separated from the lower by a horizontal line at the level of the lower margin of the orbits. The most frequent indications of defective action are seen in the frontal region.

Frontal Muscles Overacting.—These muscles usually act symmetrically, at the same time, and in similar degree; their action produces horizontal creases in the forehead, which may be deep if they act strongly. Sometimes the muscles are seen working in vermicular fashion, with an athetoid movement; in other cases the action is fine, producing minute creases, so that the skin of the forehead is thus rendered dull. This sign may be seen in children from the earliest infancy upwards. The action may be temporary. It is often more quiet when the child is at work or interested, its subsidence corresponding to a state of quiet mental attention. Of 583 boys and 145 girls with this sign, I found 16.4 per cent. of the boys and 21.7 per cent. of the girls pale, thin, or delicate; while 41.4 per cent. of the boys and 46.2 per cent. of the girls were reported as dull pupils.

Corrugation, or knitting of the eyebrows, is due to overaction or hypertonicity of the corrugator muscles drawing the eyebrows to-

---

* See "Physical Expression," International Scientific Series.

gether and making vertical creases; they may act coarsely or finely, producing dulness in this region. Corrugation may be associated with an athetoid action of the frontal muscles, producing a mass of vertical and horizontal creases. This sign alone is often associated with a status of mental stress which may be discovered on further inquiry. Of 105 boys and 22 girls with corrugation, 22.6 per cent. of the boys and 15 per cent. of the girls were delicate, while 45.7 per cent. of the boys and 52.5 per cent. of the girls were dull pupils.

Orbicularis Oculi Relaxed.—In the strong and well-toned face of a child the lower eyelid appears clean cut and well moulded, so that the rotundity of the eyeball is seen through it. When this muscle is relaxed and toneless the skin of the lower lid bulges forward and is baggy—this is removed on smiling or laughing. The relaxed condition is indicative of fatigue and exhaustion; it commonly accompanies recurrent headaches and may appear or disappear quickly. Weak balance in the hand often accompanies this sign. Of 361 boys and 224 girls with this sign, 21.4 per cent. of the boys and 32.6 per cent. of the girls were delicate, while 39.8 per cent. of the boys and 46 per cent. of the girls were dull pupils.

Grinning or Over-Smiling.—This is usually symmetrical, but may be unequal on the two sides of the face; the muscular action widens the mouth and increases the naso-labial groove, which may be duplicate. As a sign of defect it may occur without any change in the general expression and be exactly uniform in repetition on any stimulation, or may be spontaneous. Normal smiling is often accompanied by an increased color due to vasomotor relaxation and spreads all over the face. Of 52 boys and 27 girls with this sign, 18.8 per cent. of the boys and 25.5 per cent. of the girls were delicate, while 56.5 per cent. of the boys and 60.4 per cent. of the girls were dull mentally.

Mouth Open.—Some children stand with their mouth open, the jaw being drooped. This must not be considered a nerve sign unless you are sure it depends upon muscular relaxation, and not upon obstruction of the nasopharyngeal passages. Habitual drooping of the jaw depends upon want of tone in muscles supplied by the fifth cranial nerve; of this I shall speak again in referring to tooth-grinding. Of 107 boys and 38 girls with open mouth, 30.5 per cent. of the boys and ·34 per cent. of the girls were delicate; while 50.6 per cent. of the boys and 52.5 per cent. of the girls were dull.

The child's hand, when held out free and not mechanically restrained, affords in the movements of its parts, and in their balance, other valuable indications of the status of brain.

On the average, in normal children, the hands when held out in front of them at the word of command are pronated, with both upper extremities horizontal on a level with the shoulders; the metacarpal bones and the digits being all in the same plane. Two typical departures from this normal posture will serve our purpose.

Hand Balance Weak.—The wrist being drooped or flexed, the metacarpus is slightly arched or contracted laterally, while the digits are moderately flexed. The type may vary, the thumb only drooping. This posture in a limb not strongly innervated is seen in hemiplegia, in exhausted children, and during sleep, if the arm be held out by the shirt sleeve. Of 375 boys and 196 girls showing this hand balance 16 per cent. of the boys and 21.2 per cent. of the girls were delicate, while 40 per cent. of the boys and 35.3 per cent. of the girls were dull.

Hand Balance Nervous.—Here again the wrist is drooped or flexed and the metacarpus is slightly arched laterally, but the thumb is extended backwards, while the fingers at the knuckle joints are overextended, usually with some flexion of the internodal joints. The elements in this type of posture may vary in the amount of contraction of the palm of the hand, and in one or more fingers only being extended at the knuckles. This balance is usually seen in slight cases of chorea, and in children who are weak but excitable. Of 253 boys and 205 girls with this balance 20.1 per cent. of the boys and 30.6 per cent. of the girls were delicate, while 34.3 per cent. of the boys and 32.9 per cent. of the girls were dull.

Finger twitches may be seen when the hands are held out for inspection; the twitching movements may be either in flexion and extension, or lateral as produced by the small interossei muscles. It is noteworthy that while twitching fingers are about twice as frequent in boys as in girls, chorea is much more frequent in the female sex. Among 202 boys and 99 girls with finger twitches 20.2 per cent. of the boys and 36.4 per cent. of the girls were delicate, while 32.1 per cent. of the boys and 29.8 per cent. of the girls were dull pupils.

Head Balance.—In the normal condition the head balance is erect and symmetrical; it may be drooped or inclined to one side, or both. The balance was not erect and symmetrical in 151 boys and 178 girls; among whom 21 per cent. of the boys and 34.1 per cent. of the girls were delicate, while 44.2 per cent. of the boys and 45.4 per cent. of the girls were dull pupils.

Lordosis.—This arching forward of the lumbar spine and falling back of the dorsal portion is due to weakness of the spinal muscles. When the child holds out his hands in front the centre of gravity of the body is moved forward; in a strong child this is not followed by marked change of posture in the spine, but in a weak child lordosis may result, often with temporary lateral curvature and unequal balance of the shoulders, while the head is thrown back. Of 92 boys and 107 girls with lordosis 19.5 per cent. of the boys and 31.1 per cent. of the girls were delicate, while 38.9 per cent. of the boys and 30.5 per cent. of the girls were dull.

The more general and widely used indications of the brain status of a child are modes of brain action indicated and described by combinations and series of acts; their coördination and definite control through the senses. Of this class of nerve signs the following may be described:

Expression of Face.—After describing the action and tone of the facial muscles, there is still left a facial expression which baffles anatomical description, and which may be distinctly good and indicative of intelligence and mental action even in a face coarsely moved by the muscles; such is often seen in facial chorea. Defective facial expression was seen in 493 boys and 329 girls; of these 27.5 per cent. of the boys and 30.8 per cent. of the girls were delicate, while 53.1 per cent. of the boys and 53.3 per cent. of the girls were dull mentally.

General Balance Defective.—This may be indicated by asymmetry of attitude; the head, shoulders, and spine may be asymmetrically balanced, while the hands when held out are at different levels, and often the left is lower and more nearly approaches the weak type than the right; the feet may also be asymmetrically planted on the ground. Of 138 boys and 86 girls with such defective action 23.3 per cent. of the boys and 32.3 per cent. of the girls were delicate, while 49.2 per cent. of the boys and 41.5 per cent. of the girls were dull pupils.

Over-Mobile.—Constant spontaneous movement; a semi-choreic condition. Among children under seven years of age spontaneous movement is normal, especially in hands and fingers.

Children statuesque or immobile, without action except under some stimulation and wanting in spontaneity.

Response in Action Defective, Slow, or Inaccurate.—This may follow the word of command through stimulation by hearing or imitation of movements through the eye; one mode of control may act better than the other. Of these cases 69 boys and 38 girls, 25.8 per cent. of the boys and 30.3 per cent. of the girls were delicate; while 66.9 per cent. of the boys and 69.6 per cent. of the girls were dull mentally.

Speech Defective.—Speech may be absent with deafness or the child may be mute. As a mental defect, the question asked may be repeated without any reply. There may be stuttering (spasm), or defect of utterance due, not to neural defect, but to postpharyngeal growth. All forms of defect of palate, except cleft, are, I believe, consistent with good speech. Of 30 boys and 44 girls with defect of speech 8.5 per cent. of the boys and 18.5 per cent. of the girls were delicate, while 23.2 per cent. of the boys and 61.4 per cent. of the girls were dull.

Eye Movements.—When a small object is held two feet in front of the face and slowly moved in various directions, some children follow it not by movements of their eyes, but with the head, keeping the eyes fixed. In other cases fixation of the eyes is defective; they may wander irregularly, without fixing on any object indicated. Such is commonly. seen in chorea and in nervous subjects. Of 500 boys and 298 girls with defective eye movements 16.2 per cent. of the boys and 30.9 per cent. of the girls were delicate, while 41.1 per cent. of the boys and 45.7 per cent. of the girls were dull mentally.

Nystagmus, or tremor of the eyes, is almost always symmetrical; in children it is not at all necessarily accompanied by any other neural defect or by mental deficiency.

CLINICAL EXAMINATION OF THE NEURAL AND MENTAL CONDITION OF CHILDREN.

I usually let the child stand before me, and after recording any defects in development of the body and physiognomical details, proceed to observe modes of nerve-muscular action and describe any defects. It is well to proceed systematically and commence by noting the action produced by the cranial motor nerves. The third, fourth, and sixth nerves are concerned with eye movements, the examination of which has been dealt with. The size and reaction of the pupils should be examined, and it should be remembered that the pupil is minutely contracted in sleep, while a widely expanded and mobile pupil is common in the status of mental excitement. While observing the face it is convenient to fix the child's eyes by directing him to look at a small object held in the examiner's hand, thus preventing him from looking at his eyes. The zones of the face should be observed separately, as well as the expression of the face as a whole. Especially should we look for symmetry of action at the angles of the mouth in the movements of smiling and speaking; this region is most affected in chorea and in hemiplegia as well as in the grinning of imbeciles. The fifth cranial nerve, in its motor division, supplies the masseters and temporal muscles which approximate the jaws, while the pterygoids produce lateral movements. If both sets of muscles act together, tooth-grinding results, and if this has frequently occurred some of the teeth will probably be found ground or flat at their tips. It should be remembered that sensory fibres of the fifth nerve are supplied to the meninges. Tooth-grinding usually indicates a brain restless during sleep when its motor functions as well as its mental activities should be in abeyance. The same nerve-muscular apparatus is relaxed in drooping of the jaw as after a mental shock; also in biting, a bad habit not uncommon among imbecile and defective children. The hypoglossal nerve is examined when the tongue is protruded; the tongue may also be inspected as it lies on the floor of the mouth within the line of the teeth while the mouth is open for inspection. The action of the tongue may be jerky, and its muscular fibres may contract irregularly as in chorea; it may be seen in spasm as will be described in speaking of stammering. The examiner should have the child hold out his hands, and should look for normal action and coördination in finger movements, or any of the nerve-signs described, observing the exactness of imitation of movements performed by him and relations in the time of action in either hand; one side of the brain may act more slowly and feebly than the other. The hands also should be noticed as they hang by the sides; spontaneous finger twitches may be seen in the limb when it is not strongly innervated. In conducting such examination we should proceed in a regular manner. The surroundings of the child should be as natural as possible; we should not touch him and must observe him without speaking much; the aim is to see how the nerve system acts under an ordinary environment. It is necessary in placing a value on the nerve signs seen to consider the age of the child; under six or seven years constant mobility, especially of the digits, eyes, and small parts, is more clearly an indication of the normal than is coördinated action.

In a healthy infant we find movements in all parts when the brain is in full functional activity; the digits move separately, and their movements are slower than in adults, but at the earliest ages they are not controlled through the senses.* As age and cerebral evolution advance, periods of inhibition of such movement occur temporarily on any strong stimulation of sight or sound—the child is said to look at the object quietly or to attend to the sound. This period of inhibition of spontaneous movement may be followed by coördinated action, the child seizes the object presented within its view. Similarly, till say seven years or upwards, much spontaneity of movement is characteristic of healthy brain action. At older ages this is replaced by longer periods of coördinated action and mental acts.

When neural or mental defects are found in a child, their significance and prognosis are rendered more clear by examination of cranial and bodily development. When congenital defects in growth and in the proportional development of parts of the body are ap-

---

* See "Anatomy of Movement: a Treatise on the Action of Nerve-Centres and Modes of Growth," by the Author.

parent, the prognosis as to neural status is more grave; as also concerning the child's viability and physical health.

Grouping as "developmental defect cases" children with defect of cranium, palate, ears, and the features, or any of the forty-two such signs defined and enumerated in the report of the committee referred to, we find among the 2,308 boys and 1,618 girls with such defects 38.4 per cent. of the boys and 36.3 per cent. of the girls with abnormal nerve signs; 16.2 per cent. of the boys and 26.5 per cent. of the girls pale, thin, delicate; while 38.4 per cent. of the boys and 44.9 per cent. of the girls were mentally dull or backward. Such corelations vary with the different individual defects. There are two important facts concerning these "developmental defect cases:" they are more frequent among boys than girls; when, however, girls present such defects they are more apt than boys to be delicate. Vital statistics show that infant mortality falls principally on the boys, and largely under the headings "premature birth" and "congenital defects," both of which are commoner with the males. Such cases when they survive are, as shown above, predisposed to delicate health, nerve disturbance, and mental dulness.

Of all the developmental defects "cranial abnormalities" appear as the most numerous and the most important. A well-developed child at nine months has a head circumference of seventeen and a half inches; at twelve months, nineteen inches; at seven years, twenty to twenty-one inches. Heads may be too large, bossed in either frontal region or elsewhere; ridged vertically in the forehead or at the sutures, while the forehead may be otherwise ill-formed. All these conditions are more common in males. On the other hand, "small head" appears to be more than twice as frequent among girls as compared with boys. Such children are often small and delicate but by no means necessarily dull mentally.

The signs of health should be looked for in examination of the lungs, heart, skin, glands, and digestive apparatus. The mouth deserves special attention as to palate and tongue and teeth; the fauces and freedom of the nasopharyngeal passages should be examined. I have found that defect of palate and pharyngeal adenoid often coexist. The hearing and sight should be tested.

It is very desirable to make a complete clinical examination of the child before concluding that neural or mental debility depends necessarily upon permanent brain defect.

Mental Examination.

It is desirable to make some mental examination of any child with chronic neural defect or in delicate health. Among children seen to be pale, thin, delicate (boys 749, girls 770), of the boys 47.1 per cent. and of the girls 43.5 per cent. also presented "abnormal nerve signs;" while 43.1 per cent. of the boys and 40.5 per cent. of the girls were dull mentally. Among children with disorderly or tired brains indicated by nerve signs (boys 2,853, girls 2,015), of the boys 12.3 per cent., of the girls 16.6 per cent. were delicate; while 41.8 per cent. of the boys and 42.6 per cent. of the girls were dull.

In examining a child as to mental ability or potentiality, the physician should not rely solely upon questions put to the patient. We want to find out whether the child appreciates number, weight, size, and possesses the faculty of muscular sense, imitation, and power of choice, comparison, and judgment.

It is convenient to place money on the table, telling the child to count the pieces; to sort them and place them in heaps. Note if he count them best as he puts the coins one by one on the pile—*i.e.* counts his own hand movements—or whether he succeeds better as he sees you place them in piles, turning his eyes to each coin as you move it—*i.e.*, counts his eye movements. Can he name or distinguish silver coins placed in his hands, feeling their weights respectively and comparing them without closing his hands (general muscular sense), or must he feel them over with his fingers and appreciate size by movements of his digits (sense of movements of small parts)? Proportional weights—*e.g.*, one-quarter, one-half, one ounce weights—may be used. After training, the child may not only form a judgment as to proportion of weights, but also name a single weight presented—an act of memory and judgment, comparing the weight felt with the impression formerly produced by other weights.

Number may be appreciated solely by eye movements, as in counting the objects in the room by sight; or by assistance of hand movements in pointing out the objects looked at. The sense of temperature may be tested by warming a coin in hot water, then letting the child pick it up, and seeing if he appreciates its warmth.

As higher indications of mental action let him make two heaps of five objects, and place them together, saying the number thus added. I have met with lads who worked out an addition sum in money, but who could not add the coins represented. Multiplication of numbers is a higher mental faculty than addition. With a sheet of stamps or a square of twelve bricks each way, a child may count one row correctly, and add it to the second row, but fail to multiply 12×12 and thus ascertain the number present. This is sometimes found in children who can work their sums mechanically on paper; for memory of figures is sometimes good among those deficient in the sense of number.

Besides mental tests of this kind some faculty of social sense should be looked for, and ability to act correctly in social life. The child's conduct with other children and his treatment of animals are worthy of inquiry. Can he write a letter? What must you get to write a letter? How will you get a stamp if you have a shilling; what change will you receive? How does the letter get to its destination? etc., etc. Let him be asked how he would get home by himself; what he would do under certain circumstances; what it would cost.

Speech and the use of words may be defective. Utterance may be thick and indistinct; in such case the physician should look to the throat and nose as well as to the palate, there may be conditions needing active treatment. Stuttering is often coincident with other defect in the nerve system, and is more common among boys than girls. The condition is due to spasm affecting certain groups of muscles when uttering certain words or syllables and usually recurs in a uniform order. It may be seen first in the forehead producing corrugation between the eyebrows, or in muscles about the mouth. The area of spasm spreads to other muscles in the face, and even to the omohyoid in the neck. The jaw is slightly depressed, so that the tongue may be seen thrown into spasm and vibrating but not moving; sometimes it is concave with the tip elevated. On putting a question to the child, it may be long before the reply comes, or the question may be repeated without a reply. Speaking to the child may be followed by arrest of his movements or by a large number of irregular movements and asymmetrical postures, but by no verbal reply. A healthy young child tends to repeat words said to him, especially if he look at the face of the speaker. The same habit remains at older ages with some defective brains—the question is repeated or imitated without an intelligent answer. In adults a similar bad mental habit is sometimes seen: the question asked is audibly repeated; then comes a period of thinking, it may be accompanied by protrusion of the tongue, inclination of the head, fidgeting of fingers, or other extra movements and later the reply.

We should let the child talk of what he likes to do, his games, the work at school, the stories he reads, his friends, or his pocket money, and as he talks observe the expression of his face, and the movements of his body, or the signs of mental excitement or apathy. His expression of face and of body action may be better than his verbal expression. As we speak to him (auditory stimulus) we may see extra movements, a spreading area of movement; while, when in dumb show we beckon to him, pointing out objects and their parts in a picture (visual stimulus), no such signs of excitement appear; he may be better under control when directed by our action without words.

The vocabulary may be very deficient, but few words having been acquired; this is sometimes due to the child being allowed to point to things wanted instead of asking for them; just as he may become-lazy and backward from having all his wants anticipated.

Deafness is more common among girls, but deaf-mutes are more frequent among boys.

The mental dulness complained of in a child does not necessarily depend upon conditions of primary brain defect, as is illustrated in the following cases. Deafness if unobserved and neglected may lead to much mental dulness as the child passes through his education.

A boy nearly 7 years old was said to be uneducable; he had scarcely any speech, otherwise there were no abnormal nerve signs. He did not respond to a verbal direction, but was evidently deaf to a high degree. His imitation by sight was good, he made all his wants known, behaved well, and was clean. He fixed his eyes steadily, and when he handled objects showed varying expression at sight of them, making choice of what he liked best. The head and body were well developed. His mouth was kept open, he could not breathe with it shut; the tonsils were large, and adenoid growths were present. After surgical treatment he began to regain hearing and acquire speech. Probably there was no organic brain defect causing mental dulness.

A boy 13 years of age, at a private school, was preparing for a higher education; he had learned some Latin and French but was said to be so dull and backward he had to leave the school. His nerve action was fairly good. He could work out a money sum on paper and the money values corresponding with coins. He spoke well, and wrote a good letter. His head and body were well developed. He was very deaf, only hearing the watch at six inches. There was pharyngeal and nasal obstruction, which had been neglected. It may be added that other cases of deafness existed in that family.

A boy, 12 years of age, whom I saw in an elementary school was reported by the teachers as "an idiot who learned nothing." He had a weak balance of hand and spine; his face was wanting in brightness of expression with puffiness under the eyes, all these signs indicating fatigue rather than defect. His speech was good, and he was well developed in head, palate, and body. I saw no signs of organic brain defect, but several indications of exhaustion. On inquiry it appeared that the boy was kept at work after school till midnight.

A girl, 13 years of age, was said to be backward in reading, spelling, and transcription, but not dull at arithmetic. Though in most particulars rather overtrained, she had never been taught to move her eyes; there were slight congenital defects of the retina. Exercises in eye movements for five minutes twice a day were soon followed by good fixation, and an accompanying improvement in accuracy of work and better spelling.

I have seen boys, industrious and not dull at arithmetic, who could not follow a demonstration in Euclid on the blackboard, and on examination found that the pupil always looked at the teacher in place of the figure on the board, trying to remember what was said, but not following the lines of the diagram.

In describing the neural defects met with in children, it is necessary to use terms descriptive of general conditions which may be independent of structural brain changes. The terms used in describing groups of children should indicate exactly the points used as physical signs by which the group is classed or defined, *i.e.*, the single and the more general signs by which nerve-status is here described. Thus the reader, calling to mind the physiological or pathological nerve action corresponding to points in description, obtains an intelligent and scientific aspect of the status of the cases grouped. Following such methods, mental expression, functional nerve status, and neuroses may be the subjects of exact scientific analysis and study, as well as organic diseases tending to death. All attempts at grouping and describing the nerve conditions of children must take into account such a state as fatigue or exhaustion.

Fatigue, or in its further stages, exhaustion, has been shown by physiological experiment to affect the nerve centres before the muscles. After exertion in lifting a weight, when no more work can be done, the muscles still retain their contractile power to a galvanic stimulus. The nerve centres tire before the muscles. This fatigued condition is expressed by modes of muscular action in the face, limbs, and body, both in balance, movement, and defective coördination. The balance of the head, shoulders, and spine, the arms when held out, and the planting of the feet on the ground are often seen to be asymmetrical, while all the movements are slower and coördination of movements is less exact. The tone of facial expression is lessened, and there may be fulness or muscular relaxation under the eyes, while the jaw droops; the hand presents the weak balance described, especially on the left side, that arm being held at a lower level than the right, while the elbows are slightly bent. In brain fatigue the force expended in movements is lessened; at the same time there may be certain irregular and uncontrolled extra movements of face and fingers, while the eyes wander instead of remaining fixed on a given object. The weakened nerve centres send out slight spontaneous discharges, causing many small movements—just as in chorea —and the child is said to be restless, fidgety, and inattentive. Strong stimulus is required through the eye and the ear to produce coördinated action; reflex action may be excessive so that the child starts at sudden sounds, or makes reply to a question not in harmony with what is asked.

The signs of fatigue may be classed thus: (1) Lessened motor power, lessened facial expression and brightness, relaxation of the orbicularis muscles, asymmetry in attitude, head not erect, lordosis, and feeble hand balance. (2) Excess of movement in over-action of frontal muscles and corrugation; irregular eye movements and finger twitches, or general fidgetiness. (3) Slow and inaccurate responses both in movements and in mental action. Less work is accomplished both in writing and in purely mental processes. The voice, as far as it is a muscular act, is lowered and altered and monotonous, while the vocabulary is often limited. The mental power of memory, comparison, and judgment is greatly weakened; mental irritability may be shown by saying or doing the wrong thing under the circumstances. In this state head pain is apt to supervene.

Fatigue may be general or local, as indicated by the physical signs, often affecting the right side of the brain more than the left. Asymmetry is usual in chorea.

In using the term exhaustion, as distinguished from fatigue which may be removed by food, rest, and sleep, I refer to a greater degree of loss of power, applying the term to cases in which the signs given are more permanent, lasting it may be weeks or months. Frequent occurrence of fatigue may be followed by more permanent exhaustion; this, I believe, occurs more commonly in girls than boys. With both sexes, especially in cases with developmental defects of body and low nutrition, neural defects and bad habits of action, at first simply the result of environment, may become permanent.

Headaches.—The complaint is often made of a child that he suffers from recurrent headaches, while we see the signs of exhaustion; further, the association of headaches, chorea, and low nutrition of body is frequently met with. From my records of fifty-eight cases I find twenty-five boys and thirty-three girls from four to fourteen years of age, mostly between six to ten years; their own descriptions of pain and subjective symptoms are imperfect, but five others had distinct disturbance of vision accompanying headaches, the child seeing colors, sparks, or other illusions during the attacks; in all but one of these cases the mother also suffered with headaches. Sleep was generally restless and disturbed by dreams in which the child would cry out, while some were somnambulists. It is necessary to examine the heart in all these cases, and also to look for errors of refraction; it is said that the use of glasses has benefited many of these cases. Such children are usually of the "nervous type."

Nervous children are here considered apart from those with congenital brain defect. They are usually well formed in features and in bodily development, but are often under weight; they not infrequently emaciate considerably and suffer from hacking cough, though the signs over the lungs indicate that they are healthy. These children often suffer from headaches and sleep badly, as stated above; the appetite varies greatly, sometimes failing completely, while at other times the same child eats voraciously; these conditions usually pass away as the children grow towards adolescence.

The nerve signs seen are mostly those of fatigue, with over-spontaneous movement of fingers and eyes, and with the nervous balance of hand. The power of coördination remains good, showing the quality of brain which is also indicated by the facial expression; response in action and imitation is quick, and the children are, as a rule, mentally bright. Among indications of bad sleeping, the teeth are often found ground, the result of want of brain quietness during the night. The urine is usually of high specific 'gravity (1.022–1.035), laden with urea which may be crystallized out on mixture with nitric acid and cooling. These children are affectionate, but passionate and often gregarious in their associations.

GROUPING OF CHILDREN WITH NEURAL OR MENTAL DEFECTS.

Having explained the methods here adopted in describing individual cases, and the means of conducting a clinical and mental examination of children, we are in a position to proceed to the study of groups of children presenting neural or mental defects. Taking the report on 100,000 children examined in schools as a basis I am able to present the following groups:

Group 29.* *Nerve Cases.*—Including all children presenting one or more of the abnormal nerve signs described; that is, cases with any visible indications of either brain defect or brain disorderliness and incoördinated action, but not including children reported as mentally dull without nerve-signs.

Among 50,000 children seen from 1892 to 1894 the nerve cases were distributed in age-groups as follows:

Age last birthday		3	4	5	6	7	8	9–10	11–12	13	14 +
Boys	2,853	15	58	119	214	346	447	781	680	142	51
Girls	2,015	9	27	72	146	241	285	591	497	109	38
Totals	4,868	24	85	191	360	587	732	1,372	1,177	251	89

Nerve cases may roughly be divided into two classes: those in whom there is brain deficiency or congenital defect, often indicated

---

* The reference number indicating the group in the report is given.

by uniform reiterative movements, such as constant athetoid over-action of the frontal or corrugator muscles, and grinning, with defect of expression and of speech, etc.; and, secondly, a larger class in whom defective action is mainly due to incoördination, excessive spontaneous movement in small parts (twitches), and signs of fatigue. Both classes are often associated with defects in bodily development. The proportion of cases in whom abnormal nerve signs are associated with developmental defect is highest in children under seven years of age, and is then more marked among the girls. This is noteworthy, for at older ages nerve signs are more associated with developmental defect in boys.

Again, nerve cases are often pale, thin, delicate children; this is also most marked in children under seven years. We see here an indication for treatment. Nervous children are usually under the normal weight, which is the almost universal rule in chorea; high-pressure feeding combined with a period of rest will often do much to remove abnormal nerve signs. When a normal body weight has been regained physical exercises are most useful in restoring good coördinated action.

Among the nerve cases seen in schools the most uniformly associated fact was mental dulness; forty-two per cent. of these children were reported by the teachers as dull or backward pupils for their age. It appears that a brain producing slow, inactive, or ill-coördinated movements is in a status of low power for mental and intellectual action.

Group 31. *Children Mentally Dull.*—Including all whom the teachers reported as dull or backward pupils and below the average of ability for their age. This group, therefore, embraces the dull children with nerve signs, and certain groups of dull and defective children to be described later on. Any child said by the teachers to be dull was included in this group whether abnormal signs were observed or not; however, only 331 boys and 297 girls were entered as "dull only."

Among 50,000 children the mentally dull were distributed as follows:

Age last birthday		3	4	5	6	7	8	9–10	11–12	13	14 +
Boys	2,074	18	71	143	187	245	295	530	444	104	37
Girls	1,634	13	40	101	156	218	215	433	347	85	26
Totals	3,708	31	111	244	343	463	510	963	791	189	63

These dull children are often found to be delicate with signs of brain disorderliness indicated by abnormal nerve signs; this condition is also often associated with congenital developmental defects.

The proportion with developmental defect is highest at seven years and under, the association being considerably higher with girls than with boys at this age; at older ages this association of developmental defect and mental dulness is higher among the boys.

The association of mental dulness with abnormal nerve signs is greater than its corelation with developmental defects. This shows the importance of conducting educational training in such a manner as to prevent and remove any signs of brain disorderliness. The association of constitutional delicacy with mental dulness is mostly seen among children seven years old and younger, being higher among girls than boys.

I have already shown in this paper, and more fully in previous writings,[*] that there is a marked corelation and interaction between defective bodily development, abnormal nerve signs, and low physical nutrition, while each class of defect is frequently associated with mental dulness. It has been found convenient in practice to arrange a group of cases presenting all these four main classes of defect; such children usually require special care and attention.

Group 27. *Cases of Developmental Defect with Low Physical Health and Abnormal Nerve Signs Combined with Mental Dulness.*—There are grades of mental dulness from the child backward in educational ability for his age down to those congenitally defective in all mental power and ineducable, *i.e.*, the imbeciles. There are also children bright in intellectual ability yet deficient in moral sense (moral imbeciles), just as there are children of mental ability with incoördinated brain action or epilepsy. The physician, as an observer of physical facts, will prefer to class his cases mainly according to his observations; but they must often be classed according to mental capacity when advising parents and teachers as to their training and as to their probable social capacity in adult life. An important group of children is that next given.

Group 8. *Children Feebly Gifted Mentally.*—These children are distinctly deficient in mental power, but short of a degree of deficiency justifying their certification as imbecile and treatment as such. No child is included in this group unless it is believed upon evidence observed, and the teacher's report combined, to be incapable of school work in the ordinary classes. It is not possible to define what physical conditions ascertained on clinical examination, as apart from mental tests, indicate the child as unfitted in mental capacity for the usual methods of education; but the two methods

[*] See Journal of Royal Statistical Society (London), March, 1893, and March, 1896.

of observation make it possible to give good grounds for a scientific opinion. There appears to be an appreciable class of "children feebly gifted mentally" with defect of mental power short of imbecility, but still with a degree of congenital deficiency; this group includes about one per cent. of the child population. It is possible that some of these children may ultimately prove to be imbecile, while others may be capable of great improvement. Some of these cases are also epileptic or paralyzed. Diagnosis should be founded on the clinical description of physical signs observed together with a mental examination.

Group 9. *Children Mentally Exceptional.*—Children who while not necessarily mentally dull and without brain power appear deficient in certain mental characteristics and in moral sense or social instinct—such as habitual liars, thieves, and incendiaries; children liable to attacks of total mental confusion or periods of total mental inaptitude or violent passion—such cases may be described as moral imbeciles. Some of these children are the offspring of insane parents, epileptics, or criminals.

Diagnosis may be very difficult in these cases. A careful clinical examination may show no defect in development of the body and no abnormal nerve signs. A mental examination may fail to detect mental deficiency, the child answering questions brightly and correctly with indications of reasoning power. The history of the case, the history of heredity, and the actions of the child at various times may, however, indicate an absence of moral and social sense under certain circumstances if the child is carefully watched. A few cases will better indicate the class of children referred to:

The son of a clergyman heard his father say that he had arranged with a *locum tenens* to preach for him next Sunday. He searched his father's correspondence, found the address, and stealing the stamps necessary, telegraphed to the *locum tenens* not to come. The act was intelligent but immoral. In a school a girl was pointed out as bright at work, but an habitual liar and a persistent thief; she was an orphan, her father having killed her mother. A girl aged 9 years, the child of three known generations of the criminal class—well formed, good looking, bright in answering questions; she was destructive, purposely unclean, and indecent; never safe out of sight for a moment, and uninfluenced by three years of good training.

Group 12. *Children Who Appear to Require Special Care and Training.*—The group is artificial, being arranged for the purpose of indicating children unfitted for ordinary training or presenting certain difficulties, while needing more than ordinary care. The group includes idiots and imbeciles; children feebly gifted mentally or mentally exceptional; those epileptic, crippled, maimed, deformed, paralyzed, or dumb, as well as "cases of developmental defect with low physical health and abnormal nerve signs who are also dull." This group 12 includes therefore groups 8, 9, 27.

When in the course of the clinical or mental examination of a child any defect is found, it is necessary to ascertain the presence or absence of further indications of the more common forms of brain defect, especially with infants and young children in whom they are easily overlooked. Among the most important of such points we must see if there be irregularities or inequalities in the working of the two sides of the brain or hemiplegia, as well as hypertonicity, athetosis, or tremor. In infants the indications of congenital defect, damage (injury at birth) or disease of the brain may be present on one side only or more marked on one side than on the other. I referred earlier to the spontaneous movement of healthy infants (microkinesis) and its temporary inhibition and coördination through the eye or the ear leading to the performance of definite action controlled by sight or sound. Such action should be looked for separately on either side of the body.

The digits may not move as frequently or in equal degree on either side, and coördination may be more complete in one hand than in the other. A hemiplegic condition in infancy is not commonly complete, the affected limb is not usually motionless at all times, and the shoulder and elbow may move when the fingers are useless. There may be general or local hypertonicity. The limbs and the digits should be tested separately by making passive movements. We should observe any fixed or habitual attitudes or postures resulting from muscular rigidity or spasm; the more common of such postures are: (1) spasmodic talipes equinovarus with pes cavus; (2) the lower limbs may be crossed, either at the legs or at the thighs; (3) the hand often presents the closed fist, or the metacarpus is contracted, its bones being drawn together with the thumb flexed on the palm or kept approximated to the middle joint of the index finger ʼ while the fingers move. The attempt to open the hand by passive movements may cause the impression of pain, though the muscles may relax at times; the wrist is often habitually flexed, less often extended.

Athetosis or athetoid movement is usually accompanied by some degree of rigidity. While most marked in the upper extremity there is usually some accompanying athetoid movement in the foot and toes. The movements of athetosis are most marked in the small parts, as in the fingers and toes, sometimes also in the facial muscles. The chief characteristics of the movements are the uniformly repeated action, slow in time, not coördinated or controlled by varying impressions received, and therefore useless, effecting no beneficial object, while similar action recurs either spontaneously or on any stimulation by sight or sound. Athetosis may be accompanied by epilepsy; the spasm of the fit then usually commences in the part affected by athetosis, which is more useless after the fit. In athetosis the digits may move separately, the fingers being drawn into unusual positions such as are not seen in the normal child or in chorea. Among other points of detail, the fingers may be extended backward at the knuckles one or two at a time, the joints of the fingers being all bent at a right angle. The slow movement, the unusual combination of movements, and especially their uniform repetition distinguish athetosis from chorea and tremor.

In searching for indications of brain defect in older children examination by imitation of movements is most useful. I let the child stand opposite to me as I hold out my hands, telling him to look at them and to move his like mine. His coördinated movements are then controlled by the sight of mine. I observe first whether his right hand imitates best my right or left; instinctively the child imitates my right hand with his left, and vice versa. I perform slow and separate movements with my fingers, noting the while if his eyes are directed towards my hands.

(1) Are the movements imitated equally well by either hand of the child in their time, order, and in degree of movement; and is the response equally prompt on either side?

(2) Similarly the child's right hand alone is to be tested, and then his left. Is exactness in imitation and response equally good on either side? Defect on one side of the brain may often thus be detected. Such movements in imitation may be performed well by a deaf child in whom it is important to search for brain deficiency. These deaf children are more common among girls, while deaf-mutes are more frequent among boys.

Rickets has often been described as a condition affecting the skeleton and bony system, and such children have been said to be precocious. Indications of rickets are, however, frequently found in cases of epilepsy, hysteria, and migraine; while in rachitic infants the head is often large or ill-formed, and the child is liable to attacks of convulsions with laryngismus and tetanus. Rickets must then be considered as a factor in the etiology or pathology of the neural and mental defects of children. . Turning to my account of 50,000 school children examined (1888–91), I find 157 boys and 39 girls described as presenting indications of rickets in the bones. It should be said that a large and bossed cranium was not recorded as an indication of rickets unless other bones were affected. As to these 196 cases of rickets the following conditions were noted:

CONDITIONS PRESENTED BY THE RACHITIC CHILDREN.

Boys.	Girls.	Total.	
143	25	168	Cranial abnormalities arranged below in sub-classes.
79	14	93	Head large and ill-formed.
51	9	60	Cranial bosses, principally frontal and usually symmetrical.
8	1	9	Forehead misshapen.
3	0	3	Head asymmetrical; sometimes one frontal boss only developed.
1	0	1	Dolichocephalic.
1	1	2	Head small.
23	8	31	Palate defective in form.
21	6	27	Cranium and palate defective.
58	11	69	Defects in development other than of cranium and palate.
32	13	45	Rachitic children with indications of low nutrition.
54	15	69	Rachitic children with abnormal nerve signs.
64	10	74	Rachitic children reported as dull by the teachers.

Of these rachitic children 69 presented defects other than those analyzed above. They were as follows:

	Boys.	Girls.		Boys.
Small in growth	10	5	Features coarse	3
Defect of ear	23	2	Palpebral fissures small	2
Epicanthis	6	2	Mouth small	1
Deaf	2	1	Forehead hairy	1
Nasal bones wide	4	0	Congenital defect of hand	1
Prognathous	1	0	Congenital defect of eyes	2
Frontal ridge	1	1	Epilepsy	1

We have studied methods proposed for the clinical and mental examination of children and infants. In all cases the chest and the heart, the mouth and the throat, the state of digestion and the glandular system, should be examined as well as the special senses; the history of the individual and of the family is important in forming an opinion; but these points I must pass over for want of space. We proceed to consider certain defective neural and mental conditions and groups of defective children as to diagnosis, description, and classification, etiology, pathology, prognosis, and treatment. To make a diagnosis of the neural and mental condition of a child presented to the physician for examination is not an easy task; the child is referred by the observer to a class of cases. This condition in the aggregate cannot be summed up in a word, as may be done when some disease of known pathology is detected.

In place of such verbal diagnosis we indicate the type of child or the class of children corresponding to the description of the case. It is on the combination of physical signs observed that classification should depend, especially in the presence of more than one main class of defect; then we inquire as to the distribution of such class of children as to sex, age, and history under varying circumstances.

Let me point out that a child may present a neural defect or a mental fault without being classed as "a defective child" either as a social being or in educational requirements, still the condition may be important, and is in some cases remediable, while the acquisition of further defect may be avoided by due care. I have described "nerve cases," and nervous children as this term is commonly understood. It is not every child who presents a nerve sign, *e.g.*, defective fixation of the eyes, etc., who should be described as a nervous child.

The various nerve signs given may be studied as to their significance by considering the neural action corresponding. As to a motor nerve centre it is either acting or it is not acting; when it acts, stimulating a muscle, the movement which we observe is to some extent an index of the time and the quantity of the nerve act. We may see movement in an individual digit or in one angle of the mouth, noting its quantity, its duration, its frequency or rhythm in succession of movements; this indicates action in a nerve centre. Again, a number of motor nerve centres may act together, producing a combination of movements, as of the digits; and such combination of nerve centres may continue to co-act, as when the digits all open or close together on repeated occasions. When movement in several parts of the body is noted we have combinations and series of acts, making up a complex phenomenon—such series of movements may be classed as follows:

1. Uniform series of acts. 2. Augmenting series of acts. 3. Diminishing series of acts. 4. Series of acts adapted by circumstances.

1. Uniform action, occurring spontaneously or on any stimulation, and uniform in repetition is characteristic of the athetoid movements previously described. The brain centres appear incapable of acquiring new coördinated and therefore useful action.

2. An augmenting series of acts, not coördinated but spreading in the area of movement is seen in the "nervousness" of children, in expression of emotion or passion, while it often accompanies mental confusion. A smile may spread over the face followed by a burst of laughter. The face may twitch at the angles of the mouth followed by a storm of passion. The question asked may result in movements in hands, protrusion of the tongue, movements of head, vague utterances, but no reply. There is an incoördinated spreading of the area of brain action which proves both useless and exhausting.

3. A diminishing series of acts occurs as the amount of brain

action subsides, as the child becomes quiet again, or as sleep comes on.

4. Series of movements or acts adapted by the environment through eye or ear are indications of intelligent action; they are in harmony with the environment and are useful. Further, they may cause less physical brain action than an augmenting series of acts when many nerve centres are sending out force. Hence the advantages of good training in the nervous child.

A point of difference between children commonly classed as "nervous" and the larger class here grouped as "nerve cases," is that a large proportion of the latter also present deviations from the normal development of the body. Although children with a neural defect form the special subject of this essay, it is impossible to discuss their pathology without reference to other classes of defect. It has been shown that a condition of developmental defect is often followed by the child becoming pale, thin, or delicate, under the stress of circumstances, and that such state of low nutrition is often accompanied by nerve signs; hence we have fatigue of brain which may pass on to hysteria, or to permanent nerve disorder. This is specially the case with girls. The main classes of defect interact in a marked manner in producing a tendency to nerve disturbance, and affect the prognosis, so that their interaction, together with the effects of environment, are important as to pathology and treatment.

The diagnosis of a developmental defect as described in the definition depends upon observation of abnormality in size, form, or proportion of parts. Thus the palate may be narrow or arched. The external ear may be abnormal in size, proportioning, absence of parts, or texture of skin; there may be great convexity posteriorly and concavity in front; the helix or the antihelix may be absent. This test of abnormality, as distinguished from variations within the normal, gives accuracy in judgment consistent with allowance for variations in type. Defects of different parts of the body have different diagnostic and prognostic value; it is possible they differ in etiology—small head is more common among girls in towns; defective ears are more common among Irish boys.

CORELATIONS OF DEFECTS IN DEVELOPMENT AMONG 50,000 CHILDREN.

	With nerve signs.		With low nutrition.		With mental dulness.	
	Boys.	Girls.	Boys.	Girls.	Boys.	Girls.
Cranial defects..........	55.6	50.6	25.7	45.8	41.4	45.5
Palate defect...........	55.4	49.9	21.7	29.5	40.7	44.2
Ear defect	54.0	47.7	18.7	26.8	32.4	38.4
Palpebral fissures small.	62.2	68.6	22.4	19.2	41.8	47.0

It seems that inherited conditions, congenital defects, and their interaction may go wrong in a child, not only in the proportioning of parts of the body, but also, concurrently in a tendency to low vitality and nutritive power in the tissues, with a neural inaptitude for good coördination and mental power.

Mental dulness may be of various grades, and in many children is due to physical causes that the physician can deal with, or to certain deficiencies in training concerning which he may give useful advice. Some mental weaknesses correspond to modes of brain action indicated by irregular and defective motor action or "nerve signs," both depending alike upon want of cultivation of normal coördination. On this ground I think that class teachers in school should conduct some physical exercises, and adapt them like other teaching to the requirements of the pupils. The class teacher knows best the mental peculiarities of the pupil, e.g.; the child may be liable to times of mental confusion (called inattention or carelessness), the reply to a question being absurd and not sequential to (not coördinated by) the words spoken to the child. Such mental confusion may be accompanied by a number of extra movements in the limbs and fingers, while the eyes wander and the facial muscles and his words are so slightly coördinated as to have no relation to the question put. Such neural state— call it excitement or nervousness—corresponds to a spreading area of spontaneous nerve acts, incoördinated and wasting brain energy. Imitation is one of the principal means of cultivating the fine and exact modes of neural action needed for mental training. When the pupil imitates through his eye the quick movements made by the teacher, exact in the time and in the degree of movement, the nerve centres in the child's brain corresponding to those in the teacher are set in (motor) action by sight, and brain coördination is thus cultivated. Similarly, incoördinated action in the teacher, and the attitudes and movements of fatigue or listlessness, are imitated by the pupils, as I have seen in schools.

Mental action in forming a correct judgment may be cultivated by exercises in eye movements; moving the eyes from one end of a yard rule to the other, then from one corner of the table to the other enables a judgment of the length of the table to be made.

Observation of children in schools where physical exercises are much employed, and comparison with others not so trained, shows the advantages of such training, both in diminishing the number of cases of brain disorderliness (nerve signs) and in lessening the proportion of dull pupils.

Discrimination, choice, judgment are essential characteristics of mental development in young brains, as well as in those of deficient aptitude. We need to cultivate the modes of brain action corresponding to mental action before teaching verbal expression of judgment. Mental faculty may be cultivated by comparison of colors, size, weight, heat, and cold; further, by comparison of size and weight, as with coins of the same metal or with pill boxes, some empty, some filled with plaster of Paris. Speech may be more successfully cultivated after training in movements and fixation of the eyes by which the movements in the teacher's face are better seen.

The use of numbers should first be taught as corresponding to the number of similar objects seen; then as to number of successive acts or movements in the body. In counting objects at sight we must take care that the child looks at each separately; the counting results from appreciation of the number of eye movements. He may also count by touching each object, thus again appreciating the number of his movements. The appreciation• of number by movement may be taught when calculation without movement (mental arithmetic) is impracticable.

Children presenting neural and mental defects are seen under different aspects by the parent and the teacher; while the physician, as a student of living beings and of life, must look at every aspect of his case. Children with neural defects are often delicate and dull; they necessarily come under the notice of persons who see them from different points of view. The parent sees signs of ill health, and it may be restless nights and want of appetite. The teacher finds the pupil dull or inattentive at lessons. The physician notes the signs of semichorea or exhaustion, and prescribes accordingly. Still we should remember that the child with nerve delicacy often remains so for years, with periods of improvement and relapses. Thus while medical care is needed for his physical well-being, his mental development and training in action should be provided for.

Prognosis in the case of a child with neural or mental defect must vary with the diagnosis of his condition and his environment. Prognosis as to life and viability largely depends upon good or ill development of the body as well as the brain. The high mortality under five years of age falls principally on the males, and largely depends upon developmental defect, while after that age surviving cases of defect have a low probability of good health under adverse circumstances. Among children with developmental defects such as have been described, the proportion who are delicate falls as they grow up, but remains higher with girls than boys; the proportion of those who are dull rises with increasing years, especially among girls. The children with constitutional delicacy (mostly due to developmental defect) tend to acquire nerve disorder as they grow older, especially the boys.   The proportion who are dull in school life falls after ten years of age and does not vary greatly between boys and girls.

In arranging the physical care of children with developmental or neural defect certain points need to be looked to.   The clothing should be appropriate but such as does not fetter his movements.   Usually a full diet is needed, especially if the body weight is low.   If too much animal food is given, particularly in the neurotic cases, these children often fail in appetite and are constipated and have to be pressed to eat.   If the child is long in getting to sleep or wakes early, food should be placed at the bedside.

As to the mental care and the physical training of these children some points have previously been given.   In cases "mentally feeble" the labor required of the teacher[*] or attendant is great, and many hours a day need to be devoted to the child in training, occupation, and play to effect any good.   The physician having pointed out certain nerve signs it becomes the work of the teacher or trainer to remove them individually.

I have endeavored to put before the reader points for observation, and methods of description enabling large groups of children to be classified and studied, trusting in this way to bring within the scope of exact clinical research many conditions and degrees of neural and mental defect worthy of careful and minute study.   Groups of cases have been described by indicating the physical signs of their condition, just as cases are described in studying chorea, epilepsy, hemiplegia, bulbar paralysis, or general paralysis of the insane.

Knowledge of groups and classes of children concerns not only ourselves; some Departments of State in charge of children, educationalists, philanthropic workers, and teachers should also know something of the mental and physical conditions of the children for whom they are responsible.

---

[*] "The Children: How to Study Them."   F. Hodgson: 89 Farringdon Street, London, E. C.

GENERAL INDEX.

Arteries, affections of the, in gout, ii. 350, 387

    in chronic nephritis, i. 77, 89

    in myxœdema, iv. 711, 720

    in obesity, ii. 662

    in typhoid fever, xvi. 608

    aneurysms of the, iv. 586, see *Aneurysms of the Systemic Arteries*

    atheroma of the, iv. 533

    calcareous infiltration of, iv. 601

    cerebral, x. 29

        atheroma of the, iv. 537

        lesions of, in insanity, xii. 70

        syphilis of the, iv. 552, xviii. 150, 230

    chlorotic murmurs in the, vii. 346

    diseases of the, iv. 457; vi. 622

    echinococcus of the, viii. 546

    inflammation of the, iv. 529; see *Arteritis*

    lardaceous disease of, iv. 602

    obliterating endarteritis, iv. 601

    sclerosis of the, iv. 559; see *Arteriosclerosis*

    symptoms referable to the, in exophthalmic goitre, iv. 775

Arteriocapillary fibrosis, iv. 559; see *Arteriosclerosis*

Arteriometer, iv. 573

Arteriosclerosis, iv. 559

    aortic insufficiency from, iv. 258

    association of, with other morbid processes, iv. 563

    asthma associated with, iv. 579

    atheroma associated with, iv. 567

    clinical groups of, iv. 578

    dilatation of the heart associated with, iv. 566

    gouty, iv. 580

    granular kidney in, iv. 565

    hypertrophy of the heart associated with, iv. 84, 563, 571

    in diabetes, ii. 109

    in lead-poisoning, iii. 597, 601

    in obesity, ii. 675, 687, 691, 723

    in old age, xii. 440, 529

    in relation to aortic insufficiency, iv. 245

        to chronic pneumonia, vi. 686

        to myocarditis, iv. 123

        to rupture of the heart, iv. 361

Arteriosclerosis, kidney disease associated with, iv. 578

    mechanical means for determining arterial resistance, iv. 573

    mental overstrain in relation to, iv. 579

    mitral stenosis associated with, iv. 568

    morbid anatomy, iv. 560

    pathological associations, iv. 563

    pathology, iv. 569

    physical diagnosis, iv. 571

    pulmonary affections associated with, iv. 579

    syphilitic, iv. 580; xviii. 150, 230

    treatment, iv. 580

Arteritis, iv. 529

    acute and subacute, iv. 529

    bronchial, vi. 622

    chronic, iv. 533; vi. 624

        analogy of, to phlebitis, iv. 615

        clinical evidences of, iv. 534

        groups of, iv. 538

        symptoms and treatment of, iv. 538

    constricting, iv. 530

    degenerative, vi. 624

    etiology, vi. 622

    in infectious diseases, iv. 531

    in leprosy, xviii. 51

    in malaria, xix. 385

    in old age, xii. 440, 529

    nephritis associated with, i. 17, 90

    obliterans, iv. 601

    ossifying, vi. 625

    pathology, vi. 623

    relation of, to diseases of the kidneys, i. 17, 90

    symptoms, vi. 623

    syphilitic, xviii. 148

        cerebral, iv. 552; xviii. 230

    treatment, iv. 538; vi. 624

Arthaud and Butte's test for uric acid, vii. 689

Arthralgia, hysterical, x. 471

    chronic rheumatic, ii. 513, 556; see *Arthritis deformans*

    in influenza, xv. 233

    syphilitic, xviii. 205

Arthritis, ii. 331; see also *Gout*

Chemotaxis, xiii. 165, 170, 210
  influence of, on infection, xiii. 165
  negative, xiii. 172, 211, 218
  positive, xiii. 211, 217, 218
Chenzinsky's blood stain, vii. 287
Chest, barrel-shaped, in pulmonary emphysema, vi. 665
  rachitic deformities of the, vii. 540
Cheyne-Stokes respiration, iv. 348
Chicken breast, vii. 540
  cholera, bacillus of, xix. 687
Chickenpox, xiv. 191
  adenopathy in, xiv. 198
  anæmia following, xiv. 197
  and smallpox, non-identity of, xiv.
    191
  bacteriology of, not settled, xiv.
    192
  complications, xiv. 193, 195
  congenital, unknown, xiv. 192
  contagion of, xiv. 192
  definition, xiv. 191
  desquamation absent, xiv. 197
  diagnosis, xiv. 193
    from herpes zoster, xiv. 195
    from impetigo contagiosa, v.
      424
    from measles, xiv. 155
    from pemphigus, v. 381
    from scarlet fever, xiv. 196
    from smallpox, xiii. 447; xiv.
      194, 195
  encephalomyelitis following, xi.
    756
  enanthem, xiv. 194
  etiology, xiv. 192
  exanthem, xiv. 193
  gangrenous form, xiv. 193, 195
  history, xiv. 191
  incubation period, xiii. 374; xiv.
    193
  infectious period of, xiii. 374
  inoculation experiments with virus
    of, xiv. 192
  laryngitis complicating, xiv. 194
  measles complicating, xiv. 153
  mixed infection, xiv. 196
  ·nephritis following, xiv. 197
  prognosis, xiv. 197
    of laryngeal localization, xiv.
      194

Chickenpox, scars persistent after, xiv.
  195
  secondary infections in, xiv. 193, 197
  sequelæ, xiv. 197
  symptoms, xiv. 193
  temperature curve in, xiv. 193, 197
  treatment, xiv. 197
  tuberculosis following, xiv. 198
  typhoid fever associated with, xvi.
    690
  urine in, xiv. 197
Chigoe, v. 52
Chilblain, iii. 299; v. 144, 249; xii. 542,
  800
  diagnosis of, from eczema, v. 223
    from lupus erythematosus, v.
      249
    from Raynaud's disease, iii. 300
  in children, xii. 542, 800
  treatment, iii. 305
Child-bearing in relation to cancer of
  the uterus, xvii. 204, 661
Childbirth, tetanus following, xvii. 132,
  143
Childhood, insanity of, xii. 54
Child labor, evils of, iii. 322
Children Diseases of, xii. 537
  bibliographical references, xii
    829
Children, arthritis deformans in, ii. 551
  crime in, xii. 373
**Children, Neural and Mental Defects
  in, xx. 577**
Children, pneumonia in, xii. 713; xvi.
  129
  pneumothorax in, vii. 98; xii. 720
  shock in, iii. 151
  typhoid fever in, xvi. 699
Chill in anæsthetic leprosy, xviii. 538
  in appendicitis, viii. 455
  in Asiatic cholera, xiv. 368, 370, 387
  in cerebrospinal meningitis, xvi.
    166
  in dysentery, xvi. 276
  in endocarditis, iv. 168
  in lobar pneumonia, xvi. 3, 6.
  in lobular pneumonia, vi. 680, 681,
    682
  in malaria, explanation of, xix. 207
  in measles, xiv. 126
  in peritonitis, viii. 424

Freckles, diagnosis from xeroderma pigmentosum, v. 740

Freezing, iii. 289; see *Frostbite*

Freire's yellow-fever micrococcus, xx. 452

Fremitus, increased vocal, in lobar pneumonia, xvi. 23

FRENCH, JAMES M., on the Chemical and Microscopical Examination of the Urine, vii. 661
    on Treatment of the Diseases caused by Animal Parasites, viii. 629

French measles, xiv. 177; see *German measles*

Frerichs' classification of diseases of the kidney, i. 5

Friedländer's bacillus, xix. 651
    teachings concerning glomerulonephritis, i. 14

Friedlieb's apparatus for gastric lavage, viii. 183

Friedreich's disease, xi. 887; xii. 769
    phenomenon, xx. 170

Fright in relation to exophthalmic goitre, iv. 769, 795
    to scleroderma, xi. 523
    shock from, iii. 151

Frontal sinus, diseases of the, vi. 95
    foreign bodies in the, vi. 100
    tumors of the, vi. 99

Frost-bite, iii. 289, 436; v. 248; xii. 800
    bibliography, iii. 306
    chilblain, iii. 299
    definition, iii. 289
    etiology, iii. 291
    morbid anatomy, iii. 297
    resemblance of, to Raynaud's disease, iii. 300
    sequelæ, iii. 306
    symptoms, iii 294
    synonyms, iii. 289
    treatment, iii. 300

Fuchsin stains for bacteria, xix. 604

Fumigation, mercurial, in the treatment of syphilis, xviii 310
    nasal, vi. 23

Functio læsa, a symptom of inflammation, xvi 357

Functioning, retarded, in old age, xii. 462

Fungi, microscopic, xix. 542; see *Bacteria*

Fungus foot, v. 119
    bacteriology of, xix. 760
    hæmatodes, xii. 794
        of the kidney, xvii. 592
    testiculi syphiliticus, xviii. 178

Furor uterinus, old notions of the, x. 554

Furuncle, v. 457; xii. 802
    diagnosis, v. 459, 568
    due to absorption of toxins from the intestinal canal, xiii. 167
    etiology, v. 458
    following scarlet fever, xiv. 80
    in diabetes, ii. 103
    in gout, ii. 403
    in influenza, xv. 230
    in obesity, ii. 672
    in smallpox, xiii. 421, 431
    in typhoid fever, xvi. 611, 684
    of the external auditory canal, vi. 223
    of the nose, vi. 4
    oriental, v. 461
    pathology, v. 458
    sweat, v. 566
    synonyms, v. 457
    tetanus following, xvii. 134
    treatment, v. 459

GABBET's tubercle-bacillus stain, xix. 604; xx. 15

Gadinin, xiii. 17

Gafsa button, v. 461

Gait, changes in the, in syphilis of the cerebellum, xviii. 227
    de steppage, xi. 403
    in beriberi, xiv. 494
    in cerebellar disease, x. 209
    in chorea, x. 664
    in hemiplegia, x. 279
    in hereditary cerebellar ataxia, x. 212
    in paralysis agitans, x. 722
    in tabes dorsalis, xi. 830; xviii 258
    in tumors of the cerebellum, x. 333

Galactotoxismus, xiii. 49
    treatment, xiii. 56

Galacturia, i. 644; see *Chyluria*

Galette, xiii. 74

Galena, lead-poisoning among miners of, iii. 356

Galeodes araneoides, v. 64

Gall-bladder, absence of the, ix. 725

uenza, season in relation to, xv. 57
sequelæ of, gastrointestinal, xv. 187
   psychoses, xv. 219
singultus in, xv. 198
skin lesions in, xv. 228
social position in relation to, xv. 62
somnolence in, xv. 197
spasms in, xv. 198
spastic spinal paralysis in, xv. 214
spinal-cord lesions in, xv. 110
   symptoms in, xv. 214
spleen in, xv. 106, 112, 190
sputum of, xv. 65, 122, 136, 163
stomach lesions in, xv. 107
stomatitis in, xv. 108, 184
sweating in, xv. 230
symptoms, xv. 110
   articular, xv. 233
   aural, xv. 239
   bronchial, xv. 121
   bronchopneumonic, xv 127
   cardiac, xv. 115, 223
   catarrhal, xv. 112, 117
   cerebral, xv. 202
   choleraic, xv. 185
   chronic, xv. 174
   circulatory, xv. 222
   cutaneous, xv. 228
   digestive, xv. 182
   febrile, xv. 113
   gastrointestinal, xv. 182
   general, xv. 111
   genitourinary, xv. 231
   hemorrhagic, xv. 227
   hepatic, xv. 188
   initial, xv. 111
   laryngeal, xv. 118
   motor, xv. 198
   nervous, xv. 193
   neuralgic, xv. 194
   ocular, xv. 235
   osseous, xv. 233
   parotid gland, xv. 191
   peritonitic, xv. 191
   pleural, xv. 171
   pneumonic, xv. 138
   psychical, xv. 215
   pulmonary, xv. 127, 166
   referable to individual organs, xv. 116
   renal, xv. 231

Influenza, symptoms, respiratory, xv. 117
   spinal, xv. 214
   splenic, xv. 190
   tracheal, xv. 120
   vascular, xv. 225
   vesical, xv. 232
syncope in, xv. 196
telluric conditions, xv 58
temperature curve in, xv. 113
tenonitis in, xv. 237
theories of, xv. 49
thrombosis in, xv. 225
tongue in, xv. 183
toxin of, xv. 84
treatment, xv. 244
tuberculosis following, xv. 178
typhoid form, xv. 186
urticaria in, xv. 229
varieties of, xv. 116
vertigo in, xv. 195
vomiting in, xv. 184
zoster in, xv. 229
Infusion, saline, in Asiatic cholera, xiv. 370, 432
   in cholera infantum, xiv. 266
Infusoria, xix. 805
INGALS, E. FLETCHER, on Hay Fever, vii. 181
Inhalation, nasal, vi. 23
Inhaler, antiseptic, vi. 120
Initial lesion of leprosy, xviii. 468
   of syphilis, xviii. 15
Inoculation, animal, xix. 612
Inosite in the urine, vii. 698, 731, 732
Insanity, xii. 3
age in relation to, xii. 15
alcoholism in relation to, iii. 11, 116; xii 25, 95, 228
alternating, xii. 121, 138, 184
   diagnosis from general paralysis, xii. 165
anæmia in relation to, xii. 36
apoplexy in relation to, xvii. 273
arterial lesions in, xii. 70
asylum treatment, xii. 207
atrophy of the brain in, xii. 66
bacteria in the production of, xiii. 200
blood-vessel lesions in, xii. 70
brain lesions in, xii. 18, 65

iver, palpation of the, ix. 448

    parasites of the, v. 59; viii. 522, 566,
574; ix. 632; xiii. 293

    pathology of the, general, ix. 410

    physical examination of the, ix. 445

    physiology of the, ix. 401

    position of the, ix. 392, 397

    protective action of the, ix. 406, 418

    pulsations in the, ix. 447

        in tricuspid insufficiency, iv. 274

• red atrophy of the, ix. 536

    relations of the, anatomical, ix. 397

        pathological, ix. 413

    sarcoma of the, ix. 654; xvii. 522

    senile changes in the, xii. 502

    stomach in diseases of the, viii. 359

    sugar-forming function of the, ii. 38;
ix. 405

    symptoms of disease of the, ix. 443

        ascites, ix. 461

        cardiovascular, ix. 459

        digestive, ix. 460

        functional, ix. 458

        glycosuric, ix. 467

        hæmatic, ix. 474

        nutritive, ix. 475

        objective, ix. 445

        toxic, ix. 473

        urinary, ix. 462

        urotoxic coefficient, ix 469

    syphilis of the, ix. 618, xviii. 121,
282, 373

    treatment of diseases of the, ix. 508

        dietetic, ix. 509

        hydrotherapeutic, ix. 511

        mental influences in, ix. 511

      • milk diet, ix. 509

        physiological, ix. 508

        reconstituent, ix. 520

        resolvent, ix. 516

        surgical, ix. 521

        symptomatic, ix. 522

    tropical abscess of the, ix 550, xvi
253, 270, 287

        hyperæmia of the, ix. 529

    tuberculosis of the, ix. 626

    tumors of the, ix. 646· xii 661

    urea-forming function of the, ix.
403

    variegated, ix. 536

    veins of the, ix. 395

Liver. weight of the, ix. 393

    Weil's disease of the, ix. 638

Liver-fluke, v. 59, viii. 574; xiii 293

Living being, definition of the, xii. 431

LLOYD, JAMES HENDRIE, on Diseases of
Occupations, iii. 309

    on Diseases of the Cerebrospinal and
Sympathetic Nerves, xi. 1

Lobes, cerebral, x. 13

Localization, cerebral, x. 33

    arm movements, x. 37

    auditory, x. 48

    bibliography, x. 67

    deglutition, x 41

    eye movements, x. 42

    face movements, x, 39

    gustatory, x. 52

    head motions, x. 39

    in the centrum ovale, x. 52

    in the corpora quadrigemina, x.
52

    in the optic thalamus, x. 58

    in the peduncles, x. 56

    laryngeal muscles, x. 40

    leg movements, x. 38

    mastication, x. 41

    mental processes, x. 62

    motor area, x. 35

    olfactory, x. 50

    sensation, x. 59

    sensory area, x. 45

    trunk muscles, x 38

    visual, x. 45

Lockjaw, x. 688; xi. 184; xvii 138,
142

    value of, in the diagnosis of tetanus,
xvii. 147

Locomotion, instinct of, in idiots, xii. 305

Locomotive engineers and firemen, effects
of occupation upon, iii. 496

Locomotor apparatus, complications on
the part of, in rachitis, vii 544

    ataxia, xi 805; xviii. 250, 394, see
Tabes dorsalis

Loeffler bacillus, xvii. 4; xix. 672

Loeffler's blood-serum culture medium,
xix. 586

    method of staining flagella, xix 611

    methylene blue, xix. 603

Logoplegia from intracranial hemorrhage, x. 275

Melasma in a child with adrenal sarcoma, **xvii. 507**
  in Addison's disease, ii. 11, 12, 13, 14, 15
  suprarenale, ii. 8; see *Addison's disease*
Mellitagra, v. 176
Membranes, false, xvi. 376
Memory in idiots and imbeciles, xii. 335
  weakened, in influenza, xv. 221
Mendacity in chronic alcoholism, iii. 38, 48
  in idiots and imbeciles, xii. 320
Ménière's disease, vi. 245; xi. 208
  in tabes dorsalis, xi. 838
Meningeal irritation, cerebral, in syphilis, xviii. 214, 215
  spinal, in syphilis, xviii. 244
Meninges, anatomy of the, x. 357
Meninges, Diseases of the, x. 357
Meninges, hemorrhage in the, x. 275, 444
  in children, xii. 744
  inflammation of the, see *Meningitis*
  lesions of the cerebral, in idiocy, xii. 271
    in typhus fever, xv. 273
  sarcomatosis of the, x. 417
  sclerosis of the arteries of the, iv. 563
  spinal, hemorrhage into the, diagnosis of, from hæmatomyelia, xi. 666
    inflammation of the, xi. 668
    tumors of the, xi. 629
  syphilis of the, x. 418
  tuberculosis of the, x. 396
Meningitic streaks, v. 787
Meningitis, x. 358
  acute, x. 361; xii. 735
    bibliography, x. 414
    diagnosis, x. 387
    etiology, x. 369
    pathology, x. 375
    phosphaturia in, i. 632
    prognosis, x. 393
    symptoms, x. 363
    treatment, x. 394
  alcoholic, x. 386, 395
  basilar, optic neuritis in, xi. 127
  cerebral, x. 358
    in relapsing fever, xvi. 524
    syphilitic, x. 418; xviii. 219

Meningitis, cerebrospinal, x. 380; xvi. 143; see *Cerebrospinal meningitis*
  chronic, x. 417
  classification of, x. 359
  complicating measles, xiv. 140
    typhoid fever, xvi. 661
  diagnosis of, from malaria, xix. 420
    from smallpox, xiii. 450
    from typhus fever, xv. 300
  dural, x. 437
  epidemic cerebrospinal, x. 380; xvi. 143; see *Cerebrospinal meningitis*
  false, x. 385
  gummatous, xviii. 218, 241
  in criminals, xii. 398
  in idiots, xii. 359
  influenzal, xv. 108, 210; xvi. 170
    pseudo-, xv. 213
  in smallpox, xiii. 438
  lepto-, xi. 672
  of the aged, x. 385
  of the new-born, x. 385
  pachy-, x. 437
    spinal, xi. 668
  pneumonia complicated by, xvi. 69
  primary, x. 389
  pseudo-, x. 385
  rheumatic, ii. 310
  scarlet fever simulating, xiv. 53
  secondary, x. 390
  serosa, x. 385, 395
  simulated by the otitis of measles, xiv. 139
  spinal, diagnosis of, from acute alcoholic paralysis, iii. 30
    syphilitic, xviii 240
  sporadic suppurative, bacteriology of, xvi. 193
  stage of oscillations, x. 401
  suppurative, bacteriology of, xvi. 193
  symptoms of, in pernicious malarial fever, xix. 330
  syphilitic, x. 418; xi. 776; xviii. 219, 240
    cerebral, x. 418
    cerebrospinal, x. 431
    diagnosis, x. 427, 434
    of the convexities, x 425
    prognosis, x. 429, 435

Mouth, leprosy of the, viii. 62; xviii.
  491
  leukoplakia, viii. 74
  lichen ruber planus, viii. 73
  lipoma, ix. 25
Mouth, Local Diseases of the, ix. 3
Mouth, lupus of the, viii. 50; xx. 368
  lymphangioma, ix. 34
  macroglossia and macrocheilia, ix.
    40
  melanosarcoma, ix. 61
  mucous membrane of the, xvii. 51
    patches in the, viii. 39; xviii. 99
  myoma, ix. 25
  myxoma, ix. 25
  nævus, ix. 33
  neuroses of the, viii. 77
  osteoma, ix. 86
  parasites in the, viii. 71
  papilloma, ix. 53
  pemphigus, viii. 73
  phlegmon of the floor of the, ix. 15
  ranula, ix. 42, 47
  sarcoma, ix. 59, 88; xvii. 518
  scleroma of the, viii. 64
  senile changes in the, xii. 502
  symptomatology of diseases of the,
    viii. 5
  syphilitic affections of the, viii. 35;
    xviii. 96
    diagnosis, viii. 38, 40, 47; xviii.
      108
    treatment, viii. 39, 41, 46; xviii.
      299
  telangiectasis, ix. 30
  thrush of the, viii. 69
  tuberculosis of the, viii. 49; xx. 368
  tumors of the, ix. 21
    benign, ix. 22, 84
    . hour-glass, ix. 28
    malignant, ix. 59, 88
    mixed, ix. 27
    of the vessels, ix. 29
    teratoid, ix. 27
  ulcers of the, in tabes dorsalis, xi.
    837
  wounds of the, viii. 11
Movements reflecting brain action, xx.
  578
Mucin in the skin and connective tissue
  in myxœdema, iv. 721

Mucin in the urine, vii. 696, 722, 723·
Mucocele of the antrum of Highmore,
  93
  of the ethmoidal sinus, vi 104 .
  of the frontal sinus, vi. 99   .
Mucoid fever, xvi. 441; see *Simple co
  tinued fever*
Mucous membranes, erysipelas of tl
  xvi. 423
  hysterical dysæsthesia of the, x. 4
  lesions of the, in chickenpox, xi
    194
    in erythema exudativum mul
      forme, v. 150
    in German measles, xiv 18
      183
    in impetigo herpetiformis, v. 4
    in leprosy, viii. 62; xviii. 48
      496, 525, 550
    in measles, xiv. 124, 126, 12
      144
    in miliary fever, xiv. 531
    in myxœdema, iv. 707
    in pemphigus, v. 375
    in purpura hæmorrhagica, v
      486
    in scarlet fever, xiv. 13, 25, 4
      46, 50
    in smallpox, xiii. 417, 420
    in typhoid fever, xvi. 586, 59·
  pigmentation of, in Addison's d
    ease, ii. 14
  lupus of the, viii. 50; xx. 367
  lupus erythematosus of the, v. 69
  nerve terminations in, xi. 14
Mucous patches, xviii. 58
  of the anus, xviii. 118
  of the larynx, vi. 385, 393; xvi
    135
  of the mouth, viii. 39; xviii. 99
  of the nasopharynx, vi. 140; xvi
    100
  of the tonsils, vi. 303; xviii. 100
  treatment, xviii. 298
Mucus in the gastric contents, test f
  viii. 152
  in the urine a sign of renal calcul
    i. 144
Muguet, v. 116; xii. 594
Mulder's test for sugar, vii. 728
Mules (chilblains), iii. 299, 305

Normoblasts in pernicious anæmia, vii. 375

NORTON, NATHANIEL READ, on Whooping-cough, xiv. 211

Nose, acne of the, vi. 3

adenomata of the, vi. 52

affections of the, in general diseases, vi 67

in glanders, xv. 383

in hysteria, x. 466

in leprosy, xviii. 489, 551, 598

in relation to asthma, vi. 602; vii. 135

in scarlet fever, xiv. 56, 102

in smallpox, xiii. 434

in typhoid fever, xvi. 595

angiomata of the, vi. 53

cancer of the, vi. 10, 53; xvii. 465

cystomata of the, vi. 53

deformities of the, in idiocy, xii. 286

diphtheria of the, vi. 73; xvii. 66

Nose, Diseases of the, vi. 3; xii. 680

Nose, Diseases of the Accessory Sinuses of the, vi. 79

Nose, dislocation of the columnar cartilage, vi. 58

eczema of the, v. 210

enchondromata of the, vi. 52

exostoses of the, vi. 52

fibromata of the, vi. 51

foreign bodies in the, vi. 64; xii. 680

furuncle of the, vi. 4

hemorrhage from the, vi. 44; see *Epistaxis*

hypertrophy of the, vi. 4

inflammation of the, vi. 25

injuries of the, vi. 10

lupus of the, vi. 6, 73; xviii. 89; xx. 368

mucous membrane of the, xvii. 52

changes in, due to disease or injury of the fifth nerve, vi. 61

condition of, in infectious diseases, vi. 74

inflammation of the, vi. 25; see *Coryza* and *Rhinitis*

myasis of the, vi. 67

myxoma of the, vi. 48

nævus of the, vi. 5

Nose, neuroses of the, vi. 58

osteomata of the, vi. 52

papillomata of the, vi. 51

septal affections, vi. 54; xviii. 128, 133

in workers in chromium, iii. 383

polypi of the, vi. 48

pruritus of the, v. 774

reflex effects of disease of the, vi. 62

rhinoscleroma, vi. 8

rodent ulcer of the, vi. 5

sebaceous tumors of the, vi. 5

synechiæ of the, vi. 58

syphilis of the, vi. 67; xviii. 89, 126

treatment, xviii. 299

therapeutics of diseases of the, vi. 20

tipplers', vi. 3

tuberculosis of the, vi. 6, 72; xviii. 89; xx. 368

tumors of the, vi. 48

malignant, vi. 10, 53; xvii. 465

warts of the, vi. 4

worms in the, vi. 66

Nosebleed, see *Epistaxis*

Novy's apparatus for anaërobic plate cultures, xix. 599

Nucha, rigidity of the, in cerebrospinal meningitis, xvi. 150

Nuclein, xiii. 278

adenin derived from, xiii. 111

Nucleoalbumin in the urine, vii. 697

in malaria, xix. 226

Nucleohiston, vii. 261; xiii. 112

Nucleon in woman's and cow's milk, xiv. 262

Numbness in aconite poisoning, iii. 502

in arthritis deformans, ii. 545

in sore throat, xiv. 47

Nutmeg liver, ix. 536

Nutrition, disorders of, xi. 70

in children, xii. 539

in chorea, x. 665

in epilepsy, x. 610, 614

in hysteria, x. 487, 509

effects of glycosuria upon, ii. 86

in relation to beriberi, xiv. 487

to cancer, xvii. 287

to obesity, ii. 639

maintenance of, in diabetes, ii. 134

necessary in tetanus, xvii. 165

Onanism in children, xii. 679
  in idiocy, xii. 306
  in relation to asthma, vii. 173
    to hysteria, x. 456
    to insanity, vii. 622, xii. 22, 227
    to neurasthenia, x. 739
Onomotomania, x. 713
Onychatrophia, v. 620
Onychauxis, v. 619
Onychia in foot-and-mouth disease, xv.
  469
  syphilitica, xviii. 95, 298
Onychogryphosis, v. 619
Onychomycosis, v. 92; xii. 823
Onychophagia, v. 618
Onyxis, general, diagnosis from ring-
  worm of the nail, v. 94
Oöphoritis, see *Ovaritis*
Oöspora asteroides, xix. 761
    bovis, xix. 755
    farcinica, xix. 759
Ophiasis, v. 582
Ophthalmia in children, xii. 786
    complicating measles, xiv. 147, 168
    gonorrhœal, i. 458
    neuroparalytic, xi. 161
    of the new-born, xii. 785
    school, xii. 787
Ophthalmoplegia, xi. 154
    in diphtheria, xvii. 73
    in tabes dorsalis, xi. 835
    nuclear, x. 104
Ophthalmoscope, use of, in insanity, xii.
  218
OPIE, EUGENE L., on Microorganisms
  (Protozoa), xix. 765
Opisthotonos in tetanus, xvii. 138
Opium, addiction to, iii. 70
      "abstinence phenomena," iii 83
      and alcoholism contrasted, iii. 72
      cardialgia in, iii. 74
      prevalence of, iii. 80
      treatment, iii. 82
    poisoning by, iii. 70, 542
      diagnosis of, from apoplexy, x.
        291
      treatment, iii. 549
    rash caused by, v. 242
Opiumism, iii. 70
Optic nerve, diseases of the, xi. 109
    in diabetes, ii. 113

Optic nerve, myxosarcoma of the, xvii.
  509
Optic neuritis in brain tumors, x. 317
    in cerebellar disease, x. 209
    in encephalitis, x. 91
    in influenza, xv. 239
    in malaria, xix. 380
    in typhoid fever, xvi. 669
Optic thalamus, symptoms of disease in
  the, x. 58
Orbit, changes in the, in exophthalmic
    goitre, iv. 793
    echinococcus of the, viii. 553
  . epithelioma of the, xvii. 510
    sarcoma of the, xvii. 509, 603
    syphilitic lesions of the, xviii. 200,
      269
Orbital inflammation, optic neuritis in,
  xi. 132
Orchitis, i. 450
    diagnosis of, from inguinal hernia,
      ix. 289
      of the various forms of, xviii.
        178
    in gout, ii. 509
    in influenza, xv. 233
    in Malta fever, xiv. 575
    in mumps, xiii. 559, 578, 594, 601
    in smallpox, xiii. 440
    in syphilis, xviii. 175
    in typhoid fever, xvi. 681
    symptoms, i. 451
    treatment, i. 495
Organic sensations in idiocy, xii. 297
Orgies of criminals, xii. 388
Oriental boil, v. 461
    bacteriology, xix. 620
Orrhodiagnosis of Asiatic cholera, xiv.
    343, 406
    of Malta fever, xiv. 576
    of relapsing fever, xvi. 526
    of tuberculosis, xx. 234
    of typhoid fever, xvi. 705
Orrhotherapy, xiii. 235
    milk as an agent in, xiii. 273
    nature of the germicidal constituent
      of the blood serum, xiii. 277
    of anthrax, xiii. 242
    of Asiatic cholera, xiii. 254; xiv.
      428
    of avian septicæmia, xiii. 245

Sarcoma of the heart, iv. 380
  of the humerus, xvii. 579
  of the intestine, ix. 189; xvii. 521
  of the kidney, i. 107, 170, 546; xvii. 503, 592
  of the larynx, vi. 389, 474
  of the leg, xvii. 576
  of the liver, ix. 654; xvii. 522
  of the lungs, vi. 712
  of the lymph bodies, xvii. 610
  of the maxilla, ix. 88; xvii. 511, 533, 598
  of the metacarpal bones, xvii. 580
  of the mouth, ix. 59; xvii. 518, 608
  of the muscles, xvii. 513
  of the nasopharynx, vi. 173
  of the œsophagus, xvii. 520
  of the orbit, xvii. 509, 603
  of the ovaries, xvii. 527, 605
  of the pancreas, viii. 384; xvii. 524
  of the periosteum, xvii. 511, 533, 570
  of the peritoneum, viii. 492
  of the phalanges, xvii. 581
  of the pharynx, xvii. 519
  of the pia mater, x. 417; xvii. 518
  of the pineal body, xvii. 518
  of the pituitary body, xvii. 517
  of the pleura, vii. 121
  of the prostate, i. 256, 396; xvii. 532
  of the radius, xvii. 513, 579
  of the rectum, xvii. 521
  of the scapula, xvii. 513
  of the skin, xvii. 514, 609, 638
  of the skull, xvii. 512
  of the spleen, ix. 385; xvii. 523
  of the stomach, xvii. 520
  of the testis, xvii. 525, 588
  of the thigh, xvii. 570
  of the thyroid gland, iv. 814
  of the tibia, xvii. 576
  of the tongue, ix. 78; xvii. 518, 608
  of the tonsil, vi. 310; xvii. 520
  of the tympanum, xvii. 512
  of the ulna, xvii. 579
  of the urethra in the female, i. 708
  of the uterus, xvii 529, 674
  of the vagina, xvii 530, 657
  of the vertebræ, xi. 623
  of the vulva, xvii. 656

Sarcoma origin of, from benign neo-plasms, xvii. 220, 225
  pain in, xvii. 560
  pathogenesis, xvii. 487
  pathological anatomy, xvii. 497, 674
  prognosis of lingual, xvii. 608
    of mammary, xvii. 584
    of maxillary, xvii. 599, 602
    of osseous, xvii. 572
    of ovarian, xvii. 607
    of testicular, xvii. 591
    of uterine, xvii. 677
  recurrence of, after removal, xvii. 549
  reticular angioplastic, v. 683
  round-celled, xvii. 498
  sex in relation to, xvii. 559
  spindle-celled, xvii. 498
Sarcoma (Symptomatology and Treatment), xvii. 557
Sarcoma, symptoms, xvii. 559
    of mammary, xvii. 583
    of maxillary, xvii. 598, 601
    of orbital, xvii. 604
    of osseous, xvii. 571
    of ovarian, xvii. 606
    of renal, xvii. 594
    of uterine, xvii. 676
  transmission of, from man to ani-mals, xvii. 488
  traumatism in relation to, xvii. 489
  treatment of, by toxins, xvii. 611
    of mammary, xvii. 583
    of maxillary, xvii. 599, 602
    of melanotic, xvii. 565
    of orbital, xvii. 605
    of osseous, xvii. 573, 576, 580
    of renal, xvii. 597
    of testicular, xvii. 591
    of uterine, xvii. 681
  type, change in, xvii. 605
Sarcomatosis, cutaneous, xvii. 639, 642
  diffuse, of the brain and cord, x 310
  of the pia mater, x. 417
Sarcophaga carnaria, v. 63
Sarcopsylla, v. 52
Sarcoptes scabiei, v 42, 46; xii. 827
    communis, v. 50
Sarcosporidia, xix 798
Sarkin, xiii. 113
Saturnism, iii. 593

Tænia nana (v. Siebold), viii. 573
   removal of, viii. 637
   saginata, viii. 568; xii. 646
   solium, v. 58; viii. 562; xii. 646
   treatment of patient after the ex-
     pulsion of, viii. 642
   varerina, viii. 573
   water-borne, xiii. 290
Tæniacides, viii. 638
Talipes, see *Clubfoot*
Tannin, formation of cystin from, i. 620
Tapeworm, viii. 562; xii. 646; see *Tænia*
Tarantula-bites, v. 42
Tarsalgia of adolescence, xii. 586
Tarsitis syphilitica, xviii. 265
Tartar emetic, burns of the pharynx
   from, vi. 180
Taste, affections of, in diabetes mellitus,
   ii. 114
   in hysteria, x. 466
   in idiocy, xii. 293
   in malaria, xix. 385
   in ninth-nerve disease, xi. 213
   in syphilis, xviii. 272
   in tabes dorsalis, xi. 838
   in typhoid fever, xvi. 647
   in ulcer of the stomach, viii. 230
   brain centre for, x. 52
   hallucinations of, xii. 86
Tattooing among criminals, xii. 382
Taxis in strangulated hernia, ix. 342
"Tea-kettle policy" in the prevention of
   water-borne diseases, xiii. 360
Tea, poisoning by, iii. 112, 406
Tea-tasters, diseases of, iii. 406
Teeth, affections of, in diabetes, ii. 104,
   119
   in idiocy, xii. 284
   in myxœdema, iv. 707
   in relation to epilepsy, x. 623
   in scarlet fever, xiv. 80
   in syphilis, inherited, xviii. 382
   in tabes, xi. 837; xviii. 257
   carious, complicating mercurial
     treatment, xviii. 337
   discoloration of, by copper, iii. 377
   eruption of the, xii. 588
   grinding of the, in gout, ii. 363
Teichmann's hæmin test, viii. 154
Telangiectasis, v. 674
   of the mouth, ix. 30

Telangiectatic warts, v. 683
Telegrapher's cramp, iii. 478
Temperament, definition of term, ii. 449
   effect of, upon senilization, xii. 449
   in relation to inebriety, iii. 129
     to insomnia, x. 822
     to obesity, ii. 638
   venous, affecting the course of he-
     patic disorders, ix. 512
Temperature, body, at high altitudes,
   iii. 205
   during sleep, x. 817
   effect of atmospheric tempera-
     ture upon, iii. 257, 293
   effect of snake-venom upon, xx.
     514
   lowered, increasing the suscep-
     tibility to infectious disease,
     xiii. 197
   subnormal, suggestive of tuber-
     culosis, xx. 240
   changes in local, in nerve lesions, xi.
     105
Temperature curve in actinomycosis,
   xv. 490
   in Addison's disease, ii. 12
   in adenoiditis, vi 127
   in alcoholic pseudomeningitis, x.
     387
   in anæsthetic leprosy, xviii. 533
   in anthrax, xv. 451
   in apoplexy, x. 272, 273
   in appendicitis, viii. 455; ix. 162
   in arthritis deformans, ii. 545
   in athrepsia, xii. 583
   in beriberi, xiv. 499
   in bronchitis, vi. 496, 522, 533, 534;
     xii. 696
   in bronchopneumonia, vi. 680, 681,
     682; xv. 135, xii. 710
   in cancer, xvii. 368
   in capillary bronchitis, vi. 533, 534
   in cerebrospinal meningitis, xi. 382;
     xii. 738; xvi. 153
   in chickenpox, xiv. 193, 197
   in chlorosis, vii. 349
   in cholera, xiv. 365, 368, 370, 374,
     387
     infantum, xiv. 243
     nostras, xiv. 283
   in cholerine, xiv. 365

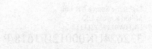

Lightning Source UK Ltd.
Milton Keynes UK
UKHW011302211118
332624UK00012B/1618/P